CASE FILES®
Emergency Medicine

Eugene C. Toy, MD
Vice Chair of Academic Affairs and
  Residency Program Director
Department of Obstetrics and
  Gynecology
The Methodist Hospital
Houston, Texas
The John S. Dunn Senior Academic Chair
St Joseph Medical Center, Houston
Clinical Professor and
  Clerkship Director
Department of Obstetrics and
  Gynecology
University of Texas Medical School
  at Houston
Houston, Texas
Associate Clinical Professor
Weill Cornell College of Medicine

Barry C. Simon, MD
Chairman, Department of Emergency
  Medicine
Clinical Professor of Medicine
Alameda County Medical
  Center/Highland Campus
University of California, San Francisco
Oakland, California

Katrin Y. Takenaka, MD
Assistant Professor, Clerkship Director
Assistant Residency Program Director
Department of Emergency Medicine
University of Texas Medical School at
  Houston
Houston, Texas

Terrence H. Liu, MD, MHP
Professor of Clinical Surgery
University of California San Francisco
  School of Medicine
San Francisco, California
Program Director, University of
  California San Francisco
  East Bay Surgery Residency
Attending Surgeon, Alameda County
  Medical Center
Oakland, California

Adam J. Rosh, MD, MS
Assistant Professor
Residency Director
Department of Emergency Medicine
Wayne State University School of Medicine
Detroit Receiving Hospital
Detroit, Michigan

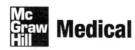

New York   Chicago   San Francisco   Lisbon   London   Madrid   Mexico City   Milan
New Delhi   San Juan   Seoul   Singapore   Sydney   Toronto

Case Files®: Emergency Medicine, Third Edition

Copyright © 2013 by The McGraw-Hill Companies, Inc. All rights reserved. Printed in the United States of America. Except as permitted under the United States Copyright Act of 1976, no part of this publication may be reproduced or distributed in any form or by any means, or stored in a data base or retrieval system, without the prior written permission of the publisher. Previous edition copyright © 2009, 2004 by The McGraw-Hill Companies, all rights reserved.

Case Files® is a registered trademark of The McGraw-Hill Companies, Inc. All rights reserved.

1 2 3 4 5 6 7 8 9 0   DOC/DOC   17 16 15 14 13 12

ISBN 978-0-07-176854-2
MHID 0-07-176854-8

Notice

Medicine is an ever-changing science. As new research and clinical experience broaden our knowledge, changes in treatment and drug therapy are required. The authors and the publisher of this work have checked with sources believed to be reliable in their efforts to provide information that is complete and generally in accord with the standard accepted at the time of publication. However, in view of the possibility of human error or changes in medical sciences, neither the editors nor the publisher nor any other party who has been involved in the preparation or publication of this work warrants that the information contained herein is in every respect accurate or complete, and they disclaim all responsibility for any errors or omissions or for the results obtained from use of the information contained in this work. Readers are encouraged to confirm the information contained herein with other sources. For example and in particular, readers are advised to check the product information sheet included in the package of each drug they plan to administer to be certain that the information contained in this work is accurate and that changes have not been made in the recommended dose or in the contraindications for administration. This recommendation is of particular importance in connection with new or infrequently used drugs.

This book was set in Goudy by Cenveo Publisher Services.
The editors were Catherine A. Johnson and Cindy Yoo.
The production supervisor was Catherine H. Saggese.
Project management was provided by Ridhi Mathur, Cenveo Publisher Services.
The designer was Janice Bielawa; the cover designer was Aimee Nordin.
RR Donnelley was printer and binder.
This book is printed on acid-free paper.

Library of Congress Cataloging-in-Publication Data

Toy, Eugene C.
    Case files. Emergency medicine / Eugene C. Toy ... [et al.].—3rd ed.
        p. ; cm.
    Emergency medicine
    Includes bibliographical references and index.
    ISBN 978-0-07-176854-2 (pbk.)
    I. Toy, Eugene C. II. Title: Emergency medicine.
    [DNLM: 1. Emergency Medicine—methods—Case Reports.   2. Emergency Medicine—methods—Problems and Exercises.   3. Diagnosis, Differential—Case Reports.   4. Diagnosis, Differential—Problems and Exercises.   5. Emergencies—Case Reports.   6. Emergencies—Problems and Exercises.   WB 18.2]
    616.02'5—dc23
                                                                                    2012024017

International Edition ISBN 978-0-07-179285-1; MHID 0-07-179285-6. Copyright © 2013. Exclusive rights by The McGraw-Hill Companies, Inc., for manufacture and export. This book cannot be re-exported from the country to which it is consigned by McGraw-Hill. The International Edition is not available in North America.

McGraw-Hill books are available at special quantity discounts to use as premiums and sales promotions, or for use in corporate training programs. To contact a representative please e-mail us at bulksales@mcgraw-hill.com.

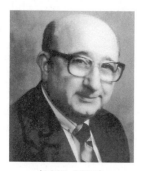

(1921-2008)

Case Files®: Emergency Medicine was the last planned book in the *Clinical Case Files* series, and now is in its third edition. It is fitting that we take this opportunity to dedicate this series to the memory of a great physician, Dr Joseph A. Lucci Jr, who has had a tremendous impact on the practice and education in medicine in Houston, particularly at CHRISTUS St Joseph Hospital. Dr Lucci was born in Morrone del Sannio, a province of Campobasso in Italy on August 21, 1921. "Dr Joe" arrived in the United States in 1930 at the age of 9 years. He obtained his medical degree from the Medical College of Wisconsin in 1946. After finishing his internship in 1947, he served as an Air Force base surgeon in Germany. He then received residency training for 2 years at the Margaret Hague Maternity Hospital in Jersey City, New Jersey. Upon his arrival to Houston, Dr Lucci received his further training in gynecologic surgery at the MD Anderson Cancer Center. He was appointed as the first academic chair over the department of obstetrics/gynecology at St Joseph Hospital, and had academic appointments at the MD Anderson Cancer Center, UTMB Galveston Medical School, and later at the University of Texas Houston Medical School. During his 31 years as academic chair, Dr Joe trained more than 100 excellent residents, revolutionized the education of gynecologic surgery, developed innovative surgical techniques, reduced maternal mortality to practically zero, and helped to coordinate medical education throughout the Houston/Galveston region. He and his wife Joan have five children: Joe, Joan Marie, Jacqueline, Regina Marie, and James, and nine grandchildren. "Dr Joe" was academic chief emeritus of the CHRISTUS St Joseph Hospital Obstetrics-Gynecology Residency. He has been a true pioneer in many aspects of medicine, touching the lives of thousands of people. We are greatly indebted to this extraordinary man and saddened by his death, which occurred peacefully on November 21, 2008 in the presence of his entire family.

To Mabel Wong Ligh whose grace, love, and commonsense bind our family together,
and in the memory of John Wong,
whose smile, integrity, and enthusiasm continue to warm our hearts.
And to their legacy, Randy and Joyce and their children Matthew and Rebekah;
and Wanda and Jerry, whose lives reflect their parents' virtue.

– ECT

To my best friend and wife Zina Rosen-Simon and
to my daughters Jamie and Kaylie
for teaching me and always reminding me what is most important in life.
I would also like to thank my faculty at Highland General Hospital and
all the residents and students who have passed through our doors
for helping make my career as an academic emergency physician challenging and
immensely rewarding.

– BS

To my parents, who continue to be my guiding light.
To my residents and colleagues,
who never fail to impress me with their dedication to our profession.
And to Clare, who remains my teacher and friend.

– KYT

To my wife Eileen for her continuous support, love, and friendship.
To all the medical students and residents
for their dedication to education and improving patient care.

– THL

A hearty thanks goes out to my family for their love and support, especially Ruby;
the dedicated medical professionals of the EDs at NYU/Bellevue Hospital and
Wayne State University/DRH;
and my patients, who put their trust in me, and teach me something new each day.

– AR

CONTENTS

Contributors / vii

Acknowledgments / ix

Introduction / xi

Section I
How to Approach Clinical Problems 1

Part 1. Approach to the Patient 2

Part 2. Approach to Clinical Problem Solving 8

Part 3. Approach to Reading 10

Section II
Clinical Cases 15

Fifty Eight Case Scenarios 17

Section III
Listing of Cases 589

Listing by Case Number 591

Listing by Disorder (Alphabetical) 592

Index / 595

Naomi Adler, MD
Resident
Department of Emergency Medicine
Alameda County Medical Center/Highland Campus
Oakland, California

Jesus Alvarez, MD
Resident
Department of Emergency Medicine
Alameda County Medical Center/Highland Campus
Oakland, California

Michael C. Anana, MD
Clinical Instructor
Department of Emergency Medicine
University of Medicine and Dentistry of New Jersey
Newark, New Jersey

Keenan M. Bora, MD
Assistant Professor
Department of Emergency Medicine
Wayne State University School of Medicine
Toxicologist, Children's Hospital of Michigan
Regional Poison Control Center
Detroit, Michigan

Christopher Bryczkowski, MD
Chief Resident
Department of Emergency Medicine
University of Medicine and Dentistry of New Jersey—Robert Wood
   Johnson Medical School
New Brunswick, New Jersey

Meigra Myers Chin, MD
Instructor
Department of Emergency Medicine
University of Medicine and Dentistry of New Jersey—Robert Wood
   Johnson Medical School
New Brunswick, New Jersey

Melissa Clark, MD
Resident
Department of Emergency Medicine
Alameda County Medical Center/Highland Campus
Oakland, California

R. Carter Clements, MD
Clinical Instructor
Department of Emergency Medicine
University of California, San Francisco
San Francisco, California
Attending Physician
Department of Emergency Medicine
Alameda County Medical Center/Highland Campus
General Hospital
Oakland, California

Andrea X. Durant, MD
Resident
Department of Emergency Medicine
Alameda County Medical Center/Highland Campus
Oakland, California

David K. English, MD, FACEP, FAAEM
Assistant Clinical Professor
Department of Emergency Medicine
University of California, San Francisco
Informatics Director
Department of Emergency Medicine
Alameda County Medical Center/Highland Campus
Oakland, California

Lauren Fine, MD
Chief Resident
Department of Emergency Medicine
Alameda County Medical Center/Highland Campus
Oakland, California

Kenneth A. Frausto, MD, MPH
Resident
Department of Emergency Medicine
Alameda County Medical Center/Highland Campus
Oakland, California

Bradley W. Frazee, MD
Clinical Professor
Department of Emergency Medicine
University of California, San Francisco
Attending Physician
Department of Emergency Medicine
Alameda County Medical Center/Highland Campus
Oakland, California

Oron Frenkel, MD, MS
Resident Physician
Department of Emergency Medicine
Alameda County Medical Center/Highland Campus
Oakland, California

Jocelyn Freeman Garrick, MD, MS
Associate Clinical Professor
Department of Emergency Medicine
University of California, San Francisco
EMS Base Director
Alameda County Medical Center/Highland Campus
Oakland, California

Krista G. Handyside, MD
Attending Physician
Department of Emergency Medicine
Tacoma General Hospital
Tacoma, Washington

Cherie A. Hargis, MD
Assistant Clinical Professor
Department of Emergency Medicine
University of California, San Francisco
Attending Physician
Department of Emergency Medicine
Alameda County Medical Center/Highland Campus
Oakland, California

H. Gene Hern, MD, MS
Associate Clinical Professor
Department of Emergency Medicine
University of California, San Francisco
Residency Director
Department of Emergency Medicine
Alameda County Medical Center/Highland Campus
Oakland, California

Kevin Hoffman, MD
Resident
Department of Emergency Medicine
The University of Texas Medical School at Houston
Houston, Texas

Kerin A. Jones, MD
Assistant Professor
Associate Residency Director
Department of Emergency Medicine
Wayne State University/Detroit Receiving Hospital
Detroit, Michigan

R. Starr Knight, MD
Assistant Clinical Professor
Department of Emergency Medicine
University of California, San Francisco
San Francisco, California

Lauren M. Leavitt, MD
Resident
Department of Emergency Medicine
The University of Texas Medical School at Houston
Houston, Texas

Eliza E. Long, MD
Resident
Department of Emergency Medicine
Alameda County Medical Center/Highland Campus
Oakland, California

David Mishkin, MD
Attending Physician
Department of Emergency Medicine
Baptist Hospital of Miami
Miami, Florida

Allison Mulcahy, MD
Assistant Professor and Attending Physician
Department of Emergency Medicine
University of New Mexico
Albuquerque, New Mexico

Arun Nagdev, MD
Assistant Clinical Professor
Department of Emergency Medicine
University of California, San Francisco
Director, Emergency Ultrasound
Department of Emergency Medicine
Alameda County Medical Center/Highland Campus
Oakland, California

Claire Pearson, MD, MPH
Assistant Professor
Department of Emergency Medicine
Wayne State University/Detroit Receiving Hospital
Detroit, Michigan

Berenice Perez, MD
Clinical Instructor in Medicine
University of California, San Francisco
San Francisco, California
Attending Physician and Co-Medical Director
Department of Emergency Medicine
Alameda County Medical Center/Highland Campus
Oakland, California

Marjan Siadat, MD, MPH
Attending Physician
Department of Emergency Medicine
Director
Emergency Medicine Residency Rotation
Kaiser Permanente South Sacramento Medical Center
Sacramento, California

Barry C. Simon, MD
Clinical Professor
Department of Emergency Medicine
University of California, San Francisco
Chairman
Department of Emergency Medicine
Alameda County Medical Center/Highland Campus
Oakland, California

Amandeep Singh, MD
Assistant Clinical Professor of Medicine
Department of Emergency Medicine
University of California, San Francisco
Attending Physician
Department of Emergency Medicine
Alameda County Medical Center/Highland Campus
Oakland, California

Randi N. Smith, MD, MPH
Resident
Department of Surgery
University of California San Francisco—East Bay
Oakland, California

Eric R. Snoey, MD
Clinical Professor
Department of Emergency Medicine
University of California, San Francisco
Vice Chair
Department of Emergency Medicine
Alameda County Medical Center/Highland Campus
Oakland, California

Aparajita Sohoni, MD
Faculty/Attending Physician
Department of Emergency Medicine
Alameda County Medical Center/Highland Campus
Oakland, California

Jennifer M. Starling, MD
Resident
Department of Emergency Medicine
Alameda County Medical Center/Highland Campus
Oakland, California

Michael B. Stone, MD
Chief, Division of Emergency Ultrasound
Department of Emergency Medicine
Brigham and Women's Hospital
Boston, Massachusetts

Anand K. Swaminathan, MD, MPH
Assistant Professor
Assistant Residency Director
Department of Emergency Medicine
New York University/Bellevue Hospital Center
New York, New York

Katrin Y. Takenaka, MD
Assistant Professor, Clerkship Director
Assistant Residency Program Director
Department of Emergency Medicine
University of Texas Medical School at Houston
Houston, Texas

Paul A. Testa, MD, JD, MPH
Assistant Professor
Department of Emergency Medicine
New York University School of Medicine
Medical Director for Clinical Transformation
NYU Langone Medical Center
New York, New York

Diana T. Vo, MD
Attending Physician
Bronx Lebanon Hospital
Bronx, New York

Brian D. Vu, MD
Resident
Department of Emergency Medicine
The University of Texas Medical School at Houston
Houston, Texas

Benjamin D. Wiederhold, MD
Assistant Medical Director
Department of Emergency Medicine
St. Joseph's Medical Center
Stockton, California

Charlotte Page Wills, MD
Assistant Clinical Professor
Department of Emergency Medicine
University of California, San Francisco
Associate Residency Director
Department of Emergency Medicine
Alameda County Medical Center/Highland Campus
Oakland, California

Ambrose H. Wong, MD
Resident
Department of Emergency Medicine
New York University/Bellevue Hospital Center
New York, New York

ACKNOWLEDGMENTS

The curriculum that evolved into the ideas for this series was inspired by two talented and forthright students, Philbert Yau and Chuck Rosipal, who have since graduated from medical school. It has been a pleasure to work with Dr Barry Simon, a wonderfully skilled and compassionate emergency room physician, and Dr Kay Takenaka who is as talented in her writing and teaching as she is in her clinical care. It has been excellent to have Adam Rosh join us. McGraw-Hill and I have had the fortune to work with Adam while he was a medical student, resident, and now an emergency medicine physician. Likewise, I have cherished working together with my friend since medical school, Terry Liu, who initially suggested the idea of this book. This third edition has eight new cases, and includes updates on nearly every case. I am greatly indebted to my editor, Catherine Johnson, whose exuberance, experience, and vision helped to shape this series. I appreciate McGraw-Hill's believing in the concept of teaching through clinical cases. I am also grateful to Catherine Saggese for her excellent production expertise, Cindy Yoo for her wonderful editing, and Ridhi Mathur for her outstanding production skills. At Methodist Hospital, I appreciate the great support from Drs Marc Boom, Dirk Sostman, Alan Kaplan, and Eric Haufrect. Likewise, without Debby Chambers and Linda Bergstrom for their advice and support, this book could not have been written. Most of all, I appreciate my everloving wife Terri, and four wonderful children, Andy, Michael, Allison, and Christina for their patience, encouragement, and understanding.

Eugene C. Toy

Mastering the cognitive knowledge within a field such as emergency medicine is a formidable task. It is even more difficult to draw on that knowledge, procure and filter through the clinical and laboratory data, develop a differential diagnosis, and finally to form a rational treatment plan. To gain these skills, the student often learns best at the bedside, guided and instructed by experienced teachers, and inspired toward self-directed, diligent reading. Clearly, there is no replacement for education at the bedside. Unfortunately, clinical situations usually do not encompass the breadth of the specialty. Perhaps the best alternative is a carefully crafted patient case designed to stimulate the clinical approach and decision making. In an attempt to achieve that goal, we have constructed a collection of clinical vignettes to teach diagnostic or therapeutic approaches relevant to emergency medicine. Most importantly, the explanations for the cases emphasize the mechanisms and underlying principles, rather than merely rote questions and answers.

This book is organized for versatility: to allow the student "in a rush" to go quickly through the scenarios and check the corresponding answers, as well as the student who wants thought-provoking explanations. The answers are arranged from simple to complex: a summary of the pertinent points, the bare answers, an analysis of the case, an approach to the topic, a comprehension test at the end for reinforcement and emphasis, and a list of resources for further reading. The clinical vignettes are purposely placed in random order to simulate the way that real patients present to the practitioner. A listing of cases is included in Section III to aid the student who desires to test his/her knowledge of a certain area, or to review a topic including basic definitions. Finally, we intentionally did not primarily use a multiple choice question (MCQ) format because clues (or distractions) are not available in the real world. Nevertheless, several MCQs are included at the end of each scenario to reinforce concepts or introduce related topics.

HOW TO GET THE MOST OUT OF THIS BOOK

Each case is designed to simulate a patient encounter with open-ended questions. At times, the patient's complaint is different from the most concerning issue, and sometimes extraneous information is given. The answers are organized with four different parts.

PART I

1. **Summary:** The salient aspects of the case are identified, filtering out the extraneous information. The student should formulate his/her summary from the case before looking at the answers. A comparison to the summation in the answer will help to improve one's ability to focus on the important data, while appropriately discarding the irrelevant information, a fundamental skill in clinical problem solving.
2. A **straightforward answer** is given to each open-ended question.

3. The **Analysis of the Case,** which is comprised of two parts:

    a. **Objectives of the Case:** A listing of the two or three main principles that are crucial for a practitioner to manage the patient. Again, the student is challenged to make educated "guesses" about the objectives of the case upon initial review of the case scenario, which help to sharpen his/her clinical and analytical skills.

    b. **Considerations:** A discussion of the relevant points and brief approach to the **specific** patient.

PART II

Approach to the Disease Process, which has two distinct parts:

    a. **Definitions or pathophysiology:** Terminology or basic science correlates pertinent to the disease process.

    b. **Clinical Approach:** A discussion of the approach to the clinical problem in general, including tables, figures, and algorithms.

PART III

Comprehension Questions: Each case contains several multiple-choice questions that reinforce the material, or introduce new and related concepts. Questions about material not found in the text will have explanations in the answers.

PART IV

Clinical Pearls: A listing of several clinically important points, which are reiterated as a summation of the text, to allow for easy review such as before an examination.

How to Approach Clinical Problems

Part 1   Approach to the Patient

Part 2   Approach to Clinical Problem Solving

Part 3   Approach to Reading

Part 1. Approach to the Patient

Applying "book learning" to a specific clinical situation is one of the most challenging tasks in medicine. To do so, the clinician must not only retain information, organize facts, and recall large amounts of data, but also apply all of this to the patient. The purpose of this text is to facilitate this process.

The first step involves gathering information, also known as establishing the database. This includes taking the history, performing the physical examination, and obtaining selective laboratory examinations, special studies, and/or imaging tests. Sensitivity and respect should always be exercised during the interview of patients. **A good clinician also knows how to ask the same question in several different ways, using different terminology.** For example, patients may deny having "congestive heart failure" but will answer affirmatively to being treated for "fluid in the lungs."

CLINICAL PEARL

▶ The **history** is usually the **single most important** tool in obtaining a diagnosis. The art of seeking this information in a nonjudgmental, sensitive, and thorough manner cannot be overemphasized.

HISTORY

1. Basic information:
   a. Age: Some conditions are more common at certain ages; for instance, chest pain in an elderly patient is more worrisome for coronary artery disease than the same complaint in a teenager.
   b. Gender: Some disorders are more common in men such as abdominal aortic aneurysms. In contrast, women more commonly have autoimmune problems such as chronic idiopathic thrombocytopenic purpura or systemic lupus erythematosus. Also, the possibility of pregnancy must be considered in any woman of childbearing age.
   c. Ethnicity: Some disease processes are more common in certain ethnic groups (such as type II diabetes mellitus in the Hispanic population).

CLINICAL PEARL

▶ The possibility of pregnancy must be entertained in any woman of childbearing age.

2. Chief complaint: What is it that brought the patient into the hospital? Has there been a change in a chronic or recurring condition or is this a completely new problem? The duration and character of the complaint, associated symptoms,

and exacerbating/relieving factors should be recorded. The chief complaint engenders a differential diagnosis, and the possible etiologies should be explored by further inquiry.

CLINICAL PEARL

▶ The first line of any presentation should include **age, ethnicity, gender, and chief complaint.** Example: A 32-year-old white man complains of lower abdominal pain of 8-hour duration.

---

3. Past medical history:
   a. Major illnesses such as hypertension, diabetes, reactive airway disease, congestive heart failure, angina, or stroke should be detailed.
      i. Age of onset, severity, end-organ involvement.
      ii. Medications taken for the particular illness including any recent changes to medications and reason for the change(s).
      iii. Last evaluation of the condition (example: when was the last stress test or cardiac catheterization performed in the patient with angina?)
      iv. Which physician or clinic is following the patient for the disorder?
   b. Minor illnesses such as recent upper respiratory infections.
   c. Hospitalizations no matter how trivial should be queried.

4. Past surgical history: Date and type of procedure performed, indication, and outcome. Laparoscopy versus laparotomy should be distinguished. Surgeon and hospital name/location should be listed. This information should be correlated with the surgical scars on the patient's body. Any complications should be delineated including, for example, anesthetic complications and difficult intubations.

5. Allergies: Reactions to medications should be recorded, including severity and temporal relationship to the dose of medication. Immediate hypersensitivity should be distinguished from an adverse reaction.

6. Medications: A list of medications, dosage, route of administration and frequency, and duration of use should be developed. Prescription, over-the-counter, and herbal remedies are all relevant. If the patient is currently taking antibiotics, it is important to note what type of infection is being treated.

7. Social history: Occupation, marital status, family support, and tendencies toward depression or anxiety are important. Use or abuse of illicit drugs, tobacco, or alcohol should also be recorded.

8. Family history: Many major medical problems are genetically transmitted (eg, hemophilia, sickle cell disease). In addition, a family history of conditions such as breast cancer and ischemic heart disease can be a risk factor for the development of these diseases.

9. Review of systems: A systematic review should be performed but focused on the life-threatening and the more common diseases. For example, in a young man with a testicular mass, trauma to the area, weight loss, and infectious symptoms are important to note. In an elderly woman with generalized weakness, symptoms suggestive of cardiac disease should be elicited, such as chest pain, shortness of breath, fatigue, or palpitations.

PHYSICAL EXAMINATION

1. General appearance: Is the patient in any acute distress? The emergency physician should focus on the **ABCs (Airway, Breathing, Circulation).** Note cachetic versus well-nourished, anxious versus calm, alert versus obtunded.

2. Vital signs: Record the temperature, blood pressure, heart rate, and respiratory rate. An oxygen saturation is useful in patients with respiratory symptoms. Height, weight, and body mass index (BMI) are often placed here.

3. Head and neck examination: Evidence of trauma, tumors, facial edema, goiter and thyroid nodules, and carotid bruits should be sought. In patients with altered mental status or a head injury, pupillary size, symmetry, and reactivity are important. Mucous membranes should be inspected for pallor, jaundice, and evidence of dehydration. Cervical and supraclavicular nodes should be palpated.

4. Breast examination: Inspection for symmetry and skin or nipple retraction, as well as palpation for masses. The nipple should be assessed for discharge, and the axillary and supraclavicular regions should be examined.

5. Cardiac examination: The *point of maximal impulse* (PMI) should be ascertained, and the heart auscultated at the apex as well as the base. It is important to note whether the auscultated rhythm is regular or irregular. Heart sounds (including S_3 and S_4), murmurs, clicks, and rubs should be characterized. Systolic flow murmurs are fairly common in pregnant women because of the increased cardiac output, but significant diastolic murmurs are unusual.

6. Pulmonary examination: The lung fields should be examined systematically and thoroughly. Stridor, wheezes, rales, and rhonchi should be recorded. The clinician should also search for evidence of consolidation (bronchial breath sounds, egophony) and increased work of breathing (retractions, abdominal breathing, accessory muscle use).

7. Abdominal examination: The abdomen should be inspected for scars, distension, masses, and discoloration. For instance, the Grey-Turner sign of bruising at the flank areas may indicate intraabdominal or retroperitoneal hemorrhage. Auscultation should identify normal versus high-pitched and hyperactive versus hypoactive bowel sounds. The abdomen should be percussed for the presence of shifting dullness (indicating ascites). Then careful palpation should begin away from the area of pain and progress to include the whole abdomen to assess for tenderness, masses, organomegaly (ie, spleen or liver), and peritoneal signs. Guarding and whether it is voluntary or involuntary should be noted.

8. Back and spine examination: The back should be assessed for symmetry, tenderness, or masses. The flank regions particularly are important to assess for pain on percussion that may indicate renal disease.

9. Genital examination:
   a. Female: The external genitalia should be inspected, then the speculum used to visualize the cervix and vagina. A bimanual examination should attempt to elicit cervical motion tenderness, uterine size, and ovarian masses or tenderness.
   b. Male: The penis should be examined for hypospadias, lesions, and discharge. The scrotum should be palpated for tenderness and masses. If a mass is present, it can be transilluminated to distinguish between solid and cystic masses. The groin region should be carefully palpated for bulging (hernias) upon rest and provocation (coughing, standing).
   c. Rectal examination: A rectal examination will reveal masses in the posterior pelvis and may identify gross or occult blood in the stool. In females, nodularity and tenderness in the uterosacral ligament may be signs of endometriosis. The posterior uterus and palpable masses in the cul-de-sac may be identified by rectal examination. In the male, the prostate gland should be palpated for tenderness, nodularity, and enlargement.

10. Extremities/skin: The presence of joint effusions, tenderness, rashes, edema, and cyanosis should be recorded. It is also important to note capillary refill and peripheral pulses.

11. Neurological examination: Patients who present with neurological complaints require a thorough assessment including mental status, cranial nerves, strength, sensation, reflexes, and cerebellar function. In trauma patients, the Glasgow coma score is important (Table I–1).

CLINICAL PEARL

▶ A thorough understanding of anatomy is important to optimally interpret the physical examination findings.

12. Laboratory assessment depends on the circumstances:
   a. CBC (complete blood count) can assess for anemia, leukocytosis (infection), and thrombocytopenia.
   b. Basic metabolic panel: Electrolytes, glucose, BUN (blood urea nitrogen), and creatinine (renal function).
   c. Urinalysis and/or urine culture: To assess for hematuria, pyuria, or bacteruria. A pregnancy test is important in women of childbearing age.
   d. AST (aspartate aminotransferase), ALT (alanine aminotransferase), bilirubin, alkaline phosphatase for liver function; amylase and lipase to evaluate the pancreas.

Table I–1 • GLASGOW COMA SCALE	
Assessment Area	Score
Eye opening	
Spontaneous	4
To speech	3
To pain	2
None	1
Best motor response	
Obeys commands	6
Localizes pain	5
Withdraws to pain	4
Decorticate posture (abnormal flexion)	3
Decerebrate posture (extension)	2
No response	1
Verbal response	
Oriented	5
Confused conversation	4
Inappropriate words	3
Incomprehensible sounds	2
None	1

Glasgow coma scale score is the sum of the best responses in the three areas: eye opening, best motor response, and verbal response

e. Cardiac markers (CK-MB [creatine kinase myocardial band], troponin, myoglobin) if coronary artery disease or other cardiac dysfunction is suspected.

f. Drug levels such as acetaminophen level in possible overdoses.

g. Arterial blood gas measurements give information about oxygenation, but also carbon dioxide and pH readings.

13. Diagnostic adjuncts:

a. Electrocardiogram if cardiac ischemia, dysrhythmia, or other cardiac dysfunction is suspected.

b. Ultrasound examination useful in evaluating pelvic processes in female patients (eg, pelvic inflammatory disease, tubo-ovarian abscess) and in diagnosing gallstones and other gallbladder disease. With the addition of color-flow Doppler, deep venous thrombosis and ovarian or testicular torsion can be detected.

c. Computed tomography (CT) useful in assessing the brain for masses, bleeding, strokes, skull fractures. CTs of the chest can evaluate for masses, fluid collections, aortic dissections, and pulmonary emboli. Abdominal CTs can detect infection (abscess, appendicitis, diverticulitis), masses, aortic aneurysms, and ureteral stones.

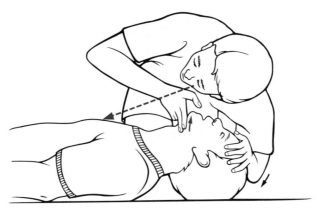

Figure I–1. Determination of breathlessness. The rescuer "looks, listens, and feels" for breath.

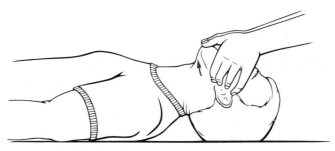

Figure I–2. Jaw-thrust maneuver. The rescuer lifts upward on the mandible while keeping the cervical spine in neutral position.

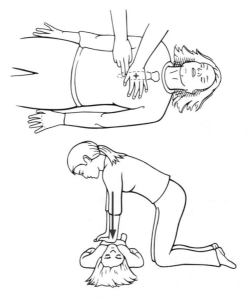

Figure I–3. Chest compressions. Rescuer applying chest compressions to an adult victim.

d. Magnetic resonance imaging (MRI) helps to identify soft tissue planes very well. In the emergency department (ED) setting, this is most commonly used to rule out spinal cord compression, cauda equina syndrome, and epidural abscess or hematoma. MRI may also be useful for patients with acute strokes.

Part 2. Approach to Clinical Problem Solving

CLASSIC CLINICAL PROBLEM SOLVING

There are typically five distinct steps that an emergency department clinician undertakes to systematically solve most clinical problems:

1. Addressing the ABCs and other life-threatening conditions

2. Making the diagnosis

3. Assessing the severity of the disease

4. Treating based on the stage of the disease

5. Following the patient's response to the treatment

EMERGENCY ASSESSMENT AND MANAGEMENT

Patients often present to the ED with life-threatening conditions that necessitate **simultaneous evaluation and treatment**. For example, a patient who is acutely short of breath and hypoxemic requires supplemental oxygen and possibly intubation with mechanical ventilation. While addressing these needs, the clinician must also try to determine whether the patient is dyspneic because of a pneumonia, congestive heart failure, pulmonary embolus, pneumothorax, or for some other reason.

As a general rule, **the first priority is stabilization of the ABCs** (see Table I–2). For instance, a comatose multitrauma patient first requires intubation to protect the airway. See Figures I–1 through I–3 regarding management of airway and breathing issues. Then, if the patient has a tension pneumothorax (breathing problem), (s)he needs an immediate needle thoracostomy. If (s)he is hypotensive, large-bore IV access and volume resuscitation are required for circulatory support. Pressure should be applied to any actively bleeding region. Once the ABCs and other life-threatening conditions are stabilized, a more complete history and head-to-toe physical examination should follow.

> ### CLINICAL PEARL
>
> ▶ Because emergency physicians are faced with unexpected illness and injury, they must often perform diagnostic and therapeutic steps simultaneously. **In patients with an acutely life-threatening condition, the first and foremost priority is stabilization—the ABCs.**

MAKING THE DIAGNOSIS

This is achieved by carefully evaluating the patient, analyzing the information, assessing risk factors, and developing a list of possible diagnoses (the differential). Usually a long list of possible diagnoses can be pared down to a few of the most likely

Table I–2 • ASSESSMENT OF ABCS		
	Assessment	**Management**
Airway	Assess oral cavity, patient color (pink vs cyanotic), patency of airway (choking, aspiration, compression, foreign body, edema, blood), stridor, tracheal deviation, ease of ventilation with bag and mask	Head-tilt and chin-lift If cervical spine injury suspected, stabilize neck and use jaw thrust If obstruction, Heimlich maneuver, chest thrust, finger sweep (unconscious patient only) Temporizing airway (laryngeal mask airway) Definitive airway (intubation [nasotracheal or endotracheal], cricothyroidotomy)
Breathing	Look, listen, and feel for air movement and chest rising Respiratory rate and effort (accessory muscles, diaphoresis, fatigue) Effective ventilation (bronchospasm, chest wall deformity, pulmonary embolism)	Resuscitation (mouth-to-mouth, mouth-to-mask, bag and mask) Supplemental oxygen, chest tube (pneumothorax or hemothorax)
Circulation	Palpate carotid artery Assess pulse and blood pressure Cardiac monitor to assess rhythm Consider arterial pressure monitoring Assess capillary refill	If pulseless, chest compressions and determine cardiac rhythm (consider epinephrine, defibrillation) Intravenous access (central line) Fluids Consider 5Hs and 5Ts: **H**ypovolemia, **H**ypoxia, **H**ypothermia, **H**yper-/**H**ypokalemia, **H**ydrogen (acidosis); **T**ension pneumothorax, **T**amponade (cardiac), **T**hrombosis (massive pulmonary embolism), **T**hrombosis (myocardial infarction), **T**ablets (drug overdose).

or most serious ones, based on the clinician's knowledge, experience, and selective testing. For example, a patient who complains of upper abdominal pain and who has a history of nonsteroidal anti-inflammatory drug (NSAID) use may have peptic ulcer disease; another patient who has abdominal pain, fatty food intolerance, and abdominal bloating may have cholelithiasis. Yet another individual with a 1-day history of periumbilical pain that now localizes to the right lower quadrant may have acute appendicitis.

CLINICAL PEARL

▶ The second step in clinical problem solving is making the diagnosis.

ASSESSING THE SEVERITY OF THE DISEASE

After establishing the diagnosis, the next step is to characterize the severity of the disease process; in other words, to describe "how bad" the disease is. This may be as simple as determining whether a patient is "sick" or "not sick." Is the patient with a urinary tract infection septic or stable for outpatient therapy? In other cases, a more formal staging may be used. For example, the Glasgow coma scale is used in patients with head trauma to describe the severity of their injury based on eye-opening, verbal, and motor responses.

CLINICAL PEARL

▶ The third step in clinical problem solving is to **establish the severity or stage of disease.** This usually impacts the treatment and/or prognosis.

TREATING BASED ON STAGE

Many illnesses are characterized by stage or severity because this affects prognosis and treatment. As an example, a formerly healthy young man with pneumonia and no respiratory distress may be treated with oral antibiotics at home. An older person with emphysema and pneumonia would probably be admitted to the hospital for IV antibiotics. A patient with pneumonia and respiratory failure would likely be intubated and admitted to the intensive care unit for further treatment.

CLINICAL PEARL

▶ The fourth step in clinical problem solving is tailoring the treatment to fit the severity or "stage" of the disease.

FOLLOWING THE RESPONSE TO TREATMENT

The final step in the approach to disease is to follow the patient's response to the therapy. Some responses are clinical such as improvement (or lack of improvement) in a patient's pain. Other responses may be followed by testing (eg, monitoring the anion gap in a patient with diabetic ketoacidosis). The clinician must be prepared to know what to do if the patient does not respond as expected. Is the next step to treat again, to reassess the diagnosis, or to follow up with another more specific test?

CLINICAL PEARL

▶ The fifth step in clinical problem solving is to monitor treatment response or efficacy. This may be measured in different ways—symptomatically or based on physical examination or other testing. For the emergency physician, the vital signs, oxygenation, urine output, and mental status are the key parameters.

Part 3. Approach to Reading

The clinical problem-oriented approach to reading is different from the classic "systematic" research of a disease. Patients rarely present with a clear diagnosis; hence, the student must become skilled in applying textbook information to the clinical scenario.

Because reading with a purpose improves the retention of information, the student should read with the goal of answering specific questions. There are seven fundamental questions that facilitate **clinical thinking.**

1. What is the most likely diagnosis?

2. How would you confirm the diagnosis?

3. What should be your next step?

4. What is the most likely mechanism for this process?

5. What are the risk factors for this condition?

6. What are the complications associated with the disease process?

7 What is the best therapy?

CLINICAL PEARL

▶ **Reading with the purpose of answering the seven fundamental clinical questions improves retention of information** and facilitates the application of "book knowledge" to "clinical knowledge."

WHAT IS THE MOST LIKELY DIAGNOSIS?

The method of establishing the diagnosis was covered in the previous section. One way of attacking this problem is to develop standard "approaches" to common clinical problems. It is helpful to understand the most common causes of various presentations, such as "the worst headache of the patient's life is worrisome for a subarachnoid hemorrhage." (See the Clinical Pearls at end of each case.)

The clinical scenario would be something such as: "A 38-year-old woman is noted to have a 2-day history of a unilateral, throbbing headache and photophobia. What is the most likely diagnosis?"

With no other information to go on, the student would note that this woman has a unilateral headache and photophobia. Using the "most common cause" information, the student would make an educated guess that the patient has a migraine headache. If instead the patient is noted to have "the worst headache of her life," the student would use the Clinical Pearl: "The worst headache of the patient's life is worrisome for a subarachnoid hemorrhage."

CLINICAL PEARL

▶ The more common cause of a unilateral, throbbing headache with photophobia is a migraine, but **the main concern is subarachnoid hemorrhage.** If the patient describes this as "the worst headache of her life," the concern for a subarachnoid bleed is increased.

HOW WOULD YOU CONFIRM THE DIAGNOSIS?

In the scenario above, the woman with "the worst headache" is suspected of having a subarachnoid hemorrhage. This diagnosis could be confirmed by a CT scan of the head and/or lumbar puncture. The student should learn the limitations of various diagnostic tests, especially when used early in a disease process. The lumbar puncture showing xanthochromia (red blood cells) is the "gold standard" test for diagnosing subarachnoid hemorrhage, but it may be negative early in the disease course.

WHAT SHOULD BE YOUR NEXT STEP?

This question is difficult because the next step has many possibilities; the answer may be to obtain more diagnostic information, stage the illness, or introduce therapy. It is often a more challenging question than "What is the most likely diagnosis?" because there may be insufficient information to make a diagnosis and the next step may be to pursue more diagnostic information. Another possibility is that there is enough information for a probable diagnosis, and the next step is to stage the disease. Finally, the most appropriate answer may be to treat. Hence, from clinical data, a judgment needs to be rendered regarding how far along one is on the road of:

(1) Make a diagnosis → (2) Stage the disease →

(3) Treat based on stage → (4) Follow the response

Frequently, the student is taught "to regurgitate" the same information that someone has written about a particular disease, but is not skilled at identifying the next step. This talent is learned optimally at the bedside, in a supportive environment, with freedom to take educated guesses, and with constructive feedback. A sample scenario might describe a student's thought process as follows:

1. Make the diagnosis: "Based on the information I have, I believe that Mr. Smith has a small-bowel obstruction from adhesive disease *because* he presents with nausea and vomiting, abdominal distension, high-pitched hyperactive bowel sounds, and has dilated loops of small bowel on x-ray."

2. Stage the disease: "I don't believe that this is severe disease because he does not have fever, evidence of sepsis, intractable pain, peritoneal signs, or leukocytosis."

3. Treat based on stage: "Therefore, my next step is to treat with nothing per mouth, NG (nasogastric) tube drainage, IV fluids, and observation."

4. Follow response: "I want to follow the treatment by assessing his pain (I will ask him to rate the pain on a scale of 1 to 10 every day), his bowel function (I will ask whether he has had nausea or vomiting, or passed flatus), his temperature, abdominal examination, serum bicarbonate (for metabolic acidemia), and white blood cell count, and I will reassess him in 48 hours."

In a similar patient, when the clinical presentation is unclear, perhaps the best "next step" may be diagnostic, such as an oral contrast radiological study to assess for bowel obstruction.

> **CLINICAL PEARL**

> ▶ Usually, the vague query, "What is your next step?" is the most difficult question because the answer may be diagnostic, staging, or therapeutic.

WHAT IS THE LIKELY MECHANISM FOR THIS PROCESS?

This question goes further than making the diagnosis, but also requires the student to understand the underlying mechanism for the process. For example, a clinical scenario may describe a 68-year-old man who notes urinary hesitancy and retention, and has a nontender large hard mass in his left supraclavicular region. This patient has bladder neck obstruction either as a consequence of benign prostatic hypertrophy or prostatic cancer. However, the indurated mass in the left neck area is suspicious for cancer. The mechanism is metastasis occurs in the area of the thoracic duct, because the malignant cells flow in the lymph fluid, which drains into the left subclavian vein. The student is advised to learn the mechanisms for each disease process, and not merely memorize a constellation of symptoms. Furthermore, in emergency medicine, it is crucial for the student to understand the anatomy, function, and how treatment would correct the problem.

WHAT ARE THE RISK FACTORS FOR THIS PROCESS?

Understanding the risk factors helps the practitioner to establish a diagnosis and to determine how to interpret tests. For example, understanding risk factor analysis may help in the management of a 55-year-old woman with anemia. If the patient has risk factors for endometrial cancer (such as diabetes, hypertension, anovulation) and complains of postmenopausal bleeding, she likely has endometrial carcinoma and should have an endometrial biopsy. Otherwise, occult colonic bleeding is a common etiology. If she takes NSAIDs or aspirin, then peptic ulcer disease is the most likely cause.

> **CLINICAL PEARL**

> ▶ Being able to assess risk factors helps to guide testing and develop the differential diagnosis.

WHAT ARE THE COMPLICATIONS TO THIS PROCESS?

Clinicians must be cognizant of the complications of a disease, so that they will understand how to follow and monitor the patient. Sometimes the student will have to make the diagnosis from clinical clues and then apply his or her knowledge of the consequences of the pathological process. For example, "a 26-year-old man complains of right-lower-extremity swelling and pain after a trans-Atlantic flight" and his Doppler ultrasound reveals a deep vein thrombosis. Complications of this process include pulmonary embolism (PE). Understanding the types of consequences also helps the clinician to be aware of the dangers to a patient. If the patient has any symptoms consistent with a PE, CT angiographic imaging of the chest may be necessary.

WHAT IS THE BEST THERAPY?

To answer this question, not only does the clinician need to reach the correct diagnosis and assess the severity of the condition, but the clinician must also weigh the situation to determine the appropriate intervention. For the student, knowing exact dosages is not as important as understanding the best medication, route of delivery, mechanism of action, and possible complications. It is important for the student to be able to verbalize the diagnosis and the rationale for the therapy.

CLINICAL PEARL

▶ Therapy should be logical based on the severity of disease and the specific diagnosis. An exception to this rule is in an emergent situation such as respiratory failure or shock when the patient needs treatment even as the etiology is being investigated.

Summary

1. The first and foremost priority in addressing the emergency patient is stabilization, then assessing and treating the ABCs (airway, breathing, circulation).

2. There is no replacement for a meticulous history and physical examination.

3. There are five steps in the clinical approach to the emergency patient: addressing life-threatening conditions, making the diagnosis, assessing severity, treating based on severity, and following response.

4. There are seven questions that help to bridge the gap between the textbook and the clinical arena.

REFERENCES

Hamilton GC. Introduction to emergency medicine. In: Hamilton GC, Sanders AB, Strange GR, Trott AT, eds. *Emergency Medicine: An Approach to Clinical Problem-Solving.* Philadelphia, PA: Saunders; 2003:3-16.

Hirshop JM. Basic CPR in adults. In: Tintinalli J, Stapczynski JS, Ma OJ, Cline D, Cydulka R, Meckler G, eds. *Emergency Medicine.* 7th ed. New York, NY: McGraw-Hill; 2010.

Ornato JP. Sudden cardiac death. In: Tintinalli J, Stapczynski JS, Ma OJ, Cline D, Cydulka R, Meckler G, eds. *Emergency Medicine.* 7th ed. New York, NY: McGraw-Hill; 2004.

Shapiro ML, Angood PB. Patient safety, errors, and complications in surgery. In: Brunicardi FC, Andersen DK, Billiar TR, et al, eds. *Schwartz's Principles of Surgery.* 9th ed., New York, NY: McGraw-Hill; 2009.

Clinical Cases

A 13-year-old adolescent boy presents to the emergency department with a chief complaint of sore throat and fever for 2 days. He reports that his younger sister has been ill for the past week with "the same thing." The patient has pain with swallowing, but no change in voice, drooling, or neck stiffness. He denies any recent history of cough, rash, nausea, vomiting, or diarrhea. He denies any recent travel and has completed the full series of childhood immunizations. He has no other medical problems, takes no medications, and has no allergies.

On examination, the patient has a temperature of 38.5°C (101.3°F), a heart rate of 104 beats per minute, blood pressure 118/64 mm Hg, a respiratory rate of 18 breaths per minute, and an oxygen saturation of 99% on room air. His posterior oropharynx reveals erythema with tonsillar exudates without uvular deviation, or significant tonsillar swelling. Neck examination is supple without tenderness of the anterior lymph nodes. Chest and cardiovascular examination is unremarkable. His abdomen is soft and nontender with normal bowel sounds and no hepatosplenomegaly. Skin is without rash.

▶ What is the most likely diagnosis?
▶ What are the dangerous causes of sore throat you don't want to miss?
▶ What is your diagnostic plan?
▶ What is your therapeutic plan?

ANSWERS TO CASE 1:

Streptococcal Pharyngitis ("Strep Throat")

Summary: This is a 13-year-old adolescent boy with pharyngitis. He has fever, tonsillar exudate, no cough, and no tender cervical adenopathy. There is no evidence of airway involvement.

- **Most likely diagnosis:** Streptococcal pharyngitis.

- **Dangerous causes of sore throat:** Epiglottitis, peritonsillar abscess, retropharyngeal abscess, Ludwig angina.

- **Diagnostic plan:** Use Centor criteria to determine probability of bacterial pharyngitis and rapid antigen testing when appropriate.

- **Therapeutic plan:** Evaluate the patient for need of antibiotics versus supportive care.

ANALYSIS

Objectives

1. Recognize the different etiologies of pharyngitis, paying close attention to those that are potentially life-threatening.

2. Be familiar with widely accepted decision-making strategies for the diagnosis and management of group A β-hemolytic streptococcal (GABS) pharyngitis.

3. Learn the treatment of GABS pharyngitis and understand the sequelae of this disease.

4. Recognize acute airway emergencies associated with upper airway infections.

Considerations

This 13-year-old patient presents with a common diagnostic dilemma: sore throat and fever. The first priority for the physician is to assess whether the patient is more ill than the complaint would indicate: **stridorous breathing, air hunger, toxic appearance,** or **drooling with inability to swallow** would **indicate impending disaster.** The ABCs (airway, breathing, circulation) must always be addressed first. This patient does not have those types of "alarms." Thus a more relaxed elicitation of his history can take place, and examination of the head, neck, and throat can be performed. In instances suggestive of epiglottitis such as stridor, drooling, and toxic appearance, examination of the throat (especially with a tongue blade) may cause upper airway obstruction in children, leading to respiratory failure. During the examination, the clinician should be alert for complications of upper airway infection; however, this patient presents with a simple pharyngitis.

Overall the most common etiology of pharyngitis is viral organisms. This teenager has several features that make group A streptococcus more likely: **age less than 15 years, fever, absence of cough,** and **the presence of tonsillar exudate.** Of note, the patient does not have "tender anterior cervical adenopathy." The diagnosis of group A streptococcal pharyngitis can be made clinically or with the aid of rapid antigen testing. Rapid streptococcal antigen testing can give a fairly accurate result immediately and treatment or nontreatment with penicillin can be based on this result. If the rapid streptococcal antigen test is positive, antibiotic therapy should be given; if the rapid test is negative, throat culture should be performed and antibiotics should be withheld. The **gold standard for diagnosis is bacterial culture**, and if positive, the patient should be notified and given penicillin therapy.

APPROACH TO:
Pharyngitis

CLINICAL APPROACH

The **differential diagnosis of pharyngitis** is broad and includes **viral etiologies** (rhinovirus, coronavirus, adenovirus, herpes simplex virus [HSV], influenza, parainfluenza, Epstein-Barr virus [EBV], and CMV [cytomegalovirus] [causing infectious mononucleosis], coxsackievirus [causing herpangina], and the human immunodeficiency virus [HIV]), bacterial causes (GABS, group C streptococci, *Arcanobacterium haemolyticum*, meningococcal, gonococcal, diphteritic, chlamydial, *Legionella*, and *Mycoplasma* species), specific anatomically related conditions caused by bacterial organisms (peritonsillar abscess, epiglottitis, retropharyngeal abscess, Vincent angina, and Ludwig angina), candidal pharyngitis, aphthous stomatitis, thyroiditis, and bullous erythema multiforme. **Viruses** are the **most common cause of pharyngitis.**

Group A streptococcus causes pharyngitis in 5% to 10% of adults and 15% to 30% of children who seek medical care with the complaint of sore throat. It is often clinically indistinguishable from other etiologies, yet it is the major treatable cause of pharyngitis. Primary HIV infection may also cause acute pharyngitis, and its recognition can be beneficial because early antiretroviral therapy can be started. Infectious mononucleosis is also important to exclude because of the risk of splenomegaly and splenic rupture. Other **bacterial etiologies** may also be treated with antibiotics. Studies suggest that certain symptoms and historical features are suggestive of streptococcal pharyngitis and may help guide the provider in generating a reasonable pretest probability of GABS. The Centor criteria, modified by age risk, is helpful in assessing for GABS (Table 1–1).

Of note, recent epidemiologic data suggest *Fusobacterium necrophorum* causes pharyngitis at a rate similar to GABS in young adults and if not treated is implicated in causing Lemierre syndrome, a life-threatening suppurative complication.

Throat cultures remain the gold standard for the diagnosis of GABS pharyngitis, but they have several limitations in use for daily practice. False-negative throat cultures may occur in patients with few organisms in their pharynx or as a result of inadequate sampling (improper swabbing method, errors in incubation or reading of plates). False-positive throat cultures may occur in individuals who are asymptomatic carriers of GABS. Throat cultures are costly and, perhaps more importantly, require 24 to 48 hours for results. Although it may be reasonable to delay therapy for

Table 1–1 • CENTOR CRITERIA FOR PREDICTING STREPTOCOCCAL PHARYNGITIS
Presence of tonsillar exudates: 1 point
Tender anterior cervical adenopathy: 1 point
Fever by history: 1 point
Absence of cough: 1 point
Age less than 15 y,[a] add 1 point to total score
Age more than 45 y,[a] subtract 1 point from total score

[a]Modifications to the original Centor criteria. See interpretation of the score in text.
Centor RM, Witherspoon JM, Dalton HP, et al. The diagnosis of strep throat in adults in the emergency room. Med Decis Making. 1981;1:239-246; and McIsaac WJ, White D, Tannenbaum D, Low DE. A clinical score to reduce unnecessary antibiotic use in patients with sore throat. CMAJ. 1998;158(1):75-83.

this period of time (delay will not increase likelihood of development of rheumatic fever), it requires further communication with the patient and perhaps an uncomfortable latency in therapy from the concerned parent. Nevertheless, a negative throat culture may prompt discontinuation of antibiotics.

The rapid-antigen test (RAT) for GABS, despite having some limitations, has been embraced by many experts and incorporated into diagnostic algorithms. The **RAT is 80% to 90% sensitive** and exceedingly specific when compared to throat cultures. Results are point-of-care and available in minutes. Many experts recommend **confirmation of negative RAT with throat culture**. Individuals with **positive RAT results should be treated**. Newer technologies, such as the optical immunoassay, may prove to be as sensitive as throat cultures while providing results within minutes; its cost-effectiveness has not been established.

If **RAT is available**, then one accepted algorithm is given in Figure 1–1.

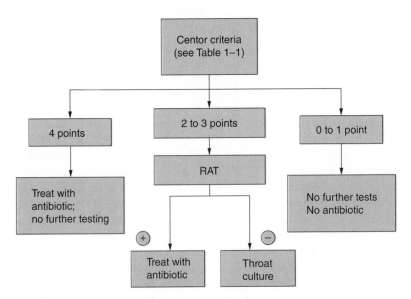

Figure 1–1. Algorithm for Centor criteria.

- Patients with 4 points from the Centor and/or McIsaac criteria should be empirically treated, because their pretest probability is reasonably high (although this practice may result in overtreatment in as many as 50% of patients).

- Patients with 0 or 1 points should not receive antibiotics or diagnostic tests (the criteria have been shown here to yield a negative predictive value of roughly 80%).

- Patients with 2 or 3 points should have RAT and those with positive RAT results should be treated. Negative RAT results should withhold antibiotics be followed with a throat culture.

If **RAT is unavailable**, then one accepted algorithm is given in Figure 1–2.

- Patients with 3 or 4 points should be empirically treated with antibiotics.

- Patients with 0 or 1 point should not receive antibiotics or diagnostic tests.

- Patients with 2 points should *not* receive antibiotics. The possible exceptions to this 2-point rule are in the setting of a GABS outbreak, patient contact with many children, an immunocompromised patient, or a patient with recent exposure to someone with confirmed GABS.

Of note, antibiotic therapy in GABS pharyngitis has been de-emphasized because complications have become increasingly rare and the data to support the efficacy of antibiotic therapy in prevention of these complications is sparse and many decades old.

The complications of GABS can be classified into nonsuppurative and suppurative processes. The **nonsuppurative complications of GABS pharyngitis** include

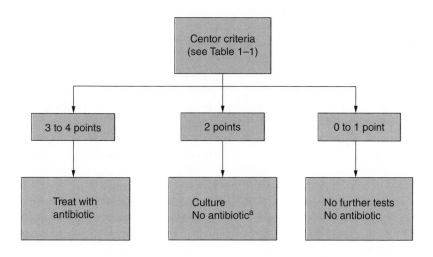

^aConsider antibiotics if in setting of GAβS outbreak, patient had contact with many children, is immunocompromised, or recent exposure to a patient with documented GAβS.

Figure 1–2. Algorithm when RAT unavailable.

rheumatic fever, streptococcal toxic shock syndrome, poststreptococcal glomerulonephritis, and PANDAS (pediatric autoimmune neuropsychiatric disorder associated with group A streptococci). Rheumatic fever is now rare in the United States (an incidence of <1 case per 100,000), and is thought to be caused by only a handful of strains of GABS. Despite its rarity, rheumatic fever can result in highly morbid cardiac and neurological sequela; it also remains the most common cause of acquired heart disease in children and adolescents in some developing countries. Published literature suggests the GABS number needed to treat (NNT) to prevent one case of rheumatic fever is between 53 and thousands depending on the endemic incidence of rheumatic fever. Streptococcal toxic shock syndrome is a very rare complication of pharyngitis. Poststreptococcal glomerulonephritis, another feared complication of GABS pharyngitis, is also very rare, and it occurs with equal frequency in both antibiotic-treated and nonantibiotic-treated groups. It is unclear if antibiotic therapy reduces the incidence of PANDAS, which is a clinical entity in development and presents with episodes of obsessive-compulsive behavior.

Prevention of the suppurative complications of GABS pharyngitis remains perhaps the most compelling reason for antibiotic therapy. These processes include **tonsillopharyngeal cellulitis, peritonsillar and retropharyngeal abscesses, sinusitis, meningitis, brain abscess, and streptococcal bacteremia.** The precise incidence of these complications is unclear, but what remains clear is that these are often preventable sequela that can have devastating consequences. Ultimately, the current practice is to treat suspected GABS pharyngitis with an appropriate antibiotic.

Treatment of GABS

Penicillin is the antibiotic of choice for GABS pharyngitis. A Cochrane review of the literature concluded that penicillin is the first choice antibiotic in patients with acute throat infections. The antibiotic is inexpensive, well-tolerated, and has a reasonably narrow spectrum. **Oral therapy requires a 10-day course,** although multiple daily doses for this duration may pose an issue with respect to compliance; penicillin V 500-mg bid dosing for 10 days in adults (as opposed to 250 mg tid or qid) is a reasonable alternative. For patients in whom compliance may be a significant issue, **a single IM shot of 600,000 units of penicillin G benzathine in patients weighing <27 kg (1.2 million units if patient weighs >27 kg)** is another option, although it requires an uncomfortable injection and, more significantly, it cannot be reversed or discontinued should an adverse reaction occur. All patients, regardless of final diagnosis, should be given adequate analgesia and reassurance. It has been shown that individuals who are perceived to want antibiotics may ultimately just want pain relief.

While somewhat controversial, some physicians recommend steroids as an anti-inflammatory agent to decrease the pain and swelling associated with GABS. A meta-analysis of over a thousand patients showed improvement 4.5 hours faster with steroids compared to placebo with a minimal reduction in pain scores. If clinically indicated, the standard agent is **dexamethasone 0.6 mg/kg up to 10 mg PO or IM.**

Airway Complications

There are several life-threatening causes of sore throat. Patients may suffer airway obstruction from acute epiglottitis, peritonsillar abscess, retropharyngeal abscess, and Ludwig angina (Table 1–2); although less frequent, airway compromise may also occur with Vincent angina and diphtheria pharyngitis; the latter requires prompt diagnosis and treatment to avoid spread of this highly infectious condition. Management of the airway in these conditions (see Table I–2 in Section I) sometimes necessitates emergency cricothyroidotomy (Figure 1–3), because the pharynx and larynx may be edematous, distorted, or inflamed. Prompt identification of acute retroviral syndrome from recent HIV infection can allow for rapid antiretroviral therapy. Infectious mononucleosis should be identified so that potentially serious sequela can be considered. These complications include splenomegaly that predisposes the patient to traumatic rupture of the spleen with relatively minor trauma; additionally, this splenomegaly can cause splenic sequestration and thrombocytopenia.

Table 1–2 • COMPLICATED UPPER AIRWAY INFECTIONS			
	Clinical Presentation	Diagnosis	Treatment
Epiglottitis	Sudden onset of fever, drooling, tachypnea, stridor, toxic appearing	Lateral cervical radiograph (thumb-printing sign)	Urgent ENT (ear, nose, throat) consultation for airway management Helium-O_2 mixture Cefuroxime antibiotic therapy
Retropharyngeal abscess	Usually child or if adult (trauma) Fever, sore throat, stiff neck, no trismus	Lateral cervical radiograph or CT imaging	Stabilize airway Surgical drainage Antibiotics (penicillin and metronidazole)
Ludwig angina	Submaxillary, sublingual, or submental mass with elevation of tongue, jaw swelling, fever, chills, trismus	Lateral cervical radiograph or CT imaging	Stabilize airway Surgical drainage Antibiotics (penicillin and metronidazole)
Peritonsillar abscess	Swelling in the peritonsillar region with uvula deviation, fever, sore throat, dysphagia, trismus	Cervical radiograph or CT imaging Aspiration of the region with pus	Abscess drainage Antibiotic therapy (penicillin and metronidazole)

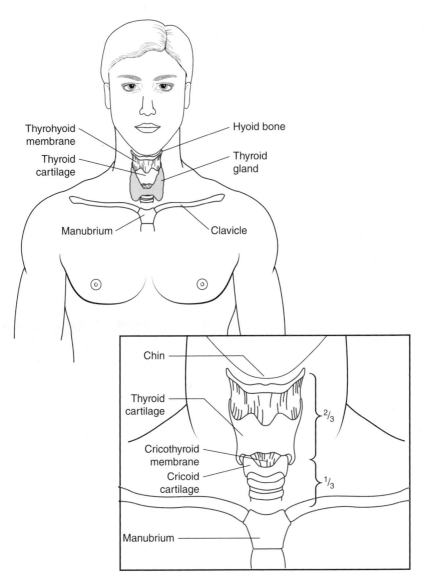

Figure 1–3. Anatomy of the neck for emergency cricothyroidotomy. Note the location of the thyroid and cricoid cartilages.

COMPREHENSION QUESTIONS

1.1 A 48-year-old man is noted to have a 2-day history of sore throat, subjective fever at home, and no medical illnesses. He denies cough or nausea. On examination, his temperature is 38.3°C (101°F), and he has some tonsillar swelling but no exudate. He has bilateral enlarged and tender lymph nodes of the neck. The rapid streptococcal antigen test is negative. Which of the following is the best next step?

   A. Oral clindamycin

   B. Treatment based on results from throat culture

   C. Observation

   D. Begin amantadine

1.2 Which of the following patients is most likely to have group A streptococcal infection?

   A. An 11-month-old male infant with fever and red throat

   B. An 8-year-old girl with fever and sore throat

   C. A 27-year-old man with a temperature of 38.9°C (102°F), pharyngitis, and cough

   D. A 52-year-old woman who complains of fever of 39.2°C (102.5°F) and sore throat

1.3 A 19-year-old college student has had a sore throat, mild abdominal pain, and fever for 5 days. He was playing football with some friends, and was tackled just short of the goal line, hitting the grass somewhat forcibly. He experiences some abdominal pain, and passes out. The EMS (emergency medical services) is called and his vital signs reveal the heart rate as 140 beats per minute and blood pressure as 80/40 mm Hg with a distended abdomen. Which of the following is the most likely etiology?

   A. Vasovagal reaction

   B. Ruptured aortic aneurysm

   C. Complications of Epstein-Barr infection

   D. Ruptured jejunum

1.4 An 18-year-old woman presents with fever and a sore throat. She is sitting up drooling, with some stridor. Her temperature is 39.4°C (103°F) and she appears ill. Which of the following is your next step?

   A. Examine the pharynx and obtain a rapid antigen test.

   B. Empiric treatment with penicillin.

   C. Throat culture and treatment based on results.

   D. Send the patient to radiology for an anteroposterior (AP) neck radiograph.

   E. Prepare for emergent airway management.

ANSWERS

1.1 **B.** This individual has a modified Centor score of 2 (history of fever, tender adenopathy, no cough, age >45 y). The rapid antigen test is negative, but a definitive culture should be performed for a Centor score of 2 or 3, and treatment should be based on culture results.

1.2 **B.** GABS is most common in patients younger than 15 years (although not in infants). McIsaac added age as a criteria because patients older than age 45 years have a much lower incidence of streptococcal pharyngitis.

1.3 **C.** This patient most likely suffered from splenic rupture caused by mononucleosis (EBV). He is hypotensive because of the massive hemoperitoneum. Aortic aneurysm is rare in teenagers.

1.4 **E.** Regardless of the etiology, this patient has a clinical presentation alarming for impending respiratory collapse, and preparations for emergent airway management is the most important next step. The drooling and stridor are suspicious for epiglottitis, which can present more insidiously in adults. Examination of the posterior oropharynx may induce laryngospasm and airway obstruction, particularly in children; a lateral neck radiograph to assess for a "thumbprinting" of epiglottitis may be helpful in making the diagnosis, but sending the patient with impending respiratory failure to radiology area is inappropriate.

CLINICAL PEARLS

▶ The most common cause of pharyngitis is viral.

▶ The Centor criteria suggestive of GABS pharyngitis include tonsillar exudate, tender anterior cervical adenopathy, history of fever, and absence of cough.

▶ GABS pharyngitis is more common in patients younger than 15 years of age, and less common in those older than 45 years of age.

▶ Overtreatment of pharyngitis with antibiotics is common and is a major source of antibiotic overuse.

▶ Glomerulonephritis is a rare complication of GABS pharyngitis (but not GABS infections of other tissues) that is not clearly prevented by antibiotic therapy.

▶ Rheumatic fever is an exceedingly rare complication of GABS pharyngitis that can be prevented by antibiotic therapy.

▶ Complicated upper airway conditions should be considered when a patient presents with "sore throat."

▶ In general, cricothyroidotomy is the safest method of surgically securing an airway in the ED.

REFERENCES

Bisno AL. Acute pharyngitis. *N Engl J Med.* 2001;344(3):205-211.

Bisno AL, Gerber MA, Gwaltney JM, Kaplan EL, Schwartz RH. Practice guidelines for the diagnosis and management of group a streptococcal pharyngitis. *Clin Infect Dis.* 2002;35:113-125.

Centor RM, Witherspoon JM, Dalton HP, Brody CE, Link K. The diagnosis of strep throat in adults in the emergency room. *Med Decis Making.* 1981;1:239-246.

Centor RM. Expand the pharyngitis paradigm for adolescents and young adults. *Ann Intern Med.* 2009; 151(11):812-815.

Cooper RJ, Hoffman JR, Bartlett, JG, et al. Principles of appropriate antibiotic use for acute pharyngitis in adults: background. *Ann Intern Med.* 2001;134:509-517.

Lee JL, Naguwa SM, Cesma GS, Gerhwin ME. Acute rheumatic fever and its consequences: A persistent threat to developing nations in the 21st century. *Autoimmunity Reviews.* 2009;9:117-123.

Linder JA, Chan JC, Bates DW et al. Evaluation and treatment of pharyngitis in primary care: the difference between guidelines is largely academic. *Arch Intern Med.* 2006; 166:1374.

McIsaac WJ, Kellner JD, Aufricht P, et al. Empiric validation of guidelines for the management of pharyngitis in children and adults. *JAMA.* 2004;291(13):1587.

McIssac WJ, Goel V, To T, Low DE. The validity of a sore throat score in family practice. *CMAJ.* 2000;163(7):811-815.

McIsaac WJ, White D, Tannenbaum D, Low DE. A clinical score to reduce unnecessary antibiotic use in patients with sore throat. *CMAJ.* 1998;158(1):75-83.

Snow V, Mottur-Pison C, Cooper RJ, Hoffman, JR. Principles of appropriate antibiotic use for acute pharyngitis in adults. *Ann Intern Med.* 2001;134:506-508.

Van Driel ML, Sutter AD, Deveugele M, et al. Are sore throat patients who hope for antibiotics actually asking for pain relief. *Ann Fam Med.* 2006;4(6):494.

Van Driel ML, De Sutter AI, Keber N, et al. Different antibiotic treatments for group A streptococcal pharyngitis. *Cochrane Database of Systematic Reviews* 2010;10. Art. No.:CD004406. DOI: 10.1002/ 14651858.CD004406.pub2.

Wing A, Villa-Roel C, Yeh B, et al. Effectiveness of corticosteroid treatment in acute pharyngitis: A systematic review of the literature. *Acad Emer Med.* 2010;17:476-483.

CASE 2

A 58-year-old man arrives at the emergency department complaining of chest pain. The pain began 1 hour ago, during breakfast, and is described as severe, dull, and pressure-like. It is substernal in location, radiates to both shoulders, and is associated with shortness of breath. The patient vomited once. His wife adds that he was very sweaty when the pain began. The patient has diabetes and hypertension and takes hydrochlorothiazide and glyburide. His blood pressure is 150/100 mm Hg, pulse rate is 95 beats per minute, respiration is 20 breaths per minute, temperature 37.3°C (99.1°F), and oxygen saturation by pulse oximetry is 98%. The patient is diaphoretic and appears anxious. On auscultation, faint crackles are heard at both lung bases. The cardiac examination reveals an S_4 gallop and is otherwise normal. The examination of the abdomen reveals no masses or tenderness. The ECG is shown in Figure 2–1.

▶ What is the most likely diagnosis?
▶ What are the next diagnostic steps?
▶ What therapies should be instituted immediately?

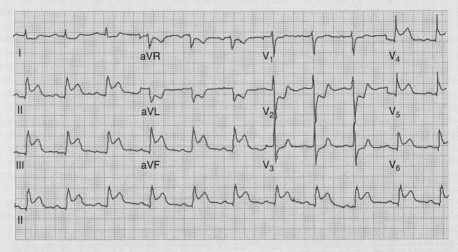

Figure 2–1. 12-lead ECG.

ANSWERS TO CASE 2:

Myocardial Infarction, Acute

Summary: This is a 58-year-old man presenting with acute severe chest pain, diaphoresis, and dyspnea. The patient has a number of risk factors for underlying coronary heart disease and the history and physical examination are typical of an acute coronary syndrome (ACS).

- **Most likely diagnosis:** Acute myocardial infarction.

- **Next diagnostic steps:** Place the patient on a cardiac monitor, establish IV access, and obtain an electrocardiogram (ECG) immediately. A chest x-ray and serum levels of cardiac markers should be obtained as soon as possible.

- **Immediate therapies: Aspirin** is the most important immediate therapy. **Oxygen** and **sublingual nitroglycerin** are also standard early therapies. Depending on the result of the ECG, emergency reperfusion therapy, such as thrombolysis, may be indicated. Intravenous β-blockers, IV nitroglycerin, low-molecular-weight heparin, and additional antiplatelet agents, such as clopidogrel, might also be indicated.

ANALYSIS

Objectives

1. Recognize acute myocardial infarction (MI) and the spectrum of acute coronary syndromes (ACSs).

2. Know the appropriate diagnostic tests and their limitations.

3. Understand the therapeutic approach to ACS.

Considerations

Chest pain accounts for more than 6 million visits every year to emergency departments in the United States. Of these 6 million visits, nearly 800,000 will end with a diagnosis of MI and 1.5 million will be given the diagnoses of unstable angina (UA) or non–ST-elevation myocardial infarction (NSTEMI). Coronary heart disease (CHD) is the leading cause of death in adults in the United States. Furthermore, missed MI accounts for the most money paid in malpractice claims in emergency medicine. Because ACS is common, treatable, and potentially catastrophic both clinically and medicolegally, emergency physicians should be thoroughly familiar with this problem.

Our understanding of the **pathophysiology** behind cardiac ischemia has evolved from a model of progressive coronary artery narrowing to a current model of plaque rupture and thrombus formation. The concept of fixed narrowing explains only stable angina brought on by increased myocardial demand. In contrast, ACS, which encompasses the spectrum of UA, NSTEMI, and ST-elevation myocardial infarction (STEMI), involves a dynamic process of inflammation and intravascular thrombosis, beginning with coronary artery plaque rupture. The fate of this plaque, in terms of location and extent of subsequent thrombosis, determines the clinical presentation and seems to correlate with the subdivisions of ACS. **STEMI** occurs when total occlusion of an epicardial vessel causes transmural infarction, classically presenting as unremitting chest pain and ST-segment elevation on the electrocardiography (ECG). It is treated with immediate reperfusion therapy.

The clinical syndromes of **NSTEMI and UA,** in contrast, are caused by subendocardial infarction or ischemia, respectively, usually caused by microemboli arising from the ruptured plaque. Chest pain is often stuttering and ECG changes such as ST-segment depression may be transient. Although often indistinguishable upon initial presentation, elevation in cardiac markers is what eventually distinguishes NSTEMI from UA. Immediate therapy for both NSTEMI and UA focuses on halting ongoing thrombosis and reducing myocardial demand. Many patients go on to have percutaneous coronary intervention (PCI), such as stent placement, directed at the unstable plaque.

APPROACH TO:
Suspected Myocardial Infarction

DEFINITIONS

MYOCARDIAL INFARCTION: Myocardial cell death caused by ischemia, as evidenced by a typical rise and fall in cardiac biomarkers.

ACUTE CORONARY SYNDROME: An ischemic chest pain syndrome, usually associated with coronary artery plaque rupture, encompassing STEMI, NSTEMI, and UA.

UNSTABLE ANGINA: An acute coronary syndrome, in which chest pain is of new onset, or increasing severity, or occurs at rest, and cardiac biomarkers are not elevated.

NON–ST-ELEVATION MYOCARDIAL INFARCTION: An acute coronary syndrome in which cardiac biomarkers are eventually elevated, but lacking new ST elevation on ECG.

ST-ELEVATION MYOCARDIAL INFARCTION: An acute coronary syndrome, in which significant ST elevation is found in two or more contiguous ECG leads, typically associated with epicardial coronary artery occlusion and transmural infarction, and resulting in Q waves if perfusion is not soon restored.

CLINICAL APPROACH

Evaluation

The cornerstone of diagnosis of acute coronary syndromes is the **ECG.** Because findings on the initial ECG form a **critical branch point in therapy,** patients presenting to the emergency department with chest pain suggestive of ACS should have an

Table 2–1 • KEY ECG FINDINGS IN ACS

STEMI: indications for immediate reperfusion therapy

- ST elevation >1 mV (1 mm) in 2 contiguous leads and <12 h since pain onset
- Left bundle-branch block not known to be old with a history suggestive of acute MI
- ST elevations in posterior leads (V7, V8, V9) or ST depression in V1-V3 with a prominent R wave and upright T wave suggestive of posterior STEMI

Typical ECG findings in NSTEMI and UA

- Horizontal ST-segment depression
- ECG findings change in accord with symptoms
- Deep T-wave inversions

Data from Hollander JE, Diercks DB. Intervention strategies for acute coronary syndromes. In: Tintinalli JE, Kelen GD, Stapczynski JS, eds. Emergency Medicine. 6th ed. New York, NY: McGraw-Hill; 2004:108-124.

ECG within 10 minutes of arrival. **Identifying STEMI by ECG as soon as possible is the first step** toward rapidly establishing reperfusion and reducing mortality (the ECG criteria for reperfusion therapy are listed in Table 2–1). In contrast to STEMI, ECG findings may be subtle or absent in NSTEMI and UA, and are not required for diagnosis and initiation of therapy. However, certain findings, such as ST-segment depression or deep T-wave inversions, particularly those that change in accord with symptoms, can rapidly establish the diagnosis of UA and NSTEMI.

Unfortunately, the **ECG is frequently nondiagnostic in ACS.** Even in patients eventually diagnosed with MI, the initial ECG is nondiagnostic in about 50% and completely normal in up to 8%. Comparing the current ECG to old tracings is crucial, because subtle changes may be seen. Serial ECGs performed at 15- to 30-minute intervals, or continuous ST-segment monitoring, may reveal the subtle dynamic changes of UA, or those of an evolving MI (Table 2–2 lists the anatomical locations of MI).

In the face of a normal or nondiagnostic ECG, the decision whether to further evaluate for ACS depends on the likelihood that the pain is actually of cardiac

Table 2–2 • FINDINGS AND ANATOMICAL CORRELATION

Coronary Artery	Location	ECG Leads
LAD	Anteroseptal	V1, V2, V3
LAD	Anterior	V2-V4
LCA	Lateral	I, aVL, V4-V6
RCA	Inferior	II, III, aVF
RCA	Right ventricular	V4R (also II, III, aVF)
RCA, LCA	Posterior	R waves in V1, V2

Abbreviations: LAD = left anterior descending artery; LCA = left circumflex artery; RCA = right circumflex artery; V4R = right-sided lead which should be placed any time an inferior MI is suspected.
Data from Hollander JE, Diercks DB. Intervention strategies for acute coronary syndromes. In: Tintinalli JE, Kelen GD, Stapczynski JS, eds. Emergency Medicine. 6th ed. New York, NY: McGraw-Hill; 2004:108-124.

Table 2–3 • RISK FACTORS FOR CORONARY HEART DISEASE

Diabetes mellitus

Hypercholesterolemia; high-density lipoprotein (HDL) cholesterol <40 mg/dL

Current tobacco use

Hypertension

Age (male ≥45 y; female ≥55 y or premature menopause)

Family history of premature CHD (MI or sudden death before age 55 y in male first-degree relative; before 65 y in female first-degree relative)

Sympathomimetics (cocaine, amphetamines)

Rheumatologic conditions (rheumatoid arthritis, systemic lupus erythematous)

Data from Hollander JE, Diercks DB. Intervention strategies for acute coronary syndromes. In: Tintinalli JE, Kelen GD, Stapczynski JS, eds. Emergency Medicine. 6th ed. New York, NY: McGraw-Hill; 2004:108-124.

origin and on the patient's overall risk profile. Inquiring about traditional risk factors for CHD remains a standard component of the chest pain evaluation. CHD risk factors are listed in Table 2–3. High risk is easily established if there is a prior history of definite CHD such as prior MI or abnormal coronary angiogram. Characteristics of the history and physical examination that alter the likelihood that the pain is of cardiac origin are listed in Table 2–4. Patients who are young, without a family history of premature CHD, and with an atypical history and a normal or nondiagnostic ECG can usually be safely discharged without further evaluation for ACS. Short-term prognosis in those with known or suspected UA or NSTEMI can be calculated with the thrombolytics in myocardial infarction (TIMI) risk score (Table 2–5).

Serum cardiac markers are used to confirm or exclude myocardial cell death, and are **considered the gold standard for the diagnosis of MI.** There are a number of markers currently in wide use, including myoglobin, CKMB, and troponin. While algorithms vary, serum levels of 1 or more cardiac markers should be obtained initially and at 4 to 12 hours after presentation. Troponin I is extremely sensitive and specific for cardiac damage; thus an elevated level confirms infarction whereas a normal level at 8 to 12 hours after the onset of pain excludes infarction. Important limitations of cardiac markers are that levels remain normal in unstable angina and

Table 2–4 • HISTORY AND PHYSICAL IN THE EVALUATION OF POSSIBLE ACS

Increases Likelihood That Chest Pain Is From CHD	Decreases Likelihood That Chest Pain Is From CHD
Pressure-like quality	Pleuritic quality
Radiation to either arm, neck, or jaw	Constant pain for days
Diaphoresis	Pain lasting less than 2 min
Third heart sound	Discomfort localized with one finger
Pain that is similar to prior MI pain	Discomfort reproduced by movement or palpation

Table 2–5 • TIMI RISK SCORE[a]
Age >65 y
Prior documented coronary artery stenosis >50%
Three or more CHD risk factors
Use of aspirin in the preceding 7 d
Two or more anginal events in the preceding 24 h
ST-segment deviation (transient elevation or persistent depression)
Increased cardiac markers

Abbreviation: TIMI = thrombolysis in myocardial infarction.
[a]One point is assigned to each of the seven components. Risk of death, MI, or revascularization at 2 wk by score: 1, 5%; 2, 8%; 3, 13%; 4, 20%; 5, 26%; 6, 41%.
Data from Antman EM, Cohen M, Bernink PJ, et al. The TIMI risk score for UA/NSTEMI. JAMA. 2000; 284(7):835-842.

serum elevations are delayed 4 to 12 hours after infarction. The trend and peak of positive biomarkers can indicate the dynamics of necrosis and infarct size.

Other studies that are routinely obtained in the workup of ACS include a **chest radiograph** (CXR), complete blood count, chemistries, coagulation studies, and blood type. The CXR serves to rule out other causes of chest pain, and to identify pulmonary edema. Although not a perfect test, a normal mediastinum on CXR makes aortic dissection least likely. For this reason, a chest radiograph should be performed prior to thrombolysis.

Treatment

When ACS is suspected based on history, treatment should be started immediately. The patient should be placed on a cardiac monitor, IV access established, and an ECG obtained. Unless allergic, affected patients should be immediately given **aspirin** to chew (162 mg dose is common). Aspirin is remarkably beneficial across the entire spectrum of ACS. For example, in the setting of STEMI, the survival benefit from a single dose of aspirin is roughly equal to that of thrombolytic therapy (but with negligible risk or cost). Other mainstays of initial treatment are **oxygen,** sublingual **nitroglycerin,** which decreases wall tension and myocardial oxygen demand, and **morphine sulfate.** Together with aspirin these three therapies make up the mnemonic **"MONA,"** which is said to "greet chest pain patients at the door." Based on results of the initial ECG, therapy then progresses in one of two directions.

ST-Elevation MI

When the ECG reveals **STEMI** and symptoms have been present for less than 12 hours, **immediate reperfusion therapy** is indicated. The saying **"time is myocardium"** is a reminder that myocardial salvage and clinical benefit are critically dependent on the time to restoration of flow in the infarct-related artery. Optimally, total ischemic time should be limited to less than 120 minutes. There are two ways to achieve reperfusion: primary PCI (angioplasty or stent placement) and thrombolysis. The choice is largely determined by the capabilities of the hospital.

Primary PCI is the treatment of choice when it can be performed rapidly by an experienced cardiologist. The standard "door-to-balloon time" goal is 90 minutes. Compared to thrombolysis, PCI leads to lower 30-day mortality (4.4% vs 6.5%), nonfatal reinfarction rate (7.2% vs 11.9%), and fewer hemorrhagic strokes. Recent studies suggest that if a patient presents to a hospital that does not offer PCI, transfer to a neighboring facility for primary PCI is superior to thrombolysis if transfer can be accomplished within 90 minutes. PCI is also used for STEMI complicated by cardiogenic shock, when there is a contraindication to thrombolysis, and in cases where thrombolysis fails to restore perfusion (rescue PCI). Administration of low-molecular-weight heparin and a glycoprotein IIB/IIIA inhibitor prior to PCI reduces the risk of reinfarction.

When PCI is not an option, intravenous thrombolytic agents may be used to achieve reperfusion. Studies of thrombolytic therapy versus placebo for STEMI show an absolute mortality reduction of roughly 3%. The benefit of thrombolysis is greatest when treatment is begun within 4 hours, and benefit approaches that of primary PCI when thrombolytics are begun within 30 minutes. However, benefit extends out to 12 hours. Adjunctive antithrombotic therapy with unfractionated or low-molecular-weight heparin is required with most thrombolytic agents. Table 2–6 lists other measures, in addition to aspirin and reperfusion therapy, that reduce mortality after MI.

Unstable Angina/Non-ST Elevation MI

Cases of ACS lacking ECG criteria for reperfusion fall into the UA/NSTEMI category. The approach to therapy for UA/NSTEMI tends to be graded, based on ECG findings, cardiac marker results, TIMI risk score, and whether the patient is likely to undergo early angiography and PCI. **Aspirin and nitroglycerin constitute the minimum therapy.** Morphine is added when chest discomfort continues despite nitroglycerin therapy. **β-blockers**, such as IV metoprolol, are usually added in cases presenting with hypertension or tachycardia. While the mortality benefit of chronic β-blocker therapy after MI is well established, in the acute setting, β-blockers should be used with caution because they can place certain patients at risk for cardiogenic shock, such as those presenting with signs of heart failure.

In high-risk patients, a more aggressive approach to halting the thrombotic process is taken, by adding **low-molecular-weight heparin** and oral **clopidogrel,** an antiplatelet agent. Patients are considered to be high risk if there are ischemic ECG

Table 2–6 • THERAPIES OF PROVEN BENEFIT FOR MI

Aspirin (162 mg, chewed immediately, then continued daily for life)

Primary percutaneous coronary intervention (angioplasty or stenting the blocked artery)

Thrombolysis (if primary PCI not available; most regimens require heparin therapy)

β-blockers (immediate IV use and started orally within 24 h; if no contraindications then continued daily)

Angiotensin-converting enzyme inhibitor (started within 1-3 d, continued for life)

Cholesterol-lowering drugs (started within 1-3 d and continued daily for life)

Enoxaparin (dosage given prior to thrombolysis or PCI, for patients less than 75 y of age)

Clopidogrel (75 mg daily with or without reperfusion therapy)

Data from American College of Cardiologists. Guidelines for managing patients with AMI, UA, and NSTEMI. J Am Coll Cardiol. 2002;40:1366-1374.

changes, elevated cardiac markers, or if the TIMI risk score is 3 or greater. Intravenous glycoprotein IIB/IIIA inhibitors, an even more potent and expensive type of antiplatelet drug, are reserved for the subset of high-risk patients who will undergo early angiography and PCI, in whom these agents have been shown to reduce subsequent CHD morbidity.

In the past, angiography was often postponed for a number of days or weeks following an episode of ACS. However, recent studies have shown that an **early invasive strategy,** where high-risk patients with UA and NSTEMI are taken for angiography and PCI within 24 to 36 h, has slightly superior efficacy to medical therapy and delayed angiography. An early invasive strategy is indicated for any of the following: refractory angina, hemodynamic instability, signs of heart failure, ventricular tachycardia, ST depressions on ECG, or elevated cardiac enzymes. Like primary PCI for STEMI, whether an early invasive strategy is chosen often depends on hospital resources and cardiology expertise.

Complications

Several life-threatening complications of acute MI may arise at any time after presentation (Table 2–7). Serious complications occur most often in the setting of anterior STEMI. MI-associated **ventricular tachycardia and ventricular fibrillation** (sudden death) are the most frequently encountered complications in the ED and prehospital setting, occurring in approximately 10% of cases. Continuous cardiac monitoring and immediate cardioversion/defibrillation has been a mainstay of cardiac care since the 1960s, and has been shown to save lives on a large scale. **Bradyarrhythmias** may also complicate MI. Heart block that occurs in the setting of anterior MI generally implies irreversible damage to the His-Purkinje system and is an indication for transvenous pacing. Inferior MI, in contrast, frequently causes arteriovenous (AV) node dysfunction and second-degree block that is transient and may respond to atropine.

Table 2–7 • POTENTIAL COMPLICATIONS FROM ACUTE MI
Ventricular fibrillation
Ventricular tachycardia
Heart block
Right ventricular infarction
Free wall rupture
Ventricular aneurysm
Hemorrhage secondary to therapy
Cardiogenic pulmonary edema
Ventricular septal defect
Cardiogenic shock
Mitral regurgitation
Pericarditis
Thromboembolism

Data from Hollander JE, Diercks DB. Intervention strategies for acute coronary syndromes. In: Tintinalli JE, Kelen GD, Stapczynski JS, eds. Emergency Medicine. 6th ed. New York, NY: McGraw-Hill; 2004:108-124.

Pump dysfunction, leading to **pulmonary edema** or **cardiogenic shock,** is an ominous complication of MI that implies a large area of myocardial injury. The left ventricular dysfunction that occurs with anterior MI usually causes recognizable pulmonary edema, with tachypnea, rales, and visible congestion on chest x-ray. A new systolic murmur may be heard when cardiogenic pulmonary edema is caused by papillary muscle dysfunction and acute mitral regurgitation. Signs of cardiogenic shock range from frank hypotension to subtle indicators of impaired perfusion such as oliguria, cool extremities, and confusion. Emergency PCI is the reperfusion strategy of choice for cardiogenic shock. Insertion of an aortic balloon pump may be indicated in addition to pressor agents. **Right ventricular infarction,** which complicates inferior MI, usually presents as hypotension without pulmonary congestion. The diagnosis is confirmed by ST elevation in lead V_4 on a right-sided ECG, and the primary treatment is aggressive volume loading. **Nitroglycerine and high-dose morphine should be avoided in these patients.**

Late complications of MI that tend to occur in the intensive care unit several hours to days after presentation include left ventricular free wall rupture causing tamponade, ventricular septal defect, pericarditis, left ventricular aneurysm, and thromboembolism. Finally, iatrogenic complications of MI therapy can occur. Emergency physicians who administer thrombolytics for STEMI must consider the risk of serious hemorrhagic complications, particularly intracranial hemorrhage, which occurs in 0.5% to 0.7% of patients and is usually fatal. Heparin and antiplatelet therapy leads to significant bleeding in up to 10% of patients, depending on what agents are given, although life-threatening hemorrhage is rare.

COMPREHENSION QUESTIONS

2.1 A 48-year-old man is being seen for chest pain. In the initial evaluation of this patient, which of the following is the most important diagnostic test?

A. Chest x-ray

B. ECG

C. Serum cardiac markers

D. Computed tomography

E. Cholesterol levels

2.2 A 58-year-old man presents to his physician's office complaining of 2 hours of substernal chest pain and dyspnea. Which of the following is the most important next step in management?

A. Administration of propranolol

B. Aspirin to chew

C. Sublingual nitroglycerin

D. Administration of a diuretic agent

E. Chest radiograph

2.3 A 45-year-old man is seen in the emergency department with 3 hours of substernal chest pain radiating to his left arm. The ECG shows only nonspecific changes. Hearing that the ECG is normal, he requests to go home. Which of the following statements is most accurate?

A. The patient may be safely discharged home.

B. If a repeat ECG in 30 minutes is normal, myocardial infarction is essentially ruled out and the patient may be safely discharged.

C. The patient should be advised that half of heart attack patients have a nondiagnostic ECG and serial cardiac biomarkers levels should be assessed.

D. The patient should undergo an immediate thallium stress test to further assess for coronary artery disease to help clarify the management.

ANSWERS

2.1 **B.** The ECG is the crucial first diagnostic test in the evaluation of chest pain. Presence versus absence of ST elevation represents a major therapeutic branch point.

2.2 **B.** While all of these therapies are useful, aspirin significantly decreases mortality, with almost no downside in nonallergic patients, and should be given immediately.

2.3 **C.** Roughly half of patients with MI, as defined by a typical rise in cardiac biomarkers, will have a nondiagnostic ECG upon presentation. Risk stratification by stress testing is sometimes ordered from the emergency department, but only after serial ECGs and cardiac biomarkers remain normal.

CLINICAL PEARLS

▶ MONA greets chest pain at the door (**m**orphine, **o**xygen, **n**itroglycerin, and, most importantly, **a**spirin).

▶ An ECG should be performed immediately in all patients with chest pain concerning for ACS.

▶ The ECG will dictate the next step in management: new ST elevation generally requires immediate reperfusion therapy. "Time is myocardium."

REFERENCES

Anderson J L, Adams C D, Antman E M, et al. ACC/AHA 2007 guidelines for the management of patients with unstable angina/non-ST-elevation myocardial infarction. *Circulation.* 2007;116:e148-e304.

Antman E M, Hand M, Armstrong P W, et al. 2007 focused update of the ACC/AHA 2004 guidelines for the management of patients with ST-elevation myocardial infarction. *Circulation.* 2008;117:296-329.

Panju A A, Hemmelgarn BR. Is this patient having a myocardial infarction? *JAMA.* 1998;280:1256-1263.

A 70-year-old man presents to the emergency department complaining of short-ness of breath for the past 2 weeks. Previously, he could walk everywhere, but now he becomes fatigued after a short stroll through the grocery store. He also notes that he has felt his heart racing even when he is at rest. His past medical his-tory is notable only for hypertension, for which he takes hydrochlorothiazide and amlodipine. On physical examination, he appears comfortable and speaks in full sentences without difficulty. His blood pressure is 130/90 mm Hg, heart rate is 144 beats per minute, respiratory rate is 18 breaths per minute, oxygen saturation is 98% on room air, and temperature is 37°C (98.6°F). His head and neck examina-tion is unremarkable. His lungs are clear to auscultation. His heartbeat is irregular and rapid, without murmurs rubs or gallops. He has no extremity edema or jugu-lar venous distension. His abdomen is soft and nontender, without masses. Labs show a normal CBC, normal electrolytes, BUN, creatinine, troponin, BNP, and thyroid stimulating hormone. A chest x-ray reveals a normal cardiac silhouette with no pulmonary edema. The ECG is shown below (Figure 3–1).

▶ What is the most likely diagnosis?
▶ What are some of the common contributing factors?
▶ What are some of the complications to this condition?

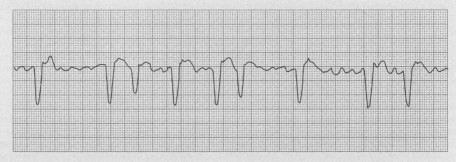

Figure 3–1. Electrocardiogram. *(Reproduced with permission from Tintinalli JE, Kelen GD, Stapczynski JS, eds.* Emergency Medicine. *6th ed. New York, NY: McGraw-Hill; 2004:185.)*

ANSWERS TO CASE 3:
Atrial Fibrillation

Summary: A 70-year-old man presents with mild dyspnea on exertion and palpitations. The physical examination reveals a heartbeat that is irregular and rapid at a rate of 144 beats per minute.

- **Most likely diagnosis:** Atrial fibrillation with rapid ventricular response

- **Common contributing factors:** Increasing age, underlying cardiopulmonary disease (such as hypertension, heart failure, and COPD), hyperthyroidism, sepsis, pulmonary embolism, and electrolyte abnormalities

- **Complications:** Early—diminished cardiac output. Late—thromboembolism and cardiomyopathy

ANALYSIS

Objectives

1. Know that atrial fibrillation is often a manifestation of serious underlying disease processes.

2. Be able to recognize atrial fibrillation on ECG.

3. Understand the approach to rate control versus rhythm control of atrial fibrillation.

4. Understand the role of antithrombotic therapy in both the acute and chronic management of atrial fibrillation.

Considerations

This individual is a 70-year-old man of fairly high function, who is brought into the emergency department because of dyspnea and palpitations. The initial approach should begin with ABCs and an assessment of any life-threatening concerns. **Upon arrival, this patient should get an IV and be placed on cardiac and pulse oximetry monitors.** The history and physical examination should focus on the patient's cardiac and pulmonary status. His pulse and the rhythm on the cardiac monitor will both reveal an irregular tachycardia, which should prompt an immediate ECG. The ECG shows an irregularly irregular tachycardia consistent with the diagnosis of atrial fibrillation (AF) with rapid ventricular response (RVR).

In this patient with symptomatic AF with RVR, an **early priority in management will be to slow the ventricular rate.** For most patients with AF, the typical symptoms of palpitations and dyspnea can be alleviated through simple rate control. In rare cases, tachycardia and loss of the "atrial kick" can lead to diminished cardiac output, hypotension, or congestive heart failure. In those cases, if the arrhythmia is thought to be the primary cause of the patients' instability, emergent electrical cardioversion is indicated. In the more stable patients, the decision of whether to convert the rhythm depends on a number of factors, including risk of thromboembolism, need for

Table 3–1 • DISEASES ASSOCIATED WITH ATRIAL FIBRILLATION	
Cardiac	Hypertension (approximately 80% of cases), coronary artery disease, cardiomyopathy, valvular heart disease, rheumatic heart disease, congenital heart disease, myocardial infarction, pericarditis, myocarditis
Pulmonary	Pulmonary embolism, chronic obstructive pulmonary disease (COPD), obstructive sleep apnea
Systemic disease	Hyperthyroidism, obesity, metabolic syndrome, inflammation
Postoperative	Cardiac surgery, any surgery
Binge alcohol drinking	"Holiday heart syndrome"
Lone AF	Approximately 10% of AF (1)

anticoagulation, and odds of recurrent AF. In all patients, a search for the underlying etiology should be undertaken because AF is often best managed by treating the underlying cause of the rhythm rather than the rhythm itself (Table 3–1).

APPROACH TO:
Atrial Fibrillation

DEFINITIONS

DYSPNEA: Difficult or labored breathing, shortness of breath, or a sensation of breathlessness

THROMBOEMBOLISM: The passage of a blood clot through the vascular system from one part of the body to another—for example, in the setting of AF, a clot forms in the heart and then embolizes through arterial circulation to the brain

CARDIOMYOPATHY: Damage to heart muscle as the result of a number of various insults causing diminished functionality, which can eventually lead to heart failure, arrhythmia, and sudden death

CLINICAL APPROACH

AF affects 1% of the general population and is the most common treatable arrhythmia seen in the emergency department. The prevalence of AF increases with age. In adults younger than 55 years old the prevalence is only 0.1%, whereas in adults greater than 80 years old the prevalence is greater than 10%. AF is more common in men than in women and more common in whites than in blacks. Among patients with AF, 80% have cardiovascular disease, most commonly hypertension, coronary artery disease (CAD), and cardiomyopathy. The remaining common underlying causes include pulmonary diseases such as pulmonary embolism, COPD, and obstructive sleep apnea and systemic diseases such as hyperthyroidism, obesity, and diabetes. The exception is lone AF, which is a term used to describe AF in patients younger than 60 years old who have no evidence of heart disease. However, increasingly the term "lone AF" has been falling out of favor because it does not have a standardized, universally-accepted definition (see Table 3–1).

Pathophysiology

It is theorized that AF is caused by a complex interaction between triggers for AF and abnormal atrial myocardium that has multiple reentrant circuits or automatic foci outside the sinoatrial (SA) node. This interplay leads to rapid electrical activity in the atria, which produces disorganized and ineffective atrial contractions. The rapid atrial electrical activity is also conducted through the atrioventriular (AV) node leading to an irregular ventricular response. The ventricular rate, which is usually around 100 to 160, depends on the AV node's ability to conduct the atrial depolarization and to recover from the previous conduction. On ECG, AF looks like an irregularly irregular, usually narrow-complex, tachcycardia without associated p waves.

AF has a number of clinical implications, most importantly cardiomyopathy and thromboembolization. Acutely, the loss of the "atrial kick" leads to a reduction in cardiac output (CO) by as much as 15%. Together with the rapid ventricular response shortening the diastolic filling time, CO may be significantly reduced, especially in those with already poor left ventricular function. This reduction in CO can result in hypotension and symptoms of heart failure including dyspnea and fatigue. Over the long term, AF causes progressive structural and elctrophysiologic changes in the atria that promote recurrent episodes of AF. Additionally, chronic low levels of tachycardia lead to global cardiomyopathy, which in turn predisposes to more AF. For this reason it is said that AF "begets" more AF.

In addition to heart failure and cardiomyopathy, another important clinical implication of AF is thromboembolization. The disorganized, ineffective atrial contractions caused by AF lead to blood stasis in the left atria, especially in the left atrial appendage. This stasis promotes the formation of a thrombus, which can then dislodge and embolize through the arterial circulation, causing problems such as stroke and limb ischemia. Patients with AF have two to threefold higher risk of stroke compared with the general population.

Treatment

The management of AF is challenging because AF, rather than being a disease unto itself, is often a symptom of underlying cardiac, pulmonary, endocrine, or toxicological pathology. Successful management begins by **initially addressing the patient's overall clinical status,** searching for treatable contributing factors, controlling the rate, and preventing thromboembolism (Figure 3–2).

In stable patients with AF, the treatment options include **rate control and/or rhythm control,** with or without anticoagulation. In the **acute setting such as the emergency department, ventricular rate control is the single most important goal of therapy.** Slowing the ventricular response to AF has a number of positive hemodynamic effects including increasing diastolic filling time, improving stroke volume and cardiac output, and stabilizing blood pressure. Drugs used to control the ventricular rate work by slowing conduction through the AV node (Table 3–2).

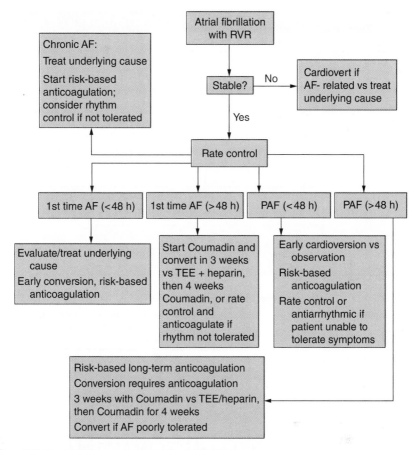

Figure 3–2. Algorithm for management of atrial fibrillation.

There are two groups of patients with AF who should not receive rate controlling agents: (1) unstable patients in whom the instability is presumed to be caused by the rhythm, (2) patients with Wolff-Parkinson-White (WPW) syndrome (Figure 3–3). **Patients who are hemodynamically unstable should get immediate electrical cardioversion** to restore sinus rhythm. Patients with WPW should not receive any AV nodal blocking agents since they can lead to accelerated conduction down the accessory pathway and potentially induce ventricular fibrillation and cardiac arrest. Patients with WPW and AF should instead get either pharmacologic or electrical cardioversion depending on their hemodynamic stability.

Cardioversion

In order to cardiovert AF, several issues must first be addressed: the need for **anticoagulation** and the **timing and method of cardioversion**. During AF, uncoordinated atrial contractions lead to intra-atrial thrombus formation. The longer the duration of AF, the greater is the likelihood of clot formation. Following cardioversion, the period of "atrial stunning" can also lead to thrombogenesis. Without anticoagulation 4% to 5% of patients will have a thromboembolic event in the first

Table 3–2 • THERAPIES FOR RATE CONTROL OF ATRIAL FIBRILLATION		
Medication	**Mechanism Of Action**	**Comment**
Calcium channel blockers (verapamil, diltiazem)	Slow AV node conduction by blocking calcium channels	Very effective Diltiazem carries the lowest risk of hypotension because it has least negative inotropic effect
β-blockers (metoprolol, propranolol, esmolol, atenolol)	Slow AV node conduction by decreasing sympathetic tone	Very effective More negative inotropic effect than diltiazem and carry a greater risk for hypotension particularly in patients with borderline low blood pressure or poor LV function
Digoxin	Slows AV node conduction by increasing parasympathetic tone via the vagus nerve	Limited role in the ED because of its slow onset of action, long half-life, and ineffectiveness at rate control in the typical high sympathetic tone ED patient Has a role in rate control in sedentary patients or those with chronic CHF
Amiodarone, (oral or IV) **Dronedarone** (oral only)	Antiarrhythmics that have some beta-blocking activity	Less effective than the pure rate control agents listed above If cardioversion is the goal, these drugs may be a single-agent approach to maintaining NSR and rate control

Abbreviations: AV = atrioventricular; LV = left ventricle; ED = emergency department; CHF = congestive heart failure; NSR = normal sinus rhythm.

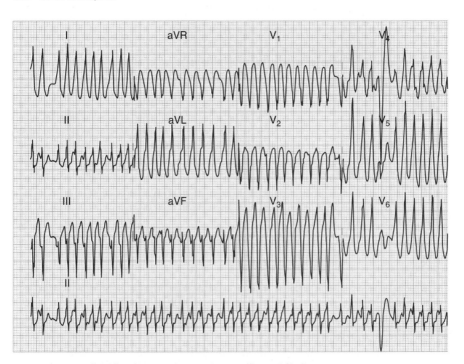

Figure 3–3. ECG of Wolff-Parkinson-White syndrome with atrial fibrillation.

month following cardioversion either from the dislodging of an existing clot or the formation of new clot caused by the "atrial stunning." This risk increases with the duration of the AF and the underlying disease processes.

Many practitioners use **the "48-hour rule"** to guide **anticoagulation**: AF of less than 48 hours duration does not generally require acute anticoagulation except when the patient has mitral valve disease, severe left ventricle dysfunction, or prior history of embolic stroke. Several recent studies have shown that it is both safe and cost-effective for patients with an uncomplicated clinical status who present to the emergency department with AF for less than 48 hours to be cardioverted and discharged directly from the emergency room.

Conversely, patients presenting with AF of greater than 48 hours duration should be anticoagulated *prior to* cardioversion. The two main approaches for pre-cardioversion anticoagulation are warfarin (Coumadin) or the combination of heparin/enoxaparin (LMWH) plus a screening transesophageal echocardiography (TEE). The conventional approach is to give warfarin therapy with an INR goal of 2 to 3 for 3 to 4 weeks before cardioversion. The alternative approach is quicker and consists of doing a TEE and, if no clot is seen, administering heparin or enoxaparin and proceeding immediately to cardioversion (Table 3–3). In both approaches, warfarin therapy (with and INR of 2-3) must be continued for at least 3 to 4 weeks post-cardioversion in order to prevent new clot formation during the "atrial stunning window." Both approaches reduce the risk of thromboembolism to less than 1% over 8 weeks.

The two methods of cardioversion are direct current (DC) cardioversion and pharmacologic cardioversion, with DC cardioversion being the more effective approach (see Tables 3–4 and 3–5). The risk of thromboembolism is similar, regardless of which method is chosen. The **likelihood of a successful cardioversion for either method** depends on the **characteristics of the patient**, the **etiology** of the AF, and, most importantly, the **duration** of the AF. New-onset AF will spontaneously convert in about 70% of cases, whereas cases of AF with a longer duration and

Table 3–3 • ANTICOAGULATION APPROACHES FOR CARDIOVERSION		
	Conventional Warfarin	**TEE plus Heparin/Enoxaparin**
Pre-cardioversion	Warfarin for 3-4 wk	If no clot on TEE, administer heparin or enoxaparin and proceed with immediate cardioversion
Post-cardioversion	Warfarin for 3-4 wk	Warfarin for 3-4 wk
Advantages	Withstood the "test of time"	Shortens period of anticoagulation, reducing the risk of bleeding complications Reduces the time in AF, increasing the chance of successful conversion to sinus rhythm
Disadvantages	Prolongs period of anticoagulation Delays cardioversion	Has no definitive guidelines Requires a highly trained physician and expensive equipment to perform TEE

Table 3-4 • DC CARDIOVERSION

Preparation	IV, O_2, cardiac and pulse oximetry monitors—following standard procedural sedation protocols, advanced cardiac life support/airway material ready and available
Synchronized DC Cardioversion	100-360 J (most patients require ≥200 J), for AF <24 h: start with 100 J; biphasic conversion offers a better success rate and fewer complications and achieves conversion at 50% of monophasic levels
Success rate	75%-93%
Complications	15% have complications including: bradycardia, ventricular tachycardia, ventricular stunning with hypotension

dilated atria may prove refractory to all attempts at cardioversion. The success rate for electrical cardioversion is between 75% and 93%, but only about 50% if the AF has been present for more than 5 years. The success rate of pharmacological cardioversion, regardless of the drug used, is between 50% and 70% for recent onset AF and about 30% for chronic AF.

Following cardioversion, 20% to 30% of patients will remain in normal sinus rhythm (NSR). The patients most likely to have recurrent AF are those with hypertension, an enlarged left atrium, heart failure, or AF for more than a year. It is generally thought that the risks of toxicity and proarrhythmic effects of antiarrhythmic therapy after cardioversion outweigh the benefits, especially in patients with no prior episodes of AF. However, in some patients who have persistent symptoms

Table 3-5 • DRUGS FOR PHARMACOLOGIC CARDIOVERSION

Drug Class	Agent	Adverse Effects	Comment
Ic	Flecainide (oral)	Dizziness, dyspnea	Contraindicated in CAD
Ic	Propafenone (oral)	Dizziness, VT	Contraindicated in CAD
III	Dofetilide (oral)	VT, torsade de pointes	Preferred if any structural heart disease is present, especially LV dysfunction
III	Amiodarone (oral or IV)	Hypotension, bradycardia, pulmonary toxicity, hepatotoxity, hyper/hypothyroidism, photo-sensitivity, ataxia, peripheral neuropathy, blurry vision	Preferred if any structural heart disease is present, especially LV dysfunction
III	Ibutilide (IV)	VT, torsade de pointes	Specifically for AF and atrial flutter
III	Vernakalant (IV)	Hypotension, bradycardia	Rapid conversion, low proarrhythmic risk

Abbreviations: CAD = coronary artery disease; IV= intravenous; VT = ventricular tachycardia; LV = left ventricle; AF = atrial fibrillation.

despite adequate rate control or who have an inability to attain adequate rate control, a rhythm control strategy may be chosen. Amiodarone and propafenone are commonly used agents to maintain sinus rhythm.

Dronedarone is a new drug approved in the United States to prevent recurrent AF. It is structurally similar to amiodarone but lacks an iodine moiety. Dronedarone has been shown to be better tolerated than amiodarone with fewer thyroid, dermatologic, neurologic and ocular side effects. The drawbacks to dronedarone are that it is less effective at decreasing recurrent AF compared with amiodarone, and that it is associated with increased mortality in NYHA class IV heart failure or recently decompensated heart failure.

An alternative therapy to maintaining sinus rhythm that has had increasing interest and investigation is radiofrequency catheter ablation. Ablation is recommended for a select patient populations with symptomatic AF and mild or no left atrial enlargement in whom a rhythm control strategy has been chosen, but who have failed treatment with one or more antiarrhythmic drugs. Given the shortcomings of chronic antiarrythmic therapy, in terms of side effects and recidivism rates, electrophysiologic interventions are likely to become more widespread.

Thromboembolic Risk Reduction

Patients with AF have a two- to threefold higher risk of stroke than the general population. The risk is the same for patients with paroxysmal, persistent or chronic AF. It was previously thought that the use of antiarrhythmic agents to maintain a sinus rhythm reduced this risk. The Atrial Fibrillation Follow-up Investigation of Rhythm Management (AFFIRM) trial, which compared rhythm control to rate control plus warfarin in 4060 patients, showed the rate control plus warfarin group had a trend toward better survival, fewer hospitalizations, and better quality of life scores. Interestingly, the rhythm control patients who were not on warfarin experienced a significantly higher incidence of stroke. This data suggest that even patients with rare or intermittent AF may benefit from antithrombotic therapy.

The type of antithrombotic therapy (either anticoagulation or antiplatelet therapy) used to prevent thromboembolism depends on the patient's individual risk of having a thromboembolic event and his risk of bleeding on antithrombotic therapy. The most validated and clinically useful risk stratification model for determining stroke risk is the CHADS2 score (Table 3–6).

Anticoagulation therapy traditionally consists of warfarin with an INR goal between 2 and 3. Dabigatran is a new oral anticoagulation agent that was shown

Table 3-6 • CHADS2	
Parameters	**Points**
Congestive heart failure	1
Hypertension	1
Age ≥75 y	1
Diabetes	1
Stroke or transient ischemic attack	2

Table 3–7 • CHADS2 SCORE AND ANTITHROMBOTIC THERAPY CHOICE			
CHADS2 Score	Stroke Risk	Stroke Risk/Year	Preferred Therapy (in order of preference)
0	Low	0.5%-1.7%	No therapy > aspirin
1	Intermediate	2%	Warfarin or dabigatran[a] > aspirin
2-6	High	>4%	Warfarin or dabigatran
Prior stoke or TIA or thromboembolic event	High	10%	Warfarin or dabigatran

[a]Annual bleeding risk on dabigatran or warfarin therapy is about 2%-3%.

to be superior to warfarin in the recent RE-LY trial. Dabigatran reduces the rate of ischemic and hemorrhagic strokes, major bleeding, and overall mortality compared to warfarin. In addition to being more effective and safer, it does not require INR monitoring, is less susceptible to diet and drug interactions, and does not have warfarin's narrow therapeutic window. However, the drawbacks to dabigatran are its higher cost, twice daily dosing, need for adjustment in patients with renal failure, lack of an antidote, and lack of long-term safety data. The dosage for dabigatran is 150 mg twice daily. The 110 mg twice daily dose is recommended for patients with increased risk of bleeding. However, the 110 mg capsule is currently not available in the United States.

Antiplatelet therapy consists of aspirin 75 to 325 mg daily, clopidogrel 75 mg daily, or both together. Aspirin has only a very small ability to reduce stroke risk. For patients with no risk factors for stroke, the current evidence shows that the risk of bleeding from aspirin likely exceeds the small benefit of decreased stroke risk. Aspirin, clopidogrel, and aspirin plus clopidogrel are all less effective in preventing stroke than warfarin. For patients who need anticoagulation but cannot take warfarin or dabigatran, the combination of clopidogrel plus aspirin is more effective than aspirin alone. However, this combination carries similar bleeding risks to formal anticoagulation (Table 3–7).

COMPREHENSION QUESTIONS

3.1 A 75-year-old man is found to have asymptomatic atrial fibrillation. Which of the following is the most common complication of his atrial fibrillation?

A. Sudden death

B. Stroke

C. Shock

D. Dyspnea

3.2 An 83-year-old woman with a history of hypertension presents to the emergency department with dyspnea, fatigue, and palpitations. Her blood pressure is 85/50 mm Hg and her heartbeat is 150 beats per minute and irregular. Which of the following is the best treatment for this patient?

A. Diltiazem

B. Metoprolol

C. Coumadin

D. DC cardioversion

3.3 A 62-year-old woman is seen in the emergency department for wrist pain after tripping and falling. She is found to have a distal radius fracture on x-ray, which is reduced and splinted. However, her heart rate is 80 beats per minute and irregular to palpation. On ECG, she is diagnosed with atrial fibrillation with a ventricular response of 114 beats per minute. She does not recall ever being told about this condition. Which of the following is the best initial treatment for this patient?

A. Diltiazem

B. DC cardioversion

C. Synthroid

D. Ibutilide

ANSWERS

3.1 **B.** Stroke is two to three times more likely in patients with AF than in the general population.

3.2 **D.** Always cardiovert any unstable patient (congestive heart failure, chest pain, hypotension) with AF if the instability is felt to be rhythm related. AF with rapid ventricular response does not allow for ventricular filling, leading to ineffective cardiac output.

3.3 **A.** Diltiazem was the only rate-controlling agent listed, and is very useful in the initial management of AF with rapid ventricular response.

CLINICAL PEARLS

▶ Treatment of atrial fibrillation (AF) begins with searching for any underlying reversible causes of the arrhythmia.

▶ In an acute setting, the most important goal of therapy is ventricular rate control, typically through the use of AV nodal blocking drugs.

▶ Unstable patients with AF or Wolff-Parkinson-White tachyarrhythmia with AF should undergo immediate electrical cardioversion.

▶ Stable patients with AF for less than 48 hours can be cardioverted in the ED provided they have no prior history of thromboembolism, mitral valve disease, or LV dysfunction.

▶ Stable patients with AF of greater than 48 hours or unknown duration can be cardioverted in two ways: (1) anticoagulation for 3-4 weeks prior to, and following cardioversion, or (2) imaging by TEE and, if no intracardiac thrombus is seen, acute anticoagulation with heparin/LMWH, followed by cardioversion, and anticoagulation for 3-4 weeks.

▶ 70% of new-onset AF will spontaneously convert to sinus rhythm.

▶ Patients with AF have a two to three times higher risk of stroke than the general population.

▶ The choice of antithrombotic therapy for long-term AF depends on an individual's CHADS2 score and risk of bleeding.

▶ Anticoagulation with either warfarin (INR goal 2-3) or dabigatran reduces the risk of thromboembolism.

REFERENCES

Association Task Force on Practice Guidelines and the European Society of Cardiology Committee for Practice Guidelines and Policy Conferences (Writing Committee to Revise the 2001 Guidelines for the Management of Patients With Atrial Fibrillation). *J Am Coll Cardiol.* 2006;48:149-246.

Connolly SJ, Ezekowitz MD, Yusuf S, et al. Dabigatran versus warfarin in patients with atrial fibrillation. *N Engl J Med.* 2009 Sep 17;361(12):1139-1151.

Connolly SJ, Pogue J, Hart R, et al. Clopidogrel plus aspirin versus oral anticoagulation for atrial fibrillation in the Atrial fibrillation Clopidogrel Trial with Irbesartan for prevention of Vascular Events (ACTIVE W): a randomised controlled trial. *Lancet.* 2006;367(9526):1903-1912.

Fuster V, Ryden LE, Cannom DS, et al. ACC/AHA/ESC 2006 guidelines for the management of patients with atrial fibrillation: a report of the American College of Cardiology/American Heart.

Fuster V, Rydén LE, Cannom DS, et al. 2011 ACCF/AHA/HRS Focused Updates Incorporated Into the ACC/AHA/ESC 2006 Guidelines for the Management of Patients With Atrial Fibrillation. A Report of the American College of Cardiology Foundation/American Heart Association Task Force on Practice Guidelines. Developed in partnership with the European Society of Cardiology and in collaboration with the European Heart Rhythm Association and the Heart Rhythm Society. *J Am Coll Cardiol.* 2011;57(11):e101-e198.

Gallagher MM, Hennessy BJ, Edvardsson H, et al. Embolic complications of direct current cardioversion of atrial arrhythmias: association with low intensity of anticoagulation at the time of cardioversion. *J Am Coll Cardiol.* 2002;40:926-933.

Manning W, Singer E, Lip G, et al. Antithrombotic therapy to prevent embolization in nonvalvular atrial fibrillation. http://www.uptodate.com/contents/antithrombotic-therapy-to-prevent-fibrillation?source= see_link&anchor=H20#H4338483. Last updated: 11/11/2010.

Michael JA, Stiell IG, Agarwal S, Mandavia DP. Cardioversion of paroxysmal atrial fibrillation in the emergency department. *Ann Emerg Med.* 1999;33(4):379-387.

Singer DE, Albers GW, Dalen JE, et al. Antithrombotic therapy in atrial fibrillation: American College of Chest Physicians Evidence-Based Clinical Practice Guidelines. *Chest.* 2008;133:556S-592S.

Stewart S, Hart CL, Hole DJ, McMurray JJ. A population-based study of the long-term risks associated with atrial fibrillation: 20 year follow-up of the Renfrew/Paisley study. *Am J Med.* 2002;113:359-364.

Stiell IG, Dickinson G, Butterfield NN, et al. Vernakalant hydrochloride: A novel atrial-selective agent for the cardioversion of recent-onset atrial fibrillation in the emergency department. *Acad Emerg Med.* 2010;17(11):1175-1182.

Weigner MJ, Caulfield TA, Danias PG, Silverman DI, Manning WJ. Risk for clinical thromboembolism associated with conversion to sinus rhythm in patients with atrial fibrillation lasting less than 48 hours. *Ann Intern Med.* 1997;126:615-620.

Wyse DG, Waldo AL, DiMarco JP, et al. A comparison of rate control and rhythm control in patients with atrial fibrillation. *N Engl J Med.* 2002;347:1825-1833.

Xavier Scheuermeyer F, Grafstein E, et al. Thirty-day outcomes of emergency department patients undergoing electrical cardioversion for atrial fibrillation or flutter. *Acad Emerg Med.* 2010;17(4):408-115.

A 25-year-old man presents to the emergency department (ED) with palpitations and lightheadedness. These symptoms started acutely about 1 hour prior to arrival while he was watching television. The patient does not have any chest pain or shortness of breath. He also denies any recent fever, upper respiratory symptoms, and hemoptysis. He does not have any significant past medical history or family history. He is not taking any medications, does not smoke, and has never used any illicit drugs.

On examination, his temperature is 98.2°F, his blood pressure is 88/46 mm Hg, his heart rate 186 beats per minute, respiratory rate is 22 breaths per minute, and oxygen saturation is 97% on room air. He is mildly anxious but otherwise in no acute distress. He does not have any jugular venous distention. His lungs are clear to auscultation, and his heart sounds are regular without any murmurs, rubs, or gallops. There is no lower extremity edema, and peripheral pulses are equal in all four extremities. The cardiac monitor reveals a regular rhythm with narrow-QRS complexes at a rate of 180 to190 beats per minute.

▶ What is the most likely diagnosis?
▶ What is the most appropriate next step?

ANSWERS TO CASE 4:

Regular Rate Tachycardia

Summary: This is a 25-year-old man with acute onset of palpitations and dizziness. He is hypotensive and has a narrow-QRS complex tachycardia at a rate of 180 to 190 beats per minute.

- **Most likely diagnosis:** Supraventricular tachycardia.

- **Most appropriate next step:** Obtain IV access and a 12-lead ECG. Prepare for synchronized cardioversion of this unstable patient with a tachyarrhythmia.

ANALYSIS

Objectives

1. Learn the differential diagnosis for regular rate tachycardias.

2. Recognize the clinical signs and symptoms to differentiate between stable and unstable patients with regular rate tachycardias.

3. Understand the diagnostic and therapeutic approach to regular rate tachycardias.

Considerations

When evaluating a patient with a tachyarrhythmia, assessment of the patient's stability is paramount. Unstable patients will require immediate synchronized cardioversion. Stable patients may be able to be managed medically. All patients will require continuous cardiac monitoring, intravenous (IV) access, and a 12-lead ECG. Regular rate tachycardias include several types of supraventricular tachycardia and ventricular tachycardia (Table 4–1). As a general rule, narrow-QRS complex tachycardias arise from above the ventricles while wide-QRS complex ones may be supraventricular or ventricular in origin.

Table 4–1 • VARIOUS TYPES OF TACHYARRHYTHMIAS		
Regular	Narrow-QRS complex	Sinus tachycardia
		Atrial tachycardia
		Atrioventricular nodal reentrant tachycardia (AVNRT)
		Atrioventricular reentrant tachycardia (AVRT)
		Junctional tachycardia
		Atrial flutter
	Wide-QRS complex	Ventricular tachycardia
		Antidromic AVRT
		Narrow complex tachycardia with aberrancy
Irregular	Narrow-QRS complex	Atrial flutter with variable block
		Atrial fibrillation
		Multifocal atrial tachycardia
	Wide-QRS complex	Polymorphic ventricular tachycardia
		Narrow complex tachycardia with aberrancy

APPROACH TO:
Regular Rate Tachycardia

CLINICAL APPROACH

Patients with tachyarrhythmias may present with a host of complaints including palpitations, fatigue, and weakness. Other symptoms may suggest a component of hypoperfusion (dizziness, near syncope, or syncope) or cardiac ischemia (chest pain, dyspnea). If the patient is stable enough for a complete history to be performed, the history should also include information about the time and circumstances surrounding symptom onset, duration of symptoms, past medical history (eg, history of coronary artery disease, congestive heart failure, dysrhythmia, valvular disease, thyroid disease), current medications (including herbal or homeopathic regimens, over-the-counter medicines, and illicit drugs), and family history (eg, sudden cardiac death, dysrhythmia, other types of heart disease).

The physical examination will initially focus on assessing the patient's stability and adequacy of the ABCs. Any evidence of hypotension, pulmonary edema, acutely altered mental status, or ischemic chest pain indicates that the patient is unstable and treatment must be initiated immediately (see treatment section below). Once the patient is stabilized, a complete head-to-toe examination can be performed. Special consideration should be given to the cardiovascular and lung components of the examination: auscultating heart sounds for gallops, murmurs, and rubs; palpating for the point of maximal impulse and any heaves; inspecting for jugular venous distention; listening for any rales or other findings of volume overload; assessing the quality of peripheral pulses. The examination may also reveal clues regarding underlying causes of tachycardia (eg, pale mucous membranes with anemia; thyromegaly or goiter with thyrotoxicosis, barrel chest or nail clubbing with chronic lung disease).

A 12-lead ECG is ostensibly the most useful diagnostic test when evaluating a patient with a tachyarrhythmia (Figures 4–1 and 4–2). These arrhythmias may be separated into regular and irregular rate tachycardias as well as narrow- or wide-QRS (>0.12 s) complex (see Table 4–1). As a general rule, narrow-QRS complex tachycardias arise from above the ventricles while wide-QRS complex ones may be supraventricular or ventricular in origin.

Table 4–2 lists the distinguishing ECG characteristics of the various types of regular rate tachycardias.

Ventricular tachycardia (VT) may be difficult to differentiate from a supraventricular tachycardia (SVT) with aberrant conduction. Certain factors favor VT, including age ≥50, history of coronary artery disease or congestive heart failure, history of VT, atrioventricular dissociation, fusion beats, QRS >0.14 second, extreme left axis deviation, and precordial concordance (QRS complexes either all positive or all negative). In contrast, age ≤35, history of SVT, preceding ectopic P waves with QRS complexes, QRS <0.14 second, normal or almost normal axis, and slowing or cessation of the arrhythmia with vagal maneuvers suggest SVT with aberrancy. If the provider cannot distinguish between VT and SVT with aberrancy with certainty, the patient should be treated as if VT is present.

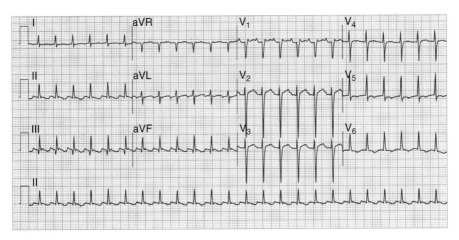

Figure 4–1. Atrial flutter with 2:1 conduction.

Chest x-rays may be useful to assess for chamber enlargement, cardiomegaly, pulmonary congestion or edema. A basic metabolic panel can rule out electrolyte abnormalities that predispose to tachyarrhythmias (eg, hypokalemia, hypocalcemia, hypomagnesemia). If the clinical scenario is suggestive, thyroid function studies (for hyperthyroidism), drug levels (eg, digoxin), or urine drug screen (for cocaine, methamphetamines, other stimulants) may be warranted.

Treatment

All patients with tachyarrhythmias require monitoring of vital signs (blood pressure, oxygen saturation, continuous cardiac monitoring) and IV access. If the patient is

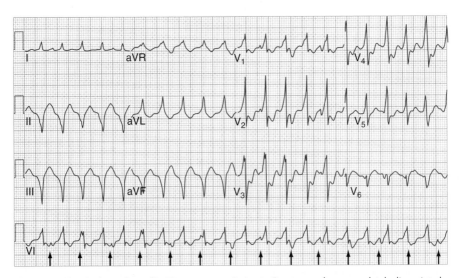

Figure 4–2. Ventricular tachycardia. Note arrows pointing to P waves and are completely dissociated from the QRS complexes.

Table 4–2 • REGULAR RATE TACHYCARDIAS

Narrow-QRS complex

Sinus tachycardia	Atrial rate 100-160 bpm. 1:1 conduction. Normal sinus P waves and PR intervals	Similar to normal sinus rhythm except >100 bpm. Treat underlying cause
Atrial tachycardia	P wave morphologically different from sinus P. 1:1 conduction	Will not convert to sinus with vagal maneuvers or adenosine. If stable, consider diltiazem, β-blockers. Treat underlying cause
Atrioventricular nodal reentrant tachycardia (AVNRT)	P wave usually buried in QRS complex. 1:1 conduction. Often preceded by premature junctional or atrial contraction. Rarely >225 bpm	Reentry within AV node. If stable, consider vagal maneuvers, adenosine, calcium-channel blockers or β-blockers
Atrioventricular reentrant tachycardia (AVRT)	Inverted retrograde P waves after QRS complex.	Retrograde reentry involving bypass tract. If stable, consider vagal maneuvers, adenosine, calcium-channel blockers or β-blockers
Junctional tachycardia	Inverted P wave before or after QRS or buried in QRS complex. Rate >100 bpm	Will not convert to sinus with vagal maneuvers or adenosine. If stable, consider diltiazem, β-blockers. Treat underlying cause
Atrial flutter	Atrial rate 250-350 bpm. "Sawtooth" flutter wave (best seen in II, III, aVF, V1-V2). 2:1 conduction common (although may be any ratio)	Will not convert to sinus with vagal maneuvers or adenosine. If stable, consider calcium-channel blockers, β-blockers. Treat underlying cause

Wide QRS-complex

Ventricular tachycardia	Dissociated P wave (if present). 100-250 bpm	If stable, consider amiodarone, procainamide, or sotalol. Lidocaine as second-line agent
Antidromic AVRT	Retrograde P waves may or may not be visible	Anterograde conduction through bypass tract, retrograde through AV node. Avoid β-blockers, calcium-channel blockers, and adenosine
Narrow complex tachycardia with aberrancy	Preceding ectopic P waves with QRS complexes. QRS usually <0.14 s. Axis normal or almost normal	If stable, adenosine

hypoxic or in respiratory distress, supplemental oxygen and airway support are indicated. If the patient is unstable (as evidenced by hypotension, pulmonary edema, altered mental status, or ischemic chest pain), synchronized cardioversion should be performed immediately. If time allows, sedation should be given prior to cardioversion.

In stable patients, a 12-lead ECG should be obtained, and medical therapy can be initiated. Potential interventions for regular narrow-complex tachyarrhythmias include vagal maneuvers (such as carotid massage and Valsalva), adenosine, β-blockers, and calcium-channel blockers. Although vagal maneuvers will not terminate tachyarrhythmias that do not involve the AV node, they may slow the rate enough to unmask the underlying rhythm abnormality. Stable patients with regular wide-complex tachycardias may benefit from amiodarone, procainamide, or sotalol. Second-line therapy for stable patients with monomorphic VT is lidocaine.

COMPREHENSION QUESTIONS

4.1 A 22-year-old baseball player comes into the ED complaining of 12 hours of intermittent chest pain and a pounding heartbeat. He denies a history of trauma. On examination, he is tachycardic. Which of the following is the best next step?

A. Synchronized cardioversion

B. Valsalva maneuver

C. Discharge home and follow up within the next 48 hours

D. Obtain an ECG

4.2 A 52-year-old healthy jogger is brought to the ED following a syncopal episode. A diagnosis of ventricular tachycardia is made, and the patient is cardioverted. She states that she has had prior episodes of VT lasting less than 30 seconds each. What is the most appropriate treatment?

A. Likely no further therapy is needed.

B. Amiodarone

C. β-blocker

D. Procainamide

4.3 All of these are AV nodal blocking maneuvers *except*:

A. Diving reflex

B. Carotid massage

C. Valsalva maneuver

D. Holding one's breath at the end of expiration

4.4 An 87-year-old woman presents with chest pain and shortness of breath. The 12-lead ECG shows a "sawtooth" pattern with a heart rate of 150 beats per minute. What is the most likely diagnosis?

A. AVNRT

B. VT

C. Atrial flutter

D. Atrial fibrillation with rapid ventricular rate

4.5 A 37-year-old woman presents with chest pain after smoking crack 2 hours ago. What are you most likely to see on the ECG?

A. Sinus tachycardia

B. SVT

C. VT

D. Atrial fibrillation

ANSWERS

4.1 **D.** One must characterize the rhythm before initiating treatment.

4.2 **A.** Nonsustained VT is by definition a self-terminating event, and therefore usually no specific treatment is indicated. Rather, treatment is directed at any existing heart condition.

4.3 **D.** AV nodal blocking maneuvers include Valsalva, diving reflex, and carotid massage. They act through the parasympathetic nervous system. If an SVT involves the AV node, slowing conduction through the node can terminate the arrhythmia. SVTs that do not involve the AV node will not usually be terminated by AV nodal blocking maneuvers. However, these maneuvers may still cause a transient AV block and unmask the underlying rhythm abnormality.

4.4 **C.** Classically atrial flutter presents with a saw tooth pattern on ECG. The rate of 150 bpm denotes that it's likely a 2:1 conduction block.

4.5 **A.** The most common regular rate tachycardia is sinus tachycardia.

CLINICAL PEARLS

▶ Regular rate tachycardias include several types of supraventricular tachycardia and ventricular tachycardia. As a general rule, narrow-QRS complex tachycardias arise from above the ventricles while wide-QRS complex ones may be supraventricular or ventricular in origin.

▶ If the patient is unstable (as evidenced by hypotension, pulmonary edema, altered mental status, or ischemic chest pain), synchronized cardioversion should be performed immediately. In stable patients, a 12-lead ECG should be obtained, and medical therapy can be initiated.

▶ If the provider cannot distinguish between VT and SVT with aberrancy with certainty, the patient should be treated as if VT is present.

▶ *Always* order an ECG in a patient with suspected tachyarrhythmia.

REFERENCES

Baerman JM, Morady F, DiCarlo LA Jr, de Buitleir M. Differentiation of ventricular tachycardia from supraventricular tachycardia with aberration: value of the clinical history. *Ann Emerg Med.* 1987;16 (1):40-43.

Brugada P, Brugada J, Mont L, Smeets J, Andries EW. A new approach to the differential diagnosis of a regular tachycardia with a wide QRS complex. *Circulation.* 1991;83(5):1649-1659.

Lau EW, Ng GA. Comparison of the performance of three diagnostic algorithms for regular broad complex tachycardia in practical application. Pacing and clinical electrophysiology: *PACE.* 2002;25(5): 822-827.

Marx, John A, Robert S. Hockberger, Ron M. Walls, James Adams, and Peter Rosen. *Rosen's Emergency Medicine: Concepts and Clinical Practice.* 7th ed. Philadelphia, PA: Mosby/Elsevier; 2010.

Mathew PK. Diving reflex. Another method of treating paroxysmal supraventricular tachycardia. *Arch Intern. Med.* 1981;141(1):22-23.

Stewart RB, Bardy GH, Greene HL. Wide complex tachycardia: misdiagnosis and outcome after emergent therapy. *Ann Intern Med.* 1986;104 (6):766-771.

Tintinalli, Judith E, and J S. Stapczynski. *Tintinalli's Emergency Medicine: A Comprehensive Study Guide.* New York, NY: McGraw-Hill; 2011.

Wellens HJ, Bar FW, Lie KI. The value of the electrocardiogram in the differential diagnosis of a tachycardia with a widened QRS complex. *Am J Med.* 1978;64(1):27-33.

A 19-year-old man is brought to the emergency department (ED) with diffuse abdominal pain, vomiting, and altered level of consciousness. The patient's symptoms began several days ago, when he complained of "the flu." His symptoms at that time included profound fatigue, nausea, mild abdominal discomfort and some urinary frequency. Today he was found in bed moaning but otherwise unresponsive. His past medical history is unremarkable, and he is currently taking no medications. On physical examination, the patient appears pale and ill. His temperature is 36.0°C (96.8°F), pulse rate is 140 beats per minute, blood pressure is 82/40 mm Hg, and the respiratory rate is 40 breaths per minute. His head and neck examination shows dry mucous membranes and sunken eyes; there is an unusual odor to his breath. The lungs are clear bilaterally with increased rate and depth of respiration. The cardiac examination reveals tachycardia, no murmurs, rubs, or gallops. The abdomen is diffusely tender to palpation, with hypoactive bowel sounds and involuntary guarding. The rectal examination is normal. Skin is cool and dry with decreased turgor. On neurologic examination, the patient moans and localizes pain but does not speak coherently. Laboratory studies: the leukocyte count is 16,000 cells/uL, and the hemoglobin and hematocrit levels are normal. Electrolytes reveal a sodium of 124 mEq/L, potassium 3.4 mEq/L, chloride 98 mEq/L, and bicarbonate 6 mEq/L. BUN and creatinine are mildly elevated. The serum glucose is 740 mg/dL (41.1 mmol/L). The serum amylase, bilirubin, AST, ALT, and alkaline phosphatase are within normal limits. A 12-lead ECG shows sinus tachycardia. His CXR is normal.

▶ What is the most likely diagnosis?
▶ What is the next step?

ANSWERS TO CASE 5:
Diabetic Ketoacidosis

Summary: This is a 19-year-old man with acute diabetic ketoacidosis. The patient has new-onset diabetes mellitus. The constellation of severe hyperglycemia, anion-gap acidosis, and ketosis (manifested by the breath odor) is diagnostic. The other findings of dehydration, hyponatremia, hypotension, altered level of consciousness, and diffuse abdominal pain, are typical of a particularly severe episode of diabetic ketoacidosis.

- **Most likely diagnosis:** Diabetic ketoacidosis

- **Next step:** Management of the ABCs, including fluid resuscitation, the initiation of insulin therapy, and a careful search for any precipitating or concomitant illness.

ANALYSIS

Objectives

1. Recognize the clinical settings, the signs and symptoms, and complications of diabetic ketoacidosis.

2. Understand the diagnostic and therapeutic approach to suspected diabetic ketoacidosis.

Considerations

This patient's clinical presentation is typical for diabetic ketoacidosis. Morbidity may result from either underlying precipitating conditions, or from delayed or inadequate treatment. Prompt recognition, effective resuscitation, and diligent attention to fluid, electrolyte, and insulin replacement are essential. (Table 5–1 lists typical laboratory values in DKA). A comprehensive and thoughtful search for associated illnesses, along with frequent reassessment of the patient, will lead to the best outcome.

Table 5–1 • TYPICAL LABORATORY VALUES IN DIABETIC KETOACIDOSIS		
	Moderate	**Severe**
Glucose (mg/dL)	<500-700	≥900
Sodium (mEq/L)	130	125
Potassium (mEq/L)	4-6	5-7
HCO_3 (mEq/L)	6-10	<5
BUN (mg/dL)	20-30	30+
pH	7.1	6.9
Pco_2 (mm Hg)	15-20	>20 (respiratory failure)

> ## APPROACH TO:
> ## Suspected Diabetic Ketoacidosis

CLINICAL APPROACH

Diabetic ketoacidosis is a metabolic emergency. A delay in treatment leads to increased morbidity and mortality. In up to one-quarter of patients, DKA is the initial presentation of type I diabetes, so lack of a diabetic history cannot exclude the diagnosis. Most cases occur in patients with type I diabetes, though some patients with type II diabetes may develop DKA during severe physiologic stress. Some patients will present with the classical symptoms of diabetes, such as polyuria, polydipsia, and fatigue. Others will complain more of dyspnea related to the metabolic acidosis, or of the idiopathic but often severe abdominal pain that frequently accompanies DKA. Patients with an underlying infection or other precipitating illness may have symptoms predominantly from that process. As in our case presentation, some patients have such an altered sensorium that a history is entirely unobtainable.

DKA results from an absolute or severe relative lack of insulin, leading to a starvation state at the cellular level. Gluconeogenesis is stimulated even as glucose utilization falls. Hyperglycemia and ketoacidosis cause a profound osmotic diuresis and massive fluid shifts. The diuresis and acidosis cause severe electrolyte disturbances, with wasting of sodium, potassium, magnesium and phosphate. Acidosis, dehydration, hyperosmolality, and insulin deficiency can lead to potassium shifts into the extracellular space, **so patients may have significant serum hyperkalemia at presentation, even with massive total body deficits of potassium.** Nausea and vomiting can be severe and further cloud the clinical picture with variable superimposed acid-base and electrolyte disturbances.

Diagnosis is based on the triad of hyperglycemia, ketosis, and metabolic acidosis. The major differential diagnosis is hyperosmolar hyperglycemic state (HHS), which can present with very high glucose but slight or no acidosis. Starvation, pregnancy, alcoholic ketoacidosis, and various toxic ingestions can present with elevated serum ketones, but the glucose is normal or low. Patients can be rapidly screened for DKA with a bedside blood glucose measurement and a dipstick urinalysis. Except for the rare anuric patient, the absence of ketones in the urine reliably excludes the diagnosis of DKA. Serum ketones are commonly measured to confirm the diagnosis, but the absolute value is not as helpful because most labs measure only one of the several ketone bodies that may be present. Table 5–2 is a guide to the differential diagnosis of DKA.

Most patients with recurrent DKA have an underlying cause of the episode, and all symptoms require a thorough investigation. In some studies, less than 10% of episodes had no underlying illness. Infection is the most frequent trigger of DKA, but it has resulted from pancreatitis, myocardial infarction, stroke, and many drugs including corticosteroids, thiazides, sympathomimetics including cocaine, and some antipsychotic drugs. In children and adolescents, voluntary cessation of insulin for psychosocial reasons is a frequent and serious cause of DKA.

Patients in DKA can have massive fluid deficits, sometimes as much as 5 to 10 L. Shock is fairly common, and must be promptly treated with crystalloid infusion to

Table 5–2 • DIFFERENTIAL DIAGNOSIS OF DIABETIC KETOACIDOSIS		
Hyperglycemia	**Acidosis**	**Ketosis**
Diabetes	Hyperchloremic acidosis	Starvation
Stress hyperglycemia	Salicylate poisoning	Pregnancy
Nonketotic hyperosmolar coma	Uremia	Alcoholic ketoacidosis
Impaired glucose tolerance	Lactic acidosis	Isopropyl alcohol ingestion
Dextrose infusion	Other drugs	
DKA	DKA	DKA

prevent further organ damage. Adults with clinical shock should receive an initial 2-L bolus of normal saline with frequent reassessment. In children, shock is treated with boluses of 20 mL/kg of normal saline. Although overaggressive hydration can present substantial complications later in the course of treatment, this concern takes a back seat to the reversal of shock. Untreated shock promotes multiple-organ dysfunction and contributes further to the severe acidosis seen in DKA.

Insulin is absolutely required to reverse ketoacidosis. Regular insulin is usually given by continuous IV infusion, though frequent IV boluses may be nearly as effective. Intramuscular injections are painful and less reliably absorbed when the patient is in shock. There is no role for long-acting insulin until the ketoacidotic state has resolved. (There are proposed protocols for treating *mild* and *recurrent* episodes of DKA with subcutaneous regular insulin, but those protocols have not yet been widely adopted.) The combination of rehydration and insulin will commonly lower the serum glucose much faster than ketones are cleared. **Regardless, insulin infusion should continue until the anion gap has returned to normal.** Dextrose should be added to the IV infusion when the serum glucose falls to 200 to 300 mg/dL (11.1-16.7 mmol/L) to prevent hypoglycemia, a common complication of treatment.

An insulin dose of 0.1 U/kg/h (5-10 U/h in the adult) is adequate for almost all clinical situations. This is sufficient to achieve maximum physiologic effect. Higher doses are no more effective, but do cause a higher rate of hypoglycemia. An initial bolus of insulin, equal to 1-hour infusion, is commonly given but has not been shown to hasten recovery or provide any other benefit. Insulin boluses are not recommended in pediatric patients. Insulin does bind readily to common medical plastics, so IV tubing should be thoroughly flushed with the drip solution at the start of therapy.

Patients in DKA generally have massive total body deficits of water, sodium, potassium, magnesium, phosphate, and other electrolytes. Specific laboratory values may vary widely depending on the patient's intake, gastrointestinal and other losses, medications, and comorbid illnesses. It is not usually necessary to calculate exact sodium and water deficits and replacements, except in cases of severe renal failure. Simply reverse shock with normal saline, and then continue an infusion of half-normal saline at two to three times maintenance. Remember that glucose should be added *before* the serum glucose falls to the normal range, usually when the glucose level reaches 250 mg/dL.

Potassium deficits are usually quite large, yet the serum potassium at presentation may be low, normal, or even high. If the potassium is elevated initially, look for and treat any hyperkalemic changes on the ECG. Give fluids without potassium until the serum K reaches the normal range, and then add potassium to the IV infusion. If the initial serum K is normal or low, potassium replacement can be started immediately. Magnesium supplementation may be necessary to help the patient retain potassium. Phosphate replacement has not been shown to improve clinical outcomes, but extremely low phosphate levels (<1.0 mg/dL) are known to cause muscle weakness and possibly rhabdomyolysis. For such patients, some of the potassium can be given in the form of potassium phosphate.

Because metabolic acidosis is such a prominent feature in DKA, some clinicians have administered substantial doses of sodium bicarbonate. Many studies have failed to demonstrate any improvement from this treatment even at surprisingly low serum pH values, but even skeptical physicians sometimes encounter a patient who is so acidotic that they feel compelled to give bicarbonate. There are multiple theoretical and observed complications from bicarbonate, including hypernatremia, hypokalemia, paradoxical CSF acidosis, and residual systemic alkalosis. Of course, in the case of hyperkalemia, bicarbonate might be lifesaving and should not be withheld.

Cerebral edema is a rare but devastating complication of DKA, seen most often and most severely in children. It almost always occurs during treatment, and is a leading cause of morbidity and mortality in pediatric DKA. It has been ascribed to the development of cryptogenic osmoles in the CNS to counter dehydration, which then draw water intracellularly during treatment, but this remains unproven. It has been variously associated with overhydration and vigorous insulin therapy, leading many pediatric centers to use extremely conservative, slow and low-dose treatment protocols for DKA. However, at least one large well-controlled study showed that the only reliable predictor of cerebral edema was the severity of metabolic derangements at presentation. Concern for cerebral edema should never be used as an excuse for the undertreatment of clinical shock. Once shock is reversed, pediatric DKA patients should be managed in consultation with an experienced pediatric endocrinologist or intensivist.

COMPREHENSION QUESTIONS

5.1 A 17-year-old adolescent boy who is a type I diabetic is brought in by his parents with concern about diabetic ketoacidosis. He has had several prior episodes of DKA. Which of the following is most diagnostic of DKA?

A. Polyuria, polydipsia, fatigue

B. Hypotension, dehydration, fruity breath odor

C. Hyperglycemia, ketosis, metabolic acidosis

D. Serum blood sugar of 600 mg/dL in the face of high concentrations of insulin

E. Elevated HCO_3 and elevated glucose

5.2 A 28-year-old insulin-requiring woman is found in her apartment by her husband. She is stuporous and cannot provide any history. EMS is called and takes the patient to the emergency center, and a diagnosis of severe DKA is made. Her blood pressure is 80/40 mm Hg and heart rate 140 beats per minute. The glucose level is 950 mg/dL, potassium level 6 mEq/L, HCO_3 4 mEq/L. Which of the following is the most appropriate initial treatment?

A. Administer 20 units regular insulin intramuscularly, and normal saline at 250 mL/h.

B. Begin an intravenous dopamine drip to raise BP above 90, then insulin at 10 U/h.

C. Initiate normal saline 2 L with KCl 20 mEq/L, insulin 10 U/h.

D. Provide an intravenous normal saline 2 L bolus, and start an insulin drip at 10 U/h.

5.3 The patient in Question 5.2 is undergoing therapy. Which of the following principles is most accurate in the treatment of DKA?

A. Isotonic saline with no dextrose should be used during the hospitalization because the patient is diabetic.

B. Typically, intravenous insulin and dextrose solution will need to be continued until the acidosis has resolved.

C. Potassium replacement is rarely necessary.

D. Sodium bicarbonate is helpful to resolve the anion gap more quickly.

5.4 The physician explains to a 25-year-old man who has recently been hospitalized with DKA that patients in DKA often have other illnesses or precipitating factors that initiated the ketoacidosis. Which of the following is the most common underlying etiology in DKA?

A. Asthmatic exacerbation

B. Cocaine use

C. Cholecystititis

D. Missed insulin doses

E. Urinary tract infection

ANSWERS

5.1 **C.** The triad of hyperglycemia, ketosis, and acidosis is diagnostic of DKA. Many other conditions cause one or two of the triad, but not all three. Although a fruity breath odor may suggest acetone, it is not reliably present and not all clinicians can distinguish it.

5.2 **D.** Fluid resuscitation via isotonic crystalloid solution to reverse shock, and IV insulin to reverse ketoacidosis, are the mainstays of therapy. Though most patients will require potassium, it should not be given while the serum K is elevated, and typically not until urine output is seen. Pressors have a limited role until the intravascular volume is restored.

5.3 **B.** The serum glucose often drops much more rapidly than the ketoacidosis resolves; insulin is necessary to metabolize the ketone bodies but dextrose prevents hypoglycemia. Potassium replacement is usually necessary, but should wait until hyperkalemia is excluded. Bicarbonate does not hasten resolution of DKA.

5.4 **E.** Many serious illnesses can precipitate an episode of DKA in the susceptible patient, including infection, stroke, myocardial infarction, pancreatitis, trauma, and surgery. Associated or precipitating illness should always be sought diligently. Urinary tract infection is the single most common underlying cause. Missed insulin doses are also common, but less common than infection.

CLINICAL PEARLS

▶ Hyperglycemia, ketosis, and acidosis confirm the diagnosis of DKA and are enough to start fluids and insulin.

▶ Patients in DKA are almost always dehydrated and have significant sodium and potassium deficits, regardless of their specific laboratory values.

▶ Abdominal pain is a common feature in DKA and is usually idiopathic, especially in younger patients.

▶ Most morbidity in DKA is iatrogenic.

REFERENCES

Charfen MA, Fernández-Frackelton M. Diabetic ketoacidosis. *Emerg Med Clin North Am.* August 2005;23(3):609-628, vii.

Kitabchi AE, Umpierrez GE, Murphy MB, Kreisberg RA. Hyperglycemic crises in adult patients with diabetes: a consensus statement from the American Diabetes Association. *Diabetes Care.* 2006;29(12):2739-2748.

Levin DL. Cerebral edema in diabetic ketoacidosis. *Pediatr Crit Care Med.* 2008;9(3):320-329.

Marcin JP, Glaser N, Barnett P, et al; American Academy of Pediatrics. Factors associated with adverse outcomes in children with diabetic ketoacidosis-related cerebral edema. *J Pediatr.* 2002;141(6):793-797.

Mazer M, Chen E. Is subcutaneous administration of rapid-acting insulin as effective as intravenous insulin for treating diabetic ketoacidosis? *Ann Emerg Med.* 2009;53(2):259-263.

Wolfsdorf J, Craig ME, Daneman D, et al; International Society for Pediatric and Adolescent Diabetes. Diabetic ketoacidosis. *Pediatr Diabetes.* 2007;8(1): 28-43.

A 73-year-old woman is brought to the emergency department (ED) from an assisted-living facility. The patient has a history of dementia, hypertension, and type II diabetes mellitus. By report, she has had chills and a productive cough for several days. In the past 24 hours she has become weaker and does not want to get out of bed. The physical examination reveals a thin, elderly woman who is somnolent but arousable. Her rectal temperature is 36.0°C (96.8°F), pulse rate is 118 beats per minute, blood pressure is 84/50 mm Hg, and respiratory rate is 22 breaths per minute. Her mucous membranes are dry. Her heart is tachycardic but regular. She has crackles at her right lung base with a scant wheeze. Her abdomen is soft and nontender. The extremities feel cool and her pulses are rapid and thready. The patient is moving all extremities, without focal deficits.

▶ What is the most likely diagnosis?

ANSWERS TO CASE 6:

Severe Sepsis

Summary: A 73-year-old woman presents from an assisted-living facility with cough, lethargy, and hypotension of unknown etiology.

- **Most likely diagnosis:** Severe sepsis due to healthcare-associated pneumonia

ANALYSIS

Objectives

1. Learn to recognize the clinical presentations of systemic inflammatory response syndrome (SIRS)/sepsis and the atypical presentations in children and the elderly.

2. Learn the pathophysiology, systemic effects, and management of sepsis and its common complications.

3. Become familiar with early goal-directed therapy in the treatment of sepsis and septic shock.

Considerations

This woman appears to be suffering from severe sepsis, a clinical entity on the continuum from systemic inflammatory response syndrome to septic shock with multiorgan system dysfunction (see below for definitions). In her case, the etiology is likely pneumonia, an extremely common cause of sepsis in elderly patients. Sepsis caused by a urinary tract infection (ie, urosepsis) is another important cause of sepsis in this population.

There are over 750,000 cases of sepsis in the United States each year. Overall mortality is 30% and, while the mortality rate has been decreasing, the rise in number of cases has led to an increase in the total number of deaths caused by sepsis: the most recent US figures attribute >215,000 deaths annually to sepsis. As this woman falls into the classification of septic shock, her risk of death may be closer to 70%, even with treatment.

The current standard of care for treating sepsis uses an algorithm known as early goal-directed therapy (EGDT), which has been shown to dramatically improve hemodynamic outcomes and mortality (see below).

APPROACH TO:

Severe Sepsis

DEFINITIONS

SYSTEMIC INFLAMMATORY RESPONSE SYNDROME (SIRS): At least two of the following:

- Temperature >38°C or <36°C

- Heart rate >90 beats per minute

- Tachypnea or hyperventilation (respiratory rate >20 breaths per minute or $Paco_2$ <32 mm Hg)

- White blood cell count >12,000 cells/mL or <4000 cells/mL, or >10% bands

SEPSIS: SIRS with an infectious source.

SEVERE SEPSIS: Sepsis in conjunction with at least one sign of organ failure *or* hypoperfusion, such as lactic acidosis (lactate ≥4 mmol/L), oliguria (urine output ≤0.5 mL/kg for 1 hour), abrupt change in mental status, mottled skin or delayed capillary refill, thrombocytopenia (platelets ≤ 100,000 cells/mL) or disseminated intravascular coagulation, or acute lung injury/acute respiratory distress syndrome.

SEPTIC SHOCK: Severe sepsis with hypotension (or requirement of vasoactive agents, eg, dopamine or norepinephrine) despite adequate fluid resuscitation in the form of a 20- to 40-cc/kg bolus.

MULTIORGAN DYSFUNCTION SYNDROME (MODS): MODS is the far end of the spectrum that begins with SIRS. It is defined as dysfunction of two or more organ systems such that homeostasis cannot be maintained without intervention.

CLINICAL APPROACH

Pathophysiology

Sepsis is usually caused by bacterial infection (see Table 6–1 for common bacterial causes of infection). However, it may be caused by viral or, increasingly, by fungal infection. In general, sepsis is a complex interaction between the direct toxic effects of the infecting organism and derangement of the normal inflammatory host response to infection.

Normally, in the setting of infection, there is concurrent local activation of the immune system and of down-regulatory mechanisms to control the reaction. The devastating effects of the sepsis syndrome are caused by a combination of (1) generalization of the immune response to sites remote from that of the infection and (2) derangement of the balance between proinflammatory and anti-inflammatory cellular regulators, as well as (3) dissemination of the infecting organism.

In general, the immune response to infection optimizes the ability of immune cells to leave the circulation and enter the site of infection. Microbial antigens trigger local cells to release proinflammatory cytokines. These molecules attract leukocytes, slow blood flow through venules and capillaries, and trigger dilation of vessels and increased "leakiness" of vessel walls. At the same time, the cytokines induce the release and production of acute-phase reactants, which fight microbes but are also procoagulants. It is when the two main effects of the inflammatory cascade— vasodilation and coagulation—spread beyond the site of local infection that the syndrome of sepsis manifests in systemic hypotension, hypoperfusion, coagulopathy, and resultant organ failure. In the face of hypoperfusion and lack of oxygen, organs are forced to use anaerobic metabolism, leading to an elevation in serum lactic acid.

Table 6–1 • COMMON BACTERIAL CAUSES OF INFECTION		
Suspected Infection	**Common Pathogens**	**Empiric Antibiotic Recommendations**
Unknown source (immunocompetent adult)	*Escherichia coli* *Staphylococcus aureus* *Streptococcus pneumoniae* *Enterococcus* spp *Klebsiella* spp *Pseudomonas aeruginosa*	Vancomycin *plus* antipseudomonal penicillin (eg, piperacillin/tazobactam) *Or* antipseudomonal cephalosporin (eg, ceftazadine, cefepime) *plus* fluoroquinolone (eg, levofloxacin, ciprofloxacin) *Or* aminoglycoside (eg, gentamicin, amikacin)
Pneumonia	*Streptococcus pneumoniae* *Mycoplasma pneumoniae* *Haemophilus influenza,* *Chlamydophila pneumoniae* *Legionella*	Antipseudomonal cephalosporin (eg, ceftazadine, cefepime) *plus* macrolide (eg, azithromycin) *Or* fluoroquinolone (eg, levofloxacin, moxifloxacin)
Urinary tract infection	*Escherichia coli* *Klebsiella* spp *Enterococcus* spp	Fluoroquinolone (eg, levofloxacin) *Or* third-generation cephalosporin (eg, ceftriaxone)
Meningitis	*Streptococcus pneumoniae* *Neisseria meningitides* *Listeria monocytogenes* (primarily in adults over 50-60 or immunocompromised patients)	Vancomycin *plus* ceftriaxone (meningeal doses) *plus* Ampicillin if listeria is suspected
Abdominal infection		Ampicillin *plus* aminoglycoside (eg, gentamicin, amikacin) *plus* metronidazole

The degree of elevation correlates strongly with prognosis: higher presenting lactate levels and slow decline of lactate during resuscitation are associated with significantly higher mortality.

Clinical Presentation

Sepsis begins with signs of a systemic inflammatory response (ie, fever, tachycardia, tachypnea, leukocytosis) and progresses to hypotension in the setting of either peripheral vasodilation ("warm" or hyperdynamic septic shock, with generalized flushing and warmth and increased cardiac output) or peripheral vasoconstriction ("cold" or hypodynamic septic shock, with cold blue or white extremities). In a patient with this presentation and physical examination findings consistent with infection, diagnosis is easy and treatment can be begun early.

It is important to remember that, especially in infants and the elderly, initial presentation may lack some of the more salient features—that is, they may present with hypothermia rather than hyperthermia, leukopenia rather than leukocytosis, and they may not be able to mount a tachycardia (as in elderly patients on β- or calcium-channel blockers) or they may have a tachycardia attributed to other causes (as in anxious infants). In a patient at the extremes of age, any nonspecific systemic complaint—vomiting, fatigue, behavioral changes—should prompt concern for sepsis, and consideration of at least initial screens for infection, such as a chest radiograph and urinalysis.

Be aware that a patient not initially meeting the criteria for sepsis may progress to full-blown sepsis even during the course of an emergency department stay, with initially only subtle changes in examination. Altered mental status is often the first sign of organ dysfunction, as it is assessable without laboratory studies, but it is easily missed in the elderly, the very young, and those with other potential causes for altered level of consciousness, such as intoxication. Decreased urine output ($\leq$0.5 mL/kg/h) is another sign that may be apparent prior to the return of laboratory values and should raise clinical concern.

Evaluation/Management

Initial Treatment Considerations The patient should immediately be placed on a cardiac and pulse-oxygenation monitor, and a manual blood pressure obtained. Supplemental oxygen by nasal canula or facemask should be titrated to keep oxygen saturation >93%, two large-bore, peripheral IVs should rapidly be inserted, and, in the absence of a fluid overload condition (eg, congestive heart failure, renal failure) a fluid bolus of 20 to 40 mL/kg (2-4 L in adults) crystalloid administered (Table 6–2). If available, a point of care lactic acid should be obtained without delay. Ideally, it should be obtained prior to the initial fluid bolus; however, this should under no circumstances cause a delay resuscitation. If the patient clearly has severely increased work of breathing or cannot protect her airway, the patient should be intubated, with care taken with selection of induction agents, as many cause hypotension.

Table 6–2 • Initial Management of Patient with Suspected Sepsis
Two large-bore IVs
Lactic acid
Initial fluid bolus of 20-40 mL/kg or 2-4 L in adults
CBC
CMP
Blood cultures from two sites
Urinalysis with culture
Pregnancy test in women of childbearing age
Chest radiograph
Empiric antibiotics (goal is <1 h from initial presentation)

Blood should be drawn for a complete blood count (with differential), comprehensive metabolic panel, blood cultures (two sets), and lactic acid (if not already obtained). A urinalysis with culture and chest x-ray should be ordered immediately as part of what must be an aggressive search for the source of the infection (the majority of sepsis in this country is caused by either pneumonia or urinary tract infections). An ECG should also be ordered early in the workup, to evaluate for cardiac ischemia secondary to hypoperfusion.

Broad-spectrum intravenous antibiotics should be started rapidly—ideally after the cultures have been drawn, but antibiotic infusion should not be delayed if cultures cannot be obtained in a timely fashion (<1 h after presentation), particularly in a patient like this one, who is extremely ill and hemodynamically unstable. Initial therapy should be empiric, with good coverage for all possible sites and organisms, as there is good evidence that inappropriate antibiotic selection doubles mortality (see Table 6–1 for suggested antibiotics).

Subsequent Priorities Immediately upon termination of the first fluid bolus, the patient should be reassessed. If the patient continues to be hypotensive *or* has a lactate level greater than 4 mmol/dL *or* has other signs of continued hypoperfusion, then early goal-directed therapy (EGDT) should be initiated. EGDT is a method of continual assessment and reassessment of clinical and laboratory markers, with interventions aimed at normalizing those markers. The overarching goal of EGDT is to eliminate mismatch between oxygen demand and oxygen supply (the hallmark of sepsis) by increasing supply and—where possible—by decreasing demand.

Early Goal-Directed Therapy

Goal 1: central venous pressure (CVP) 8-12 mm Hg: CVP should be kept between 8 and 12 mm Hg (or >12 mm Hg if mechanically ventilated), with continued fluid boluses (which may total as much as 6 to 10 L of crystalloid over the first hours) to maintain an adequate CVP. In practice, 500 cc of normal saline can be bolused every 15 to 30 minutes until the CVP goal is met.

Goal 2: mean arterial pressure (MAP) ≥65 mm Hg: If the patient's MAP remains <65 mm Hg despite adequate fluid resuscitation, vasopressors should be initiated, with either norepinephrine or dopamine usually recommended as the starting agents. They should be titrated to a goal of MAP ≥65 mm Hg. If blood pressure is unresponsive to the first vasopressor, a second agent may be added. Low-dose vasopressin can be used as a second- or third-line agent.

Goal 3: central venous oxygen saturation ($Scvo_2$) ≥70%: On placement of the central line, blood obtained should be sent for an oxygen saturation. If the $Scvo_2$ is ≤70% (meaning the tissues are extracting as much oxygen as possible from the blood, and therefore that tissue demand is not being met), then oxygen delivery should be optimized by

- Transfusing packed red blood cells to a hematocrit ≥30%.

- If the $Scvo_2$ continues to be <70% despite achieving CVP 8 to 12 mm Hg, MAP ≥65 mm Hg, and HCT ≥30%, then dobutamine infusion should be started to boost cardiac output.

- If all of the above measures are taken and $ScvO_2$ continues to be <70%, then patient can be intubated to maximize oxygenation and sedated in an attempt to decrease oxygen demand.

Additional goal: lactate clearance of ≥10%: An initial lactate should be sent in every patient with suspected sepsis. After a minimum of 2 hours of resuscitation a repeat lactate should be checked to ensure that at least 10% of the lactate has been cleared. If the lactate clearance is not at least 10% then oxygen delivery should be optimized in much the same way that is described in the $ScvO_2$ section by

- Transfusing packed red blood cells if the hematocrit is <30%.

- If there is not a lactate clearance of at least 10% after transfusion then dobutamine infusion should be started and titrated to achieve a 10% clearance.

If a 10% clearance is not achieved, lactate levels should be checked at 1 to 2 hour intervals and repeat clearance calculated each time. New data show that in hospitals where $ScvO_2$ cannot easily be monitored, lactate can be used in lieu of $ScvO_2$ monitoring.

A patient in severe sepsis or septic shock should be admitted to an intensive care unit. Throughout her stay in the emergency department, she should be frequently reassessed, using measurements of blood pressure, central venous pressure, oxygen saturation, central venous saturation, urine output, and lactate to direct therapy. If severe sepsis progresses to multiorgan dysfunction syndrome, therapy includes support or replacement of the affected organs/systems as indicated below under complications.

Other Therapies/Interventions

Ultrasound: Is a noninvasive method that can be used to monitor CVP that does not require placement of a central venous catheter thus avoiding the time delay and catheter-associated complications. Studies have looked at using compression ultrasound of the forearm or measurement of the internal jugular vein to approximate CVP. In the hands of a well-trained sonographer this can be used as a noninvasive way to estimate central venous catheter.

Steroids: While historically steroids have been used in sepsis, their role is becoming more limited. Recent published data suggest that even "physiologic doses" of steroids do not improve overall mortality in severe sepsis. It is not recommended that they be used in sepsis without shock unless there is a recent history of prolonged steroid use or history suggesting adrenal suppression. In the case of septic shock unresponsive to fluid resuscitation *and* vasopressors, steroids may be considered.

Activated protein C: Protein C is an enzyme produced in the liver that inhibits thrombosis and promotes fibrinolysis. A patient's native ability to activate protein C appears to be impaired in sepsis. Given the contribution of coagulopathy and impaired microvascular circulation to mortality in sepsis, it was theorized that exogenous activated protein C might be helpful. There is some evidence that it may decrease mortality in patients who have severe sepsis *and* have a high risk of death, but it does not benefit patients at low risk of death. Therefore, it should only be given to patients with sepsis-induced organ dysfunction that are deemed to be at a high risk of death. It should *not* be given if there are contraindications to antico-agulation (ie, active bleeding, risk of bleeding, history of intracranial bleeding, etc). The use of activated protein C is never recommended in children.

Glucose control: This is an area of recent controversy. For a period of time it was thought that there was benefit to maintaining tight control of blood glucose in the range of 80 to 120 mg/dL. However, more recent studies have shown that glucose control this tight leads to significantly more severe hypoglycemia. Therefore, we rec-ommend that in sepsis a patient's glucose goals should be between 140 and 180 mg/dL.

Intravenous immunoglobulin: In children, administration of intravenous immu-noglobulin (IVIG) in both neonates and older children has been shown in some studies to result in improvement in mortality and fewer complications, although a recent meta-analysis was inconclusive as to IVIGs benefit in sepsis. Its presumed mechanism of action is augmented clearance of pathogenic organisms and feedback inhibition of inflammatory cytokines.

Extracorporeal membrane oxygenation: Extracorporeal membrane oxygenation (ECMO), a form of mechanical heart-lung bypass, has been used in septic shock in children with unclear results. It may be tried, when available, to treat a patient in cardiorespiratory failure that is refractory to traditional means of support.

HMG-CoA reductase inhibitors ("statins"): HMG-CoA reductase inhibitors, or statins, are lipid-lowering agents that are thought to have a significant anti-inflammatory component. Animal studies have shown increased survival from sepsis with administration of statins, and there is evidence from observational studies that being on a statin lowers human patients' likelihood of death from sepsis. Statins are relatively safe and inexpensive drugs. If forthcoming studies show benefit, statins may become a standard component of the treatment of sepsis.

Complications

ALI and ARDS (acute lung injury and acute respiratory distress syndrome): The inflammatory milieu of sepsis is especially damaging to the lungs. Buildup of inflam-matory fluid in the alveoli impairs gas exchange favors lung collapse, and decreases compliance, with the end result of respiratory distress and hypoxemia. ALI/ARDS is a common complication of severe sepsis and is often visible on chest x-ray, in the form of bilateral pulmonary opacities consistent with pulmonary edema. A septic patient who did not initially require mechanical ventilation may later require it if she develops ALI/ARDS after fluid resuscitation. In such cases, low tidal volumes (ie, tidal volume set initially to 8 mL/kg then titrated down to 6 mL/kg in the first couple hours of therapy) should be used, with measures taken to limit peak inspira-tory pressures and thus limit barotrauma to the lung—a significant risk.

DIC (disseminated intravascular coagulation): In DIC caused by sepsis, the coagu-lation cascade is diffusely activated as part of the inflammatory response. At the same time, the fibrinolytic system, which normally acts to keep the clotting cascade in check, is activated. These factors begin a feedback spiral in which both systems are constantly and diffusely activated—new clots always being formed, then broken down. A large proportion of the body's clotting factors and platelets are consumed in such clots. Thus, patients are at risk for complications from both thrombosis and hemorrhage. In this setting, platelets may be given if the platelet count is <5000 cells/mm^3 without signs of bleeding, or <30,000 cells/mm^3 with active bleeding. Fresh-frozen plasma should be given *if* there is active bleeding. The development of any coagulopathy in sepsis correlates with a worse outcome.

Cardiac failure: Myocardial depression is an early complication of septic shock, with the mechanism thought to be direct action of inflammatory molecules rather than decreased perfusion of coronary arteries. Supporting the heart's function involves careful attention to preload (hydration with close monitoring of CVP), afterload (vasopressors), and contractility (supported with dobutamine). Sepsis places an unprecedented workload on a heart, which can precipitate acute coronary syndrome or a myocardial infarction, especially in the elderly. Thus inotropic agents and vasopressors (most of which can result in tachycardia) must be used with care when necessary but never when unwarranted.

Hepatic failure: Liver failure usually manifests as cholestatic jaundice, with increases in bilirubin, aminotransferases, and alkaline phosphatase. Synthetic function is usually not affected unless patients are hemodynamically unstable for long periods.

Renal failure: Hypoperfusion appears to be the main mechanism for renal failure in the setting of sepsis, which is manifested by oliguria, azotemia, and inflammatory cells on urinalysis. The treatment is first to adequately support perfusion with hydration and vasopressors. However, if the renal failure is severe or the kidneys cannot be adequately perfused, then renal replacement therapy (eg, hemodialysis or continuous veno-venous hemofiltration) is indicated.

Multiorgan dysfunction syndrome: Dysfunction of two or more organ systems such that intervention is required to maintain homeostasis.

- Primary—in which failure of organs is directly caused by infection or injury of them; that is, heart/lung failure in the setting of severe pneumonia

- Secondary—in which failure of organs is caused by generalized inflammatory response to an insult; that is, ALI or ARDS in the setting of urosepsis

COMPREHENSION QUESTIONS

6.1 A 32-year-old woman is noted to have persistent hypotension from suspected toxic shock syndrome despite 6 L of normal saline given intravenously. Which of the following is the best next step?

　A. Use colloid (albumin) for the next bolus.

　B. Initiate norepinephrine infusion.

　C. Administer corticosteroid therapy.

　D. Transfuse with fresh-frozen plasma.

　E. Activated protein C.

6.2 A 45-year-old man with acute cholecystitis is noted to have a fever of 38.3°C (101°F), hypotension, and altered sensorium. His HCT is noted to be 24%. Broad-spectrum antibiotics and intravenous saline are administered, and, although his CVP is 10 and his MAP is 80, his Scvo$_2$ remains <70%. Which of the following is most likely to be beneficial?

A. Initiate corticosteroids

B. Tight glucose control

C. Acetaminophen 500 mg PR

D. Transfusion

E. Lithotripsy

6.3 A 32-year-old woman is admitted to the hospital for acute pyelonephritis. The patient is treated with oral ciprofloxacin. After 4 days of therapy, she returns to the ED with persistent fever to 38.9°C (102°F) and flank tenderness. The urine culture reveals *E coli* greater than 100,000 colony-forming units per mL susceptible to ciprofloxacin. When you arrive to examine her, you note that she is tachypneic, tachycardiac, and appears lethargic. Which of the following is the next step?

A. Order an intravenous pyelogram.

B. Obtain IV access and administer a fluid bolus.

C. Initiate a workup for fictitious fever.

D. Consult a surgeon for possible appendicitis.

E. Add antifungal therapy.

6.4 A 66-year-old woman is noted to have acute pneumococcal pneumonia and is being treated with antibiotics, and with norepinephrine and dobutamine to maintain her BP and urine output. Which of the following is a bad prognostic sign?

A. Urine output of 1 mL/kg/h

B. Mean arterial blood pressure of 80 mm Hg

C. Lactic acid level of 6 mmol/dL

D. Serum bicarbonate level of 22 mEq/L

E. Hematocrit 35%

ANSWERS

6.1 **B.** A vasopressor agent such as norepinephrine (or dopamine) is the treatment of choice for hypotension that is unresponsive to intravenous saline infusion. The use of colloids during resuscitation has not been shown to improve outcome compared to crystalloids. Fresh-frozen plasma is not indicated. There is not enough information provided to asses if activated protein C is indicated.

6.2 **D.** This patient has met two of the three goals of EGDT, but fails to meet the third goal of $ScvO_2$ >70%. In the setting of HCT <30%, transfusion with PRBCs is indicated. Tight glucose control and steroids have not been shown to consistently improve mortality in all comers with severe sepsis.

6.3 **B.** This patient is progressing to severe sepsis, and possibly septic shock. While an intravenous pyelogram may be needed eventually to rule out mechanical obstruction (eg, an infected stone) as a cause of this patient's refractory UTI, the urgent need here is prompt fluid resuscitation.

6.4 **C.** The elevated serum lactate is evidence that oxygen supply is not meeting systemic oxygen demand. A lactate level ≥4 is a poor prognostic sign. The other parameters are normal.

CLINICAL PEARLS

▶ The most common causes of severe sepsis are urosepsis and pneumonia.

▶ Older, younger, or immunocompromised individuals may present with subtle signs such as lethargy, decreased appetite, or hypothermia.

▶ Early goal-directed therapy for sepsis includes careful monitoring of multiple markers of organ perfusion, with aggressive measures to restore any imbalance between oxygen supply and demand.

▶ Initially, large volumes of fluid administered in multiple boluses may be necessary (and in some cases sufficient) to maintain perfusion.

▶ An early and thorough search for a source must be undertaken, with immediate measures taken to control it. Whether or not an operable source is found, broad-spectrum antibiotics should be started immediately. If an operable source is found, it should be surgically treated as soon as the patient can tolerate it.

▶ A vasopressor agent such as norepinephrine or dopamine is the next step in treating hypotension that persists despite intravenous fluids.

REFERENCES

Dellinger RP, Levy MM, Carlet JM, et al. Surviving sepsis campaign: international guidelines for management of severe sepsis and septic shock: 2008. *Crit Care Med.* 2008;36(1):296-327.

Finfer S, Chittock DR, Su SY, et al. Intensive vs conventional glucose control in critically ill patients. *NEJM.* 2009:360:1283-1297.

Gao F, Linhantova L, Johnston AM, et al. Statins and sepsis. *Br J Anaesth.* 2008;100(3):288-298.

Ibrahim EH, Sherman G, Ward S, et al. The influence of inadequate antimicrobial treatment of bloodstream infections on patient outcomes in the ICU setting. *Chest.* 2000;118:146-155.

Jones AE, Shapiro NI, Trzeciak S, Arnold RC, Claremont HA, Kline JA. Lactate clearance vs central venous oxygen saturation as goals of early sepsis therapy: a randomized clinical trial. *JAMA.* 2010;303 (8):739-746.

Laterre P. Clinical trials in severe sepsis with drotrecogin alpha (activated). *Crit Care Med.* 2007;11 (suppl 5):S5.

Laupland KB, Kirkpatrick AW, Delaney A. Polyclonal intravenous immunoglobulin for the treatment of severe sepsis and septic shock in critically ill adults: a systematic review and meta-analysis. *Crit Care Med.* December 1, 2007;35(12):2686-2692.

Nagdev AD, Merchant RC, Tirado-Gonzalez A, et al. Emergency department bedside ultrasonographic measurement of the caval index for noninvasive determination of low central venous pressure. *Ann Emerg Med.* 2010;55(3):290-295.

Rivers E, Nguyen B, Havstad S, et al. Early goal-directed therapy in the treatment of severe sepsis and septic shock. *N Engl J Med.* 2001;345(19):1368-1377.

Trzeciak S, Cinel I, Dellinger RP, et al. Resuscitating the microcirculation in sepsis: the central role of nitric oxide, emerging concepts for novel therapies, and challenges for clinical trials. *Acad Emerg Med.* 2008;15:399-413.

A 23-year-old man is transported to your emergency department (ED) from the scene of a rollover motor vehicle collision (MVC). He was found approximately 1 hour after the accident had occurred. At the scene, the patient was awake and complained of pain in his back and legs. In the ED, he is awake, his speech is clear and appropriate, and he has normal breath sounds over bilateral lung fields. He has palpable, equal bilateral femoral pulses. His temperature is 35.6°C (96.1°F) (rectally), pulse rate is 106 beats per minute, blood pressure is 110/88 mm Hg, respiratory rate is 24 breaths per minute, and Glasgow coma scale is 15. Multiple abrasions are noted over the neck, shoulders, abdomen, and legs. His chest wall is nontender. His abdomen is mildly tender. The pelvis is stable, but he has extensive swelling and tenderness of the right thigh. He has a deep scalp laceration over his right temporal area that continues to ooze. A focused abdominal sonographic examination trauma (FAST) is performed revealing free fluid in Morison pouch and no other abnormalities. The patient's initial complete blood count (CBC) reveals a white blood cell count (WBC) of 14,800 cells/mm^3, hemoglobin of 11.2 g/dL, and hematocrit of 34.4%.

▶ What is the next step in the evaluation of this patient?
▶ If this patient becomes hypotensive, what is the most likely cause?

ANSWERS TO CASE 7:
Hemorrhagic Shock

Summary: A healthy 23-year-old man presents following a motor vehicle accident with mild tachycardia, scalp laceration, femur fracture, and a tender abdomen with a positive FAST examination.

- **Next step: The Emergency Medicine approach to every critically ill patient begins with evaluation and stabilization of the airway, breathing, and circulation (ABC). This approach is also advocated by** Advanced Trauma Life Support (ATLS) guidelines. Once the ABCs are stabilized, a thorough secondary survey, consisting of a detailed physical examination, should follow. In this patient, the ABCs are stable and the secondary survey reveals abdominal pain and a likely right femur fracture with intact pulses. Immediately subsequent to the secondary survey, the ultrasound examination demonstrates free fluid in the hepatorenal potential space known as Morison pouch. Presence of fluid in the hepatorenal space indicates intra-abdominal hemorrhage likely secondary to solid organ injury. Since this patient is hemodynamically stable, a computed tomography (CT) scan of the abdomen and pelvis should be done to identify and grade the severity of the injuries. In addition to estimating the amount of intraperitoneal free fluid, the CT scan can aid in identifying the source of bleeding and the presence of other injuries that may have not been appreciated on clinical examination. The limitations of CT scans in blunt trauma—mainly the lower sensitivity for hollow organ injuries and bowel wall hematomas—should be kept in mind when reviewing a CT scan in this setting.

- **Most likely cause of hypotension:** Hemorrhagic shock. The probable sources of blood loss in this patient are thigh, abdomen, and scalp laceration. Other possible causes or contributors to his hypotension are cardiogenic shock secondary to myocardial contusion or spinal shock secondary to injury to the spinal cord. The latter can easily be ruled out by performing a neurologic examination during the secondary survey, or even as part of the disability evaluation during the primary survey.

ANALYSIS

Objectives

1. Learn the basics of initial assessment of a trauma patient (Figure 7–1).

2. Learn the definitions and pathophysiology of shock and hemorrhagic shock.

3. Learn the advantages and disadvantages of base deficit, serum lactate, hemoglobin/hematocrit, and pulmonary artery catheter application for shock identification and patient resuscitation.

4. Learn the initial approach to managing and treating the patient with hemorrhagic shock.

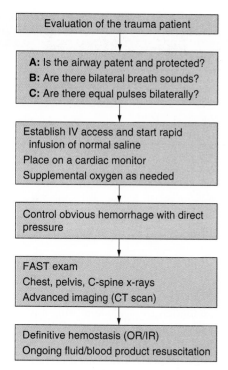

Figure 7–1. Algorithm for assessment/management of the trauma patient.

Initial Assessment of the Trauma Patient

The **first priorities in the evaluation of any trauma patient are the ABCs.** Airway is assessed by asking the patient to state his or her name, followed by noting the presence or absence of tracheal deviation. If the patient is unable to protect his airway because of confusion, loss of consciousness, or an extrinsic threat to the airway (ie, expanding neck hematoma), the patient should be intubated with an endotracheal tube. Next, breathing is assessed by listening to the chest for the presence of equal bilateral breath sounds and by observing the symmetry of chest wall expansion. The unstable patient with clinical signs of pneumothorax or tension pneumothorax should be treated with immediate needle decompression followed by placement of a chest tube. Finally, circulation is assessed via the vital signs and by palpation of bilateral femoral, radial, or pedal pulses. Any suggestion of cardiovascular instability requires immediate crystalloid or colloid resuscitation through two large bore peripheral IVs.

Next, the patient's ability to follow commands should be evaluated and an overall assessment of his/her level of functioning should be made. This consists of assigning a score on the Glasgow coma scale, ranging from 3 to 15 (see also Table I–1 in Section I). Subsequently, a focused history should be quickly elicited. The mnemonic "AMPLE" is useful for guiding the history taking (Table 7–1).

Based on the capability of your hospital and trauma or emergency services, bedside ultrasound can be incorporated into the initial evaluation of the trauma patient.

Table 7–1 • "AMPLE" GUIDE TO HISTORY-TAKING IN THE TRAUMA PATIENT	
A	Does the patient have any allergies?
M	Does the patient take any medications?
P	Does the patient have any significant past medical history?
L	When was the patient's last meal?
E	Does the patient recall events leading up to, or involving, the accident?

Aside from the FAST examination (assessment for free fluid in Morison pouch, splenorenal and supra-splenic space, pelvis, and pericardial space), ultrasound can be used for rapid identification of pneumothorax, hemothorax, cardiac activity, and central line placement if needed. The use of ultrasound in the trauma patient is operator-dependent.

The secondary survey follows, in which the patient is examined from head to toe. In the presence of severe, obvious injuries, it is appropriate to start the examination at the affected sites. However, one must be cautious and diligent to complete a thorough physical examination to preclude missing any less obvious but equally important or potentially life-threatening injuries. Additional history from paramedics, and emergency medical technicians (EMTs) should also be elicited.

In this patient, the entire history is very concerning. In addition to being ejected from a vehicle involved in a collision at high speed, and therefore at risk for multisystem injuries secondary to a high kinetic energy transfer, the patient was found 1 hour following the incident. The risk for hypothermia and a diminished ability to respond to hemorrhagic shock is great.

APPROACH TO:
Hemorrhagic Shock

DEFINITIONS

SHOCK: Insufficient cellular perfusion/inability to deliver sufficient oxygen to the tissues.

HEMORRHAGIC SHOCK: Inadequate tissue oxygenation resulting from a blood volume deficit. In this situation, the loss of blood volume decreases venous return, cardiac filling pressures, and cardiac output. End-organ perfusion is subsequently decreased as blood flow is preferentially preserved to the brain and heart.

CLINICAL APPROACH

In shock, the lack of oxygen available to cells results in an inability of mitochondria to generate adequate ATP. Instead, anaerobic metabolism dominates, leading to an accumulation of pyruvate that is converted to lactate.

Shock is divided into three stages: Compensated, progressive, and irreversible. Shock is initially compensated by control mechanisms that return cardiac output and arterial pressure back to normal levels. Within seconds, baroreceptors and chemoreceptors elicit powerful sympathetic stimulation that vasoconstricts arterioles and increases heart rate and cardiac contractility. After minutes to hours, angiotensin constricts the peripheral arteries while vasopressin constricts the veins to maintain arterial pressures and improve blood return to the heart. Angiotensin and vasopressin also increase water retention, thereby improving cardiac filling pressures. Locally, vascular control preferentially dilates vessels around the hypoxic tissues to increase blood flow to injured areas. The **normal manifestations of shock do not apply** to **pregnant** women, **athletes,** and individuals with **altered autonomic nervous systems** (older patients, those taking β-blockers).

As shock evolves into the *progressive stage*, **arterial pressure falls.** This leads to cardiac depression from decreased coronary blood flow, and, in turn, further decreases arterial pressure. The result is a feedback loop that becomes a vicious cycle toward uncontrolled deterioration. Inadequate blood flow to the nervous system eventually results in complete inactivation of sympathetic stimulation. In the microvasculature, low blood flow causes the blood to sludge, amplifying the inadequate delivery of oxygen to the tissues. This ischemia results in increased microvascular permeability, and large quantities of fluid and protein move from the intravascular space to the extravascular compartment, which exacerbates the already decreased intravascular volume. The **systemic inflammatory response syndrome caused by severe injury and shock may progress to multiorgan failure.** Pulmonary edema, acute respiratory distress syndrome (ARDS), poor cardiac contractility, loss of electrolyte and fluid control, and inability to metabolize toxins and waste products set in. Cells lose the ability to maintain electrolyte balance, metabolize glucose, maintain mitochondrial activity, and prevent lysosomal release of hydrolases. Resuscitation during this progressive stage of tissue ischemia can cause reperfusion injury from the burst of oxygen-free radicals.

Finally, the patient enters the *irreversible stage* of shock, and any therapeutic efforts become futile. Despite transiently elevated arterial pressures and cardiac output, the body is unable to recover, and death becomes inevitable.

Pathophysiology and Stages of Hemorrhagic Shock

Hemorrhagic shock is the most common cause of death in trauma patients aside from traumatic brain injury. A high level of suspicion for hemorrhage and hemorrhagic shock should dominate evaluation of a trauma patient, especially as vital signs may not become abnormal until a significant amount of hemorrhage has occurred. Hemorrhagic shock is classified by the advanced trauma life support (ATLS) into four categories to further emphasize the progression of vital sign instability in response to blood loss (Table 7–2). Additional clinical signs that indicate hemorrhagic shock include skin pallor/coolness, delayed capillary refill, weak distal pulses, and anxiety.

As demonstrated by the ATLS classification of stages of hemorrhagic shock, the clinician must not rely solely on vital signs for determination of extent of hemorrhage. This patient obviously has had some blood loss from his femur fracture, and the **focused abdominal sonography for trauma (FAST) examination suggests intra-abdominal solid organ injury associated with additional hemorrhage.**

Table 7–2 • ATLS CLASSIFICATION OF HEMORRHAGE				
Class Of Hemorrhage	Class I	Class II	Class III	Class IV
Blood loss (mL)	<750	750-1500	1500-2000	>2000
Pulse (beats per minute)	<100	>100	>120	>140
Blood pressure	Normal	Normal	Decreased	Decreased
Pulse pressure (mm Hg)	Normal	Decreased	Decreased	Decreased
Respiratory rate (breaths per minute)	14-20	20-30	30-40	>40
Urine output (mL/h)	>30	20-30	5-15	Negligible
Central nervous system (mental status)	Slightly anxious	Mildly anxious	Anxious, confused	Lethargic

Additionally, his scalp laceration must be evaluated as a potential source for serious exsanguination. Despite these multiple sources of hemorrhage, our patient has a normal blood pressure and only a slightly elevated heart rate, which places him in Class II hemorrhagic shock.

DIAGNOSTIC APPROACH

Identify the Source of Bleeding

A trauma patient should be carefully screened to locate the source of blood loss. In this patient, the possibility of bleeding should be assessed in **five areas**: (1) **external bleeding** (eg, scalp/extremity lacerations); (2) **thorax** (eg, hemothorax, aortic injury); (3) **peritoneal cavity** (eg, solid organ lacerations, large vessel injury); (4) **pelvis/ retroperitoneum** (eg, pelvic fracture); and (5) **soft-tissue compartments** (eg, long-bone fractures). Adjunctive studies that should be obtained in blunt trauma patients early during their evaluation include chest and pelvic roentgenograms and computed tomography (CT) scans of the head, chest, abdomen, and pelvis. Chest roentgenograms can identify a hemothorax and potential mediastinal bleeding. Pelvic films can demonstrate pelvic fractures as a source of pelvic blood loss. Films of any affected extremity, in this case the femur, should also be obtained. Fractures are not only associated with blood loss from the bone and adjacent soft tissue, but their presence indicates significant energy transfer (often referred to as a significant mechanism of injury) and should increase the clinical suspicion for intra-abdominal and retroperitoneal bleeding. Typically, tibial or humeral fractures can be associated with 750 mL of blood loss (1.5 units of blood), whereas femur fractures can be associated with up to 1500 mL of blood (3 units of blood) in the thigh. Pelvic fractures may result in even more blood loss—up to several liters can be lost into a retroperitoneal hematoma.

Laboratory Evaluation

Laboratory studies that aid (but are not necessary) in evaluating acute blood loss are hemoglobin, hematocrit, base deficit, and lactate levels. In the setting of acute hemorrhage, hemoglobin and hematocrit levels may or may not be decreased. These values measure concentration, not absolute amounts. Hemoglobin is measured in grams of red blood cells per deciliter of blood; hematocrit is the percentage of blood volume that is red blood cells. Loss of whole blood will not decrease the red blood cell concentration or the percentage of red cells in blood. The initial minor drops in hemoglobin and hematocrit levels are the results of mechanisms that compensate for blood loss by drawing fluid into the vascular space. To see significant decreases in these values, blood loss must be replaced with crystalloid solution; therefore, most decreases in hemoglobin and hematocrit values are not seen until patients have received large volumes of crystalloid fluid for resuscitation.

With the ongoing metabolic acidosis of hemorrhagic shock, an increased base deficit and lactate level will be seen. Both lactate and base deficit levels are laboratory values that indicate systemic acidosis, not local tissue ischemia. They are global indices of tissue perfusion and normal values may mask areas of under perfusion as a consequence of normal blood flow to the remainder of the body. These laboratory tests are not true representations of tissue hypoxia. It is, therefore, not surprising that lactate and base deficit are poor prognostic indicators of survival in patients with shock. Although absolute values of these laboratory results are not predictors of survival in patients with shock, the baseline value and trends can be used to determine the extent of tissue hypoxia and adequacy of resuscitation. Normalization of base deficit and serum lactate within 24 hours after resuscitation is a good prognostic indicator of survival. Of note, given that lactate is hepatically metabolized, it is not a reliable value in patients with liver dysfunction.

Central Monitoring

The approach to central monitoring in the trauma patient has changed dramatically. The benefit of central monitoring is to most accurately determine cardiac preload, given that preload, or end-diastolic sarcomere length, is the driving force behind the cardiac output as defined by the Starling Curve. Previously, placement of a pulmonary artery catheter was used to measure the pulmonary capillary occlusion (wedge) pressure. This number was used as an approximation of left atrial pressure, which in turn was an indirect measurement of left ventricular end-diastolic pressure and volume. **Left-ventricular end-diastolic volume is considered the best clinical estimate of preload.** However in recent years, the invasive nature of PA catheters has raised concern about their placement. Clinical practice varies, but in general has shifted towards the use of central venous catheters recording central venous pressure (CVP) to estimate volume status. Even more recently, ultrasound has been used to assess intravascular volume status by examining the respiratory variation of the inferior vena cava (more variation signifying low intravascular volume), or by calculation a ratio of the diameter of the IVC to the aorta. The adoption of these techniques is highly institution-specific.

Management of Hemorrhagic Shock

Resuscitation The **most common and easily available fluid replacements are isotonic crystalloid solutions** such as normal saline or lactated Ringer solution. For each liter of these solutions that is infused, approximately 300 mL stays in the intravascular space while the remainder leaks into the interstitial space. This distribution has led to the guideline of **3 mL crystalloid replacement for each 1 mL of blood loss.** A blood transfusion is indicated if the patient persists in shock despite the rapid infusion of 2 to 3 L of crystalloid solution, or if the patient has had such severe blood loss that cardiovascular collapse is imminent. When possible, typed and cross-matched blood is optimal; however, in the acute setting, this is often unfeasible. Type-specific unmatched blood is the next best option, followed by O-negative blood in females and O-positive blood in males. Blood is generally administered as packed erythrocytes or packed red blood cells (PRBCs). Crystalloids, fresh-frozen plasma (FFP), and/or platelets may need to be transfused if massive blood volumes have been given. Transfusion protocols differ by institution regarding the ratio of FFP to platelets to PRBCs that should be administered. Colloid solutions such as albumin and hetastarch or dextran are not superior to crystalloid replacement in the acute setting and have the potential for large fluid shifts and pulmonary or bowel wall edema. Hypertonic solutions such as 7.5% saline have the advantage of retaining as much as 500 mL in the intravascular space and may be useful in trauma situations with no access to blood products, such as in military settings.

The concept of permissive hypotension is now more widely accepted in trauma care. The central tenet is that patients suffering from hemorrhagic shock (excluding intracranial hemorrhages) may benefit from judicious fluid administration. In permissive hypotension, the patient's blood pressure is not resuscitated to their normal blood pressure, or to what physicians consider a normal blood pressure. Instead, the blood pressure is allowed to remain low (mean arterial pressures of 60-70 mm Hg or a systolic blood pressure of 80-90 mm Hg). Permissive hypotension is thought to be effective in hemorrhagic shock because it is thought that post-hemorrhage, the artificially increased blood pressure by aggressive fluid resuscitation may disrupt endogenous clot formation and promote further bleeding. Also, crystalloid is often administered at room temperature, which is actually colder than the body temperature and can result in hypothermia following excessive administration. Crystalloid can also dilute the endogenous clotting factors and erythrocyte concentration, resulting in poorer control of bleeding and also diminished oxygen carrying capacity. Though shown to have great benefits in animal models, human studies of permissive hypotension are few. However, this concept is becoming more accepted in trauma centers. Patients in whom permissive hypotension should not be practiced are: patients with traumatic brain injuries who require maintenance of their cerebral perfusion pressure; patients with a history of hypertension, congestive heart failure, or coronary artery disease, in whom hypotension will be poorly tolerated and may produce other medical problems such as strokes or myocardial infarctions.

Controlling Hemorrhage Achieving hemostasis is paramount in managing the trauma patient with hemorrhagic shock. Wounds amenable to local tamponade with direct pressure, dressings, or tourniquet application should be managed as such. For other injuries that require operative repair, such as intra-abdominal injuries, or for pelvic fractures that require advanced therapies such as interventional radiology (IR)–guided embolization, the appropriate specialists should be contacted immediately.

While contacting and arranging for further definitive care, appropriate resuscitation of the patient should be initiated.

COMPREHENSION QUESTIONS

7.1 A 32-year-old man was involved in a knife fight and had stab injuries to his abdomen, although it is unclear how deep these injuries are. He is brought into the emergency room with a heart rate of 110 beats per minute and blood pressure of 84/50 mm Hg. Based on the clinical assessment, which of the following is the amount of acute blood loss he has experienced?

A. 250 mL

B. 500 mL

C. 1000 mL

D. 1500 mL

7.2 Which of the following is an advantage of the FAST examination in a patient with hemorrhagic shock?

A. Can identify retroperitoneal hematomas

B. Can be performed quickly at bedside

C. Can identify the specific site of injury

D. Can quantify the exact amount of blood loss

7.3 A 20-year-old man involved in a motor vehicle accident is brought into the emergency room having lost much blood at the accident scene. His initial blood pressure is 80/40 mm Hg and heart rate 130 beats per minute. He is given 3 L of normal saline intravenously and is still hypotensive. Which of these statements most accurately describes the pathophysiology of his condition?

A. Insufficient cardiac preload

B. Insufficient myocardial contractility

C. Excessive systemic vascular resistance

D. Excessive IL-6 and leukotrienes

7.4 A 35-year-old man has been involved in a motor vehicle accident, and is found to be hypotensive. Which of the following locations of bleeding can cause significant complications but does not explain the hypotension?

A. Chest and abdomen

B. Pelvic girdle and soft-tissue compartments

C. External bleeding

D. Intracranial bleeding

ANSWERS

7.1 **D.** Blood pressure at rest typically does not decrease until class III hemorrhagic shock, when 1500 to 2000 mL of blood is lost (30%-40% of blood volume). Class I hemorrhagic shock is well compensated associated with 750 mL EBL or less, with no effect on blood pressure and minimal effect on heart rate. Class II shock, associated with 750 to 1500 mL EBL, is associated with tachycardia but normal blood pressure at rest, and low urine output.

7.2 **B.** DPL and FAST cannot rule out retroperitoneal injury or identify the specific site of injury, but they can be performed quickly at bedside on unstable trauma patients. To find the specific site of injury and rule out retroperitoneal injury, a CT scan can be done; however, the trauma patient must be hemodynamically stable to be transported to the CT scan suite.

7.3 **A.** In situations of trauma and hemorrhage, persistent hypotension is caused by blood loss unless otherwise proven. Hypotension is caused by lack of preload. Preload is end-diastolic sarcomere length, and insufficient circulating volume does not allow for sufficient venous return or cardiac output.

7.4 **D.** It is important to systematically check for bleeding sources in the chest, abdomen, pelvic girdle, soft-tissue compartments (long-bone fractures), and external bleeding. Intracranial bleeding, although a significant injury, is usually not the cause of hypotension. The exception to this is the patient who is moribund secondary to a head injury.

CLINICAL PEARLS

▶ Evaluation of a trauma patient begins with assessment and stabilization of the ABCs.

▶ Hypotension in a trauma patient is hemorrhage until proven otherwise.

▶ A trauma patient should be assessed systematically for the source of hemorrhage.

▶ Laboratory evaluation is not as sensitive as the combination of history, clinical examination, physical examination findings, and vital sign abnormalities for the diagnosis of hemorrhagic shock.

▶ Therapy must be initiated promptly with fluid and/or blood product administration.

▶ Definitive therapy for control of hemorrhage should be arranged as soon as possible.

REFERENCES

Holcroft JW. Shock—approach to the treatment of shock. In: Wilmore DW, Cheung LY, Harken AH, et al, eds. *ACS Surgery.* New York, NY: Webmed Professional Publishers; 2003:61-74.

Mullins RJ. Management of shock. In: Mattox KL, Feliciano DV, Moore EE, eds. *Trauma.* New York, NY: McGraw-Hill; 1999:195-234.

Rossaint R, Bouillon B, Cerny V, et al. Management of bleeding following major trauma: an updated European guideline. *Crit Care* Med. (London, England). 2010;14:R52.

Spahn DR, Cerny V, Coats TJ, et al. Management of bleeding following major trauma: a European guideline. *Crit Care.* 2007;11(1):R17.

Wilson M, Davis DP, Coimbra R. Diagnosis and monitoring of hemorrhagic shock during the initial resuscitation of multiple trauma patients: a review. *J Emerg Med.* 2003;24(4):413-422.

An intoxicated 25-year-old man was brought to the emergency department (ED) by paramedics after he was involved in an altercation and sustained several stab wounds to the torso and upper extremities. His initial vital signs in the ED showed pulse rate of 100 beats per minute, blood pressure of 112/80 mm Hg, respiratory rate of 20 breaths per minute, and Glasgow coma scale of 13. A 2-cm stab wound is noted over the left anterior chest just below the left nipple. Additionally, there is a 2-cm wound adjacent to the umbilicus, and several 1- to 2-cm stab wounds are noted in right arm and forearm, near the antecubital fossa. The abdominal and chest wounds are not actively bleeding and there is no apparent hematoma associated with these wounds. However, one of the wounds in the right arm is associated with a 10-cm hematoma that is actively oozing.

▶ What are the next steps in the evaluation of this patient?
▶ What are the complications associated with these injuries?

ANSWERS TO CASE 8:

Penetrating Trauma to the Chest, Abdomen, and Extremities

Summary: A 25-year-old hemodynamically stable, intoxicated man presents with stab wounds to the chest, abdomen, and upper extremities.

- **Next step:** Assess ABCDE: airway, breathing, circulation, disability, and exposure. After completing this survey, consider probing knife wounds (except chest wounds) to see whether they are superficial or deep.

- **Potential complications from injuries:**

  - Chest wound: Pericardial effusion/tamponade, pneumothorax, hemothorax, diaphragmatic injury

  - Abdominal wound: Hollow viscus, vascular, or urinary tract injury

  - Extremities: Vascular, nerve, or tendon injury

ANALYSIS

Objectives

1. Be able to classify penetrating injuries by location, including chest, thoracoabdominal region, abdomen, flank, back, and "cardiac box."

2. Learn the priorities involved in the initial management of penetrating injuries.

3. Become familiar with the treatments of penetrating truncal and extremity injuries.

Considerations

A systematic approach must be undertaken in the evaluation of this patient. **The clinician must guard against being distracted by injuries not immediately threatening to loss of life or limb.** Likewise, young healthy individuals, particularly those who are intoxicated, may have significant injuries and not manifest many physical examination findings or hemodynamic changes. Advanced trauma life support (ATLS) guidelines stress the initial primary survey to identify and address potentially life-threatening injuries. The primary survey consists of the **ABCDEs (airway, breathing, circulation, disability, and exposure).** Exposure (removing all of the patient's clothing and rolling the patient to examine the patient's backside) is particularly important in a patient with penetrating trauma because puncture wounds may be hidden in axillary, inguinal, and gluteal folds.

Following the primary survey, preliminary labs, plain x-rays, and a bedside ultrasound should be obtained as clinically indicated. In this case, an upright chest x-ray (CXR), preferably at end expiration will be needed to assess for pneumothorax and hemothorax. A focused abdominal sonogram for trauma (FAST) examination should be performed to evaluate for pericardial and intraperitoneal free fluid. This patient is hemodynamically stable and possesses minimal abdominal examination findings. Therefore, a reasonable strategy is to perform local wound exploration to determine the depth of the puncture wound. A wound that does not penetrate the abdominal fascia may be irrigated and closed without further diagnostic requirement. However, it is important to note that in an intoxicated patient, the physical examination may not be very sensitive.

APPROACH TO:
Penetrating Trauma

DEFINITIONS

CHEST: Area from clavicles to costal margins, 360 degrees around.

"CARDIAC BOX": Anatomical region bordered by the clavicles superiorly, bilateral midclavicular lines laterally, and the costal margins inferiorly. This box includes the epigastric region between the costal margins. Eighty-five percent of penetrating cardiac stab wounds originate from a puncture to the "box."

THORACOABDOMINAL: Area from the inframammary crease (women) or nipples (men), down to the costal margins, 360 degrees around. The clinical significance of a penetrating wound to this region is that there is a risk of injury to the intrathoracic and intra-abdominal contents, as well as to the diaphragm.

ANTERIOR ABDOMEN: Area bordered by the costal margins superiorly, the bilateral midaxillary lines laterally, and by the inguinal ligaments inferiorly.

FLANK: Area from the coastal margin down to the iliac crest, and between the anterior and posterior axillary lines.

BACK: Area between the posterior axillary lines. Because of thick musculature over the back, only about 5% of stab wounds to the back lead to significant injuries.

CLINICAL APPROACH

Initial Management

The primary survey, or ABCDEs, should be addressed first (see Table I–2 in Section I). The clinician should not be distracted by eye-catching but not immediately life-threatening injuries. In an unstable patient, treatment decisions often need to be made before obtaining diagnostic tests. For example, a patient with a stab wound to the chest and rapidly dropping oxygen saturations will require tube thoracostomy ("B" breathing) prior to confirmatory CXR. Bleeding, even if profuse, is most effectively controlled by direct hand pressure to the bleeding site. Gauze and pressure dressings are generally less effective. All patients should have immediate placement of large-bore IV access at two sites. Volume repletion should be initiated with warm IV fluids. After completion of the primary survey, a systematic search for other injuries (secondary survey) should be undertaken. Diagnostic tests should be performed expeditiously after the primary survey and often concurrent with the secondary survey (Table 8–1).

Table 8–1 • IDENTIFICATION OF INJURIES			
Location	Complications	Signs and Symptoms	Further Studies/ Interventions
Chest	Pericardial effusion/ tamponade Pneumothorax or hemothorax	Distant heart sounds, hypotension, JVD Decreased breath sounds, low oxygen saturation, hypotension	CXR may detect air or fluid in the pleural cavity. FAST is sensitive in detecting fluid within the pericardial sac ED ultrasound is useful in detecting an occult pneumothorax Chest tube thoracostomy may yield a rush of air or blood
Abdomen or pelvis	Hollow viscus injury Liver laceration Splenic laceration Vascular injury	Peritonitis Shock (hypotension, altered mental status) Bowel evisceration	Local wound exploration CT scan may reveal path of injury and grading of solid organ injuries Angiography may be useful for both diagnosis and treatment FAST—free intraperitoneal fluid Exploratory laparotomy Diagnostic laparoscopy
Back/flank	Retroperitoneal hematoma Urinary tract injury	Hematuria Hypotension	CT is the best diagnostic tool for evaluating retroperitoneal bleeding CT with delayed imaging and intravenous pyelography
Extremities	Vascular injury Nerve damage Tendon disruption	6 Ps (pain, pulselessness, poikilothermia, paresthesias, pallor, paralysis)	Ankle-brachial indexes (ABIs) CT angiography Angiography Wound exploration in the OR

In general, gunshot wounds are more likely to cause greater tissue destruction and life-threatening injuries than stab wounds. This is due to the unpredictable path of the bullet which can lead to significant tissue destruction. Hence, it is not safe to assume that a bullet has taken a direct path between the entrance and exit wounds.

The management of patients with penetrating injuries has undergone significant evolution over the past two decades. During the 1980s and 1990s, most patients underwent invasive diagnostic evaluations, including exploratory laparotomy and angiography based solely on mechanism and location. Currently, selective treatment for some penetrating injuries is acceptable. Selective treatment may involve close observation, and additional minimally invasive diagnostic studies such as ultrasonography, laparoscopy, and thoracoscopy. This option has led to a significant reduction in unnecessary operations. However, selective treatment must be tailored to the clinical situation and balanced against the risk of delay to diagnosis and definitive operative intervention. The decision to proceed with selective treatment is best determined by a qualified surgeon, after the initial evaluation.

Specific Anatomical Regions

Chest Injuries Generally, 10% to 15% of patients with penetrating chest trauma require urgent operative intervention. Fortunately the majority of these patients can be identified within the first minutes by initial hemodynamic instability, the presence of a large hemothorax on CXR, or high chest tube output. The remaining 85% to 90% of patients may require only close observation, diagnostic imaging, and tube thoracostomy.

The upright **chest x-ray (CXR)** has adequate sensitivity to evaluate for pneumothorax and hemothorax. Obtaining an end-expiratory film may increase the likelihood of detecting a small pneumothorax. In a patient with a high risk mechanism, the absence of a pneumothorax should be confirmed by a repeat upright CXR in 4 to 6 hours or by computed tomography (CT). CT of the chest is highly sensitive for the detection of pneumothorax. A small pneumothorax visualized by CT and missed by CXR is referred to as an "occult pneumothorax." An occult pneumothorax should be reevaluated for progression in 4 to 6 hours by CXR.

Local wound exploration of a chest injury is not recommended because the procedure itself can penetrate the pleura and cause a pneumothorax. Pneumo- or hemothorax found by CXR is treated by placement of a 36- or 40-French chest tube. Smaller tubes clot easily with blood and are not indicated in the setting of trauma. If the pneumo- or hemothorax does not resolve with one chest tube, then a second chest tube should be placed. There has not been a consensus on the size of traumatic pneumothorax that warrants tube thoracostomy, although recent literature has shown a push towards more invasive procedures especially when the pneumothorax is 20% or greater. However, if the injury requires mechanical ventilation then a chest tube should be placed, regardless of size, to prevent a worsening of the pneumothorax or a tension physiology from the positive pressure ventilation. **The best initial treatment of a tension pneumothorax** is **needle decompression** followed immediately by the placement of a chest tube. Considerations for operative thoracotomy include initial output of 1500 mL of blood, or 200 mL/h over the next 4 hours.

Any patient with an injury within the cardiac box should undergo prompt **FAST** examination of the heart by an experienced sonographer. The subxiphoid view may be complemented by a parasternal view. The experienced sonographer can detect pericardial blood with up to 100 percent sensitivity (Figure 8–1). Hemopericardium is an indication for pericardial exploration in the operating room.

Resuscitative (or so-called emergency department) thoracotomy is reserved for patients who are *in extremis* or who have **lost vital signs in the ED or within a few minutes prior to arrival.** This procedure is associated with a great deal of controversy. The practitioner must bear in mind that mortality exceeds 97%. In addition, this intervention may expose healthcare providers to unnecessary accidental injury and infectious agents. The best outcomes occur when this procedure is performed in properly selected patients by an experienced physician and in a medical center with the capability to provide definitive treatment.

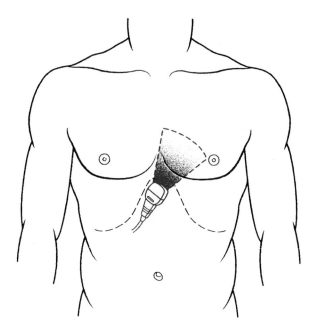

Figure 8–1. FAST examination imaging the subxiphoid region for pericardial fluid.

Thoracoabdominal   Thoracoabdominal wounds are of particular interest because injuries to the diaphragm are difficult to detect. Unless the diaphragmatic defect is large, herniation of stomach or intestines is rarely visualized by CXR in the ED. Moreover, CT is not sensitive enough to detect small diaphragmatic injures. Surgical consultation should be obtained when diaphragmatic injury is suspected because the definitive diagnostic study is surgical evaluation by **laparoscopy or thoracoscopy**. If these injuries go untreated, herniation of intra-abdominal contents into the chest may eventually occur due to the presence of negative intrathoracic pressure.

Anterior Abdomen   Immediate indication for **laparotomy** includes evidence of **shock** (hypotension, tachycardia, cold and clammy skin, or diaphoresis), **peritonitis, gun-shot wound** with a suspected course through the abdominal cavity, or **evisceration** of abdominal contents. In the absence of these findings, further radiographic evaluation or observation is indicated.

Local wound exploration is the best initial evaluation for a stable patient with an abdominal stab wound. This procedure is performed after preparing the skin with an antiseptic agent, creating a sterile field and anesthetizing the skin and soft tissues. The skin laceration is enlarged, and the wound tract is gently followed until either its termination or its violation of the anterior abdominal fascia. An intact fascia makes it highly unlikely that there is an intra-abdominal injury, and therefore the wound may be irrigated and closed.

If the anterior abdominal fascia has been penetrated, then it is critical that a surgeon becomes involved in the patient's care in order to help facilitate observation with serial abdominal examinations or surgical intervention. Historically, **diagnostic peritoneal lavage (DPL) was performed at the bedside to further investigate potential intra-abdominal injuries.** However, DPL has been largely replaced by CT scan or diagnostic laparoscopy in the hemodynamically stable patient and by laparotomy in the unstable patient.

Back/Flank The physical examination, FAST, and DPL are insensitive in diagnosing injuries to the retroperitoneum, including the colon, kidneys, and ureters. The only clue to a retroperitoneal process irritating the psoas muscles may be the patient's need to flex their hips. Hematuria is the most reliable sign of injury to the kidneys, ureters, and bladder. If gross or microscopic hematuria is present or if a high degree of suspicion exists for possible injury, further evaluation is needed. CT with delayed images, intravenous pyelography (**IVP**), and perhaps retrograde cystography are useful imaging modalities. Recent literature suggests that most renal injuries without associated hemodynamic compromise or urinary collection system leaks do not mandate exploration. These patients require hospital admission, bedrest, and serial laboratory studies. Laparotomy may be necessary for high-grade renal lacerations in an unstable patient.

Extremities The six Ps of arterial insufficiency (pain, paralysis, parasthesias, pallor, pulselessness, and poikilothermia) and the hard signs of vascular injury (pulsatile bleeding, expanding hematoma, absent distal pulses, palpable thrill, or audible bruit) should be evaluated. Their presence is an indication for immediate operative or angiographic evaluation. A careful pulse examination should be performed to look for a deficit. If pulses are not palpable, then Doppler can be used to identify arterial flow. Sites of injury should be auscultated for a bruit that can represent a traumatic arteriovenous fistula. Ankle-brachial indexes (ABI) can be a useful measurement for evaluating lower extremity vascular trauma. An ABI value of <0.9 may represent vascular injury and, therefore, warrants further investigation. However, in long-standing diabetics, ABIs are less sensitive due to stiffened diseased vasculature leading to spurious values. Additionally, a motor or sensory deficit can represent nerve or tendon injury that is best evaluated and treated in the operating room.

COMPREHENSION QUESTIONS

8.1 A 23-year-old man is involved in an altercation in the parking lot after a baseball game. He suffers a single stab wound 2-cm medial and superior to the left nipple. His blood pressure is 110/80 mm Hg and heart rate is 80 beats per minute. Which of the following management options is most appropriate for this patient?

A. CXR, wound exploration, and ECG

B. CXR and CT scan of the abdomen

C. CXR and echocardiography

D. CXR, echocardiography, and laparoscopy

8.2 For which of the following patients is CT imaging an appropriate diagnostic option?

A. A 38-year-old man with diffuse abdominal pain, involuntary guarding, and a 6-in knife impaled just below the umbilicus

B. A 22-year-old man with a single stab wound to the back, pulse rate of 118 beats per minute, blood pressure of 94/80 mm Hg, and gross hematuria

C. A 16-year-old adolescent boy with a single stab wound 2 cm above the left inguinal crease, with heart rate of 120 beats per minute and blood pressure of 90/78 mm Hg

D. A hemodynamically stable, 34-year-old woman, who is 26 weeks pregnant and has a single stab wound to the back and no other abnormalities on physical examination

8.3 A 34-year-old man is brought into the emergency department after a motor vehicle accident. He complains of dyspnea and initially had an oxygen saturation of 88%. On examination, he has decreased breath sounds of the right chest and now has an oxygen saturation of 70% on room air. Which of the following is the most appropriate next step?

A. Chest radiograph

B. CT of the chest

C. Tube thoracostomy

D. Heparin anticoagulation

ANSWERS

8.1 **C.** CXR is sensitive in identifying hemothorax and pneumothorax, while echocardiography is useful in identifying pericardial fluid. Wound exploration of the chest wound is not recommended because the information gained is limited and the procedure is associated with the potential of producing pneumothorax. An ECG provides limited information regarding cardiac injury and is generally not done. A stab wound above the nipple line is rarely associated with intraabdominal injury, therefore, CT scan of the abdomen or diagnostic laparoscopy is unnecessary.

8.2 **D.** CT of the abdomen may be useful in identifying injuries to the retroperitoneal structures in a patient with a stab wound to the back. That the patient is 26-week pregnant does not contraindicate CT scan. Further diagnostic study would not be beneficial in patients listed in choices A, B, and C because these patients are exhibiting signs of significant injury that would necessitate urgent exploratory laparotomy.

8.3 **C.** The constellation of clinical signs points toward a pneumothorax. The presence of significant hypoxia requires immediate placement of a chest tube prior to chest radiograph confirmation as further delay may progress to cardiovascular collapse.

CLINICAL PEARLS

▶ The systematic approach to the trauma patient is ABCDE (airway, breathing, circulation, disability, exposure).

▶ A wound that does not penetrate the abdominal fascia may be irrigated and closed without further diagnostic studies.

▶ Penetrating trauma to the chest below the nipple line may cause thoracic, intra-abdominal, and occult diaphragmatic injuries.

▶ The FAST (focused abdominal sonogram for trauma) is fairly accurate in assessing intraperitoneal free fluid.

▶ Approximately 85% of penetrating cardiac stab wounds originate from a puncture to the "cardiac box."

REFERENCES

Cameron JL, ed. *Current Surgical Therapy.* 7th ed. St. Louis, MO: Mosby; 2001.

Townsend CM, Beauchamp RD, Evers BM, Mattox KL, eds. *Sabiston Textbook of Surgery.* 16th ed. Philadelphia, PA: W.B. Saunders; 2001.

Trunkey DD, Lewis FR, eds. *Current Therapy of Trauma.* 4th ed. St. Louis, MO: Mosby; 1999.

A 26-year-old waiter was serving food at a social function when he tripped and fell down a flight of stairs. He did not lose consciousness following the event but complains of severe neck pain and right wrist and hand pain. He was placed in a C-collar and transported by EMS to the emergency department (ED) with appropriate C-spine precautions. His vital signs and cardiopulmonary examinations are within normal limits, Glasgow coma scale (GCS) is 15, and he is able to move all extremities. Palpation of his neck reveals tenderness at the midline, and his right distal forearm/wrist/hand is swollen and exquisitely tender to touch.

▶ What are the appropriate steps in the evaluation of his neck pain?
▶ What are the important elements in the evaluation of his right upper extremity?

ANSWERS TO CASE 9:
Extremity Fracture and Neck Pain

Summary: A young man tripped and fell down some stairs and now complains of neck and right upper extremity pain. His history and presentation are concerning for cervical spine and right upper extremity injuries.

- **Evaluation of neck pain:** Obtain computed tomography (CT) of the cervical spine. If the CT does not demonstrate any bony fractures or dislocation and his midline tenderness persists, then obtain flexion/extension x-rays or MRI of the C-spine to help differentiate ligamentous injury/spinal instability from soft tissue contusion.

- **Evaluations of upper extremity:** Given the soft tissue swelling and the location of pain, physical examination of the affect extremity should include detailed evaluation of the hand, wrist, and forearm, and this should include clinical assessments of tissue perfusion and functionality. Although, vascular injuries are uncommon with this patient's injury mechanism, arterial inflow need to be evaluated based on capillary refill and presence or absence of pulses. If the perfusion status is in doubt, Doppler evaluation of pulse quality and pressures should be obtained. X-rays of the humerus, radius, ulna, wrist, and hand should be obtained to assess for possible bone injuries.

ANALYSIS

Objectives

1. Learn the common cervical spine injuries associated with the various injury mechanisms.

2. Learn the decision rules that guide the use of cervical spine radiography in trauma patients.

3. Learn the current role of corticosteroids in patients with spinal cord injuries.

4. Learn the emergency department management of elbow, forearm, wrist, and hand injuries.

Considerations

The neck pain associated with midline tenderness on palpation in this patient raises the concern for C-spine injury; therefore, radiographic evaluations must be obtained for further assessment. Either three views of the C-spine (AP, lateral, and odontoid views) or CT can be performed. CT is preferable over three views as the preferred diagnostic study in many centers because it is associated with much lower rates of false-negative examinations than plain radiography. CT would be especially helpful in this patient who exhibits concerning symptoms and physical findings. If the neck pain and midline C-spine tenderness persist despite negative CT, additional imaging to determine C-spine stability or to identify ligamentous injuries should be obtained. C-spine precautions should be maintained until the possibility of unstable injury can be eliminated based on imaging. Only when imaging studies indicate the absence of flexion/extension instability or the absence of ligamentous injuries can the patient be assumed to have neck pain related to soft tissue injuries only.

This patient also exhibit findings in the right distal forearm/wrist/hand that suggest the possibility of bony injuries. The initial evaluation should be directed toward evaluations of hand and digits functions; namely, motor/sensory functions and ligamentous integrity. Careful palpation of the hand, wrist, and forearm should also be performed to localize areas of concern for bony injuries. Two-view radiographs should be obtained to assess the bony integrity of the humerus, radius, ulna, carpal bones, and phalanges. When identified, fractures and dislocations should be reduced to minimize neurovascular compromises. Further assessments and management of all bony, ligamentous injuries and functional abnormalities should be discussed with an orthopedic or hand specialist.

APPROACH TO:

Cervical Spine and Upper Extremity Orthopedic Injuries

DEFINITIONS

NEXUS LOW-RISK CRITERIA: This C-spine clearance approach was derived based on a 1998 publication by Hoffman et al (*Ann Emerg Med* 1998;32:461-469). The recommendations are that C-spine radiography is indicated for asymptomatic trauma patients unless they meet all of the following criteria: (1) No posterior midline cervical tenderness. (2) No evidence intoxication. (3) Normal level of alertness. (4) No focal neurologic deficits. (5) No painful distracting injuries. The major limitation of this approach is that no precise definition for painful distracting injuries was provided.

THE CANADIAN C-SPINE RULE (CCR): This is a guideline to determine the need for radiographic evaluations of **alert and stable trauma patients.** In comparison to the NEXUS criteria, the CCR has been shown to have slightly greater sensitivity and specificity for identification of patients who do not have C-spine injuries. (See Figure 9–1.)

PARTIAL CORD SYNDROMES: Compression or contusions to the spinal cord can develop with or without concomitant bony injuries. Compression of the **anterior cord** can produce complete motor paralysis, loss of pain and temperature perceptions. **Posterior cord** syndrome (Brown-Sequard) causes paralysis loss of vibratory sensation and proprioception ipsilaterally and loss of pain and temperature sensations contralaterally. **Central cord** syndrome is produced by injuries to the corticospinal tract, which produces great upper extremities weakness in comparison to the lower extremities.

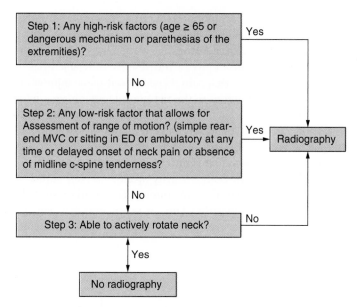

Figure 9-1. Sample algorithm for assessing neck injury.

CLINICAL APPROACH

Millions of adults at risk for cervical spine injuries and/or upper extremity orthopedic injuries are evaluated in emergency departments throughout the United States and Canada every year. Among patients presenting with intact neurological status to the emergency department, the incidence of acute C-spine fracture or spinal injury is less than 1%. Even though spinal injury incidences are low, there are great consequences associated with mismanagement. Similarly, mismanagement of upper extremity injuries can lead to potential employment and functional compromises.

Clearing the C-spine in the Blunt Trauma Patient

The goal of C-spine clearance is to establish that injuries are not present, and based on statistics, probabilities for injuries are low. The approach to patients is based on patient classifications, where individuals are classified as **asymptomatic, temporarily non-assessable, symptomatic,** and **obtunded. Asymptomatic patients** can be approached using the CCR, which has been shown to lead to the reduction in unnecessary radiography and has been demonstrated to be superior in comparison to the NEXUS criteria. For **temporarily non-assessable patients (either due to intoxication or distracting injuries)**, the approach is to assess the patient as an obtunded patient or reassess the individual after treatments of distracted injuries or return of normal mentation. **Symptomatic patients** are recognized by the presence of neck pain, midline tenderness, or neurologic signs and symptoms; symptomatic patients need to be initially evaluated with either 3-view C-spine x-rays or preferably CT; symptomatic patients with negative CT who are suspected of having ligamentous injuries need to be further evaluated with MRI of the C-spine, and if both CT and

MRI are negative, then the patients can be discharged with a collar for comfort; however, if the patient has persistent neck pain after 2 weeks, flexion/extension films are recommended to assess C-spine stability. All symptomatic patients should be evaluated by a spine specialist prior to discharge from the ED. For **obtunded trauma patients** (altered mental status or prolonged intubation or psychiatric disturbances or uncooperative), the initial evaluation is CT of the C-spine. If this is negative, there are two options; one option is to clear the C-spine, and the second option is to perform MRI to rule out ligamentous injuries. The major argument for option one is that isolated ligamentous injuries are rare, and the major argument for option two is that the negative predictive value of CT for ligamentous injuries is only 78%. It should be pointed out that the American College of Radiology recommends that CT and MRI are the most appropriate modalities for C-spine evaluation in the obtunded trauma patient. All obtunded trauma patients should be evaluated by trauma and/or spine specialists.

Emergency Department Management of C-spine Injuries

The initial management of any patient with C-spine injuries is to prioritize the ABCs, as most C-spine injuries do not occur as isolated injuries. Early definitive airways may be required for some patients who develop soft tissue swelling of the neck that lead to airway compromise. Similarly, definitive airway and mechanical ventilation may be required in patients with paralysis or muscle weakness associated with C-spine injuries. Definitive airway management in these patients is best accomplished by in-line C-spine stabilization and orotracheal intubations, following rapid-sequence induction. It is important to bear in mind that most of the respiratory accessory muscles receive their motor innervations from the thoracic level, and the diaphragm receives its innervations from C3-C5; therefore, patients with compromised ventilation secondary to C-spine injuries generally do not exhibit any external signs of respiratory distress, and the most reliable way to detect hypoventilation is by $Paco_2$ measurements on arterial blood gas. Estimation of neurologic deficits can be determined based on physical examinations and radiographic evidence of fracture and/or dislocation. From C1 to C7, nerve root exit above the level of the vertebrae, and from C8 and below, the nerve roots exit below the vertebrae.

If possible, it is always preferable to be able to perform a thorough motor-sensory examination prior to intubation. For patients with spinal cord injuries, it is always preferable to maintain a mean arterial pressure of 85 to 90 mm Hg to maximize spinal cord perfusion. If needed, patients with isolated spinal cord injuries may benefit from initiation of vassopressors such as dopamines or norepinephrine. Bradycardia associated with neurogenic shock can be addressed with atropine.

The priorities for any spinal cord injury patients are to address the life-threatening injuries first followed by management of the limb and quality-of-life threatening injuries.

Role of Corticosteroids for Spinal Cord Injuries

Corticosteroids had been a mainstay of therapy in the early management of spinal cord injury patients; however, more recent publications suggest that high-dose corticosteroids administration had only some benefits for individuals when the treatment was initiated within 3 hours of the injury. Unfortunately, the treatments with high-dose corticosteroids are associated with increased rates of sepsis and other steroid-associated medical complications. In light of these published data, the application of corticosteroids for spinal cord injured patients have been dramatically reduced, and steroids should not be initiated for patients in the emergency department prior to discussions with the trauma and/or spine specialists who will ultimately manage the patient after ED discharge.

Management of Upper Extremity Injuries

Upper extremity injuries are commonly encountered in the ED. Inappropriate diagnosis and management in the ED can lead to chronic pain, and threat to recreational and vocational activities. Orthopedic injuries to the upper extremities are categorized by the bone, location (proximal, midshaft, or distal), presence or absence of joint involvement, degree of angulation, extent of comminution, and whether the fracture is open or closed.

Forearm fractures: Rotation of the forearm is crucial for hand function and activities of daily living. Normally, the radius rotate around the fixed ulna, and the ability of these bones to rotate around each other depends on the shape of the bones and their positions in relationship to each other. Initial evaluations of patients require careful determination of neurovascular status of the extremity followed by x-rays. Injuries that involve only one of the two bones are generally stable and are treated by closed manipulation, cast immobilization under conscious sedation or ultrasound-guided regional nerve blocks. Most displaced, fractures that involve both the ulna and radius are considered unstable fractures and are less amendable to closed fixations; therefore, many of these fractures are managed by open-reduction and internal fixations.

Distal radius fractures: This is one of the most common fractures encountered in children and adults. The bimodal distribution of this injury demonstrates a peak in late childhood (predominantly males) and after the sixth decade of life (predominantly females). The most common mechanism associated with this injury is a ground-level fall with outstretched hand. The **Colles-Pouteau fracture** is a fracture of the distal radial metaphysic with dorsal displacement of the distal fragment, and this represents the most commonly encountered distal radial fracture. In children, distal radius fractures are grouped as metaphyseal and physeal fractures, with the physeal fractures demonstrating involvement of the growth plate and can be further classified by the Salter-Harris classifications. Most of distal radius fractures in children are treated by closed reduction and cast fixation. The goals of a management in adults are to restore bone alignment and avoid shortening of the radius. The decision to treat patients by closed reduction and fixation versus operative reduction and fixation are determined by the degree of alignment, age, and functional status of the patients. Common complications associated with these injuries are malunion, nerve injury, tendon injury, stiffness, and chronic pain.

Carpal bone fractures: There are eight carpal bones in the hand. Carpal bones in general have limited blood supply and are susceptible to avascular necrosis following injuries. Often, details of fractures and/or dislocations of the carpal bones are difficult to visualize by plain radiography, therefore CTs or MRIs are sometimes used to determine the location and extent of injuries. Most displaced fractures are managed by operative reduction and fixation. Some of the stable, non-displaced carpal fractures can be initially approach with cast fixation. The management of any carpal injuries should be discussed with an orthopedic or hand specialist.

Metacarpal and phalangeal fractures: These fractures can be sometimes over-looked especially in a patient with multisystem injuries. The failure to identify and treat these injuries could lead to potential finger misalignement, pain, and functional loss. The goals of management of metacarpal fractures are to preserve bone length, rotational functions, and articular functions, which can be accomplished by either immobilization or internal fixation. The goals of managing phalangeal fractures are to minimize angulation and rotational deformities. Functional recoveries in most cases require patients' participation in rehabilitation programs. Early involvement of a hand or orthopedic specialist is vital in the management of these patients.

COMPREHENSION QUESTIONS

9.1 A 78-year-old man is brought to the emergency center from an extended care facility. The patient reportedly was found to have fallen down in the bath room. He has contusions over his face and is confused. According to reports by his caretakers, this is his baseline mental status. How would you clear his C-spine?

A. Palpation of his C-spine for tenderness, if not tender than ask him to turn his head and if no pain is reported, the C-spine is cleared.

B. Keep him in C-spine precaution and reexamine him later when his mental status is improved.

C. Obtain CT, MRI, if these are negative, obtain flexion/extension films.

D. CT of the C-spine.

E. Remove the collar if he denies neck pain.

9.2 Which of the following approaches is most appropriate for the clearance of the C-spine in a 25-year-old man who the driver of a car struck from behind? He is hemodynamically stable, nonintoxicated, and has a GCS of 15.

A. NEXUS criteria

B. Canadian C-spine rule

C. CT of the C-spine

D. 3-view x-ray of the C-spine

E. Remove the collar because he does not have any pain

9.3 Which of the following is the most appropriate next step in the management of a 22-year-old man with C5 fracture and C5-C6 subluxation, absence of motor or sensory functions below the C4 level, heart rate of 45, and BP 100/60?

A. Maintain mean arterial pressure >85 to 90 mm Hg

B. Surgical airway

C. Orotracheal intubation with rapid sequence induction

D. Blind nasotracheal intubation

E. Administer atropine 1mg intravenously

9.4 Which of the following patient's presentation is most compatible with the Brown-Sequard syndrome?

A. A 20-year-old man with absence of all motor/sensory functions in all extremities

B. A 20-year-old man with greater weakness in the upper extremities than the lower extremities

C. A 20-year-old man with complete motor paralysis, loss of vibratory sensation and proprioception on the ipsilateral side, and contralateral loss of pain and temperature sensation.

D. A 20-year-old man with fracture/dislocation of C5-C6 and intact motor/sensory functions throughout

E. A 20-year-old man with normal CT of the C-spine and motor and sensory deficits below the C6 level

ANSWERS

9.1 **D.** For this patient with chronic altered mental status due to underlying medical conditions; therefore, the approach to clear his C-spine is one directed toward obtunded patients. His C-spine can be cleared based on a normal CT of the C-spine alone, which is sufficient to identify greater than 99% of all vertebral bony fractures/dislocations. An MRI can be added to identify the rare instances of isolated ligamentous injuries if the CT is normal. There is no consensus on whether MRI is indicated in this setting.

9.2 **B.** The Canadian C-spine rule (CCR) is an approach developed for the clearance of C-spines in asymptomatic patients following low mechanism events. The CCR has been compared to the NEXUS criteria and found to be more specific and sensitive in clearance of the C-spine.

9.3 **C.** This patient has signs consistent with neurogenic shock following a high spinal cord injury. The first concerns are his airway and ventilation. The airway appears to be clear but he needs a definitive airway to maintain optimal ventilation. Orotracheal intubation with rapid sequence induction and in-line C-spine stabilization is the optimal airway strategy for this patient. Maintenance of adequate pulse and blood pressure are important to maintain spinal cord perfusion, but these steps should be delayed until a secured airway is established.

9.4 **C.** The Brown-Sequard syndrome is caused by posterior spinal cord injury, characterized by paralysis, loss of vibratory sensation and proprioception on the ipsilateral side, and loss of pain and temperature sensation on the contralateral side. Patient described in A is compatible with complete cord injury. The patient described in B is compatible with central cord injury. The patient in D appears to have vertebral fractures/dislocation without neurologic compromises. The patient in E has a spinal cord injury without radiographic abnormality (SCIWORA); SCIWORAs occur more commonly in children than adults.

CLINICAL PEARLS

► The Canadian C-spine rule is an effective evaluation system to clinically clear C-spines in asymptomatic patients.

► Cervical spine injuries occur in 1% to 3% of all victims following blunt trauma.

► Distal radius fractures have a bimodal pattern with peaks in late childhood and after the sixth decade of life.

REFERENCES

Abraham MK, Scott S. The emergent evaluation and treatment of hand and wrist injuries. *Emerg Med Clin N Am*. 2010;28:789-809.

Anderson PA, Gugala Z, Lindsey RW, et al. Clearing the cervical spine in the blunt trauma patient. *J Am Acad Orthop Surg*. 2010;18:149-159.

Heggeness MH, Gannon FH, Weinberg J, et al. Orthopedic Surgery. In: Brunicardi FC, Andersen DK, Billiar TR, et al, eds. *Schwartz's Principles of Surgery*. 9th ed. New York, NY: McGraw-Hill; 2010:1557-1608.

Lifchez SD, Sen SK. Surgery of the hand and wrist. In: Brunicardi FC, Andersen DK, Billiar TR, et al, eds. *Schwartz's Principles of Surgery*. 9th ed. New York, NY: McGraw-Hill; 2010:1609-1645.

Pimentel L, Diegelmann L. Evaluation and management of acute cervical spine trauma. *Emerg Med Clin N Am*. 2010; 28:719-738.

A 35-year-old woman is brought to the emergency department (ED) by ambulance after collapsing at home. She had been seen by her regular doctor earlier in the day and prescribed amoxillin for sinusitis. Paramedics report field vital signs remarkable for a blood pressure of 70/30 mm Hg, heart rate of 140 beats per minute, respiratory rate of 40 breaths per minute, and an oxygen saturation of 76%. Intravenous fluids and oxygen were administered during transport. Paramedics are assisting the patient's breathing with bag-valve mask ventilation, but oxygen saturations remains low. On physical examination, the patient is obtunded with perioral cyanosis, tongue swelling, stidor, wheezing, and labored breathing. Her skin is cool and clammy with large urticarial lesions.

▶ What are the next steps?
▶ What treatments should be instituted?

ANSWERS TO CASE 10:

Anaphylaxis

Summary: This patient is demonstrating signs and symptoms of anaphylaxis. Anaphylaxis is rapidly progressive severe allergic reaction which compromises a patient's airway, breathing, and circulation. Patients may also exhibit flushing, hives, and swelling of mucous membranes. Successful treatment of anaphylaxis requires early recognition of the symptoms of anaphylaxis, support of the airway, and administration of epinephrine.

- **Next step:** In the presence of symptoms meeting the diagnostic criteria for anaphylaxis, epinephrine should be administered immediately. The first dose should be administered intramuscularly. In the setting of a severe reaction like the one described above, moving quickly to intravenous infusion of epinephrine is recommended.

- **Further treatments:** This patient requires rapid resuscitation and stabilization. Airway, breathing, and circulation (ABCs) should be managed appropriately and in that order, which will mean both procedural and pharmacological intervention. A **definitive airway** will need to be immediately established in the face of impending airway obstruction (see Case 1), and the patient's cardiovascular compromise must be supported with epinephrine. Experts have referred to the ABCs of anaphylaxis as A E B C; the E is for epinephrine.

In addition to airway management and early administration of epinephrine, pharmacologic therapy is tailored to the other systemic manifestations of the anaphylactic response. These include volume resuscitation with crystalloid, nebulized beta agonists, nebulized racemic epinephrine, corticosteroids, antihistamines (including H_2 blockers), and removal of any remaining antigen (ie, the bee stinger).

ANALYSIS

Objectives

1. Rapidly recognize the characteristic clinical features of anaphylaxis.

2. Understand the underlying pathophysiology of anaphylaxis.

3. Become familiar with the available treatment options; most importantly the correct administration of epinephrine.

Considerations

This patient is brought into the ED with swelling of the tongue and labored breathing. The perioral cyanosis, diffuse wheezing, stridor, and hypoxia all indicate **impending respiratory failure.** A delay of even a minute may be life-threatening. The most important intervention in addition to administration of epinephrine is **securing an airway.** This patient likely has edema of the pharynx and larynx making intubation technically difficult. Airway management in a patient like this often requires a **cricothyroidotomy**.

Intravenous access with administration of **epinephrine** is the most important pharmacologic intervention. Epinephrine should first be given intramuscularly; if that route fails, an intravenous drip should be initiated. Dosing of epinephrine will be covered below. Identification of the inciting agent is not essential for treatment of anaphylaxis, but is helpful in preventing further exposures and recurrence of symptoms.

APPROACH TO:
Anaphylaxis

CLINICAL APPROACH

Epidemiology

Millions of people present to emergency departments every year complaining of allergic symptoms ranging from the minor rashes to multisystem anaphylaxis. Most of the time, it is difficult if not impossible to identify the trigger. Many reactions may occur in response to medical therapies such as antibiotics and radiologic contrast agents. Because the spectrum of allergic responses is so broad, anaphylaxis is likely underreported. As a result it is difficult to calculate a precise incidence of this disease. There are an estimated 30,000 ED visits every year for adverse food reactions. However, there are far more visits for more vague complaints and unknown exposures that may be difficult to identify as anaphylaxis. In the emergency department the goal is rapid diagnosis, symptomatic treatment, and prevention of further episodes.

Pathophysiology

True anaphylaxis is a **type 1 hypersensitivity** reaction occurring after a previous sensitizing exposure. In its purest form, this is an immune-mediated **activation of basophils and mast cells with subsequent release of prostaglandins, leukotrienes**, and **histamine**. From a clinical standpoint, an anaphylactoid reaction also includes release of these compounds but through non–immune-mediated pathways. The only clinical significance of this difference is that anaphylactoid reactions can occur without prior sensitization. Regardless of the underlying mechanism, their effects are similar, and early recognition will determine successful clinical management in these patients (see Table 10–1 for pitfalls).

When first exposed to a substance, binding antibodies trigger class switching and regulatory changes in gene expression, effectively priming the immune system for its next encounter with the offending agent. In certain cases, this leads to **immunoglobulin (igE) binding mast cells and basophils**. In the classically defined anaphylactic reaction, the antigen again encounters the immune system, binds to the IgE on the mast cells and basophils, and releases a flood of cytokines that set the clinical response in motion. In an anaphylactoid reaction, the antigen causes direct release

Table 10–1 • PITFALLS IN ANAPHYLAXIS
Failure to recognize the symptoms of anaphylaxis
Underestimating the severity of laryngeal edema and failure to secure the airway early
Reluctance to administer epinephrine early in the course of illness
Forgetting to remove the allergen; eg, the IV drip of penicillin or bee stinger
Lack of appropriate patient education
Failure to prescribe an epinephrine auto-injector prior to discharge

of cytokines by mast cells and basophils, without need for prior sensitization. In both cases, the end result is the same, and clinically indistinguishable.

The early stages of some anaphylactic reactions involve increased secretion by mucous membranes. In addition to **watery eyes and rhinorrhea, increased bronchial secretions and increased smooth muscle tone cause wheezing** and increase the work of breathing. Decreased vascular tone and **increased capillary permeability** lead to **cardiovascular compromise and hypotension.** Patients may lose over 30% of their blood volume to extravasation in the first ten minutes of their allergic reaction. Other cytokines, specifically histamine, can cause **urticaria and angioedema.** There are numerous cytokines involved in the immunologic cascade following exposure, but no one major substance is felt to be primarily responsible. Leukotriene C_4, prostaglandin D_2, histamine, and tryptase are known key components in the reaction. Elevated tryptase levels confirm the diagnosis.

Causes

Some of the most common causes of anaphylaxis are healthcare related, most notoriously allergies to penicillin and sulfa-containing medications. Some studies suggest as many as 1 in 500 exposures to penicillin will result in anaphylaxis. Radiographic intravenous contrast agents can also cause anaphylaxis. This reaction is not IgE mediated, and is more common in patients receiving the less-expensive hyperosmolar agents. Overall, there are an estimated 0.9 fatal reactions per 100,000 patients exposed to intravenous contrast. This number skyrockets to 60% in patients who have had a prior exposure and reaction.

Hymenoptera, or bee and wasp, stings are another cause of anaphylaxis. Anaphylaxis from stings results in an average of 50 deaths per year in the United States. Overall, the number of cases of arthropod anaphylaxis seen by physicians is small compared to the number of iatrogenic cases, but because exposures often occur miles from medical treatment, they can have serious outcomes.

Food sources round out the major causes of serious allergic reactions. **Peanuts** are easily the **most common cause of serious allergies,** but any food can be responsible. Other common food allergens include eggs and shellfish.

Diagnosis

The diagnosis of anaphylaxis is made clinically. The most commonly affected system is the skin, which manifests with **angioedema, urticaria, erythema, and pruritus** in at least 80% of patients with anaphylaxis. The cardiovascular system is also affected, primarily as a result of decrease vasomotor tone and capillary leakage.

This leads to **hypotension and tachycardia.** Respiratory compromise is common. **Bronchospasm and bronchorrhea** in the lower respiratory tract in combination with edema of the upper respiratory tract are the most feared and difficult to manage aspects of anaphylaxis. After administration of epinephrine, control of the airway the most important therapeutic intervention, as **nearly all deaths caused by anaphylaxis are a result of airway compromise.** Early and aggressive airway management—surgical if needed—is indicated in these patients. Gastrointestinal symptoms including nausea, cramping, and diarrhea may be seen, and are associated with particularly severe anaphylactic reactions.

Clinical Criteria for Diagnosis of Anaphylaxis

Clinical criteria were developed from a multidisciplinary symposium to best identify anaphylaxis early and accurately. Anaphylaxis is highly likely if any one of the following three diagnostic criteria exist.

1. **Acute onset** (minutes to hours) with reaction of the skin and/or mucosal tissue **in addition** to *respiratory symptoms* or **hypotension.** Skin symptoms include itching, redness, hives, generalized urticaria, and mucosal edema, Respiratory manifestations include laryngeal stridor, bronchospasm, bronchorrhea, and hypoxia. Hypotension results from extravasation of fluid from the vasculature and loss of vasomotor tone.

2. Two or more of the following occurring rapidly (minutes to hours) *after exposure to a likely allergen:* involvement of the **skin-mucosal** tissue, **respiratory symptoms, hypotension,** or **gastrointestinal symptoms.** Gastrointestinal symptoms include abdominal pain, cramping, and diarrhea.

3. **Hypotension occurring rapidly (minutes to hours)** *after exposure to known allergen* **for that patient. Hypotension may present as faintness or altered mental status.**

Treatment

The primary initial therapy for anaphylaxis is **epinephrine** (Table 10–2). Epinephrine will act as a pressor for hemodynamic support, a bronchodilator to relieve wheezing, as well as to counteract released mediators and prevent their further release. Epinephrine can be dosed intramuscularly or intravenously. Subcutaneous administration of epinephrine is no longer recommended as it has been proven less effective than intramuscular administration. Initial administration is intramuscular in the anterior thigh with the more concentrated 1:1000 dose at 0.3 to 0.5 mL every 5 minutes. If there is no response or if the patient is already demonstrating cardiovascular compromise, intravenous administration should be started immediately.

IV epinephrine dosing can be confusing and potentially dangerous by provoking cardiac dysrhythmias. In general, all **ampules of epinephrine have 1 mg of medication** (1 mL of 1:1000 = 1 mg of medication; 10 mL of 1:100,000 = 1 mg of medication). **One method of administration is to place 1 mg (1 ampule) of epinephrine into 1 L of intravenous fluid (equivalent to 1 μg/mL) and infuse to 1 to 4 cc/min (1-4 μg/min).** This allows for precise titration of dosing to desired effect, and

Table 10–2 • TREATMENT FOR ANAPHYLAXIS

Drug	Adult Dose	Pediatric Dose
Epinephrine	IV single dose: 100 µg over 5-10 min; 1:100,000 dilution given as 0.1 mg in 10 mL at 1 mL/min IV infusion: 1-4 µg/min IM: 0.3-0.5 mg (0.3-0.5 mL of 1:1000 dilution)	IV infusion: 0.1-0.3 mcg/kg/min; maximum 1.5 µg/kg/min IM: 0.01 mg/kg (0.01 mL/kg of 1:1000 dilution)
IV fluids: NS or LR	1-2-L bolus	10-15-mL/kg bolus
Diphenhydramine	25-50 mg q6h IV, IM, or PO	1 mg/kg q6h IV, IM, or PO
Ranitidine	50 mg IV over 5 min	0.5 mg/kg IV over 5 min
Cimetidine	300 mg IV	4-8 mg/kg IV
Hydrocortisone	250-500 mg IV	5-10 mg/kg IV (max: 500 mg)
Methylprednisolone	125 mg IV	1-2 mg/kg IV (max: 125 mg)
Albuterol	Single treatment: 2.5-5.0 mg nebulized (0.5-1.0 mL of 0.5% solution) Continuous nebulization: 5-10 mg/h	Single treatment: 1.25-2.5 mg nebulized (0.25-0.5 mL of 0.5% solution) Continuous nebulization: 3-5 mg/h
Ipratropium bromide	Single treatment: 250-500 µg nebulized	Single treatment: 125-250 µg nebulized
Magnesium sulfate	2 g IV over 20 min	25-50 mg/kg IV over 20 min
Glucagon	1 mg IV q5min until hypotension resolves, followed by 5-15 µg/min infusion	50 µg/kg q5min
Prednisone	40-60 mg/day PO divided bid or qd (for outpatients: 3-5 days; tapering not required)	1-2 mg/day PO divided bid or qd (for outpatients: 3-5 days; tapering not required)

Reprinted, with permission, from Tintinalli JE, Kelen GD, Stapczynski JS, eds. Emergency Medicine. 6th ed. New York, NY: McGraw-Hill; 2004:250.

provides more rapid administration of epinephrine than intramuscular dosing. Caution should be exercised in the elderly and in those with known cardiovascular disease. Intravenous administration of epinephrine can cause hypertension, tachycardia, dysrhythmias, and myocardial ischemia.

Inhaled beta agonists are indicated for wheezing, and nebulized racemic epinephrine has been hypothesized to decrease laryngeal edema. Intravenous **glucagon** has been proposed for individuals on **β-blockers** in the event they are unresponsive to epinephrine. Glucagon may overcome hypotension by activating adenyl cyclase independent of the beta receptor.

Other adjuvants include systemic **steroids**, specifically methylprednisolone and prednisone. Steroids will not take action for at least 6 hours, but will blunt further immune responses. Steroids should be continued for days after the reaction and gradually tapered. H_1 and H_2 blockers should also be administered. Again, the goal of therapy is to mitigate the effects of as many cytokines as possible. Diphen-hydramine and ranitidine are the most commonly employed agents. It should be remembered that these other medications, while safe and easy to administer, are not first-line agents, and will not counteract respiratory and cardiovascular compromise.

COMPREHENSION QUESTIONS

10.1 An 18-year-old woman is brought to the ED with suspected anaphylaxis. Which of the following most suggests anaphylaxis rather than a simple allergic reaction?

A. Itching

B. Watery eyes

C. Blood pressure of 80/40 mm Hg

D. Hives

E. Anxiety

10.2 A 6-year-old girl with a known peanut allergy is brought to the ED by ambu-lance after accidentally eating a cookie made with peanut butter at a school party. She is wheezing with hives. Which of the following should be the first intervention?

A. Endotracheal intubation

B. Normal saline 20 cc/kg IV

C. Examination of the skin

D. Epinephrine 0.15 mg intramuscular

E. Nebulized albuterol

10.3 Which of the following management options is the greatest determinant of patient outcome in anaphylaxis?

A. Timely administration of steroids

B. Administration of diphenhydramine

C. Early identification of the allergen

D. Early administration of epinephrine

E. Aggressive resuscitation with intravenous fluids

10.4 A 32-year-old man collapses in the emergency room after being brought in by paramedics. He was stung by a bee and known to be highly allergic. He appears cyanotic and had extreme stridor in the ambulance. Severe laryngeal edema is notable. Which of the following is the best treatment?

A. Nebulized albuterol, H_1 and H_2 antagonists, corticosteroids, and crystalloids

B. Subcutaneous epinephrine, H_1 and H_2 antagonists, and corticosteroids

C. Rapid sequence intubation, subcutaneous epinephrine, and corticosteroids

D. Intramuscular epinephrine, rapid sequence intubation, and corticosteroids

E. Intravenous epinephrine, rapid sequence intubation with preparation for a surgical airway, corticosteroids, nebulized albuterol, and H_1 and H_2 antagonists

ANSWERS

10.1 **C.** Hypotension indicates a systemic reaction and cardiovascular compromise, thereby classifying this allergic reaction as anaphylaxis. The other option may all be part of an anaphylactic response, but may also just be simple allergic reactions.

10.2 **D.** Intramuscular epinephrine should be administered immediately. If there is significant respiratory or airway compromise, then the patient should be controlled.

10.3 **D.** Again, early recognition of anaphylaxis and immediate dosing of epinephrine is most important.

10.4 **E.** This patient has severe anaphylaxis, and it would be appropriate to move straight to intravenous epinephrine. If intravenous dosing is not immediately available, then intramuscular epinephrine should be given. Attention should then be turned to managing the airway. Because of the significant laryngeal edema, endotracheal intubation will be nearly impossible; hence, cricothyroidotomy may be required. After securing the airway, steroids, beta agonists, H_1 and H_2 antagonists should be administered.

CLINICAL PEARLS

▶ The airway should be secured early and often. It is much easier to extubate a patient without severe laryngeal edema than to intubate a patient with an occluded posterior oropharynx.

▶ Epinephrine should be given at the first sign of cardiovascular compromise.

▶ Look for causes of anaphylaxis after you have started your initial resuscitation.

▶ Steroids, antihistamines, and beta agonists are all helpful pharmacologic adjuvants for managing the many symptoms of anaphylaxis.

REFERENCES

Braunwald E, Fauci AS, Kasper DL, et al, eds. *Harrison's Principles of Internal Medicine.* 15th ed. New York, NY: McGraw-Hill; 2001.

Rowe BH, Carr S. Anaphylaxis and acute allergic reaction. In: Tintinalli JE, Kelen GD, Stapczynski JS, eds. *Emergency Medicine.* 6th ed., New York, NY: McGraw-Hill: 2004:108-124.

Sampson HA, Munoz-Furlong A, Campbell RL, et al. Second symposium on the definition and management of anaphylaxis: Summary report—Second National Institute of Allergy and Anaphylaxis Network Symposium. *J Allergy Clin Immunol.* 2006.

Soar J, Pumphrey R, Cant A, et al. Emergency treatment of anaphylactic reaction: Guidelines for healthcare providers. *Resuscitation.* 2008;77:157-169.

At 3 AM the paramedics call to inform you that they are en route to the emergency department with a 33-year-old asthmatic. As she is brought in, you immediately notice that she is struggling to breathe. Sweat pours from her face and body as her neck and chest heaves in an attempt to inhale another breath. Her efforts are ultimately futile as consciousness slips away and she becomes apneic.

▶ What are your initial priorities in the management of this patient?
▶ What are your standard treatment options in managing her emergency medical condition?

ANSWERS TO CASE 11:

Acute Exacerbation of Asthma

Summary: This is a case of a 33-year-old woman experiencing a severe asthma attack. Respiratory arrest is imminent.

- **Initial Priorities:** The first priority in this patient's management is addressing the ABCs (airway, breathing, circulation). Based on this presentation, immediate protection of her airway with rapid-sequence endotracheal intubation is indicated. Simultaneously, this patient should be placed on a cardiac monitor with automated blood pressure measurement, establishment of IV access, and continuous pulse oximetry.

- **Standard treatment options:** Basic treatment options include adrenergic agonists (eg, albuterol, terbutaline), anticholinergic agents, and corticosteroids. Intravenous magnesium sulfate is often given to patients with severe asthma exacerbations.

ANALYSIS

Objectives

1. Understand the pathophysiology of respiratory distress caused by acute asthma exacerbation.

2. Describe the key historical and physical examination features.

3. Be able to discuss treatment options for the patient with acute bronchospasm caused by asthma.

Considerations

This 33-year-old asthmatic patient has progressive respiratory difficulty until she becomes apneic. Regardless of the underlying etiology, airway and breathing are the most important initial concerns in any patient. Attention to the airway is critical, and in this case, rapid-sequence endotracheal intubation is the best option. Because airway issues may arise at any given time, the emergency room physician must be skilled, rehearsed, and have equipment to perform endotracheal intubation at any given time. Protection of the airway and mechanical ventilation is the best therapy in this instance. Administration of beta-agonist agents, corticosteroids, anticholinergic agents, and search for the trigger are likewise important.

APPROACH TO:

Asthma

Epidemiology and Pathophysiology

In the United States, asthma accounts for more than 2 million emergency department (ED) visits, 456,000 hospitalizations, and 3500 deaths each year. Overall, between 4%

and 8% of all adults carry a diagnosis of asthma, with a higher prevalence reported in children, the elderly, and in Hispanic and African Americans. It is the most common chronic disease in children and adolescents and the third leading cause of preventable hospitalizations in the United States. Asthma results in more than 10 million lost school and workdays per year, and results in $30 billion of medical expenses per year.

Asthma is considered a chronic inflammatory disorder of the airways. It consists of narrowing of the airway leading to reduced airflow and can be induced by smooth muscle contraction, thickening of the airway wall, and the presence of secretions within the airway lumen in response to an inciting allergen. In susceptible individuals, these changes result in recurrent episodes of wheezing, breathlessness, chest tightness, and cough.

Two distinct phases of asthma have been described. The early (or immediate) phase of asthma consists of acute airway hyperresponsiveness and reversible bronchoconstriction. Following allergen challenge, the lungs begin to constrict within 10 minutes. Peak bronchoconstriction occurs at 30 minutes and either spontaneously or with treatment resolves within 1 to 3 hours. With continued allergen challenge or with refractory bronchoconstriction, this initial phase can progress into the late phase of asthma. This late (or delayed) phase of asthma begins 3 to 4 hours after the allergen challenge and constitutes the inflammatory component seen with acute asthma. Inflammatory cell recruitment, bronchial edema, mucoserous secretion, and further bronchoconstriction all play key roles in the development and propagation of late-phase asthma. Whereas beta-2 agonists target the immediate phase of asthma, corticosteroids target the delayed phase.

Diagnosis

The typical asthma exacerbation is characterized by cough, chest tightness, dyspnea, and wheezing in a patient with a known asthma history. Formal diagnosis is made by spirometry with 75% of asthmatics diagnosed before age 7. Although wheezing characterizes airway obstruction and is often thought of as the hallmark finding in asthma, it is not specific to asthma, and can be absent during severe asthma exacerbations. The history and physical examination should focus on excluding other diagnoses while evaluating the severity of the current asthma exacerbation. Key features to elicit are the nature and time course of the symptoms, precipitating triggers (Table 11–1), use of medication prior to arrival, and any high-risk historical features (Table 11–2).

The evaluation of an asthmatic patient begins with the general appearance of the patient. Those who are extremely anxious or drowsy, unable to speak in full sentences secondary to respiratory distress, or are using accessory muscles of inspiration (tripod position/inability to lay supine) are at significant risk for rapid decompensation. Additional worrisome features are signs of central cyanosis, hypoxia (pulse oximetry <90%), significant tachypnea (>30 breaths per minute), tachycardia, diaphoresis, diffuse or absent wheezing, and poor air entry on pulmonary examination.

Although extremely helpful, physical examination findings are not sensitive indicators of a clinically severe exacerbation. Since asthmatics have a propensity for deteriorating quickly, an objective measure of severity should be sought whenever possible. Bedside testing that measures peak expiratory flow rate (PEFR) or

Table 11-1 • ASTHMA TRIGGERS
Exercise
Cold air
Emotional stress
Allergen exposure (dust, mold, pollen, animal dander, etc)
Infection (primarily viral)
GERD
Hormonal fluctuations

fractional expiratory volume at 1 second (FEV_1) are simple, inexpensive ways of measuring the severity of airway obstruction and are commonly used to monitor response to treatment in the ED. Severe asthma is defined as an FEV_1 of less than 50% of predicted (typically <200 L/min in an adult) or one's own personal best measurement.

Routine laboratory investigations (eg, complete blood count, basic metabolic panel), arterial blood gas (ABG) analysis, chest radiography, and cardiac monitoring are not required in the uncomplicated asthmatic. Table 11–3 suggests indications for each of these modalities.

MANAGEMENT

Immediate priorities in the management of all asthma patients include an initial assessment of the patient's airway, breathing, and circulation status. Patients in extremis require placement of peripheral intravenous lines, continuous supplemental oxygen therapy, and cardiac monitoring. While these interventions are underway, the physician should ascertain a history, perform a physical examination, and initiate appropriate therapy.

Oxygen, Compressed Air, and Heliox

Oxygen should be provided to maintain a pulse oximetry reading of at least 90% in adults and at least 95% in infants, pregnant women, and patients with coexisting heart disease. Oxygen is often used as the delivery vehicle for nebulized medications, although compressed air and helium-oxygen mixtures (heliox) can also be used.

Table 11-2 • HIGH-RISK HISTORICAL FACTORS
Prior intubation for asthma
Prior hospitalization or ICU admission
Frequent ED visits
Frequent albuterol metered-dose inhaler (MDI) use
Use of inhaled or oral corticosteroids at home
Comorbid conditions (CAD, COPD, psychiatric)
Low socioeconomic status
Illicit drug use, especially inhaled cocaine

Table 11–3 • SUGGESTED INDICATIONS FOR ANCILLARY TESTING
ABG
• To determine degree of hypercapnea or assess degree of deterioration in tiring patient not yet sick enough to warrant endotracheal intubation.
CXR
• Temp >38°C
• Unexplained chest pain
• Leukocytosis
• Hypoxemia
• Comorbidities/alternative diagnosis
ECG
• Persistent tachycardia
• Comorbidities/alternative diagnosis

Heliox mixtures produce a more laminar airflow and potentially deliver nebulized particles to more distal airways, but they have not been shown to consistently lead to improved ED outcomes for all asthmatic patients. A systematic review concluded that heliox may be beneficial only in patients who present with severe asthma that is refractory to initial treatment.

Adrenergic Agents

Inhaled albuterol, through nebulization or metered-dose inhaler (MDI) with spacer device, is the mainstay of treatment for acute asthma. Typically 2.5 to 5 mg of albuterol is intermittently nebulized every 15 to 20 minutes for the first hour of therapy and then repeated every 30 minutes thereafter for 1 to 2 more hours. Continuous nebulization with higher doses (10-20 mg/h) of albuterol benefits severe asthmatics. Beta-2 agonists bind pulmonary receptors and activate adenyl cyclase which results in an increase in intracellular cyclic adenosine monophosphate (cAMP). This results in a drop in myoplasmic calcium and subsequent bronchial smooth-muscle relaxation. In addition, beta-2 agonists are thought to have some anti-inflammatory properties by inhibiting inflammatory mediator release. Side effects of these agents are generally mild and include tachycardia, nervousness, and shakiness or jitteriness.

Alternatively, albuterol can be administered with an MDI and spacer device. In the ED, patients can receive 4 to 8 puffs every 15 to 20 minutes for the first hour of therapy and then every 30 minutes thereafter for 1 to 2 more hours. MDI with spacer device therapy is therapeutically equivalent to nebulizer therapy in adults and may be more efficacious than nebulizer therapy in children as less medication is lost to the environment. Implementation of MDI with spacer device therapy for asthmatics in the ED is also associated with decreased health care cost.

Although inhalation therapy is optimal, occasionally patients with severe obstruction or who cannot tolerate inhalation therapy (eg, children) are given subcutaneous administration of epinephrine or terbutaline. Epinephrine is given in a dose of 0.3 to 0.5 mg subcutaneously every 20 minutes to a maximal combined total dose of 1 mg. Terbutaline is given 0.25 mg subcutaneously every 20 minutes up to a maximum of three doses. Generally, terbutaline is preferable because of its beta-2 selectivity and fewer cardiac side effects.

Levalbuterol, the R-isomer of racemic albuterol, was developed because in vitro studies suggested that the S-isomer may have deleterious effects on airway smooth muscle. However, randomized trials have not shown a significant clinical advantage of levalbuterol over racemic albuterol for the treatment of acute asthma in the emergency department. National asthma treatment guidelines currently consider levalbuterol equally safe and effective to racemic albuterol and endorse its use for the treatment of acute asthma exacerbations.

Anticholinergic Agents

When added to albuterol, anticholinergic agents lead to a modest improvement in pulmonary function and decrease the admission rate in patients with moderate to severe asthma exacerbations. Anticholinergics decrease intracellular cyclic guanosine monophosphate (cGMP) concentrations, which reduce vagal nerve-mediated bronchoconstriction on medium- and larger-sized airways. Additionally, anticholinergic agents may have some minor anti-inflammatory properties that help to stabilize capillary permeability and inhibit mucous secretion. The typical dose for ipratropium bromide is two puffs from a MDI with spacer device, or 0.5 mL of the 0.02% solution. Anticholinergics can be combined with beta agonists in nebulization devices and should be given to those not responding to initial beta-agonist therapy and those with severe airway obstruction. Since there is little systemic absorption, inhaled anticholinergics are associated with few side effects.

Corticosteroids

Corticosteroids have been used to treat chronic asthma since 1950 and acute exacerbations of the disease since 1956. Although a tremendous amount of research has been done on the value of corticosteroids in asthma, many fundamental issues have yet to be resolved, such as the optimal dose, route, and timing of steroids. It is generally agreed that corticosteroids should be initiated early in the treatment of the following cases:

- Acute asthma in patients with moderate/severe asthma attack

- Worsening asthma over many days (>3 days)

- Mild asthma not responding to initial bronchodilator therapy or asthma that develops despite daily inhaled corticosteroid use.

Some authors believe that more liberal use of corticosteroids is warranted and advocate steroids for any patient whose symptoms fail to resolve with a single albuterol treatment. Even more liberal asthmatologists prefer that steroids be given for every asthma patient who is sick enough to warrant ED evaluation.

Steroids act on the delayed phase of asthma and modulate the inflammatory response. They have been shown to improve pulmonary function, decrease the rate of hospital admission, and decrease the rate of relapse in patients that receive them early in their ED treatment course. Oral administration of prednisone (dose 40-60 mg) is usually preferred to intravenous methylprednisolone (dose 125 mg), because it is less invasive and the effects are equivalent. Intravenous steroids, however, should be administered to patients with severe respiratory distress who are too dyspneic to swallow, patients who are vomiting, or patients who are agitated or drowsy. For patients who will be discharged, a single intramuscular dose of methylprednisolone (dose 160 mg) may be given when there is a history of medication noncompliance. A 2-day course of oral dexamethasone (dose 16 mg) is also an option because it has been shown to be equivalent to five days of prednisone. Alternative steroids include hydrocortisone 150 to 200 mg IV, dexamethasone 6 to 10 mg IV, or oral dexamethasone 0.6 mg/kg (maximum dose 16 mg) in pediatric patients.

Leukotriene Antagonists

The development of leukotriene antagonists represents an important advancement in the treatment of chronic asthma. Studies involving zileuton (Zyflo Filmtab), zafirlukast (Accolate), and montelukast (Singulair) demonstrate that their daily use over the course of several months can lead to improvement in pulmonary function and decrease in asthma symptomatology. However, the role of leukotriene antagonists in the treatment of acute asthma exacerbations remains unclear. A randomized study of intravenous montelukast showed that it significantly improved FEV_1 when added to standard asthma therapy, but this improvement in lung function did not translate to lower hospitalization rates. At this time, asthma treatment guidelines recommend the use of leukotriene antagonists only in the management of chronic asthma.

Magnesium

Although no benefit has been shown in mild to moderate asthmatics, magnesium sulfate given intravenously at dosages of 2 to 4 g benefits asthmatics with severe airway obstruction. Magnesium is thought to compete with calcium for entry into smooth muscle, inhibit the release of calcium from the sarcoplasmic reticulum, prevent acetylcholine release from nerve endings, and inhibit mast cell release of histamine. Additionally, there is some evidence that magnesium may directly inhibit smooth muscle contraction, but this is controversial. The onset of magnesium is quick and effects can be seen 2 to 5 minutes after initiation of therapy. The effects are short lived and diminish quickly when the infusion is stopped. The dose of magnesium is 2 to 4 g IV in adults and 30 to 70 mg/kg IV in children given over 10 to 15 minutes. Magnesium has minimal side effects. The most commonly reported are hypotension, a flushing sensation, and malaise. It is contraindicated in renal failure and in cases of hypermagnesemia as it can cause significant muscle weakness.

Other Agents—Methylxanthines, Antibiotics

The marginal benefit, significant side effects, and difficulty achieving a therapeutic dose of theophylline argue against its routine use in acute asthma. A systematic review concluded that the addition of aminophylline to treatment with beta agonists and glucocorticoids improved lung function, but did not significantly reduce symptoms or length of hospital stay. Therefore, methylxanthines are not recommended in the treatment of acute asthma exacerbations. The routine administration of antibiotics has also not been shown to decrease symptomatology in asthma patients without concurrent bacterial lower respiratory infection or sinusitis.

Positive Pressure Ventilation

Positive pressure ventilation (PPV), with either invasive or noninvasive methods, is indicated for patients with respiratory failure or impending failure who are not responsive to therapy. Several studies have suggested that bi-level positive airway pressure (BiPAP) may be beneficial in severe asthma exacerbations. For example, a randomized trial enrolled severe asthmatics (defined as FEV_1 <60% and RR>30) to receive BiPAP and found significant improvements in pulmonary function and reduced rates of hospitalization. Severe asthmatics with impending respiratory failure should receive a trial of BiPAP prior to being intubated. The BiPAP machine should be set at inspiratory pressure 8 to 15 cm H_2O and expiratory pressure 3 to 5 cm H_2O. Patients who fail to improve over 30 to 60 minutes will likely require intubation. Furthermore, contrary to prior teaching, a short trial (30 minutes) of BiPAP is considered acceptable for mild to moderate altered level of consciousness attributed to hypercapnea.

Immediate rapid-sequence endotracheal intubation should be reserved for unconscious or near-comatose patients with respiratory failure. In an awake patient, an appropriate induction agent (eg, ketamine) and paralytic agent (eg, succinylcholine) should be used prior to intubation. Ketamine is the induction agent of choice because it stimulates the release of catecholamines and causes relaxation of bronchial smooth muscle, leading to bronchodilation. Numerous case reports have also demonstrated that a ketamine infusion may be useful when severe asthmatics fail to respond to conventional treatments. Ketamine is given as an intravenous bolus of 1 mg/kg, followed by a continuous infusion of 0.5 to 2 mg/kg/h.

Once an asthmatic patient is intubated, the ventilator should be set to promote the goal of permissive hypercapnea which aims at minimizing dynamic hyperinflation (ie, breath stacking or auto-PEEP [positive end-expiratory pressure]) with low tidal volumes, and increased time for expiration, while limiting plateau pressures. It is critical to recognize that mechanically ventilated asthmatic patients are at high risk for hyperinflation and auto-PEEP which can result in life threatening complications such as tension pneumothorax or cardiac arrest. Suggested initial settings are Assist Control mode at a respiratory rate of 8 to 10 breaths per minute, tidal volume 6 to 8 mL/kg, no extrinsic PEEP, inspiratory-to-expiratory (I/E) ratio of 1:4, and an inspiratory flow rate of 80 to 100 L/min. To prevent barotrauma, plateau pressures should not exceed 30 cm H_2O. Following initiation of PPV, blood-gas analysis can be used to modify ventilator or BiPAP settings.

ADMISSION/DISCHARGE CRITERIA

Acute asthma is a heterogeneous condition and as such patients should be individualized when it comes to disposition decisions. Patients who respond well to therapy by improved subjective and objective criteria (eg, symptoms resolved, normal or near-normal pulmonary examination) are suitable candidates for discharge. Patients should be on room air and moving about the emergency department before finalizing the decision to discharge the patient. An improvement of PEFR or FEV_1 to greater than 70% predicted or personal best can also be used as a sign of objective improvement. Hospital admission should be considered in patients that fail to respond to therapy (ie, PEFR or FEV_1 < 50% predicted) after 4 to 6 hours of treatment or patients with partial response to therapy (ie, PEFR or FEV_1 between 50% and 70% predicted) and one or all of the following:

1. New-onset asthma

2. Multiple prior hospitalizations or ED visits

3. Have comorbidity from coronary artery disease

4. Have significant medical or social issues that impair access to health care, personal judgment, or understanding of their disease.

Asthmatics who are discharged from the ED should receive albuterol, an MDI spacer device, and a 5- to 10-day course of oral steroids. Most patients should be treated for at least 1 week, but can stop their oral steroids based on resolutions of their symptoms and self-monitored peak flow values. Tapering is not necessary if the duration of steroid treatment is less than 3 weeks, if inhaled steroids are concomitantly prescribed for preventative ongoing therapy, or as long as the patient has not recently been on steroid therapy.

Inhaled corticosteroids (ICS) should be prescribed to anyone with frequent beta-agonist MDI use and is symptomatic enough to warrant urgent medical evaluation. Several studies have demonstrated that ICS improve lung function, diminish symptoms, and decrease "rescue use" of beta agonists. Beneficial effects of ICS can be observed after a single dose and therapeutic effects are achieved with chronic administration. Furthermore, one can initiate treatment alongside oral steroids without fear of added systemic toxicity. Recent studies have documented a significant reduction in relapse rates when combining oral and inhaled steroids. For patients who continue to have poorly controlled asthma and recurrent exacerbations despite maximal therapy, other medications may be added such as long-acting inhaled beta agonists, oral leukotriene antagonists, and omalizumab (a monoclonal anti-IgE antibody).

While awaiting discharge, MDI with spacer device technique should be reviewed with the patient, and the patient should be instructed on how to monitor peak flow readings at home. Additionally, patients should be educated about the common asthma precipitants and how to avoid them, as well as receive written and verbal instructions on when to return to the ED. Finally, patients should be referred for a follow-up medical appointment in a timely manner. Arranging ongoing care with an asthma specialist or a clinic focusing on asthma patients is more likely to reduce subsequent emergency department visits. Patients who are unable to follow up with their primary physician can be instructed to return to the ED for a recheck of their symptoms.

COMPREHENSION QUESTIONS

11.1 A 24-year-old man is brought into the ED complaining of an exacerbation of his asthma. Which of the following is the most appropriate method of assessing the severity of his disease?

A. Spirometry

B. Measurement of the diffusion capacity of the lungs

C. Measurement of the peak expiratory flow

D. Measurement of the alveoli oxygen tension

11.2 A 19-year-old woman is admitted to the hospital for an exacerbation of asthma likely precipitated by pollen and colder weather. Her inpatient regimen includes both intravenous and inhalant medications. Which of the following medications is most likely to be used as part of discharge plan?

A. Theophylline

B. Antibiotics

C. Magnesium

D. Histamines

E. Corticosteroids

11.3 Which of the following initial ventilator settings is appropriate for intubated asthmatics?

A. IMV mode, rate 16, tidal volume 6 to 8 mL/kg

B. IMV mode, rate 16, tidal volume 10 to 12 mL/kg

C. AC mode, rate 8 to 10, tidal volume 6 to 8 mL/kg

D. AC mode, rate 8 to 10, tidal volume 10 to 12 mL/kg

E. AC mode, rate 16, tidal volume 6 to 8 mL/kg

ANSWERS

11.1 **C.** The peak expiratory flow is a reliable and fairly accurate method of assessing asthma severity. Spirometry, although providing important information, is rarely available in the ED.

11.2 **E.** Corticosteroids are often used after a hospitalization. Other standard medications include beta-agonists and oral leukotriene antagonists. None of the other medications are used routinely for discharged asthma patients.

11.3 **C.** The initial settings for patients with obstructive lung disease should be AC mode, rate 8 to 10, tidal volume 6 to 8 mL/kg. Low volumes and small tidal volumes are used to prevent air stacking and barotrauma.

CLINICAL PEARLS

▶ Initiate therapy with albuterol while obtaining history and performing a physical examination for patients with significant asthma.

▶ Glucocorticosteroids should be administered early for asthmatic exacerbations and continued for at least 1 week.

▶ Measure peak flow to help assess asthma severity and monitor progression during treatment.

▶ Use lower than traditional ventilator settings to prevent barotrauma in the intubated asthmatic.

▶ Most asthmatics should be discharged from the ED with inhaled corticosteroids for ongoing preventative therapy.

▶ The individual who presents with an initial episode of "wheezing" may have etiologies other than asthma, for example, foreign body, pneumonia, or congestive heart failure.

▶ Absence of wheezing can sometimes be misleading in the individual in extremis because of very little air movement.

REFERENCES

Akinbami LJ, Moorman JE, Liu X. Asthma prevalence, health care use, and mortality: United States, 2005-2009. National Health Statistics 2011:32.

Camargo CA, Rachelefsky G, Schatz M. Managing asthma exacerbations in the emergency department: Summary of the National Asthma Education and Prevention Program Expert Panel Report 3 guidelines for the management of asthma exacerbations. *J Allergy Clin Immunol.* 2009;124:S5-S14.

Keenan SP, Sinuff T, Cook DJ, et. al. Does noninvasive positive pressure ventilation improve outcome in acute hypoxemia respiratory failure? A systematic review. *Crit Care Med.* 2004;32(12):2516-2523.

Krishnan JA, Davis SQ, Naureckas ET, et al. An umbrella review: Corticosteroid therapy for adults with acute asthma. *Am J Med.* 2009;122(11):977-991.

National Heart, Lung, and Bood Institute, National Asthma Education Prevention Program. Expert Panel Report 3: guidelines for the diagnosis and management of asthma: full report 2007. Available at: http://www.nhlbi.nih.gov/guidelines/asthma/asthgdln.pdf). Accessed March 1, 2011.

Rodrigo GJ, Castro-Rodriguez JA. Anticholinergics in the treatment of children and adults with acute asthma: A systematic review with meta-analysis. *Thorax.* 2005;60:740-746.

Schatz M, Rachelefsky G, Krishnan JA. Follow-up after acute asthma episodes: What improves future outcomes? *J Emerg Med.* 2009;37:S42-S50.

A 32-year-old man, involved in a motor vehicle collision (MVC), is brought to the emergency department (ED). He lost control of his car and hit a utility pole with the front end of his car, while traveling at approximately 35 MPH. He was thrown against the windshield of the car, hitting his face and forehead against the windshield. There was no loss of consciousness. His blood pressure is 125/79 mm Hg, heart rate is 92 beats per minute, respiratory rate is 16 breaths per minute, and pulse oxygenation is 99% on room air. On examination, he has a 7-cm laceration on the right side of his face that courses from his right ear to just below the lower lip. He is alert and has no focal neurologic deficits on examination. When he is asked to smile, the right side of his mouth droops.

▶ What is the most likely diagnosis?
▶ What is the most appropriate therapy?

ANSWERS TO CASE 12:

Facial Laceration

Summary: A 32-year-old man presents to the ED after a motor vehicle collision. There is no evidence of injury except for a 7-cm laceration on the right side of his face, which courses from his ear, to across the cheek, and ends just below the right lower lip. His neurologic examination is normal except for the inability to smile on the right side.

- **Most likely diagnosis:** Right facial nerve laceration

- **Most appropriate therapy:** Microsurgical repair of right facial nerve and closure of skin laceration

ANALYSIS

Objectives

1. Understand the critical structures that can be injured in facial lacerations.

2. Understand the need for tetanus immunization in trauma patients.

3. Know the basic principles of facial laceration repair.

Considerations

This patient suffered a laceration across his right cheek after being involved in a motor vehicle collision. The **mainstay in trauma management includes managing the airway, breathing, and circulation (ABCs).** Once the primary survey is complete, the physician then performs the secondary survey, which includes a head-to-toe physical examination that evaluates for non–life-threatening injuries. **Any trauma to the head, face, or neck should raise concern for a cervical spine (C-spine) injury.** If there is suspicion for a C-spine injury, the patient should be placed in a rigid cervical collar until either appropriate imaging can be performed or appropriate clinical evaluation completed. Facial trauma often results in bony injuries to the orbits and mandible. Injury to cranial nerves V and VII are common. The facial nerve (CN VII) exits the stylomastoid foramen and branches into motor and sensory branches to the temporal, zygomatic, buccal, and mental regions. Lacerations to the **buccal branch** are associated with injury to the **parotid duct**. Identification of a **facial nerve injury** is critical because **delayed diagnosis results in poor outcome.** Microsurgical techniques give fairly good results. After repair of the injury, the patient needs a **tetanus immunization** if the last time the patient received a tetanus vaccine was longer than 5 years ago.

APPROACH TO:
Facial Lacerations

DEFINITIONS

FACIAL TRAUMA: Any soft or deep tissue injury secondary to physical force, burns, or foreign objects to the following structures: the scalp, forehead, nose, eyes, lips, cheeks, tongue, oral cavity, and jaw.

VERMILLION BORDER: The junction between the lip and facial skin. An injury to this area can result in a significant cosmetic defect if not repaired correctly.

AURICULAR HEMATOMA: Collection of blood in the ear that results from the traumatic interruption of the perichondrium and cartilage. If left untreated, it can evolve into a fibrous mass leaving the affected ear with a cauliflower-like appearance.

SADDLE NOSE DEFORMITY: Nasal injury secondary to the necrotic breakdown of the septal cartilage. It is caused by a traumatic injury to the nose resulting in a nasal septal hematoma. If the hematoma is left untreated, it separates the septal cartilage from its perichondrium depriving it of its nutrient supply.

TETANUS: An often fatal infectious disease caused by the bacteria *Clostridium tetani*, which usually enters the body through a puncture, cut, or open wound.

CLINICAL APPROACH

The basic approach to wound care includes assessment for other injuries, probing the depth of the wound, irrigation, a neurovascular examination, and deciding on whether primary closure is advisable (ie, leave open if infection is likely such as contamination or delay in presentation). The length of time the suture stays in place and the type of suture depends on the body location (Table 12–1). Additionally, the need to update the patient's tetanus vaccination should be assessed.

Irrigation

When the decision to suture is made, a stepwise preparation must take place. All wounds must first be irrigated and explored for foreign bodies and environmental debris. Proper irrigation can significantly reduce the risk of wound infection. High-pressure and large-volume irrigation remains the gold standard to reduce or eliminate particulate matter and bacterial loads from the wound. This is usually established with a 35- to 60-mL syringe and 16- to 19-gauge catheter using constant hand pressure. This generates a pressure of 5 to 8 psi, which is adequate to irrigate a wound. Sterile saline is the most commonly used irrigant. Application of povidone iodine, hydrogen peroxide, and detergents should be avoided because of their toxic effects on tissue.

Table 12–1 • SUTURE SIZE FOR CORRESPONDING ANATOMIC REGION	
Anatomic Region	Suture Size
Face	5-0 to 6-0
Scalp	3-0 to 5-0
Chest	3-0 to 4-0
Back	3-0 to 4-0
Abdomen	3-0 to 4-0
Extremities	4-0 to 5-0
Joints	3-0 to 4-0
Oral	3-0 to 5-0 absorbable

Anesthesia

Once irrigation is complete and the wound is examined, anesthesia should be administered. Delaying anesthesia until irrigation is completed allows the patient to reveal any sensation of a retained foreign body that might dislodge during irrigation. Local anesthetics are divided into two major groups, amides and esters. Although it is rare, some patients are allergic to anesthetics. However, if a patient is allergic to one class, the other class can be safely administered. It is thought that the allergy is to the preservative in the anesthetic, rather than the anesthetic itself (Table 12–2).

Local anesthesia can be attained in many ways including injection directly into the wound, topical application, or by a nerve block. The most common method is local infiltration. Several techniques are available to reduce pain experienced by the patient during injection. These include using smaller gauge needles, injecting at a slow rate, infiltrating the wound edge instead of surrounding skin, adding sodium bicarbonate to the anesthetic solution at a 1:10 dilution, and warming the solution. Some authors recommend first applying topical anesthetic. This is particularly useful in the pediatric population. Initially TAC (tetracaine, 0.25%-0.5%; adrenaline, 0.025%-0.05%; cocaine, 4%-11%) was commonly used, but was associated with seizure, arrhythmia, and cardiac arrest. LET (lidocaine, 4%; epinephrine, 0.1%; tetracaine, 0.5%) is generally safer than TAC and is used for anesthesia of the face and scalp. EMLA (eutectic mixture of local anesthetics) consists of lidocaine and prilocaine and is also commonly used. Because of the possibility for systemic absorption of lidocaine and tetracaine, these anesthetics should be avoided in large wounds and mucus membranes.

Epinephrine is added to many anesthetic solutions. This augments hemostasis and prolongs the duration of action of the anesthetic by decreasing systemic absorption through local vasoconstriction. Although it is controversial, it is recommended to **avoid injecting solutions with epinephrine into sites such as digits, the tip of the nose, ears, and penis due to the risk of necrosis.**

Table 12–2 • COMMONLY USED LOCAL ANESTHETICS

Class	Name	Onset	Duration of Action (h)	Maximal Dose (mg/kg)
Amides	Bupivacaine	Slow	4-5	2
	(w/epinephrine)		7-8	3
	Ropivacaine	Medium	3-4	3
	(w/epinephrine)		6-7	3
	Mepivacaine	Rapid	2-3	5
	(w/epinephrine)		5-6	7
	Lidocaine	Rapid	1-2	5
	(w/epinephrine)		2-4	7
Esters	Procaine	Slow	0.5-1	8
	(w/epinephrine)		1-1.5	10
	Tetracaine	Slow	3-4	1.5
	(w/epinephrine)		9-10	2.5
	Prilocaine	Medium	0.5-1	5
	(w/epinephrine)		5-6	7.5
	Chloroprocaine	Rapid	0.5-1	10
	(w/epinephrine)		1-1.5	15

Suture Placement

To reduce scarring, sutures on the face should be placed approximately 1 to 2 mm from the wound edge and 3 mm apart. Cosmesis is less of a concern with other body areas.

Wound Closure

Once the wound is irrigated, explored, and anesthetized, closure can begin. Below are several methods and approaches for wound closure depending on the site of injury; addressing proper methods to examine specific areas and appropriate closure techniques.

Scalp and Forehead

These lacerations are usually caused by a combination of blunt and sharp trauma. Careful inspection of the wound is critical, with care to palpate for depressed skull fractures, and assess the integrity of the galea aponeurosis, which covers the periosteum. Repair usually follows the skin lines for the best cosmetic result. The **scalp should be closed with a 4-0 monofilament suture of different color than the patient's hair** or **staples** can be used. Sutures and staples should be **removed after 7 to 10 days**. Because scalp lacerations can be associated with significant hemorrhage, rapid closure with staples may decrease the blood loss. If the galea is involved, it should be repaired with long-lasting absorbable suture material (eg, Vicryl, Monocryl). **Closing the galea helps to control heavy bleeding associated with scalp wounds and limits the spread of potential infection.** **Forehead** lacerations should be repaired in layers. The skin should be approximated with **6-0 nonabsorbable interrupted sutures, and removed after 5 days.** Care should be taken to precisely approximate hair lines.

Eyelids

The eyelid is thin and delicate and is functionally and cosmetically important. Because of the risk of periorbital trauma, the emergency physician should have a **low threshold to refer to an oculoplastic specialist or ophthalmologist** for evaluation and repair. This includes **lacerations to upper and lower lid margins** and those **involving the lacrimal duct.** Any laceration **medial to the puncta** should be highly concerning for a **canicular system injury.** Staining the laceration with fluorescein dye can be used to determine damage to the canaliculus. In addition, damage to the levator palpebrae superioris muscle should be ruled out with traumatic lacerations of the upper lid. This commonly manifests as ptosis. A majority of eyelid lacerations can be managed without suture repair, including lacerations that are superficial and involve less that 25% of the eyelid. When sutures are indicated, repair is generally undertaken **with 6-0 or 7-0 interrupted sutures, with care to stay superficial; the suture is removed after 3 to 5 days.**

Nose

The nose is commonly injured, and is the most common fracture in victims of domestic violence. It is the focal point of the face, thus it is important to ensure proper management of nasal lacerations for optimal cosmesis. Inspection for the depth of injury is important. Infection can occur when all of the layers are penetrated or when cartilage is exposed. **Septal trauma may lead to hematoma formation, which can lead to necrosis of the septum** or **chronic obstruction of the nasal passageway.** Untreated hematoma separates the septal cartilage from its perichondrium depriving it from the nutrient supply. The septal cartilage can necrose resulting in a **saddle nose deformity.** Therefore, septal hematomas require drainage. Anesthesia in this area is difficult because of the tightness of skin over the cartilage, but can be obtained via a dorsal nerve block. Injection directly into a wound can distort wound edges for repair and is extremely uncomfortable, as well. Epinephrine must be avoided in this area. Topical lidocaine is generally helpful. Cartilage lacerations should be repaired with 4-0 or 5-0 absorbable sutures, and the skin closed with 6-0 nonabsorbable suture for 3 to 5 days. Lacerations to the nasal alae are usually complex and difficult to anesthetize; these wounds often require consultation of a plastic or ear, nose, and throat (ENT) surgeon.

Lips

The junction between the skin and the red portion of the lip, the vermillion border, is of vital cosmetic importance. Additionally, the orbicularis oris muscle that surrounds the mouth is critical for facial expression, speech formation, and the retention of saliva. Lacerations involving the lip that do not cross the vermillion border can be closed in layers with **6-0 nonabsorbable suture and left in place for 5 days.** If the vermilion border is disrupted, the first stitch in repair should exactly approximate the border using 6-0 nonabsorbable suture. This first suture needs to be precise, **because even a 1-mm discrepancy is noticeable** (Figure 12–1). A plastic surgeon can be consulted for these injuries. Regional anesthesia is helpful, because local anesthetic infiltration can obscure the anatomy. The most common regional blocks include the mental nerve block and infraorbital block for the lower and upper lip, respectively. All intraoral wounds are dirty wounds and are at high risk for infection. Therefore, prophylactic penicillin or clindamycin is indicated.

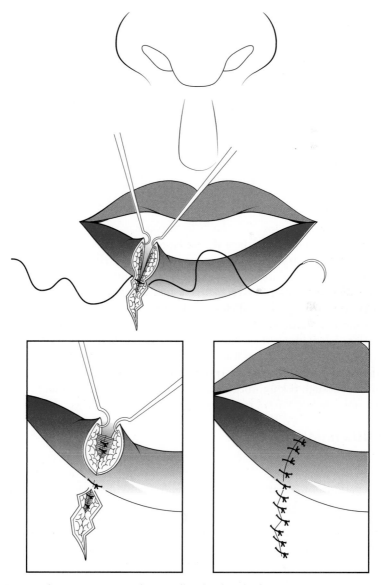

Figure 12–1. Lip laceration crossing the vermillion border. The first step is to approximate the vermillion-skin junction, the orbicularis muscle is then approximated and, finally, the skin is repaired.

Ears

In patients with trauma to the ear region, the physician should evaluate the patient for a **basilar skull fracture** or tympanic membrane rupture. After inspection, cotton can be placed into the ear canal during irrigation of any lacerations. Regional auricular block is effective, and again, epinephrine should be avoided. Lacerations of the ear should be approached with the following goals: cosmesis, avoidance of hematoma, and prevention of infection. Repair of lacerated ear tissue should mirror its symmetric counterpart as much as possible for the best cosmetic results. Superficial lacerations should be repaired with 6-0 nonabsorbable sutures, and removed in 5 days. Meticulous hemostasis is important to prevent hematoma formation. If an auricular hematoma is present, and is left unaddressed, the ear is prone to abnormal cartilage production and subsequent calcification commonly referred to as a "cauliflower ear." Auricular hematoma, avulsed tissue, or crushed cartilage is probably best handled by a plastic surgeon or otolaryngologist. Any cartilage that is exposed should be covered to reduce infection, erosive chondritis, and subsequent necrosis. If a plastic surgeon or otolaryngologist are unavailable, small superficial lacerations should be repaired with uninterrupted sutures. Sutures should be placed in the skin surrounding these wounds paying special attention to avoid suturing the ear cartilage, which could lead to avascular necrosis. After the laceration is repaired, a pressure dressing should be applied to help prevent the formation of an auricular hematoma.

Cheeks and Face

Lacerations of the **cheek and face** should be repaired after investigating the vital structures in the region such as the facial nerve and parotid duct (Figure 12–2). Generally, a **6-0 monofilament interrupted suture technique is appropriate for repair. Sutures are removed after 5 days. Simple lacerations (<2 cm) isolated to the buccal cavity typically do not need closure. These areas are highly vascularized and heal well without sutures. Proper irrigation is important to prevent complications of infection. Lacerations in the buccal cavity greater than 2 cm have the propensity to collect food, which can lead to infection. These typically require closure. Absorbable 5-0 sutures are preferred.** As stated above, all intraoral wounds are dirty and are at high risk for infection. Therefore, prophylactic penicillin or clindamycin is indicated.

TETANUS IMMUNIZATION

Tetanus is an acute, often fatal, but preventable disease caused by the gram-positive bacterium *Clostridium tetani*. The **spores are ubiquitous in soil** and animal manure. Contamination of a wound with *C tetani*, particularly in **devitalized, crushed, or infected tissue,** can lead to its proliferation and expression of the neuroexotoxin **tetanospasmin.** This powerful exotoxin acts on the motor endplates of skeletal muscle, the spinal cord, the sympathetic nervous system, and the brain, leading to generalized muscle rigidity, autonomic nervous system instability, and severe muscle contractions. **The most common presentation of tetanus is muscle spasm of the masseter muscles, "lockjaw,"** but the back, arms, diaphragm, and lower extremities can also be affected. The diagnosis is made clinically. In up to 10% of tetanus cases,

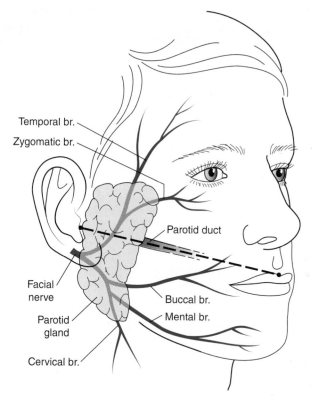

Figure 12–2. Anatomic structures of the cheek.

the patient does not recall a wound. The usual incubation period varies from 7 to 21 days, but can extend from 3 to 56 days.

Patients with tetanus should be **admitted to the intensive care unit.** Wound debridement, respiratory support as needed, and muscle relaxants or neuromuscular blockade may be helpful. **Patients with tetanus should receive passive immunization with tetanus immunoglobulin (TIG) 3000 to 6000 units IM on the side opposite of the tetanus toxoid injection.** It clearly reduces morbidity and mortality. Penicillin is usually given, but is of questionable efficacy.

Prevention of tetanus is accomplished with regular active immunization of all individuals. The dose of tetanus toxoid (TT) or diphtheria/tetanus toxoid (dT) is 0.5 mL IM regardless of age. **Tetanus immunoglobulin (TIG) is given in patients with a possible tetanus exposure and have incomplete tetanus immunization** (<3 injections). The dosage varies with age **(Table 12–3).** Tetanus immunoglobulin and tetanus toxoid should be administered in different body sites with different syringes.

History of Absorbed Tetanus Toxoid (# of doses)	Clean, Minor, Wound		All Other Wounds	
	TDaP, TD or DTaP	TIG	TDaP, TD or DTaP	TIG
Unknown or <3	Yes	No	Yes	Yes
≥3	No^a	No	No^b	No

Table 12–3 • A GUIDE TO TETANUS PROPHYLAXIS IN BASIC WOUND MANAGEMENT

Abbreviations: TDaP = tetanus, diphtheria, acellular pertussis; DTaP = diphtheria, tetanus, acellular pertussis; Td = tetanus, diphtheria; TIG = tetanus immunoglobulin.
^aYes, if > 10 years since the last tetanus toxoid containing vaccine dose.
^bYes, if >5 years since the last tetanus toxoid containing vaccine dose.
Note: Please refer to CDC guidelines for more complete recommendations (CDC Health Information for International Travel 2008, Chapter 4: Prevention of Specific Infectious Diseases).

COMPREHENSION QUESTIONS

12.1 An 18-year-old man was involved in an altercation at a local bar. He suffered a laceration of the scalp, neck, forehead, and upper lip. Which of the following is likely to be most challenging to repair from a cosmetic perspective?

A. Scalp

B. Neck

C. Forehead

D. Cheek

E. Upper lip

12.2 A 24-year-old woman was the victim of domestic violence and received treatment at the local emergency department for multiple contusions and lacerations of the face. Six months after treatment, she notices a defect of the nasal septum with communication between the right and left nasal passage way. Which of the following is the most likely diagnosis?

A. Physician use of epinephrine on the nasal septum

B. Patient use of cocaine

C. Hematoma of the nasal septum

D. Post-traumatic stress syndrome

12.3 A 48-year-old man was rock climbing when he slipped and suffered a laceration to his right lower leg. He put pressure on it, wrapped the area, and made his way to the ED. He recalls getting "all his shots" when he was a child, but doesn't recall the last tetanus booster. Which of the following is the best choice regarding tetanus prevention?

A. Diphtheria toxoid/tetanus toxoids (DT) vaccine 0.5 mL IM

B. DT 0.5 mL IM and tetanus immune globulin (TIG) 250 units IM

C. DT 0.5 mL IM, TIG 250 units IM, and intravenous penicillin 600,000 units every 6 hours

D. Admit to the ICU to observe for muscle spasm and administer 2500 units TIG IM and 0.5 mL tetanus toxoid IM in the opposite deltoid muscles

12.4 An 18-year-old man presents to the emergency department complaining of right ear pain after sustaining a cut on his ear during a wrestling match. On examination, you note some swelling and exposed cartilage of the right upper ear. Which of the following is a correct statement?

A. Exposed cartilage should be left undressed and the patient should be discharged with follow-up.

B. Hemostasis and evacuation of an auricular hematoma should not be performed because it promotes infection.

C. When repairing an ear laceration, make sure to avoid placing sutures in the cartilage and only include the perichondrium when approximating the skin edges.

D. Tetanus toxoid is not recommended for these types of injuries.

12.5 A 5-year-old boy is brought to the ED by his mom for a forehead laceration after hitting his head on the jungle gym. There was no loss of consciousness. The child is alert and active. He has a 3-cm forehead laceration which crosses the hairline. Which of the following is the most appropriate method of wound closure in this patient?

A. Shave the hair surrounding the laceration and close with interrupted sutures.

B. Close with staples.

C. Close with steri-strips.

D. Close with interrupted sutures.

ANSWERS

12.1 **E.** Lining up the vermillion border is by far the most challenging to repair because even a 1-mm discrepancy is noticeable. Injuries to the scalp usually can be repaired with sutures or staples, and are rarely cosmetically debilitating. Injuries to the neck, forehead, and cheek require approximation of wound edges to ensure appropriate wound healing; however, these lacerations do not require meticulous approximation as seen in repair of the vermillion boarder. It is important to point out to your patients that all laceration repairs will leave a scar.

12.2 **C.** The patient likely developed a septal hematoma, which caused necrosis to the septum and the subsequent communication between the nasal passageways. Cocaine is associated with septal perforation secondary to its vasoconstrictive properties. There is no indication that this patient used cocaine. The use of epinephrine on the nose is contraindicated because of the potential for necrosis. However, epinephrine is not associated with septal perforation. Although post-traumatic stress syndrome can be debilitating for patients, it does not cause septal perforation.

12.3 **A.** Because the patient likely received a full series of immunizations, but does not remember the last booster, he should receive tetanus toxoid 0.5 mL IM. TIG should be reserved for the following patients: those who do not know their immunization status or know that they never received the full series of three shots and sustained a contaminated wound. Admission to the ICU should be considered if the patient has signs of tetanus, such as muscle spasm or lockjaw.

12.4 **C.** Small superficial ear lacerations should be repaired with uninterrupted sutures. Do not place sutures in lacerated ear cartilage. Sutures placed in the skin surrounding these wounds in the cartilage should include the perichondrium (thin tissue layer overlying the cartilage). This method allows the approximation at the cartilage edges. Exposed cartilage should be covered or dressed to prevent infection and necrosis. Hemostasis and evacuation of an auricular hematoma is recommended to prevent the development of "cauliflower ear." All patients with interruptions in the skin should be offered tetanus prophylaxis if their immunization status is not current.

12.5 **D.** Facial lacerations should be closed with a **6-0 nonabsorbable suture** in interrupted fashion. Staples do not provide the desired cosmesis for a facial wound repair. Staples are more appropriate for scalp lacerations. Steri-strips can be used in very small skin openings with minimal tension. They will not provide the tensile strength required for this patient's wound closure. Shaving surrounding hair increases the risk of infection and is not recommended.

CLINICAL PEARLS

▶ The vermillion border must be precisely approximated because of its important cosmetic characteristics. Even a small discrepancy in lining up of the tissue is noticeable.

▶ The facial nerve courses from the mastoid region across the cheek area and is prone to injury in facial lacerations. Care must be taken to identify an injury to the nerve to prevent permanent deformity.

▶ Complex lacerations of the face, eye, ear, nose, and mouth, including lacerations associated with focal neurologic deficits (eg, facial droop or ptosis) should be cared for with expert consultation such as an ENT surgeon or ophthalmologist.

▶ Meticulous hemostasis is important in repairing ear lacerations to avoid "cauliflower ear."

▶ Tetanus is an acute disease of wound contamination, which is largely preventable with immunization. All patients at risk for tetanus and not up-to-date on their tetanus vaccination should receive tetanus immunoglobulin or tetanus toxoid.

REFERENCES

Brown DJ, Jaffe JE, Henson JK. Advanced laceration management. *Emerg Med Clin N Am.* 2007:25; 83-99.

Brunicardi FC, Anderson DK, Billiar TR, et al, eds. *Schwartz's Principles of Surgery.* 9th ed. New York, NY: McGraw-Hill; 2009.

Kretsinger K, Broder KR, Cortese MM, et al. Preventing tetanus, diphtheria, and pertussis among adults: use of tetanus toxoid and acellular pertussis vaccine recommendations of the Advisory Committee on Immunization Practices (ACIP) and recommendation of ACIP, supported by the Healthcare Infection Control Practices Advisory Committee (HICPAC), for use of TDaP among health-care personnel. *MMWR Recomm Rep.* Dec 15, 2006 Dec 15:55 (RR-17): 1-37.

Roberts JR, Hedges JR. *Clinical Procedures in Emergency Medicine.* 5th ed. Philadelphia, PA: Saunders; 2010.

Tintinalli JE, Kelen GD, Stapczynski JS, eds. *Emergency Medicine.* 7th ed. New York, NY: McGraw-Hill; 2004:302-304.

Updated recommendatioms for use of tetanus toxoid, reduced diphtheria toxoid and acellular pertussic (TDaP) vaccine from the Advisory Committee on Immunization Practices, 2010. MMWR. January 14, 2011;60(01)13-15.

A 15-year-old adolescent boy was cleaning some items in the shed in his backyard, when he saw a bat in middle of the shed. The bat bit the boy on his dominant hand, after which the teenager ran into the house. His parents brought the boy to the emergency department. His vital signs on arrival were a blood pressure of 115/70 mm Hg, heart rate of 105 beats per minute, respiratory rate of 14 breaths per minute, pulse oximetry of 99% on room air, and a temperature of 37.1°C (98.9°F). Inspection of the wound shows deep bite marks with a laceration close to the proximal interphalyngeal joint. The bat escaped after the boy was bitten and was not found.

▶ What is the most likely diagnosis?
▶ What is the next step in treatment?

ANSWERS TO CASE 13:

Rabies/Animal Bite

Summary: A teenager complains of a deep bite to his dominant hand by a bat acting strangely. The bite is fresh and the bat cannot be located.

- **Most likely diagnosis:** Unprovoked attack by a rabies-infected bat.

- **Best initial treatment:** Notify animal control to locate the animal, then clean the wound and administer both passive and active rabies immunization to the patient. Administer tetanus toxoid if not received within the last 5 years.

ANALYSIS

Objectives

1. Recognize that bat bites are a common vector for rabies.

2. Know the treatment of common bite injuries.

3. Know the clinical presentation of rabies.

4. Know the treatments for rabies and when treatment should be given.

5. Understand the basic principles of snakebite management.

Considerations

This 15-year-old teenager encountered a **bat exhibiting abnormal behavior.** The bat, normally a nocturnal animal, is active in the afternoon. This is suspicious for a rabies-infected bat. Other important considerations in this case are that the patient was **bit near a joint space,** the patient's **tetanus status,** and the possibility of **retained teeth.**

In this patient's case, postexposure prophylaxis for rabies and delayed primary closure to observe for infection are reasonable. **Postexposure prophylaxis** for rabies should include a combination of immediate, **passive (rabies immunoglobulin)** immunization and **active immunization** (human diploid cell vaccine). **Tetanus vaccine** should be administered if the patient has not received it **within the last 5 years.**

APPROACH TO:

Animal Bites

DEFINITIONS

HYDROPHOBIA: The violent contraction of respiratory, diaphragmatic, laryngeal, and pharyngeal muscles initiated by consumption of liquids.

VENOM: A specialized form of saliva that is rich in proteins, polypeptides, peptidases, and nucleases. Its effects can range from paralysis, digestion, or incapacitation to death.

CLINICAL APPROACH

General Bite Management

Good wound care is the mainstay of bite management. A detailed history of the bite including type of animal, whether provocation occurred, location of bite, and time since the bite, should be followed by a careful physical examination. Physical examination should focus on the patient's neurovascular status, the potential for tendon involvement, any evidence of cellulitis, and the potential for joint space violation. **The wound should be irrigated, tetanus booster updated if more than 5 years has elapsed since the last administration (see Case 12), and antibiotics administered if the bite is high risk for infection or already infected.** A radiograph should also be obtained to evaluate for a fracture and retained teeth. For bites with potential tendon injury, the involved extremity should be splinted. Simple bites of the trunk and extremities (except for hands and feet) less than 6 hours old can generally be closed primarily. Simple bites of the head and neck area less than 12 hours old also can be repaired primarily. However, puncture wounds, bites of the hand or foot, wounds more than 12 hours old, and infected tissues, are usually left open.

With any bite injury, the appropriate authorities should be notified to find the animal and observe it for abnormal behavior. Prior to arriving to the ED, any open wound or bite should be thoroughly washed with soap and water. In the ED, **irrigation of the wound with saline removes debris and lowers bacterial counts.** There is no added benefit to the addition of hydrogen peroxide or povidone iodine to the irrigant. Any foreign body or devitalized tissue should be removed. Administering prophylactic antibiotics in the case of simple bites is left to physician preference, as there is no conclusive evidence that it reduces infection rates.

The clenched-fist injury, also called a **"fight bite,"** is especially important to assess because a small bite injury may deeply embed bacteria into the joint spaces or tendon sheaths of the hand. This can lead to a serious infection. A radiograph to assess for fracture or foreign body should be performed. The wound should be irrigated, the tendons examined, and antibiotics administered. In cases of delayed evaluation, look for signs of infection including cellulitis, abscess formation, or tenosynovitis. Due to the high risk of infection, these cases typically require admission to the hospital for IV antibiotics or surgery.

Bacterial Infections

Dogs, cats, and humans account for almost all mammalian bite injuries. Oral flora in dogs and cats include *Staphylococcus aureus*, **Pasteurella spp,** *Capnocytophaga canimorsus*, *Streptococcus*, and oral anaerobes. Humans usually have mixed flora, including *S aureus*, *Haemophilus influenzae*, **Eikenella corrodens** and beta-lactamase–positive oral anaerobes. In cat bite wound infections, *P multocida* is the most commonly isolated bacteria. Human bite infections are typically polymicrobial. Good initial-choice antibiotics include amoxicillin–clavulanic acid, ticarcillin–clavulanic acid, ampicillin–sulbactam, or a second-generation cephalosporin. Duration of administration for established infections is **10 to 14 days and 3 to 5 days for prophylaxis**. Failed outpatient treatment of wound infections is an indication for admission and IV antibiotics.

Rabies

Rabies is a single-stranded ribonucleic acid (RNA) **rhabdovirus** that attacks the central nervous system causing an encephalomyelitis that is almost always fatal. It has a variable incubation period, averaging 1 to 2 months, but may be as short as 7 days or as long as 1 year. Clinical presentation begins with a **1- to 4-day prodrome** with fever, headache, malaise, nausea, emesis, and a productive cough. An encephalic stage follows with hyperactivity, excitation, agitation, and confusion. Brain stem dysfunction follows with cranial nerve involvement, excessive salivation, followed by coma and respiratory failure. **Hydrophobia** (the violent contraction of respiratory, diaphragmatic, laryngeal, and pharyngeal muscles initiated by consumption of liquids) is a late sign of infection.

A bite is the most common means of transmission of rabies. Although, animal vaccination programs have decreased the incidence of rabies, they have not completely eliminated it. Risk factors for transmission include unprovoked attacks, unknown or unobserved animals, or animals displaying unusual behavior. Animals with increased lacrimation, salivation, dilated irregular pupils, unusual behavior, or hydrophobia are particularly suspected. Bites to the face or hands confer the highest risk of rabies transmission, but any breakage of the skin can transmit the virus. Worldwide, in locations with incomplete animal vaccination, dogs are the most frequent vector for rabies transmission to humans. In the United States, dogs are largely rabies free. No cases have been recorded in animals having received two injections, but animals only receiving one vaccine have been infected. **Healthy dogs, cats, or ferrets that bite humans should be confined and observed for at least 10 days for signs of illness;** with any sign of illness, the animal should be euthanized and its head shipped refrigerated to a laboratory qualified to assess for rabies.

Rabies Prophylaxis

A thorough history and physical examination in the context of the geographical location will give important clues for treatment. Identification of the animal and observation will help guide treatment as described above. Preexposure prophylaxis with active vaccination may be given to individuals at risk (animal trainers, animal control field workers, etc). This does not obviate the need for postexposure prophylaxis. **Postexposure prophylaxis is indicated for any person possibly exposed to a rabid animal.** Postexposure prophylaxis is a medical urgency, not an emergency, but time is essential. Rabies immunoglobulin can give a rapid, **passive immunity that will last for 2 to 3 weeks.** Passive immunization with human rabies immunoglobulin 20 IU/kg should be injected around the wound site as soon as possible. Active immunization should then be given intramuscularly with a different syringe at a different site. The active vaccines include human diploid cell vaccine (HDCV), purified chick embryo cell vaccine (PCEC), and rabies vaccine adsorbed (RVA), and should be administered on days 0, 3, 7, and 14. Active immunization will lead to antibody formation in about 1 week and should last for several years.

Snakebites

Venomous snakes are found throughout the United States except in Maine, Alaska, and Hawaii. There are two main families of venomous species; the Crotalinae and the Elapidae. The Crotalinae, also called pit vipers because of the presence of a pitlike depression on their face, include rattlesnakes, copperheads, and water moccasins. The Elapidae includes the coral snakes.

Not every snakebite results in the release of venom into the victim; "dry bites" occur up to 20% of the time. When venom is injected, it usually occurs in subcutaneous tissue and is absorbed via the lymphatic and venous system. Clinical manifestations of envenomation will vary depending on the toxin, depth of envenomation, location of the bite, and size and underlying health of the victim. Pit viper envenomation ranges from minor local swelling and discomfort at the injection site to marked swelling, pain, blisters, bruising, and necrosis at the incision site; and systemic symptoms such as fasiculations, hypotension, and severe coagulopathy. In contrast, Elapid envenomation usually begins as minor pain at the incision with a delayed serious systemic reaction that may lead to respiratory distress secondary to neuromuscular weakness.

The primary objectives in snakebite management are to determine if envenomation occurred, to provide supportive therapy, to treat the local and systemic effects of envenomation, and to limit tissue loss and disability. If the species can be identified, the appropriate antivenin can be administered if required. Treatment of envenomations is also varied. If it is a "dry bite," general wound care is usually sufficient. Radiographs should be performed to evaluate for retained teeth. Signs of envenomation can be broadly classified into either **hematologic or neurologic.** Hematologic effects of envenomation include **disseminated intravascular coagulopathy, ecchymosis, and bleeding disorders.** If there are signs of envenomation, then laboratory studies including, but not limited to, clotting studies, liver enzymes, and complete blood counts with platelets are necessary. Giving blood products to an envenomated patient with a coagulopathy will not correct the problem. The circulating venom responsible for the coagulopathy is still present and will likely inactivate the blood products. Therefore, the mainstay in treatment in venom-induced coagulopathy is antivenin, preferably type specific, not blood products. Nonetheless, if the patient is bleeding, it is prudent to administer both antivenom and blood products. The most commonly available antivenom for treatment of North American Crotalid envenomations is **Crotalidae polyvalent immune Fab CroFab. Surgical debridement or fasciotomy in the setting of envenomation should not be done** as this may lead to further bleeding. Neurologic effects include weakness, **paresthesia, paralysis, confusion, and respiratory depression.** Asymptomatic patients who were bit by a pit viper should be observed for 8 to 12 hours after the bite. This should be extended to 24 hours for coral snakebites because of the absence of early symptoms. The local poison control center should be contacted early in all symptomatic snakebites and will be able to help with management and location of antivenin. The national phone number for the **poison control center is 1-800-222-1222.** While the American

Heart Association has recommended the use of pressure dressings in the treatment of snakebites, correct application of these is extremely difficult and incorrect application may result in harm. Their position is still being debated at this time.

COMPREHENSION QUESTIONS

Match the single best therapy (A to E) to the clinical scenarios in Questions 13.1 to 13.4.

A. Identify the species, clean and immobilize the site, and administer antivenin.

B. Clean bite site and treat with prophylactic antibiotics.

C. Clean site, observe animal, and watch for signs of secondary infection.

D. Clean the site and begin rabies prophylaxis with active and passive immunization.

E. Admit for radical surgical debridement in the operating room.

13.1 Your dog, who was immunized against rabies within the last year, bites your neighbor.

13.2 A woman arrives in your ED with a human bite to her breast that occurred earlier in the day. There is a small puncture wound and no signs of cellulitis.

13.3 A scoutmaster brings a boy scout to the ED with a snakebite to his left foot. He says he heard the snake's rattle just before it bit him. His entire foot is purple, swollen to his mid-calf, and very painful to the touch.

13.4 While raking leaves under his fruit tree at dusk, a man says a bird flew into his face. When he checked his face in the mirror he saw a bite mark under blood streaks.

ANSWERS

13.1 **C.** This is a low-risk bite. The dog is your housedog with a low risk of ever contracting rabies. You have it immunized every year and can observe it for 10 days. As always, clean the bite thoroughly and consider radiographs to be sure no broken teeth are in the wound or that the bone has been penetrated. Administer tetanus if indicated and watch for secondary bacterial infection. Prophylactic antibiotics are indicated.

13.2 **B.** Human bites have high rates of infectivity. This wound does not appear to be infected. Nonetheless, the wound should be cleaned and 3- to 5-day course of prophylactic antibiotics should be initiated. Human bites rarely lead to retained teeth so a radiograph is not indicated. If this bite occurred on the hand or across a joint space, a radiograph should be performed. Tetanus toxoid should be given if indicated. TDaP has now been approved for use in patients over 65 years old.

13.3 **A.** This is a high-risk snakebite. The authorities should immediately be notified to search for the snake. Although some percent of venomous snakebites fail to inject venom, this bite is clearly envenomed. The rapid swelling, pain, and discoloration demands immediate attention. First responders should immobilize the site and place constriction bands that *do not* obstruct arterial flow. The swelling is not a compartment syndrome unless elevated pressures are measured. **Avoid incisions and fasciotomies** or packing in ice. Immediate antivenin injection in and around the site should be a priority. Remember that species-specific antivenin is important and that administration time is critical. Best results are obtained within 4 hours. Mark the swelling every 15 minutes, evaluate coagulation profiles, electrocardiogram (ECG), renal function, and liver function, and consider ICU admission to ensure adequate perfusion and to avoid disseminated intravascular coagulation (DIC). An index of antivenin can be obtained from the American Zoo and Aquarium Association (301-562-0777) as well as your local poison control center (**800-222-1222**).

13.4 **D.** This injury is at high risk for rabies transmission. Dusk is the usual time for bat activity, and although this man did not feel a bite, he discovered bite marks under his injury site. Bats carry high rates of rabies and this man was bitten on the face. Because the animal cannot be examined, immediate passive and active immunization should be initiated and tetanus administered, if indicated. As always, watch for secondary bacterial infection and update his tetanus status if it has been more than 5 years since his last immunization.

CLINICAL PEARLS

▶ In the United States, rabies transmission by dogs is nearly zero whereas transmission by bats is more often seen. Worldwide, dog transmission is still common.

▶ Rabies prophylaxis is indicated for uncaught wild animals and animals that start behaving abnormally.

▶ Bites that are more than 6 hours old are, in general, left open, because of the risk of infection.

▶ Snakebites should be treated like other bites with special attention paid to species identification and rapid administration of antivenin if required.

REFERENCES

Ball V, Younggren BN. Emergency management of difficult wounds: part I. *Emerg Med Clin North Am.* 2007;25:101-121.

Campbell BT, Corsi JM, Boneti C, et al. Pediatric snakebites: lessons learned from 114 cases. *J Pediatr Surg.* 2008;43(7):1338-1341.

Gold BS, Dart RC, Barish RA. Bites of venomous snakes. *N Engl J Med.* 2002;347(5):347-356.

Leung AK, Davies HD, Hon KL. Rabies: epidemiology, pathogenesis, and prophylaxis. *Adv Ther.* 2007;24(6):1340-1347.

Markenson D, Ferguson JD, Chameides L, et al. Part 13: First aid: 2010 American Heart Association and American Red Cross International consensus on first aid science with treatment recommendations. *Circulation.* 2010;122(16 Suppl 2):S582-S605.

Riley BD, Pizon AF, Ruha A. Snakes and other reptiles. In: *Goldfrank's Toxicologic Emergencies.* 9th ed. New York, NY: McGraw-Hill; 2010.

Rupprecht CE, Briggs D, Brown CM, et al. Use of a reduced (4-dose) vaccine schedule for postexposure prophylaxis to prevent human rabies. *MMWR Recomm Rep.* 2010; 59(RR-2):1-9.

Schalamon J, Ainoedhofer H, Singer G, et al. Analysis of dog bites in children who are younger than 17 years. *Pediatrics.* 2006;117(3):e374-e379.

A 59-year-old man with a history of hypertension presents to the emergency department (ED) with right-sided paralysis and aphasia. The patient's wife states he was in his normal state of health until one hour ago, when she heard a thud in the bathroom and walked in to find him collapsed on the floor. She immediately called emergency medical services, who transported the patient to your ED. En route, his fingerstick blood sugar was 108 mg/dL. On arrival in the ED, the patient is placed on monitors and an IV is established. His temperature is 36.8 °C (98.2°F), blood pressure is 169/93 mm Hg, heart rate is 86 beats per minute, and respiratory rate is 20 breaths per minute. The patient has a noticeable left-gaze preference and is verbally unresponsive, although he will follow simple commands such as raising his left thumb. He has a normal neurologic examination on the left, but on the right has a facial droop, no motor activity, decreased deep tendon reflexes (DTRs), and no sensation to light-touch.

► What is the most likely diagnosis?
► What is the most appropriate next step?
► What is the best therapy?

ANSWERS TO CASE 14:

Stroke

Summary: This is a 59-year-old man with acute onset of aphasia and right-sided paralysis 70 minutes prior to arrival in the ED.

- Most likely diagnosis: Stroke

- Most appropriate next step: CT scan of the head

- **Best therapy:** Thrombolytics

ANALYSIS

Objectives

1. Recognize the clinical findings of an acute stroke.

2. Understand the diagnostic and therapeutic approach to suspected stroke patients.

3. Be familiar with the National Institutes of Health (NIH) Stroke Scoring system.

Considerations

This 59-year-old man presents with an acute onset of focal neurologic deficits, which are typical for a cerebrovascular accident (CVA). Management priorities include: ABCs, stabilization of vitals, and a careful history and physical to distinguishing CVA from other etiologies which may present similarly, such as hypoglycemia. Non-enhanced CT is used to quickly determine whether the CVA is ischemic or hemorrhagic. If the event is ischemic, the patient may be a candidate for thrombolytic administration. The goal is to complete an evaluation and, if the patient is eligible, initiate treatment within 60 minutes of the patient's arrival to the ED.

APPROACH TO:

Suspected Stroke

DEFINITIONS

STROKE: The rapid development of the loss of brain function due to a disturbance in the blood vessels supplying the brain. It is also referred to as a cerebrovascular accident (CVA).

TRANSIENT ISCHEMIC ATTACK (TIA): Occurs when the blood supply to a particular area of the brain is interrupted. Often referred to as a "mini stroke," the symptoms of a TIA typically last minutes to hours, but resolve within 24 hours.

THROMBOLYTICS: Medications that act to degrade clots and are used in the treatment of myocardial infarctions, pulmonary embolisms, and strokes.

NATIONAL INSTITUTES OF HEALTH STROKE SCALE: A bedside assessment tool that provides a reproducible, quantitative measurement of the stroke-related neurologic deficit.

CLINICAL APPROACH

Stroke is a serious and common disorder, which affects over 795,000 persons in the United States each year. It remains the **third leading cause of death in the United States and the number one cause for disability.** Twenty percent of persons affected will die within 1 year. Many of the surviving victims are left with neurologic deficits and may be unable to care for themselves.

Stroke is a term that describes the loss of perfusion to a territory of the brain, resulting in ischemia and a corresponding loss of neurologic function. Symptoms vary widely depending on the type of infarct, the location, and the amount of brain involved (Tables 14–1 and 14–2). Strokes are classified as either **ischemic** or **hemorrhagic.** Eighty percent of strokes are ischemic—due to the blockage of a blood vessel secondary to thrombosis or embolism. They are generally seen in patients older than the age of 50 and present with the sudden onset of focal neurologic deficits. Hemorrhagic strokes are typically seen in younger patients and are due to intraparenchymal or subarachnoid cerebral vessel bleeding.

The **history and physical examination remains the cornerstone to evaluating stroke patients.** The symptoms may include weakness, numbness, or discoordination of the limbs or face, cranial nerve palsies, dysarthria, or cognitive impairments such as aphasia or neglect. It is *critical* to find out the **exact onset of stroke symptoms**

Table 14–1 • ISCHEMIC STROKE SYNDROMES	
Syndrome	Symptoms
Transient ischemic attack (TIA)	Neurological deficit resolving within 24 h; highly correlated with future thrombotic stroke
Dominant hemisphere	Contralateral numbness and weakness, contralateral visual field cut, gaze preference, dysarthria, aphasia
Nondominant hemisphere	Contralateral numbness and weakness, visual field cut, contalateral neglect, dysarthria
Anterior cerebral artery	Contralateral weakness (leg > arm); mild sensory deficits; dyspraxia
Middle cerebral artery	Contralateral numbness and weakness (face, arm > leg); aphasia (if dominant hemisphere)
Posterior cerebral artery	Lack of visual recognition; altered mental status with impaired memory; cortical blindness
Vertebrobasilar syndrome	Dizziness, vertigo; diplopia; dysphagia; ataxia; ipsilateral cranial nerve palsies; contralateral weakness (crossed deficits)
Basilar artery occlusion	Quadriplegia; coma; locked-in syndrome (paralysis except upward gaze)
Lacunar infarct	Pure motor or sensory deficit

Table 14–2 • HEMORRHAGIC STROKE SYNDROMES	
Syndrome	Symptoms
Intracerebral hemorrhage	May be clinically indistinguishable from infarction; contralateral numbness and weakness; aphasia, neglect (depending on hemisphere); headache, vomiting, lethargy, marked hypertension more common
Cerebellar hemorrhage	Sudden onset of dizziness, vomiting, truncal instability, gaze palsies, stupor

as thrombolytics can only be given **within a 4.5-hour window from the onset of symptoms.** If the patient is unable to communicate or awoke with symptoms, the physician must determine when the patient was last awake and "normal."

Strokes are more common in the elderly (75% occur in patients older than 75 years), males, and African Americans. Other **risk factors** for stroke include a history of **transient ischemic attack (TIA)** or **previous stroke, hypertension, atherosclerosis, cardiac disease** (eg, atrial fibrillation, myocardial infarction, valvular disease), **diabetes, carotid stenosis, dyslipidemia, hypercoagulable states, tobacco** and **alcohol use.**

It is possible, although challenging, to **clinically infer the location of the anatomic insult** to the clinical presentation by correlating symptoms with circulatory region (Figure 14–1). For instance, aphasia usually corresponds to a left hemispheric stroke; neglect generally indicates a right hemispheric stroke; crossed signs (eg, right-sided facial droop with left-sided extremity weakness) typically indicate brainstem involvement.

The evaluation should include the use of **the NIH Stroke Scale (NIHSS)** (Table 14–3), a standardized system that measures the level of impairment caused

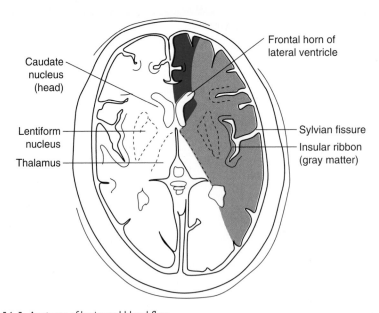

Figure 14–1. Anatomy of brain and blood flow.

Table 14–3 • NATIONAL INSTITUTES OF HEALTH STROKE SCORE

Category	Patient Response	Score
Level of consciousness questions (know month and age?)	Answers both questions correctly	0
	Answers one correctly	1
	Answers none correctly	2
Level of consciousness commands (patient instructed to open & close eyes and then to grip and release nonparetic hand)	Obeys both correctly	0
	Obeys one correctly	1
	Obeys none correctly	2
Best gaze (horizontal gaze tested)	Normal gaze	0
	Partial gaze palsy	1
	Forced deviation or total gaze paresis	2
Best visual (visual fields tested by confrontation)	No visual loss	0
	Partial hemianopsia	1
	Complete hemianopsia	2
	Bilateral hemianopsia (blind including cortical blindness)	3
Facial palsy (patient instructed to show teeth or raise eye brows or close eyes)	Normal symmetric movement	0
	Minor paralysis	1
	Partial paralysis	2
	Complete paralysis of one or both sides	3
Best motor arm Right _____ Left _____	No drift	
	Drift <10 s	
	Falls <10 s	
	No effort against gravity	
	No movement	
Best motor leg Right _____ Left _____	No drift	
	Drift <10 s	
	Falls <10 s	
	No effort against gravity	
	No movement	
Limb ataxia (finger-nose-finger and heel-toe bilaterally)	Absent	0
	Ataxia in one limb	1
	Ataxia in two limbs	2
Sensory (sensation or grimace to pinprick)	No sensory loss	0
	Mild sensory loss	1
	Severe sensory loss	2
Best language (describe picture, name items on sheet)	No aphasia, normal	0
	Mild to moderate aphasia	1
	Severe aphasia	2
	Mute, global aphasia	3
Dysarthria (read or repeat words from a sheet)	Normal	0
	Mild to moderate	1
	Severe	2

(Continued)

Table 14–3 • NATIONAL INSTITUTES OF HEALTH STROKE SCORE (CONTINUED)		
Category	Patient Response	Score
Extinction and Inattention	No abnormality	0
	Visual, tactile, spatial, or personal inattention or extinction to bilaeral simultaneous stimulation	1
	Profound hemi-attention or hemi-attention to more than one modality	2

Reproduced from the National Institutes of Health, 2000.

by stroke. It measures several aspects of brain function such as consciousness, vision, sensation, movement, speech, and language. A score above 20 to the maximal score of 42 represents a severe stroke. Current guidelines allow strokes with scores above 4 to be treated with tPA.

Many hospitals have a **"Stroke Team"** or a **"Code Stroke" protocol** that facilitates the prompt diagnosis and treatment of stroke patients as the treatment of stroke is highly time sensitive. The National Institute of Neurological Disorders and Stroke (NINDS) has established door-to-treatment time frames in responding to acute stroke. These include a physician evaluation within 10 minutes of arrival, specialist/neurologist notification within 15 minutes, CT of head within 25 minutes and CT interpretation within 45 minutes. For ischemic strokes, the guideline for the administration of rtPA (recombinant tissue-type plasminogen activator) in eligible patients is within 60 minutes, within the "golden hour" of stroke care (See Table 14-4).

Diagnostic Studies:

Most of the **diagnostic studies in acute stroke patients are used to exclude other etiologies for neurologic impairments** and identify possible contraindications to tPA administration. An oxygen saturation is needed to exclude hypoxia as etiology of neurologic impairments. Because cardiac abnormalities are common among stroke patients, an ECG should be obtained. The most common dysrhythmia is atrial fibrillation. Although further cardiovascular studies will ultimately be performed, they should be done as an inpatient so that the acute care of the patient is not delayed. Another critical bedside test that should be performed is a capillary blood glucose (CBG). **Hypoglycemia is a known mimicker of acute stroke** and this condition can be rapidly ruled out with a normal glucose level.

Blood tests usually include a complete blood count including platelets (platelets should also be above 100,000 per mm^3 to administer thrombolytics), coagulation studies, and cardiac markers. Coagulation studies are important on patient with anticoagulation who are supratheraputic and at higher risk for an intracerebral bleed.

Patients with suspected strokes should undergo **diagnostic imaging,** commonly a **non-contrast head CT scan.** Because of the difficulty in *clinically* differentiating a hemorrhagic from an ischemic stroke—the CT is vital for ruling out an intracerebral

Table 14–4 • CRITERIA FOR INTRAVENOUS THROMBOLYSIS[a] IN ISCHEMIC STROKE
INCLUSIONS
• Age 18 years or older
• Clinical criteria of ischemic stroke
• Time of onset well-established, <3 h
EXCLUSIONS
• Minor stroke symptoms
• Rapidly improving neurological signs
• Prior intracranial hemorrhage or intracranial neoplasm
• Arteriovenous malformation or aneurysm
• Blood glucose <50 mg/dL or >400 mg/dL
• Seizure at onset of stroke
• Gastrointestinal or genitourinary bleeding within preceding 21 days
• Arterial puncture at a noncompressible site or lumbar puncture within 1 week
• Recent myocardial infarction
• Major surgery within preceding 14 days
• Sustained pretreatment severe hypertension (systolic blood pressure >185 mm Hg, diastolic blood pressure >110 mm Hg)
• Previous stroke within past 90 days
• Previous head injury within past 90 days
• Current use of oral anticoagulant or prothrombin time >15 s or INR >1.7
• Use of heparin within preceding 48 h or prolonged partial thromboplastin time
• Platelet count <100,000/mm³

[a]*Recombinant tissue plasminogen activator (rtPA) should be used with caution in individuals with severe stroke symptoms, NIHSS > 22.*
Data from Adams HP, Brott TG, Furlon AJ, et al. Guidelines for thrombolytic therapy for acute stroke, Circulation. 1996;94:1167.

bleed, which is an absolute contraindication to thrombolytic therapy. **An early CT finding** in ischemic stroke is **loss of the grey-white differentiation** due to increased water concentration in ischemic tissues—leading to a loss of distinction among the basal ganglia nuclei, gyri swelling, and sulcal effacement. Another early CT finding is **increased density within the occluded vessel,** which represents the thrombus.

Other imaging modalities such as contrast-enhanced CT and MRI may equal CT's efficiency in detecting intracerebral hemorrhage. MRI is superior to CT for the demonstration of subacute and chronic hemorrhage, and gradient-echo MR can also detect other vascular lesions such as malforations and amyloid angiopathy. However, the length of these studies may delay the time-sensitive administration of tPA.

Differential Diagnoses

The differential for stroke is broad and may include:

Neurologic entities such as seizure/Todd's paralysis, complicated migraine headaches, nonconvulsive status epilepticus, flares of demyelinating disorders such as multiple sclerosis, or spinal cord lesions.

Toxic/metabolic abnormalities such as hypo- and hyperglycemia, hypo- or hypernatremia, drug overdose, and botulism.

Infectious etiologies such as systemic infection, Bell palsy, meningitis/encephalitis, Rocky Mountain spotted fever, and brain abscess.

Cardiac or vascular causes such as hypertensive encephalopathy, carotid/aortic/vertebral artery dissection, subarachnoid hemorrhage, cerebral vasculitis.

Other etiologies such as tumor, sickle cell cerebral crisis, depression or psychosis, and heat stroke.

Treatment

Stroke patients are managed as critically ill patients. Management imperatives include: assessment and stabilization of the **ABCs,** formal evaluation for possible **thrombolytic administration,** and addressing **comorbid conditions** such as hypertension.

Alteplase (intravenous recombinant tissue-type plasminogen activator: rtPa) may help restore tissue perfusion in ischemic stroke and is the only FDA approved thrombolytic for stroke. The NIH/National Institute of Neurological Disorders and Stroke (NINDS) study in 1995 found that **Alteplase improved functional outcomes at 3 months compared to placebo** if given within three hours of symptoms onset. In May 2009, the American Heart Association/American Stroke Association (AHA/ASA) guidelines for the administration of rtPA following acute stroke were revised to expand the window of treatment from 3 hours to 4.5 hours to provide more patients with an opportunity to receive benefit from this effective therapy.

Recent studies have suggested that there may be a longer therapeutic window for the administration of thrombolytics. However, **earlier administration is always better as "time is brain"—nervous tissue is lost as the stroke progresses.** rtPa is usually administered 0.9 mg/kg with a maximum dose of 90 mg, with 10% of the dose administered as an IV bolus and the remainder infused over 60 minutes. Furthermore, neither heparin nor aspirin is used during the initial 24 hours. However, thrombolytics should not be withheld from a patient who has recently taken aspirin. Additionally, endovascular therapies such as intra-arterial and mechanical thrombolysis are being used for a subset of patients with acute ischemic stroke. See Table 14–4.

Elevated blood pressures are generally left untreated to maintain cerebral perfusion pressure. However, systolic blood pressure >220 mm Hg and diastolic blood pressures >120 mm Hg are best treated with easily titratable agents such as IV labetalol and nitrates. The blood pressure should not be lowered more than 25 percent of the presenting mean arterial blood pressure. The treated blood pressure should be below 185/110 mm Hg for rTPA administration.

Treatment of hemorrhagic stroke is different and includes blood pressure control with antihypertensives such as nimodipine, possibly reversing any anticoagulation with cryoprecipitate or platelets, and consultation with a hematologist and neurosurgeon.

COMPREHENSION QUESTIONS

14.1 A 58-year-old man experienced a neurologic deficit and is diagnosed as having a stroke. Which of the following is the most likely etiology?

A. Ischemic

B. Hemorrhagic

C. Drug-induced

D. Trauma-induced

E. Metabolic-related

14.2 An 80-year-old man is being evaluated for possible thrombolytic therapy after presenting with 2 hours of right arm weakness and aphasia. Which of the following is a contraindication for thrombolytic therapy?

A. Bilateral cerebral infarct

B. Hemorrhagic stroke

C. Hypertension-related stroke

D. Age of 80 years

14.3 An otherwise healthy 65-year-old woman is taken to the ED with probable stroke. Which of the following are the most urgent diagnostic studies?

A. Coagulation studies

B. ECG and cardiac enzymes

C. Bedside blood glucose and CT scan of the head

D. MRI of the head with and without contrast

14.4 A 67-year-old woman is seen in the emergency room with left arm weakness and right facial droop. Her blood pressure is 180/105 mm Hg. Which of the following is the best management for the hypertension?

A. Lower the blood pressure to less than 160/80 mm Hg by giving a small dose of labetalol.

B. Lower the blood pressure to less than 120/80 mm Hg.

C. No intervention for her blood pressure, but continue to monitor.

D. Lower the blood pressure to below 160/80 mm Hg if she is eligible for tPA.

ANSWERS

14.1 **A.** Ischemia is the most common etiology of stroke (due to thrombosis, embolism, or hypoperfusion) and is responsible for up to 80% of strokes.

14.2 **B.** Indications for tPA administration include an ischemic stroke with a clearly defined time of onset, measurable neuralgic deficit, and a baseline CT with no evidence of intracranial hemorrhage. Contraindications for tPA therapy vary and include: seizure at the time of stroke, history of intracranial hemorrhage, persistent blood pressure >185/110 mm Hg despite antihypertensive therapy, recent surgery or GI bleed, recent MI, pregnancy, or elevated aPTT or INR due to heparin or warfarin use, platelet count <100,000, etc.

14.3 **C.** Bedside blood glucose and CT scan of the head are the most urgent diagnostic studies in evaluating possible stroke patients. Coagulation studies, a complete blood count or platelet count should not delay tPA administration unless the patient is taking anticoagulation or has suspected thrombocytopenia. Non-contrast head CT is generally the initial imaging study, not MRI, to exclude hemorrhage or tumor as a cause of neurologic deficits. Though MRI provides more information, its cost, limited availability, restricted patient access, and other contraindications such as patient claustrophobia or metal implants limit its use.

14.4 **C.** Emergency administration of antihypertensive agents should be withheld in acute stroke to maintain cerebral perfusion pressure, unless the blood pressure is greater than 220/120 mm Hg. Patients are eligible for tPA with BP < 185/110 mm Hg. If patients have concurrent conditions that require acute lowering of blood pressure such as aortic dissection, hypertensive encephalopathy, acute renal failure, or congestive heart failure, a reasonable goal is to lower their mean arterial pressure 15% to 25% within the first 24 hours.

CLINICAL PEARLS

▶ Strokes may present in a variety of ways, and the differential diagnosis of stroke is broad. Clinicians must take a careful history, including the time of onset of symptoms. The NIHSS measures the impairment due to stroke.

▶ A bedside glucose measurement and a CT scan of the head are the most urgent diagnostic studies in suspected stroke.

▶ Treatment is aimed at stabilizing the ABCs, evaluating for possible thrombolytic administration, and addressing comorbid conditions such as hypertension.

REFERENCES

Adams HP Jr, del Zoppo G, et al. American Heart Association; American Stroke Association Stroke Council; Clinical Cardiology Council; Cardiovascular Radiology and Intervention Council, and the Atherosclerotic Peripheral Vascular Disease and Quality of Care Outcomes in Research Interdisciplinary Working Groups. Guidelines for the early management of adults with ischemic stroke. *Stroke.* 2007;38:1655-1711.

Asimos AW. Code stroke: a state-of-the-art strategy for rapid assessment and treatment. *Emerg Med Prac.* 1999;1(2):1-24.

Del Zoppo GJ, Saver JL, Jauch EC, Adams HP Jr. Expansion of the time window for treatment of acute ischemic stroke with intravenous tissue plasminogen activator: a science advisory from the American Heart Association/American Stroke Association. *Stroke.* Aug 2009;40(8):2945-2948.

Diedler J, Ahmed N, Sykora M, et al. Safety of intravenous thrombolysis for acute ischemic stroke in patients receiving antiplatelet therapy at stroke onset. *Stroke.* Feb 2010;41(2):288-294.

Hacke W, Kaste M, Bluhmki E, et al. Thrombolysis with alteplase 3 to 4.5 hours after acute ischemic stroke. *N Engl J Med.* 2008;359(13):1317-1329.

Huang P, Khor GT, Chen CH, et al. Eligibility and rate of treatment for recombinant tissue plasminogen activator in acute ischemic stroke using different criteria. *Acad Emerg Med.* 2011;18(3):273-278.

Latchaw R, Alberts M, Lev M. Recomendations for imaging of acute ischemic stroke: a scientific statement from the American Heart Association. *Stroke.* 2009;40;3646-3678.

Lewandowski C, Barsan W. Treatment of acute ischemic stroke. *Ann Emerg Med.* 2001;37(2):202-216.

The National Institute of Neurological Disorders and Stroke rt-PA Stroke Study G. Generalized efficacy or tPA for acute stroke. *Stroke.* 1997;28:2119-2125.

The National Institute of Neurological Disorders and Stroke rt-PA Stroke Study G. Tissue plasminogen activator for acute ischemic stroke. *N Engl J Med.* 1995;333(24):1581-1587.

Tintinalli JE, Kelen GD, Stapczynski JS, eds. *Emergency Medicine.* 5th ed. New York, NY: McGraw-Hill; 2000:1430-1439.

U.S. Centers for Disease Control and Prevention and the Heart Disease and Stroke Statistics—2007 Update, published by the American Heart Association. Available at: http://www.strokecenter.org/patients/stats.htm. Accessed April, 2011.

A 64-year-old man is brought into the emergency department (ED) by his family after fainting at home. He was standing, dusting a bookshelf, when he fell backward onto the couch. He was noted to be pale and clammy during the incident, and recovered spontaneously in approximately 30 seconds. He does remember the moments just prior to and after the incident. He felt lightheaded and had palpitations just prior to falling, but does not describe any shortness of breath, chest pain, headache, nausea, diplopia, or loss of bowel or bladder control. His history includes a myocardial infarction 2 years prior. The patient has been taking his regular medicines as directed, which include aspirin, a β-blocker, and a cholesterol-lowering agent. His primary medical doctor has not recently started any new medicines or changed his doses. On presentation to the ED, the patient's vitals are blood pressure 143/93 mm Hg, heart rate of 75 beats per minute, respiratory rate of 18 breaths per minute, temperature of 37.1°C (98.8°F), and oxygen saturation of 97% on room air. His examination is significant for a cardiac gallop. No carotid bruits, neurological abnormalities, rectal bleeding, or orthostatic changes are noted. A 12-lead electrocardiogram (ECG) demonstrates a normal sinus rhythm at 75 beats per minute with no significant changes from a prior study 6 months earlier; the ECG reveals Q waves in leads II, III, and aVF. The patient now states he feels fine and would like to go home.

▶ What is the most likely diagnosis?
▶ What is your next step?

ANSWERS TO CASE 15:

Syncope

Summary: This is a 64-year-old man with a medical history that includes a myocardial infarction who presents with an episode of syncope. The patient has an ECG with inferior Q waves, but no acute changes at the time of presentation.

- **Most likely diagnosis:** Syncope, most likely caused by a cardiac dysrhythmia with spontaneous resolution

- **Next step:** Management of ABCs, intravenous access, and initiation of continuous cardiac monitoring

ANALYSIS

Objectives

1. Recognize worrisome historical and physical features of syncope.

2. Understand the emergency physician's (EP's) role in evaluation of patients with syncope, and the role of selective diagnostic testing.

3. Learn to recognize which patients need to be admitted to the hospital.

Considerations

Syncope has many etiologies that are often difficult to identify with certainty in the ED. The goal of the EP is to identify and treat any life threats. If there is no critical immediate treatment needed, the goal is then to risk stratify patients for the likelihood of an adverse outcome. The patient in this case is at high risk for a cardiac etiology of his syncope. This patient should be immediately placed on a cardiac monitor and receive an intravenous line. The physician should treat any abnormal findings. If the patient appears dehydrated, he should receive intravenous fluids. If a dysrhythmia exists (eg, ventricular tachycardia), it should be immediately addressed with either cardioversion or defibrillation. If the patient appears stable, the workup should proceed with the patient maintained on the cardiac monitor. The decision to admit or discharge the patient depends on many factors. However, if there is suspicion that there is a cardiac etiology for syncope, this patient should be admitted to a monitored hospital bed.

APPROACH TO:

Syncope

DEFINITIONS

SYNCOPE: A transient loss of consciousness with a corresponding loss of postural tone, with a spontaneous and full recovery.

PRESYNCOPE: A sensation that one is about to lose consciousness, usually with nonspecific symptoms consistent with a prodrome of syncope such as lightheadedness, weakness, dizziness, blurred vision, or nausea.

VASOVAGAL SYNCOPE: A form of neurocardiogenic syncope, which occurs in the setting of increased peripheral sympathetic activity and venous pooling.

CLINICAL APPROACH

Syncope is an extremely common presenting symptom to the ED, accounting for approximately 5% of all ED visits in this country. Between 1% and 6% of hospitalized patients are admitted for an evaluation of syncope. The list of potential etiologies of syncope is extensive; causes include cardiac, reflex-mediated, orthostatic (eg, postural hypotension caused by volume depletion, sepsis-related peripheral vasodilation, or medications), psychiatric, hormonal, neurologic, and idiopathic. Unnecessary or inappropriate ancillary testing can consume thousands of dollars per patient and increase ED length of stay. With a carefully taken history and physical examination, clinicians can better risk stratify patients and determine who needs to be admitted to the hospital for further evaluation and who can be safely discharged for outpatient workup.

Etiologies

Cardiac syncope refers to the loss of postural tone secondary to a sudden and dramatic fall in cardiac output. **Bradydysrhythmias, tachydysrhythmias,** heart block, and mechanisms that **disrupt outflow or preload** are the functional physiologic abnormalities that cause these sudden changes in blood flow and ultimately inadequate perfusion of the brain. Patients with various forms of organic heart disease (eg, aortic stenosis and hypertrophic cardiomyopathy), and those with coronary artery disease, congestive heart failure, ventricular hypertrophy, and myocarditis are at highest risk. Causes of bradydysrhythmias include sinus node disease, second/third-degree heart block, and pacemaker malfunction. Tachydysrhythmias include ventricular tachycardia, ventricular fibrillation, torsades de pointes, and supraventricular tachycardia of both nodal and atrial origin, some of which may be associated with conditions such as Wolfe-Parkinson-White syndrome, Brugada syndrome, or long QT syndrome. When syncope is precipitated by a tachydysrhythmia, patients may complain of palpitations. Mechanical etiologies such as pericardial tamponade and aortic dissection should be considered in causes of cardiac syncope as both entities will result in a significant fall in functional cardiac output. Massive pulmonary embolism must also be considered, as it can lead to syncope caused by right ventricular outflow obstruction which, in turn, leads to a fall in left-sided filling pressure. Right-sided ventricular strain and dilatation can also lead to dysrhythmia.

Reflex-mediated syncope, also known as situational syncope, includes **vasovagal, cough, micturition, defecation, emesis, swallow, Valsalva, and emotionally** (eg, fear, surprise, disgust) related syncope. Loss of consciousness and motor tone is caused by stimulation of the **vagal reflex,** resulting in transient bradycardia and hypotension. Warmth, nausea, lightheadedness, and the impending sense that often precedes loss of consciousness are common complaints of those affected by vagal syncope.

Carotid sinus disease or stimulation of overly sensitive baroreceptors in the neck (a tight collar) are other causes of sudden reflex-related syncope. These patients will often note a specific activity that is temporally related to their syncopal episodes (turning the head in a certain direction). A recent examination of the Framingham cohort found that patients who were clearly identified to have syncope of vasovagal etiology were not at any increased risk of cardiovascular morbidity or mortality. Unfortunately, making a firm diagnosis of vasovagal syncope in the setting of the ED is difficult, and it should be a diagnosis of exclusion.

Orthostasis (ie, a drop in systolic blood pressure of 20 mm Hg or more resulting from a **rapid change in body position** from a supine to more upright posture) is another common cause of syncope. Diaphoresis, lightheadedness, and graying of vision may suggest orthostatic syncope, and recurrence of these symptoms on standing is more significant than the actual numeric change in blood pressure. However, orthostasis may be present in up to 40% of patients older than the age of 70 who are asymptomatic. Orthostatic hypotension can be related to volume depletion, sepsis-related peripheral vascular dilation, medications, and autonomic instability, which can develop in a number of chronic illnesses such as diabetes, Parkinson disease, multiple sclerosis, and other neuromuscular disorders. Volume depletion secondary to sudden blood loss needs to be considered in all patients with syncope. Patients of all ages can develop a sudden gastrointestinal (GI) bleed and the initial blood flow can be occult because it is confined to the lower GI tract. Elderly patients can lose massive amounts of blood from a leaking or ruptured abdominal aortic aneurysm, with abdominal or flank pain as common associated complaints, but syncope alone can also be the presenting complaint. In the female patient of childbearing age, normal intrauterine or ruptured ectopic pregnancy may present with syncope. The former may cause orthostasis as a result of the normal cardiovascular changes associated with pregnancy, and the latter as the only manifestation of life-threatening hemorrhage.

Hypotension leading to syncope is not necessarily related to volume loss. Patients, particularly the elderly, may present with syncope as the first overt manifestation of sepsis. Hypotension in these patients is caused by relative lack of intravascular volume secondary to decreased vascular tone as part of the inflammatory response. Patients with a history of hypertension may have what appears to be a "normal" blood pressure when they are actually in a state of relative hypotension.

Medication, especially polypharmacy, a common problem in the elderly, is another important cause of syncope. **Antihypertensives, antidepressants, antianginals, analgesics, central nervous system depressants**, medications that can **prolong the QT interval** (eg, erythromycin, clarithromycin, haloperidol, amiodarone, droperidol, and others), **insulin, oral hypoglycemics, and recreational polypharmacy** are common culprits. Geriatric patients with complicated medical histories are particularly at risk, although a detailed ingestion history should be obtained from all patients presenting with syncope. One should look closely for recent additions or changes to a medication regimen, including over-the-counter medications.

Neurologic causes of **syncope** are **rare**, unless seizure is included in the differential diagnosis; seizure and syncope should be differentiated and thought of as discrete diagnoses. Seizure can usually be quickly identified by the history of witnessed seizure activity, especially if accompanied by a history of seizures in the past. It is also suggested by physical examination findings (eg, tongue biting, loss of bowel/bladder control) and especially the observation of a postictal state, which commonly resolves over a period from several minutes to many hours. **Brief tonic-clonic activity,** resulting not from a seizure focus, but from the transient hypoxia of the brain stem, which leads to loss of consciousness, may be associated with syncope. However, the duration of confusion or lethargy following the episode is short lived. The sudden onset of a severe headache associated with loss of consciousness suggests a subarachnoid hemorrhage as the cause of syncope. Other neurological causes of syncope include migraines, subclavian steal, and transient ischemic attack or stroke of the vertebrobasilar distribution.

Sometimes patients with **psychiatric disease** will present with the complaint of sudden loss of consciousness. The history of these patients may include several prior episodes of syncope. Typically, these incidents will present with **minimal physical trauma** and none of the signs or symptoms that are commonly associated with cardiac syncope. Anxiety, with or without hyperventilation, conversion disorder, somatization, panic attacks, and breath-holding spells are all manifestations of psychiatric illness that can cause syncope. However, psychiatric and emotional etiologies of syncope are considered a diagnosis of exclusion. This diagnosis should be considered only after appropriate laboratory or ancillary testing has ruled out more serious etiologies. Furthermore, it must be recognized that many of the most commonly prescribed **neuroleptics** cause **QT prolongation,** which in turn, can lead to ventricular dysrhythmia.

Diagnosis

Much to the frustration of patients and providers, the **underlying cause of the syncopal presentation is not elucidated in approximately half of patients who present to the ED with syncope.** Unfortunately, patients in this category represent a mixed population in which it is estimated that anywhere between 45% and 80% may have had a cardiac cause. Most of the young and otherwise healthy patients will be discharged home without a clearly defined cause for their loss of consciousness. Many of the elderly patients will be admitted for additional testing and observation. Of all the diagnostic tools available to physicians in the evaluation of syncope, a good thorough history, a physical examination, and ECG are the only level A recommendations from the American College of Emergency Physicians (ACEP). The information gathered from the history and physical examination alone will identify the potential cause of syncope in 45% of cases.

The goal of the initial evaluation is to find out exactly what happened to the patient. It is critical to ascertain a step-by-step history of the event. This includes getting a detailed account from any bystanders or family members, which can be valuable in making the correct diagnosis. The **history and complete physical examination,** combined with the **electrocardiogram,** form the preliminary workup of patients with syncope. Orthostatic blood pressure measurements should be obtained if orthostasis is likely.

This approach is often suggestive of a diagnosis in cases of vasovagal, situational, orthostatic, polypharmacy, and some cardiac-related syncope. Although vasovagal and situational syncope may be strongly suspected based upon the history, a true diagnosis of vasovagal syncope requires additional testing not available in the ED. While vasovagal/situational syncope does occur in elderly patients, it is a diagnosis that cannot be safely relied upon in the ED unless the history is completely indicative (ie, syncope at the sight of blood) and there are no physical or diagnostic test findings that raise concern for more ominous causes. Elderly patients are also at risk for serious injuries such as hip fractures from even relatively benign causes of syncope. Although older patients admitted with a story consistent with vasovagal syncope may ultimately leave the hospital with that diagnosis, the risk profile of elderly patients as a whole almost always makes this a diagnosis that cannot be determined within the confines of the ED. However, young, healthy patients with histories consistent with vasovagal syncope may be approached with less diagnostic testing. Younger patients should be questioned regarding a family history of early cardiac or sudden death; although rare, certain genetic conditions such as Brugada syndrome, hypertrophic cardiomyopathy, and long QT syndrome may present with syncope.

Laboratory Tests

Although laboratory testing rarely elucidates the cause of the syncope, it can be helpful in a **limited number of situations.** Inexpensive laboratory tests include complete blood count (CBC) for blood loss, glucometer for hypoglycemia, and electrolytes and blood urea nitrogen/creatinine levels for dehydration. Toxicology screening for drug-related syncope is rarely helpful for the immediate evaluation and stabilization of the patient. Furthermore, assumption of a toxicologic cause should not deter the physician from performing a complete evaluation. A urinalysis is an inexpensive and useful screening test that can provide information about glucose, infection, the patient's state of hydration, and the presence or absence of ketones. **A urine pregnancy test should always be obtained in women of childbearing age,** because early pregnancy and ectopic pregnancy can present as syncope.

Management

Patients with history or examination findings suggestive of a particular pathology should undergo continuous **cardiac monitoring, echocardiography, Doppler vascular studies,** or contrast **computed tomography (CT) imaging.** Those patients with unexplained syncope and high-risk clinical features (eg, advanced age, abnormal electrocardiogram, previous cardiac history, exertional syncope) require admission for further investigation such as tread-mill testing, tilt-table testing, CT imaging of the head, cardiac enzymes, cardiac catheterization, and electrophysiologic studies.

While diagnosis and treatment are the goals in the evaluation of syncope, the decision tree for EM physicians is more focused than that of the specialist or outpatient physician (Figure 15–1). Unstable patients presenting after a syncopal episode, including those with persistent hypotension, life-threatening dysrhythmias, active blood loss, acute coronary syndromes, hemodynamically significant pulmonary emboli, and cardiac tamponade must be managed emergently. **The "ABC" (airway, breathing, circulation)** approach to the unstable patient applies in this scenario as in all presentations with unstable vital signs. History and physical examination in

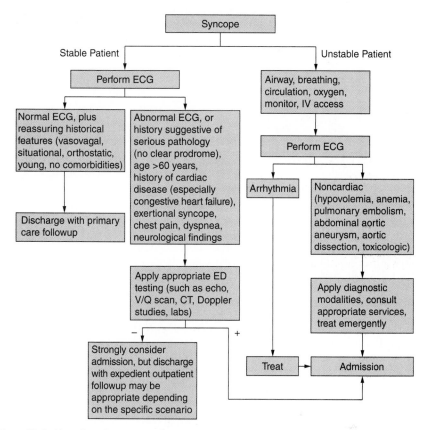

Figure 15–1. Algorithm of syncope evaluation.

the context of syncope should guide diagnostic thinking, but should not substitute for emergent management considerations.

Disposition

For the patient who presents after syncope but is hemodynamically normal at the time of presentation, the decision to admit versus discharge from the ED with outpatient follow-up is dependent on other clinical features suggesting that the patient is at high risk for a short-term adverse outcome.

Several studies have tried to aid the EM physician in identifying high-risk patients by using clinical decision rules (Table 15–1). The **San Francisco Syncope Rule,** the **OESIL** (Osservatorio Epidemiologico sulla Sincope nel Lazio), and the **ROSE** (Risk Stratification of Syncope in the Emergency Department) are decision rules that attempt to provide clinicians with patient characteristics associated with an increased likelihood for an adverse outcome The San Francisco Syncope rule uses five criteria: history of CHF, abnormal ECG, hematocrit <30, shortness of breath, and/or systolic BP of <90 mm Hg at triage, to predict who requires hospitalization. The OESIL score is based upon abnormal ECG, history of cardiac disease, age >65, and syncope without prodrome. The **ROSE** predictors are: BNP >300, positive fecal

Table 15–1 • SYNCOPE RULES						
	Symptoms	ECG	Laboratory	PMH	Vital Signs	Age
SFSR	SOB	Abnormal **ECG**	HCT<30	CHF	SBP <90	
OESIL	No prodrome	Abnormal **ECG**		Cardiac disease		>65
ROSE		Abnormal **ECG**	Hb<9 Fecal occult blood BNP>300		O_2 sat <94%	

Abbreviations: OESIL = Osservatorio Epidemiologico sulla Sincope nel Lazio; ROSE = Risk stratification of syncope in the emergency department.
Based on data from SFSR: San Francisco Syncope Rules.

occult blood, hemoglobin <9.0, oxygen saturation <94%, and Q waves present on ECG. The Rose rule is the first to incorporate a biochemical marker, BNP, into the criteria and claims a sensitivity and negative predictive value of 87.2% and 98.5%, respectively. An abnormal ECG is the only common thread in all three rule sets (Figure 15–2), although "abnormal" may be defined in a variety of ways. If the biochemical marker BNP in the ROSE criteria is considered a surrogate for a history of CHF, this reinforces that known cardiac disease is a factor associated with high-risk patients. Regardless of which rule set one considers, it should be recognized that decision tools and algorithms should never be used as a substitute for a full evaluation and individualized clinical judgment of all aspects of the patient's presentation. Many of these decision rules are still undergoing evaluation in an effort to gain validation. In fact, a recent analysis comparing the efficacy of risk stratification using the San Francisco and OESIL rule sets versus clinical judgment on short-term prognosis found that both rule sets had relatively low sensitivities. Having to use both rule sets would be needed to identify all patients who subsequently died, and the best results were obtained if a clinician used a combination of clinical knowledge with a rule set.

The **American College of Emergency Physicians (ACEP) clinical policy guidelines** emphasizes risk stratification of patients presenting with syncope in a similar fashion to those presenting with chest pain. It is generally accepted that historical or physical examination findings consistent with heart failure, structural or coronary heart disease, as well as an abnormal ECG are linked with high risk of poor outcome. Advancing age is coupled with a continuum of growing cardiovascular risk and should also be a consideration. It also bears mentioning that in the high-risk groups, however they are defined, presyncopal events should be evaluated and managed as syncope, because the etiologies are the same and are distinguished only by the degree of hypoperfusion of the brain. The younger patient with no comorbidities, reassuring first-time symptoms, and a normal electrocardiogram can usually be discharged from the ED. Referral to a primary medical doctor should be made for coordination of any outpatient studies that may be warranted in the evaluation of recurring syncope. Patients with specific job-related concerns, such as heavy machine operators, pilots, or physicians, may require more expeditious referral and notification of the appropriate State authorities. **Even benign causes of syncope, such as vasovagal syncope, can be fatal when the patient is driving.**

Predictor Variables of Risk Rules

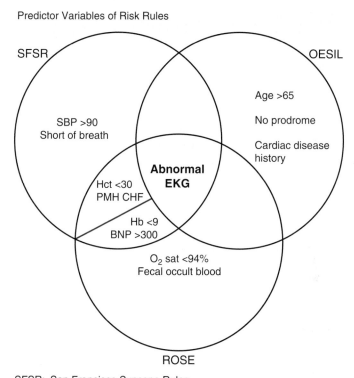

SFSR

OESIL

SBP >90
Short of breath

Age >65

No prodrome

Cardiac disease
history

**Abnormal
EKG**

Hct <30
PMH CHF

Hb <9
BNP >300

O₂ sat <94%
Fecal occult blood

ROSE

SFSR: San Francisco Syncope Rules
OESIL: Osservatorio Epidemiologico sulla Sincope nel Lazio
ROSE: Risk Stratification of Syncope in the Emergency Department

Figure 15–2. Predictor variables of risk rules.

COMPREHENSION QUESTIONS

15.1 A 37-year-old man is brought into the ED because he passed out at work. He denies any prodromal symptoms. Family history is negative for sudden cardiac death. In the ED, his BP lying down is 125/75 mm Hg, heart rate is 75 beats per minute, and respiratory rate is 14 breaths per minute. The patient's blood pressure and heart rate standing are 120/75 mm Hg and 77 beats per minute, respectively. His ECG shows a sinus rhythm with a rate of 72. Physical examination does not reveal any abnormal findings. Currently, he is lucid and has no neurologic abnormalities. After a complete evaluation of this patient, which of the following is the most common etiology of syncope?

A. Dysrhythmia

B. Orthostasis

C. Idiopathic

D. Situational

15.2 A 35-year-old woman presents to the ED complaining of feeling light-headedness. She noticed some vaginal bleeding earlier in the day. Her blood pressure is 85/53 mm Hg, heart rate is 130 beats per minute, and respiratory rate is 18 breaths per minute. Which of the following is the most appropriate next step in management?

A. Obtain a urine pregnancy test.

B. Obtain a serum quantitative beta human chorionic gonadotropin (β-hCG).

C. Obtain immediate IV access and begin fluid resuscitation.

D. Obtain **stat** OB/GYN consult.

15.3 A 21-year-old man is brought to the ED after collapsing to the ground while playing basketball. He is alert and oriented, denies chest pain, difficulty breathing, or any other physical complaints. There was no trauma. He denies any past medical problems. Physical examination is unremarkable. Which of the following elements on his ECG is concerning for a life-threatening cause of syncope?

A. Heart rate of 55

B. P-wave inversion in lead aVR

C. Sinus arrhythmia

D. QTc of 495 msec

15.4 A 72-year-old man is brought to the ED by paramedics after passing out at the supermarket. His syncopal episode was witnessed by shoppers who stated the patient collapsed, hitting his head. The patient is currently alert and oriented, and denies any persistent symptoms. His past medical history is significant for carotid stenosis, for which he takes aspirin and clopidogrel. What is most appropriate next step in the management of this patient?

A. Head CT scan

B. Order a carotid duplex ultrasound

C. Obtain an ECG

D. Chest radiograph

ANSWERS

15.1 **C.** Idiopathic. Approximately 50% of all patients with a presenting complaint of syncope will not have a definitive cause. Cardiac causes of syncope (eg, dysrhythmia) are the most worrisome, because patients are at increased risk for sudden cardiac death. Situational syncope is a rare cause of syncope. It is a result of an abnormal autonomic reflex response to a physical stimulus. Some triggers of this response include coughing, swallowing, defecation, and micturition. The patient does not have evidence for orthostatic hypotension as demonstrated by his vital signs.

15.2 **C.** Obtain IV access and begin fluid resuscitation. Investigating the possibility of pregnancy, specifically ectopic pregnancy, is critical. However, initial stabilization of the patient takes precedence. Hypotension must be treated emergently with fluids. Obtaining a consult early in the patient's course is important. Definitive management will be in the operating room.

15.3 **D.** The upper level of normal for the corrected QT interval is approximately 440 msec for men and 460 msec for women. A finding of a prolonged QT interval should prompt a more thorough investigation into this patient's medications, family history, and potential electrolyte imbalances. Prolonged QT syndrome is associated with sudden death, especially in young athletes. Mild bradycardia alone in a young, healthy patient who has fully recovered from an episode of syncope is of little concern. P-wave inversion in lead aVR is a normal finding. Sinus arrhythmia is a normal variation in the RR interval with respiration.

15.4 **C.** Obtain an ECG. This patient has a high probability for a cardiac cause of his syncope. Initial management includes placing the patient on a cardiac monitor and obtaining an ECG to monitor for dysrhythmias. A head CT scan should be performed after an ECG is obtained. A carotid duplex ultrasound and chest radiograph may aid in the workup for syncope, but it is most important to first rule out a dysrhythmia.

CLINICAL PEARLS

▶ The primary goal of the EP in the evaluation of patients with syncope is to be able to identify those who are at high risk for morbidity and mortality.

▶ The causes of syncope are varied, and a successful diagnosis hinges on diligent history collection and appropriate use of diagnostic tools.

▶ Even the most experienced clinician will be unable to determine the cause of syncope in up to 50% of patients.

▶ Reassuring clinical signs in syncope are youth, a normal ECG, absence of comorbidities, and reassuring historical features.

▶ Unstable patients should be treated emergently and stabilized, first addressing the ABCs.

REFERENCES

American College of Emergency Physicians. Clinical policy: critical issues in the evaluation and management of patients presenting with syncope. *Ann Emerge Med.* 2007;49:431-444.

Carlson, MD. Syncope. In: *Harrison's Principles of Internal Medicine.* 17th ed. New York, NY: McGraw-Hill; 2008.

Colivicchi F, Ammirati F, Melina D, et al. Development and prospective validation of a risk stratification system for patients with syncope in the emergency department: the OESIL risk score. *Eur Heart J.* 2003;24:811.

De Lorenzo RA. Syncope. In: *Rosen's Emergency Medicine: Concepts and Clinical Practice.* 6th ed. St Louis, MO: Mosby; 2005.

Dipaola FCG, Perego F, Borella M, et al. San Francisco Syncope Rule, Osservatorio Epidemiologico sulla Sincope nel Lazio risk score, and clinical judgment in the assessment of short-term outcome of syncope. *Am J Emerg Med.* 2010;28:432-439.

Dovgalyuk J, Holstege C, Mattu A, Brady WJ. The electrocardiogram in the patient with syncope. *Am J Emerg Med.* 2007;25(6):688-701.

Huff JS, Decker WW, Quinn JV, et al; American College of Emergency Physicians. Clinical policy: critical issues in the evaluation and management of adult patients presenting to the ED with syncope. *Ann Emerg Med.* 2007;49:431-434.

Kessler C, Tristano JM, DeLorenzo R. The emergency department approach to syncope: evidence-based guidelines and prediction rules, *Emerg Med Clin N Am.* 2010; 28:487-500.

Linzer M, Yang EH, Estes NA, et al. Diagnosing syncope part 1: value of history, physical examination, and electrocardiography. *Ann Intern Med.* 1997;126(12):989-996.

Linzer M, Yang EH, Estes NA, et al. Diagnosing syncope part 2: unexplained syncope. *Ann Intern Med.* 1997;127(1):76-84.

Quinn, J. Syncope. In: *Tintinalli's Emergency Medicine: A Comprehensive Study Guide.* 7th ed. McGraw-Hill; 2011.

Quinn JV, Stiell IG, McDermott DA, et al. Derivation of the San Francisco syncope rule to predict patients with short-term serious outcomes. *Ann Emerg Med.* 2004;43:224-232.

Reed MJ, Newby DE, Coull AJ, et al. The ROSE (Risk Stratification of Syncope in the Emergency Department) Study. *J Am Coll Cardiol.* 2010;55 (8):713-721.

Schipper JL, WN Kapoor. Cardiac arrhythmias: diagnostic evaluation and management of patients with syncope. *Med Clin North Am.* 2001;85(2):423-456.

Serrano LA, Hess EP, Bellolio MF, et al. Accuracy and quality of clinical decision rules for syncope in the emergency department: a systematic review and meta-analysis. *Ann Emerg Med.* 2010;56(4):362-373.

Soteriades ES, Evans JC, Larson MG, et al. Incidence and prognosis of syncope. *New Engl J Med.* 2002;347:878-885.

Sun BC, Emond JA, Camargo CA Jr. Direct medical costs of syncope-related hospitalizations in the United States. *Am J Cardiol.* 2005;95(5):668-671.

A 34-year-old man presents to the emergency department (ED) complaining of shortness of breath and chest pain that he describes as right sided and increased with deep breathing. He states it started suddenly when he woke up and was worse with activity. He denies fever, chills, nausea, vomiting, or cough. He has a recent history of multiple gunshot wounds resulting in ongoing pain in his upper back and T-10 paraplegia. One week ago, he was discharged from the hospital to a rehabilitation facility. He is currently taking acetaminophen/hydrocodone and ibuprofen for his pain, which has increased with his physical therapy and occupational therapy. He is also taking hydrochlorothiazide and lisinopril for hypertension and fluoxetine for depression. He recently quit smoking tobacco since he was hospitalized and denies any alcohol or illicit drug use. On physical examination, he is an otherwise fit young man who appears slightly short of breath and uncomfortable. His heart rate is 101 beats per minute, his blood pressure is 110/78 mm Hg, and his respiratory rate is 26 breaths per minute. His pulse oximetry is 96% on 2 L of O_2 by nasal canula. His lungs are clear to auscultation. There is mild swelling of his left calf. He has no sensation in his lower extremities. Laboratory studies reveal a white blood cell count (WBC) of 10,000/mm^3. Hemoglobin, hematocrit, electrolytes, and renal function are all within normal limits. A 12-lead electrocardiogram (ECG) reveals a sinus rhythm at a rate of 103 beats per minute. His chest radiograph reveals minimal bibasilar atelectasis but no evidence of infiltrates or effusions.

▶ What is the most likely diagnosis?
▶ What is your next diagnostic step?

ANSWERS TO CASE 16:
Pulmonary Embolism

Summary: A 34-year-old man with hypertension, depression, and recent gunshot wounds resulting in T-10 paraplegia presents with dyspnea, pleuritic and right-sided chest pain, tachypnea, tachycardia, left calf swelling, and bibasilar atelectasis on chest radiography.

- **Most likely diagnosis:** Pulmonary embolism (PE) secondary to deep venous thrombosis (DVT) in the left lower extremity.

- **Screening and confirmatory studies:** For evaluation of PE, D-dimer level, venous duplex ultrasonography, ventilation-perfusion scan (V/Q scan), pulmonary CT angiography, and catheter pulmonary angiography are available and may be applied on a selective basis.

ANALYSIS

Objectives

1. Learn the clinical presentations of PE.

2. Learn to formulate reasonable diagnostic strategy for the diagnosis of pulmonary embolism in the emergency department setting.

3. Learn the sensitivity, specificity, and limitations of the D-dimer test and the contrast-enhanced helical computed tomography angiogram for the diagnosis of DVT and PE.

Considerations

This 34-year-old patient who has been immobilized has a primary risk factor for venous thromboembolism. The presentation of acute dyspnea, chest pain, borderline tachycardia, and unilateral lower extremity swelling in the absence of identifiable alternative cardiopulmonary disease place him in the high-risk category for a pulmonary embolism. An ECG in patients with suspected PE is generally helpful for identifying other etiologies of his symptoms such as ischemic heart disease, pericarditis, and dysrhythmias. In some instances, the ECG may reveal right-heart strain patterns that are more specific for the diagnosis of PE. Although nonspecific, sinus tachycardia is still the most frequent presenting ECG finding among patients with PE. Even 25% of patients with identified PE may have a normal ECG. The relatively normal chest radiograph is valuable in eliminating alternative diagnoses, such as pneumonia, pneumothorax, and congestive heart failure. An arterial blood gas can be used to assess patients with shortness of breath, but it is non-specific in the diagnosis of PE. Taking into consideration the clinical, radiographic, and ECG data, a presumptive diagnosis of PE can be made. The next steps in management include maintenance of cardiopulmonary stability, consideration of empiric anticoagulation therapy, and confirmation of the diagnosis.

APPROACH TO:
DVT and PE

DEFINITIONS

DEEP VENOUS THROMBOSIS: Formation of clot (thrombus) in a deep vein (a vein that accompanies an artery). Eighty to ninety percent of diagnosed PEs arise from a DVT of the lower extremity. However, thrombi of deep veins in the calf (tibial veins) are difficult to detect, but also much less likely to embolize than more proximal thrombi.

PULMONARY EMBOLISM: Blockages of the pulmonary arteries, most often caused by blood clots originating from deep veins in the legs or pelvis. In rare circumstances, air bubbles, fat droplets, amniotic fluid, clumps of parasites, or tumor cells may also cause a PE. Risk factors for thrombosis are related to Virchow triad of hypercoagulability, venous stasis, and venous injury.

D-DIMER ASSAY: Fibrin D-dimer is released into the circulation following degradation of cross-linked fibrin by plasmin. Multiple commercial assays are available that use a monoclonal antibody to detect the D-dimer fragment. The two most commonly used assays are the whole blood immunoagglutination test (less accurate) and the quantitative plasma ELISA assay (more accurate). Elevated levels may indicate the presence of concurrent thrombus formation and degradation. Other conditions in which D-dimer elevation occurs include sepsis, recent myocardial infarction or stroke (<10 days), recent surgery or trauma, disseminated intravascular coagulation, collagen vascular disease, metastatic cancer, pregnancy, hospitalized patients and liver disease. The D-dimer may be falsely negative if clot formation is greater than 72 hours before the blood is assayed. Conversely, it may be falsely positive since levels may remain elevated for as long as 2 years. In pregnancy, the upper limits of normal are increased with each trimester, but a true normal D-dimer should never be greater than 1000 µg/L.

VENOUS DUPLEX ULTRASONOGRAPHY: Ultrasound imaging modality combining direct visualization of veins with Doppler flow signal to assess luminal patency and compressibility of the deep venous system in the extremities and the presence of thrombosis. This imaging modality is most accurate for assessment of the iliac, femoral, and popliteal veins.

PERFUSION AND VENTILATION (V/Q) SCAN: Radioisotope used to identify ventilation-perfusion mismatches. Results are categorized into probability-ranked groups after taking into account of coexisting pulmonary pathology and the patient's overall clinical picture. Radiologists interpret V/Q scans as normal, low, intermediate or high probability for V/Q mismatch or PE in the right clinical setting. Unfortunately, many patients with known PE have nondiagnostic V/Q scans, and these low to intermediate probability scans have significant disagreement among interpreters. Current literature indicates its benefits primarily in renal failure when contrast may precipitate renal failure. V/Q scans may also be the test of choice for pregnant patients. It is reported that multidetector CT (MDCT) scanning has higher radiation exposure for the mother but lower fetal radiation exposure, whereas V/Q scan has lower maternal and higher fetal radiation exposure. Remy-Jardin recommends perfusion scintigraphy (Q) without ventilations scintigraphy (V), which significantly decreases fetal radiation exposure.

COMPUTED TOMOGRAPHY PULMONARY ANGIOGRAPHY (CTPA): Magnified CT imaging of the pulmonary vasculature obtained during the arterial phases of venous contrast injection. While highly specific for PE, the reported sensitivity is variable and ranges from 50% to 90%. The diagnostic sensitivity is higher for centrally located PE but reduced for subsegmental clots. The Prospective Investigation of Pulmonary Embolism Diagnosis II (PIOPED II) study suggests that CTPA identifies more PE than V/Q scanning, but these may be false-positives or clots that do not require anticoagulation. The diagnostic accuracy is also related to observer expertise. The initiation of multidetector CT scanning has greatly improved imaging of central, segmental, and subsegmental arteries. An advantage of this modality is its ability to detect alternative diagnoses. Pulmonary MDCT angiography has a reported sensitivity of 83% and a specificity of 96% in PIOPED II.

PULMONARY ANGIOGRAPHY: Imaging involving intravascular contrast injection and fluoroscopy to determine patency of the pulmonary arterial vasculature. Although once considered the gold standard for diagnosing PE, this test has largely been replaced by pulmonary CT angiography (CTA). Baile et al showed that these two tests had no difference in the detection of subsegmental sized PE. They concluded that pulmonary CTA and pulmonary angiography are comparable for detecting PE. Pulmonary angiography is invasive and is associated with increased morbidity and mortality when compared to CTA.

CLINICAL APPROACH

Deep Venous Thrombosis

Up to **60% of patients with untreated proximal DVT will develop PE;** consequently, accurate diagnosis of this condition is critical for emergency physicians. **Unfortunately, the clinical features of DVT are frequently nonspecific,** and may include pain, tenderness, swelling, edema, and erythema. The physical examination and thromboembolic risk factors (Table 16–1) are important in assessing the clinical suspicion (ie, pretest probability), and based on the pretest probability, clinical algorithm for the diagnosis of lower extremity DVT may be formulated (Figure 16–1).

Duplex ultrasound is the most common test used to evaluate for the presence of DVT. Its accuracy approaches 98% for proximal DVT detection, when an experienced operator performs the test. ELISA D-dimer can serve as a screening tool for DVT. In practice, a positive ELISA D-dimer is not of any clinical value. However, due to its high sensitivity, **a negative ELISA D-dimer suggests the absence of an acute thrombus.** In patients with low pretest probability and a negative ELISA D-dimer, the diagnosis of DVT can be ruled out. Venography is the traditional gold standard for DVT. However, due to its invasiveness, risk of reaction to contrast dye, and the advent of newer technologies that are just as accurate, venography is rarely used in clinical practice.

All patients diagnosed with a DVT at or above the popliteal level should be treated with anticoagulation. Treatment goals are directed toward the prevention

Table 16–1 • RISK FACTORS FOR VENOUS THROMBOEMBOLISM DISEASE		
Acquired Disorders	**Medical Conditions**	**Inherited Disorders**
Prior history of venous thromboembolism	Congestive heart failure	Factor V Leiden
Immobilization	Nephrotic syndrome	Protein C and S deficiency
Malignancy—active	Myocardial infarction	Antithrombin III deficiency
Obesity	Stroke	Other blood factor deficiencies
Trauma	Hyperviscosity syndrome	
Surgery—recent <4 wk	Crohn disease	
Pregnancy		
Smoking		
Central venous catheters		
Estrogen use		
Lupus anticoagulant		

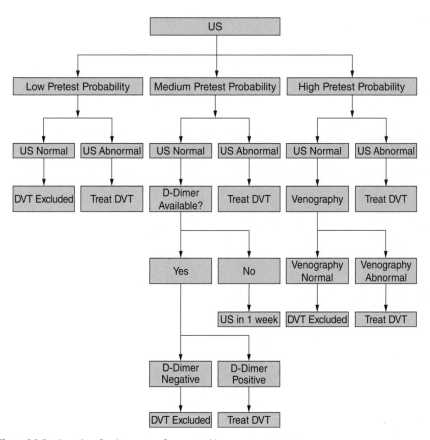

Figure 16–1. Algorithm for diagnosis of suspected lower extremity DVT.

of thrombus propagation and embolization. In patients with extensive DVT that involves the iliac and femoral veins, the use of thrombolytic therapy should be considered to help minimize the postphlebitic sequelae. For most patients, acute management consists of anticoagulation with unfractionated heparin (UFH) or low-molecular-weight heparin (LMWH). When UFH therapy is selected, it is vital to achieve therapeutic levels rapidly. When this is accomplished within 24 hours, the DVT recurrence rate is 4% to 6%, compared to 23% when therapeutic levels are delayed. LMWH can be administered for the treatment of DVT with or without PE. **Enoxaparin is a commonly used LMWH** (Table 16–2). Patients developing recurrent DVT during optimal anticoagulation therapy should undergo evaluation for hypercoagulability conditions and be considered for inferior vena cava (IVC) filter placement (eg, Greenfield filter). **IVC filters are also useful for individuals with contraindications to anticoagulation. However, these filters present their own risks for developing thrombosis and PE and have limited effect over time.**

Pulmonary Embolism

Few common medical conditions are as difficult to diagnose as PE. The majority of patients have dyspnea and chest pain at presentation, whereas cardiovascular collapse is observed in 10% of the patients. Symptoms of PE include sudden onset **cough** (3%-55%), blood-streaked sputum (3%-40%), sudden onset of **dyspnea at rest or with exertion** (75%), splinting of ribs with breathing, **chest pain** (50%-85%), and **diaphoresis** (25%-40%). Nonspecific signs of PE include **tachypnea** (50%-60%), **tachycardia** (25%-70%), **rales/crackles** (50%), and **low-grade fever** (7%-50%), the latter of which is suggestive of pulmonary infarction. Tachypnea is the most commonly reported sign in patients diagnosed with PE. Chest pain associated with PE is commonly pleurtitic in nature. The "classic triad" for PE (hemoptysis, dyspnea,

Table 16–2 • TREATMENT OPTIONS FOR DVT/PE			
Agent	**Loading Dose**	**Maintenance Dose**	**Monitoring of Levels**
Unfractionated Heparin (UFH)	5000 units (80 U/kg)	1000 units/h (18 U/kg/h)	Yes target PTT 50-90
Low-molecular-weight heparin's (LMWH)			
Enoxaparin	None	1.5 mg/kg SQ qd or 1 mg/kg SQ bid	None
Dalteparin	None	200 IU/kg SQ qd or 100 IU/kg SQ bid	None
Fondaparinux	None	<100 lbs 5 mg daily 110-220 lb 7.5 mg daily >220 lb 10 mg daily	None
Long-term oral therapy			
Warfarin[a]	5 mg PO qd	Varies	INR 2-3

[a]*Warfarin should always be administered in conjunction with either unfractionated or low molecular weight heparin until a therapeutic INR level is achieved.*

and chest pain) occurs in fewer than 20% of patients in whom PE is diagnosed. PE is occasionally diagnosed in young, active patients presenting to the ED complaining only of pleuritic chest pain. Such patients are often dismissed inappropriately with inadequate workups and nonspecific diagnoses such as musculoskeletal chest pain or pleurisy. Spontaneous onset of chest wall tenderness without a history of trauma is worrisome, because this may be the only physical finding of PE. In a recent study by Courtney et al, non–cancer-related throbophilia, pleuritic chest pain and family history of VTE increased the probablility of PE or DVT. Unusual clinical presentations of PE also include seizure, syncope, abdominal pain, high fever, productive cough, adult-onset asthma, new-onset supraventricular arrhythmias, or hiccups.

Diagnosis

The diagnosis of PE remains a difficult task despite the multitude of resources. Routine tests obtained in the ED, such as radiographs, ABGs, and ECG provide limited and nonspecific information. In an effort to make the correct diagnosis, EPs must calculate a pretest probability for PE. There are multiple scoring systems available that attempt to classify patients into low, intermediate, and high-risk categories. A commonly used scoring system is the **Wells criteria** (Table 16–3). Based on findings from the PIOPED study, clinicians correctly excluded pulmonary embolism 91% of the time in low-clinical-probability patients; however, in the intermediate- and high-probability patients, clinicians correctly diagnosed PE only 64% to 68% of the time. Because **clinical variables alone lack power to permit treatment decisions,** patients with intermediate to high probability must undergo further testing until the diagnosis is proven, ruled out, or an alternative diagnosis is identified.

The Pulmonary Embolism Rule-Out Criteria (PERC) is another commonly used clinical decision rule (Table 16–4). This rule only applies to those who are low risk for PE. If eight of the clinical criteria are met, then there is less than a 2% risk that the patient has a PE and no further work-up is needed.

Table 16–3 • WELLS CRITERIA FOR ASSESSMENT OF PRETEST PROBABILITY OF PULMONARY EMBOLISM		
Criterion		**Points**
Suspected DVT		3
An alternate diagnosis is less likely than PE		3
HR >100 beats/min		1.5
Immobilization or surgery in the previous 4 weeks		1.5
Previous DVT/PE		1.5
Hemoptysis		1
Malignancy (being treated currently or in the last 6 months)		1
Score Range (Points)	**Mean Probability of PE**	**Interpretation of Risk**
0-2	4%	Low
3-6	21%	Moderate
>6	67%	High

Data from Wells PS, Anderson DR, Rodger M, et al. Derivation of a simple clinical model to categorize patient's probability of pulmonary embolism: increasing the model's utility with the simpliRED D-dimer. Thromb Haemost. 2000;83:416-420.

Table 16–4 • PERC RULE CRITERIA
Age < 50 years
Pulse > 100 bpm
SaO$_2$ > 94%
No unilateral leg swelling
No hemoptysis
No recent trauma or surgery
No prior PE or DVT
No hormone use

The initial chest radiograph (CXR) in a patient with PE is abnormal in 76% to 90% of patients. However, there is no finding on chest radiograph that is diagnostic of PE. Rarely, the classic **Westermark sign** (peripheral lung vasoconstriction) and **Hampton hump** (pleural wedge-shaped density associated with pulmonary infarction) are seen. Serial CXRs obtained in a patient with PE are frequently associated with progression suggestive of atelectasis, pleural effusion, and elevated hemidiaphragm. After 2 to 3 days, the CXR in one-third of patients with PE demonstrates focal infiltrates mimicking pneumonia. Because of the variability in these findings, chest radiography is of limited use in diagnosing PE.

Interpretation of nuclear scintigraphic **ventilation-perfusion scanning (V/Q scan)** may **group patients into four result types: normal, low probability, indeterminant, and high probability.** Similar to the diagnosis of DVT, the clinical suspicion determines the pretest probability and the accuracy of V/Q scans. Therefore, the subsequent management following V/Q scans should be formulated on the basis of clinical impression and V/Q scan interpretations. One study reported that V/Q scan combined with chest radiography had the same diagnostic accuracy as pulmonary CTA and V/Q scanning.

High-resolution CT angiography has become the standard initial diagnostic test for the evaluation of high risk patients for PE. Additionally, MDCTA has largely replaced single-detector CT scanners. MDCTA, according to PIOPED II, has a sensitivity of 83% and a specificity of 96% for diagnosing PE. A negative pulmonary MDCTA can safely exclude a PE. It has a positive predictive value of 86% and a negative predictive value of 95%. Due to limitations of PIOPED II, these results may not apply to patients with renal failure, pregnant women, and critically ill patients.

The addition **of indirect CT venography (CTV)** was also investigated in PIOPED II. Although they reported a statistically insignificant increase in sensitivity (83%-90%), specificity was not changed. CTV increases the radiation exposure and has the equivalent diagnostic results as lower-extremity sonography. It should be used with caution in **younger patients** who have the greatest long-term risk of radiation exposure. It has the advantage of having the patient only undergo one test and getting information on the pulmonary and venous system. Remy-Jardin reported that the greatest benefit from the addition of CTV to CTA has been shown in sicker patients, in centers with less experience, and with older equipment.

In high pre-test clinical probability patients who have a negative MDCTA test for PE, further testing is recommended. These patients represent a discordant group—high risk but with a negative test. Options include repeat pulmonary MDCTA if there were technical problems with the first test, pulmonary angiography, V/Q scan, or lower extremity venous sonography.

Pulse oximetry and ABG measurements are insensitive in identifying PE and should never be used to direct diagnostic workup. Despite the common practice of obtaining ABGs in the workup of PE, multiple studies demonstrate that a normal PaO_2, normal PCO_2, and normal A-a oxygen gradient does not exclude the diagnosis of PE.

Many recent investigations have focused on the use of the D-dimer assay for PE and DVT diagnosis. D-dimer **is a cleavage product created by the degradation of cross-linked fibrin strands** by the fibrinolytic system. **The power of the** D-dimer **test is in its negative predictive value rather than its positive predictive value, provided a highly sensitive assay is chosen.** A normal D-dimer value is helpful for the exclusion of PE in patients with low pretest probability; however, because intravascular thrombosis may occur in conditions other than PE and DVT, the specificity of elevated D-dimer is limited. It is important to bear in mind that a combination of clinical history, physical examination findings, laboratory studies, and diagnostic investigations are frequently needed for the evaluation of high-risk patients. **In high-risk individuals, negative** D-dimer **assay alone cannot effectively rule out PE,** therefore imaging studies such as venous duplex ultrasonography, V/Q scan, CTPA, or pulmonary angiogram are needed to exclude the diagnosis.

Clinical Decision Making

Ultimately, it is the clinician's burden to combine the imaging and laboratory test results with clinical impression to determine whether treatment for DVT/PE is indicated. Figure 16–2 is a clinical pathway utilizing the Wells criteria for pretest probability to evaluate for PE. The treatment for pulmonary embolism is generally intravenous heparin therapy in conjunction with initiation of warfarin therapy (see Table 16–2). **Thrombolytic therapy** has been advocated for those individuals with a massive PE, such as those with **hypotension for whom mortality is as high as 20% to 30%. There are no conclusive studies that prove** a survival advantage for thrombolytic therapy in PE.

Clinical Characteristics	Score
Signs of DVT (leg swelling, pain, tenderness with palpation of deep veins)	3
Heart rate >100	1.5
Immobilization or surgery in previous 4 weeks	1.5
Previous DVT/PE	1.5
Hemoptysis	1
Malignancy	1
An alternative diagnosis less likely than PE	3
(Total Score: Low clinical suspicion <2; Moderate clinical suspicion 2-6; High suspicion ≥6)	

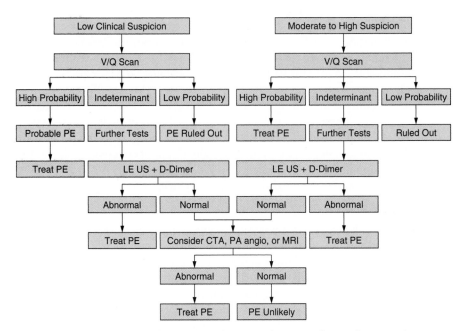

Figure 16–2. Diagnostic strategy for patients with suspected PE. (Data from Wells PS, Ginsberg JS, Anderson DR, et al. Use of a clinical model for safe management of patients with suspected pulmonary embolism. *Ann Intern Med. 1998;129(12):997-1005.*)

COMPREHENSION QUESTIONS

16.1 Which of the following statements regarding DVT is most accurate?

   A. A patient with thrombosis of the superficial femoral vein is never at risk for PE.

   B. Venography is the definitive test for the diagnosis of DVT.

   C. Thrombosis of the vena cava, subclavian veins, and right atrium are frequent sources of PE.

   D. Venous duplex ultrasonography is most useful in diagnosing DVT in the pelvic veins.

   E. Cancer successfully treated 5 years ago is associated with a higher risk for DVT.

16.2 A 52-year-old healthy man presents with a 3-day history of a pleuritic chest pain and SOB. He has normal vital signs and physical examination. Which test is most useful in ruling out this patient for pulmonary emboli?

   A. Electrocardiogram (ECG)

   B. Chest x-ray

   C. Arterial blood gas (ABG)

   D. D-dimer level

   E. Oxygen saturation

16.3 Which of the following patients with shortness of breath has the lowest clinical probability for PE?

   A. A 67-year-old man who underwent bilateral total knee replacements 2 weeks ago

   B. A 38-year-old man who underwent an uncomplicated open appendectomy 3 weeks ago

   C. A 35-year-old woman with a history of ovarian cancer

   D. A 35-year-old man with a history of a DVT 15 years ago, which occurred after an accident

   E. A 26-year-old woman who had an uncomplicated vaginal delivery 10 days ago

16.4 A 57-year-old man presents to the ED complaining of shortness of breath. The onset was sudden, and is associated with pleuritic chest pain. He was recently released from the hospital after being diagnosed with lymphoma. He had an indwelling catheter placed in his left subclavian vein the day before for chemotherapy administration. He was previously healthy without significant medical history. His vital signs are heart rate of 105 beats per minute, blood pressure 126/86 mm Hg, respiratory rate of 28 breaths per minute, O_2 saturation 100% on room air. The breath sounds are clear bilaterally. His heart sounds are normal without an S_3 or S_4 gallop. His left arm is mildly edematous, but otherwise painless, with a normal pulse examination. There is no swelling of his lower extremities and he has no pain with palpation of his calves. His catheter incision site is clean and intact. Which of the following studies is inappropriate for this patient?

A. Chest x-ray

B. ECG

C. Contrast CT scan of the chest

D. D-dimer assay

E. Duplex ultrasonography of the deep veins of the upper and lower extremities

ANSWERS

16.1 **B.** Venography is the gold standard for diagnosing thromboses of the deep veins of the extremities and is useful when duplex studies are inconclusive in high-risk, high-probability patients. Duplex ultrasonography combines direct visualization of the vein with Doppler flow signals. Part of the study relies on the examiner's ability to visualize compression of the veins to rule out an occluding thrombus. Because intra-abdominal and pelvic veins are difficult to compress, their evaluation by this method is limited. Most clinically significant PE derives from the large veins of the lower extremity, especially the iliofemoral veins that can embolize large clots to the pulmonary vasculature with disastrous hemodynamic consequences. Infrequent sources of PE can be central veins of the upper extremity, the vena cava, or even the right atrium. Despite its name, the superficial femoral vein is considered a deep vein (it accompanies the superficial femoral artery), and can be the source of clinically significant thromboemboli. Active cancer, rather than a history of treated cancer (>5 years) is associated with a higher risk of DVT.

16.2 **D.** ECG findings are often normal or nonspecific in patients with PE. ST-segment and T-wave abnormalities are the most common, but occasionally signs of right-heart stain may be noted, including peaked P waves in lead II (P pulmonale), right-bundle-branch block, supraventricular arrhythmias, and right-axis deviation. The classic ECG findings of PE are S wave in lead I, Q wave in lead III, and inverted T wave in lead III (S1Q3T3); however, this is rarely seen. ECGs may help to diagnose other etiologies of chest pain and shortness of breath such as pericarditis or tachydysrhythmias.

Chest radiographs are also usually normal. In severe PE, dilation of proximal pulmonary vessels with collapse of distal vasculature is noted (Westermark sign). Twenty-four to seventy-two hours after a PE, atelectasis and a focal infiltrate may be seen as a consequence of loss of surfactant. Pleural effusions may be noted, and, rarely, a triangular or rounded pleural-based infiltrate with its apex pointed to the hilum (Hampton hump) may be seen in the case of an infarction. ABG findings are often confusing, and abnormalities are usually a result of underlying pathology such as chronic obstructive pulmonary disease (COPD) or pneumonia. A low Po_2 in an otherwise healthy patient at risk for DVT/PE is more useful. O_2 saturation is rarely depressed and not very useful in the workup of PE. High sensitivity D-dimer levels are most useful for their negative predictive value in helping to rule out PE in low to moderate pretest-probability patients. It is a very sensitive, but non-specific test. A normal high sensitivity D-dimer level in a low to moderate pretest probability patient makes PE unlikely and further diagnostic workup is not indicated.

16.3   **B.** Malignancy, acquired or inherited hypercoagulable states, previous DVT or PE, immobility, and pregnancy are all risk factors for DVT and PE. Although surgery is a known risk factor, the length of the operation and time of post-operative immobility are factors that contribute to thrombosis. The patient who underwent a noncomplicated appendectomy is at minimal risk for a DVT. Patient with the bilateral knee replacement would have very limited mobility for a long period time putting him at risk for DVT and PE. Patient with ovarian cancer is at risk because of her malignancy. A patient with a previous DVT certainly has a greater lifetime risk for recurrence of a DVT. Patient had a normal vaginal delivery 10 days previously would have a higher risk of DVT than the general population.

16.4   **D.** This patient may very well have a PE, but other sources of his chest pain and shortness of breath must also be considered. An ECG will aid in the diagnosis of cardiac etiologies including heart attacks or arrhythmias. A chest x-ray will show other possible pulmonary processes, including pneumonia or a pneumothorax from the central line placement (as well as confirm the position of the line). Duplex ultrasonography will help examine the venous system for thromboses and possible sources of PE, including the deep veins of the upper extremity, because this patient now has an indwelling catheter that can be a source of thrombus formation. A D-dimer assay is not useful in this patient because he is a high-probability patient and this test should only be ordered in low-probability patients. CTA would be an appropriate test to order in this patient as it can diagnose a PE as well as other etiologies of his symptoms. Also, pulmonary angiography is not yet indicated in this patient until further diagnostic workup leads one to suspect a PE as the source of his symptoms with an otherwise negative workup. Pulmonary angiography is invasive, costly, time consuming, and not without its own complications, and should therefore be used judiciously.

CLINICAL PEARLS

▶ High clinical suspicion is the most important factor in determining the workup of PE, as its presentation is often elusive.

▶ High-sensitive D-dimer study is useful for its negative predictive value in excluding DVT and PE.

▶ V/Q scan is useful in risk-stratifying renal failure and possibly the pregnant patient with suspected PE.

▶ MDCTA has become the initial test of choice for patients with a high pre-test probability for PE and no contraindications.

▶ Eighty percent of PEs develop from DVTs involving the iliac, femoral, or popliteal veins.

REFERENCES

Anderson DR, Kahn SR, Rodger MA, et al. Computed tomographic pulmonary angiography vs. ventilation perfusion lung scanning in patients with suspected pulmonary embolism: a randomized controlled trial. *JAMA.* 2007;298(23):2743-2753.

Baile EM, King GG, Muller NL, et al. Spiral computed tomography is comparable to angiography for the diagnosis of pulmonary embolism. *Am J Respir Crit Care Med.* 2000;161(3 Pt 1):1010-5.

Courtney M, Kline J, et al. Clinical features from the history and physical examination that predict the presence of absence of pulmonary emobolism in symptomatic emergency department patients: results of a prospective, multi-center study. *Ann Emerg Med.* 2010; 55 (4):307-315.

Kline JA, et al. Prospective multicenter evaluation of the pulmonary embolism rule-out criteria. *J Thromb Haemost.* 2008;6:772-780.

Kline, JA, Runyon, MS. Pulmonary embolism and deep vein thrombosis. In: Marx JA, Hockberger RS, Walls RM, eds. *Rosen's Emergency Medicine: Concepts and Clinical Practice.* 6th ed. Philadelphia, PA: Mosby Elsevier; 2006.

Kline, JA. Pulmonary embolism. In: Tintinalli JE, Kelen GD, Stapczynski JS, eds. *Emergency Medicine: A Comprehensive Study Guide.* 6th ed. New York, NY: McGraw-Hill; 2004.

Rogers RL, Winters M, Mayo D. Pulmonary embolism: remember that patient you saw last night? *Emerg Med Pract.* 2004;6(6):1-20.

Rosen CL, Tracy JA. The diagnosis of lower extremity deep venous thrombosis. *Emerg Med Clin North Am.* 2001;19:895-912.

Sadigh G, Kelly A, Cronin P. Challenges, controversies, and hot topics in pulmonary embolism imaging. *AJR.* 2011:196(3);497-515.

Sadosty AT, Boie ET, Stead LG. Pulmonary embolism. *Emerg Med Clin North Am.* 2003;21(2):363-384.

Wells PS, Anderson DR, Rodger M, et al. Excluding pulmonary embolism at the bedside without diagnostic imaging: management of patients with suspected pulmonary embolism presenting to the emergency department by using a simple clinical model and D-dimer. *Ann Intern Med.* 2001;135(2):98-107.

A 55-year-old man is brought in to the emergency department (ED) by his wife for altered mental status (AMS). She states that for the past day, he has been confused and unsteady when he walks. The patient has a history of hypertension (HTN) and hyperlipidemia. He complains of headache and blurry vision. On examination, he is alert and oriented to person only. On fundoscopy, the optic discs appear hyperemic and swollen, with a loss of sharp margins. His neurologic examination is nonfocal and otherwise has a normal physical examination. The patient's vital signs are a blood pressure of 245/140 mm Hg, heart rate of 95 beats per minute, respiratory rate of 18 breaths per minute, oxygen saturation of 98% on room air and he is afebrile.

▶ What is the most likely diagnosis?
▶ What is the best management?

ANSWERS TO CASE 17:
Hypertensive Encephalopathy

Summary: 55-year-old man with a history of hypertension that presents with AMS, headache, and blurry vision with a blood pressure of 245/140 mm Hg. His physical examination is significant for bilateral papilledema and AMS.

- **Most likely diagnosis:** Hypertensive encephalopathy.

- **Best management:** Confirm the diagnosis by ruling out ischemic or hemorrhagic stroke, infection, and mass lesion. Lower blood pressure with intravenous (IV) medications and check for evidence of other end-organ damage.

ANALYSIS

Objectives

1. Identify the presentation of various hypertensive emergencies.

2. Recognize the difference between a hypertensive urgency and emergency.

3. Understand how to manage blood pressure in hypertensive emergencies.

Considerations

This is a 55-year-old man with AMS, papilledema, and severe hypertension. This presentation is most likely hypertensive encephalopathy, which is defined as the presence of neurologic abnormalities secondary to acute elevation in blood pressure. In the past, hypertensive encephalopathy and malignant hypertension have been used interchangeably. The latter term, however, was removed from the national blood pressure guidelines. Hypertensive encephalopathy is one of many forms of hypertensive emergency. It is critical for the physician to **manage the patient's blood pressure** if there is evidence of end-organ dysfunction. This is in contrast to blood pressure management in hypertensive urgency.

Once the patient's airway, breathing, and circulation (ABCs) are addressed, the first step in management is to **obtain a noncontrast head computed tomography (NCHCT)** to rule out the presence of mass lesion and hemorrhagic or ischemic stroke. Once these diagnoses are eliminated and the diagnosis of hypertensive encephalopathy is established, the focus should turn to lowering the blood pressure. **Intravenous antihypertensives should be administered to lower the patient's blood pressure.** The goal is not to normalize the blood pressure because this can lead to cerebral ischemia secondary to hypoperfusion. Instead, the goal is to **reduce the MAP by 20% to 25% over the first hour. Various antihypertensive agents are available to manage this disorder.** This is in contrast to typical blood pressure management in patients with long-standing hypertension who do not have acute end-organ damage. **Sodium nitroprusside, labetalol, and nicardipine are the first-line agents** for lowering blood pressure in the setting of hypertensive encephalopathy. Sodium nitroprusside is administered as an IV infusion starting at a rate of 0.25 µg/kg/min and can be increased to a maximum of 10 µg/kg/min. Labetalol is administered as an IV bolus of 20 mg, which can be repeated. It can also be administered as an IV infusion at a rate of 0.5 to 2.0 mg/min. Nicardipine is administered at 5 mg/h, and can be increased by 2.5 mg/h every 5 minutes to a maximum of 30 mg/h.

APPROACH TO:
Hypertensive Emergencies

DEFINITIONS

HYPERTENSION: Defined as blood pressure greater than or equal to 140/90 mm Hg.

HYPERTENSIVE EMERGENCY: The presence of acute end-organ damage in the setting of elevated blood pressure.

HYPERTENSIVE URGENCY: The presence of elevated blood pressure, without evidence of acute, ongoing end-organ damage. It requires urgent, but not emergent, blood pressure reduction.

HYPERTENSIVE ENCEPHALOPATHY: Transient neurologic symptoms associated with elevated blood pressure.

PREECLAMPSIA: Elevated blood pressure (140 mm Hg systolic or 90 mm Hg diastolic) in a pregnant patient accompanied by proteinuria, edema, or both occurring after 20 weeks of gestation. Preeclampsia in a patient with preexisting essential hypertension is diagnosed if systolic BP has increased by 30 mm Hg or if diastolic BP has increased by 15 mm Hg.

SEVERE PREECLAMPSIA: Severe hypertension, excess proteinuria, oliguria, cerebral or visual disturbances, pulmonary edema, impaired liver function, epigastric or right upper quadrant pain, thrombocytopenia or fetal growth restriction.

ECLAMPSIA: Seizure activity or coma unrelated to other cerebral conditions in a pregnant patient with preeclampsia.

CLINICAL APPROACH

Hypertension is found in 20% to 30% of adults in developed countries. Hypertension is more common in men than in women, and blood pressure seems to increase with age. The incidence of hypertension is 1.5 to 2.0 times greater in African Americans than in Caucasians. Hypertension is defined as two readings of greater than 140/90 mm Hg on two different occasions. Hypertensive emergencies will occur in approximately 1% of these individuals and account for approximately 2% to 3% of all ED visits. The most common risk factor in hypertensive emergencies is a history of hypertension.

Hypertensive urgencies are acute elevations in blood pressure **without** the **signs or symptoms of acute end-organ damage.** Previously, it was believed that hypertensive urgencies required immediate, aggressive blood pressure reduction.

However, no studies demonstrated a benefit of this management and the potential for harm exists. The elevated blood pressure in this circumstance should be reduced over days to weeks and the patient can be discharged from the ED and followed up in 24 to 48 hours as an outpatient.

The pathophysiology of hypertensive end-organ damage is not completely understood. Current theory holds that the acute rise in blood pressure leads to a series of vascular events, which causes end-organ damage. In hypertensive encephalopathy it is believed that the **acute rise in blood pressure causes endothelial cell dysfunction in the brain's vascular supply leading to cerebral edema.** Hypertensive encephalopathy can manifest clinically as visual changes, papilledema, focal neurologic deficits, and seizure. Hypertensive encephalopathy is an uncommon clinical entity. In order to establish the diagnosis, **more common causes of altered mental status must be ruled out,** including, but not limited to, meningitis, encephalitis, ischemic or hemorrhagic stroke, mass lesion, and toxic ingestion.

The diagnosis of **hypertensive emergency requires evidence of acute end-organ dysfunction that is attributable to an elevation in blood pressure.** This dysfunction can manifest through **multiple organ systems** and includes **acute myocardial infarction, aortic dissection, acute left ventricular failure,** acute pulmonary edema, **cerebral infarction or hemorrhage, acute renal failure, preeclampsia/eclampsia, symptomatic microangiopathic hemolytic anemia, and hypertensive encephalopathy.**

It is critical to **differentiate a hypertensive emergency from urgency.** This is accomplished through a focused history, physical examination, and appropriate ancillary tests. A detailed medical history must be obtained to determine if the patient has underlying renal, cardiac, or endocrine manifestations. The patient's current medications must be known and the possibility of ingestion of illicit drugs or other substances must be considered. In particular, obtaining history about the use of cocaine or other sympathomimetic substances (phenylephrine, monoamine oxidase inhibitors) is crucial as it significantly alters the treatment regimen (β-blockers must be avoided in the setting of sympathomimetic use). Elucidate any symptoms related to end-organ damage such as chest pain (myocardial infarction, aortic dissection), dyspnea (congestive heart failure, pulmonary edema), anuria (renal failure), visual changes (papilledema, retinal hemorrhages), altered mental status, and seizures. For patients more than 20 weeks pregnant or who recently gave birth, investigate symptoms of preeclampsia.

The physical examination should also assess for signs of end-organ damage. Fundoscopy can reveal papilledema, retinal hemorrhages, and exudates. Cardiovascular examination can identify signs of heart failure such as jugular venous distension, an S_3 gallop, pulmonary rales, and extremity edema. Neurologic examination should evaluate the mental status and signs of focal deficits.

Ancillary testing varies in the patient with hypertensive emergency depending on the patient's symptoms and which end-organ is affected. An ECG and cardiac enzymes should be obtained in patients suspected of having a myocardial infarction. Electrolytes including creatinine (Cr) and blood urea nitrogen (BUN), hemoglobin, and proteinuria and red blood cell casts on urinalysis may point toward renal failure or glomerulonephritis. A chest radiograph may aid in the diagnosis of congestive heart failure, pulmonary edema, and aortic dissection. A head CT scan should be obtained in all patients who present with altered mental status or a focal neurologic deficit in order to rule out a mass lesion, ischemic and hemorrhagic stroke.

Hypertensive Disease in Pregnancy

Preeclampsia is a unique form of hypertensive emergency, which occurs in pregnant patients. The exact pathophysiology is unknown but it is characterized by an abnormal vascular response to placental implantation. It is associated with increased systemic vascular resistance, activation of the coagulation system, platelet aggregation, and endothelial cell dysfunction. Predicting which patients will develop preeclampsia or eclampsia is difficult but epidemiologic studies have identified several risk factors including chronic hypertension and nulliparity.

Various organ systems can be affected, especially with severe elevation in blood pressure. Damage to the renal glomerular system leads to proteinuria and eventually, renal failure. Hepatic function is compromised and can lead to periportal hemorrhagic necrosis, subcapsular hematoma, or hepatic rupture. Disorders of coagulation may occur as hemolytic-uremic syndrome. A percentage of women suffering from preeclampsia go on to develop **HELLP syndrome** characterized by **H**emolytic anemia, **E**levated **L**iver enzymes and **L**ow **P**latelet count. Eclampsia is characterized by tonic-clonic seizures in addition to the above multiorgan system involvement. Vasospasm and impairment of the autoregulation system in the brain can cause cerebral edema, thrombosis, hemorrhage, blindness, seizure, or coma.

Management primarily focuses on stabilization of the mother through control of blood pressure and progression to eclampsia. Hydralazine is the antihypertensive agent of choice in preeclampsia and eclampsia. The goal should **not** be to normalize the blood pressure because this can lead to placental insufficiency (inadequate blood flow to the fetus). Target blood pressure is approximately 160/100 mm Hg. When hydralazine is ineffective, labetalol is the second-line medication for treating hypertension. **Delivery is the only definitive treatment for preeclampsia.** The gestational age and the severity of the disease must be considered so the risks and benefits of delivery versus expectant management can be assessed.

Management of Hypertensive Emergencies

Hypertensive emergency is a true medical emergency. Immediate evaluation and management is critical to limit morbidity and mortality. The patient should be placed on a cardiac monitor and an intravenous line should be started. After the ABCs are assessed and stabilized, treatment begins by making the patient comfortable, consequently eliminating contributing factors that may exacerbate hypertension such as pain, urinary retention, and hypoxia. Patients require immediate administration of antihypertensive medications to prevent irreversible end-organ damage (except in the case of acute ischemic stroke). As the elevation in blood pressure is being addressed, definitive measures should be taken to address any complications.

Understanding the concept of autoregulation is essential in the management of hypertensive emergencies. **Autoregulation** serves to maintain a constant, effective blood flow and perfusion to end organs, despite large variations in pressure. In the brain, autoregulation acts by adjusting cerebral blood flow within the brain microcirculation. Extensive studies of cerebral circulation demonstrate that cerebral blood flow (CBF) is maintained across wide variations of systemic blood pressure by vasoconstriction and vasodilatation in normotensive patients. Because it is difficult to measure CBF accurately, especially regional differences and requirements, the cerebral perfusion pressure (CPP) is used as a surrogate indicator for monitoring. The CPP is the pressure gradient required to perfuse the cerebral tissue. CPP is calculated as the difference between the mean arterial pressure (MAP) and the intracranial pressure (ICP):

$$MAP - ICP = CPP$$

where MAP can be approximated as: diastolic blood pressure + ([systolic blood pressure − diastolic blood pressure]). Local cellular oxygen demands can be met and regional cerebral blood flow maintained over a wide range of CPP (between 50 and 150 mm Hg in a normally functioning system).

In individuals with chronic hypertension, the CBF remains constant at higher CPP. However, if MAP, and thus CPP, drops into normal ranges, CBF precipitously declines leading to cerebral hypoperfusion. Although not as well studied, it is theorized that rapid, large declines in blood pressure in chronically hypertensive patients would lead to hypoperfusion of other end organs as well.

Common Antihypertensive Agents Used in Hypertensive Emergencies (Table 17–1)

Sodium nitroprusside: It is a potent peripheral vasodilator that decreases preload and afterload by dilating both arteries and veins that cause an immediate decrease in blood pressure. The recommended starting IV dose is 0.25 µg/kg/min and titrated to desired clinical response and blood pressure. Because of its rapid action and potency, intra-arterial monitoring is recommended when starting an infusion. Some drawbacks to this medication include its metabolism to a toxic cyanide compound. It is also associated with reflex tachycardia and coronary steal in the setting of acute coronary syndrome.

Labetalol: It is a selective alpha-1 adrenergic and nonselective beta-adrenergic blocker. It lowers systemic vascular resistance while maintaining renal, coronary, and cerebral blood flow. Unlike other vasodilators, labetalol causes minimal reflex tachycardia. It is contraindicated in patients with acute asthma, COPD, and heart failure, heart block, and sympathomimetic drug abuse (eg, cocaine). Intravenous boluses of labetalol require 2 to 5 minutes to begin lowering the blood pressure. If a single bolus of 20 mg does not achieve the desired blood pressure reduction after 10 minutes, either repeated boluses at twice the original dosage can be given or an IV infusion can be started and titrated to the desired blood pressure.

Esmolol: It is a short-acting selective beta-1 adrenergic blocker. It has a rapid onset and short duration of action. These properties make it easy to titrate. Esmolol is effective in blunting the reflex tachycardia induced by nitroprusside. It carries the same contraindications as other β-blockers (see Labetalol). Standard dosing is an IV bolus of 500 µg/kg followed by a continuous infusion of 50 µg/kg/min, which can be increased by 50 µg/kg/min every 4 to 5 minutes until the desired blood pressure is obtained.

Table 17–1 • COMMON ANTIHYPERTENSIVE AGENTS

Antihypertensive	Preferred Use in	Recommended Starting Dose	Side Effects and Contraindications
Sodium nitroprusside	Hypertensive encephalopathy, aortic dissection[a]	0.25-10 µg/kg/min IV gtt	Reflex tachycardia, coronary steal, methemoglobinemia, metabolized to cyanide
Nitroglycerin	Myocardial infarction, congestive heart failure, left ventricular dysfunction	5-100 µg/min IV gtt	Hypotension: contraindicated in severe aortic stenosis, left ventricular outflow obstruction, and inferior myocardial infarction
Nicardipine	Hypertensive encephalopathy, myocardial infarction, congestive heart failure, cerebral infarction/hemorrhage	5 mg/h IV gtt, increasing by 2.5 mg/h IV every 5 min to a max of 30 mg/h IV gtt	Hypotension: contraindicated in severe aortic stenosis. Reflex tachycardia
Labetalol	Hypertensive encephalopathy, myocardial infarction, preeclampsia/eclampsia, cerebral infarction/hemorrhage	20-80 mg IV bolus every 10 min, 0.5-2 mg/min IV gtt	Hypotension: contraindicated in acute asthma, COPD, acute CHF, heart block and sympathomimetic intoxication (eg, cocaine)
Esmolol	Hypertensive encephalopathy, myocardial infarction, eclampsia, cerebral infarction/hemorrhage	Loading dose 500 µg/kg IV over 1 min, 25-50 µg/kg/min IV gtt titrate every 10-20 min	See labetalol
Fenoldopam	Acute renal failure, congestive heart failure	0.1-0.6 µg/kg/min IV gtt	Contraindicated in increased intraocular pressure
Enalaprilat	Congestive heart failure, active renin-angiotensin system	1.25-5 mg IV every 6 h	Contraindicated in pregnancy and ACE I–related angioedema
Hydralazine	Preeclampsia/eclampsia	5-10 mg IV bolus can be repeated every 10-15 min	Reflex tachycardia, CNS, and myocardial ischemia

[a] Should be administered with a ß-blocker to avoid reflex tachycardia.

Nicardipine: It is a dihydropyridine calcium channel blocker (CCB). It may have unique benefits in hypertensive encephalopathy as it crosses the blood-brain barrier (BBB) to vasorelax cerebrovascular smooth muscle and minimizes vasospasm, especially in subarachnoid hemorrhage. Nicardipine is contraindicated in patients with advanced aortic stenosis. The main adverse effect is abrupt reduction in blood pressure and reflex tachycardia, which can be harmful in patients with coronary heart disease. The initial infusion rate is 5 mg/h, increasing by 2.5 mg/h every 5 minutes to a maximum of 30 mg/h. Once the target BP is reached, downward adjustment by 3 mg/h should be attempted as tolerated.

Nitroglycerin: It is a potent vasodilator that acts mainly on the venous system. It decreases preload and also increases coronary blood flow to the subendocardium. Nitroglycerin can be administered as a paste, sublingual spray, dissolvable tablet, or an infusion. It has a rapid onset and is considered the drug of choice in hypertensive emergencies in patients with cardiac ischemia, left ventricular dysfunction, and pulmonary edema. The recommended starting IV infusion dose is 5 to 15 mcg/min and titrated to desired clinical response. It is not recommended in patients with severe aortic stenosis, left ventricular outflow obstruction, or inferior wall myocardial infarction because of the chance of precipitating cardiovascular collapse.

Fenoldopam: It is a selective peripheral dopamine type 1 (D_1) agonist that has recently been added to the list of medications used in the treatment of hypertensive emergencies. It causes both vasodilation and natriuresis. Fenoldopam is administered as an IV infusion with a starting dose of 0.1 to 0.3 µg/kg/min and can be increased in increments of 0.05 to 0.1 µg/kg/min every 15 minutes to targeted effect. It has the advantage of increasing renal blood flow and improving creatinine clearance. As a result, fenoldopam may be the drug of choice in treating hypertensive emergencies in the setting of impaired renal function. It is contraindicated in patients with increased intraocular pressure.

Hydralazine: It lowers blood pressure by a direct vasodilatory effect on arteriolar smooth muscle. The exact mechanism of this effect is unknown. It is the preferred treatment by obstetricians in treating preeclampsia/eclampsia for decades, but has fallen out of favor for treatment of hypertension in other conditions. Hydralazine can cause reflex tachycardia and CNS and myocardial ischemia. Another downside of hydralazine is that while the half life is 3 to 6 hours, the total duration of effect is up to 36 hours and can be unpredictable. The recommended starting dose is 5 to 10 mg IV bolus, which can be repeated every 10 to 15 minutes.

Enalaprilat: It is the active IV form of enalapril, an angiotensin-converting enzyme (ACE) inhibitor. Enalaprilat lowers systemic vascular resistance, pulmonary capillary pressure, and heart rate while increasing coronary vasodilation. It has minimal effect on cerebral perfusion pressure. Some studies have found enalaprilat to be particularly useful in hypertensive emergency with acute pulmonary edema (APE). ACE inhibitors are contraindicated in pregnancy. The dose of enalaprilat is 1.25 mg IV bolus over 5 minutes and can be repeated every 6 hours. Enalaprilat cannot be titrated to effect.

Conditions Associated With Hypertensive Emergencies

Hypertensive encephalopathy: The **initial goal** is to rapidly lower the blood pressure **by no more than 20% to 25% of the MAP.** More aggressive lowering of the blood pressure can lead to hypoperfusion and ischemia as discussed above. More normalization of the blood pressure may be contemplated over 24 to 48 hours. The preferred medication is nitroprusside, labetalol, or nicardipine.

Acute cerebral infarction or hemorrhage: There is continued controversy as to when and how much elevated blood pressure should be lowered in patients with ischemic stroke. In fact, a recent multicenter, randomized control trial in Europe failed to demonstrate any benefit of lowering blood pressure in acute stroke and showed a trend towards harm. For patients who are candidates for thrombolytic therapy, blood pressure should be lowered to less than 185/110 mm Hg and maintained to less than 180/105 mm Hg for the next 24 hours. Otherwise, for patients who are not thrombolytic candidates, cautious lowering of pressure greater than 220/120 mm Hg is generally accepted, being careful to avoid lowering it too much or too rapidly as to induce drops in cerebral perfusion and cause greater ischemia. The preferred medications include labetalol, nitroprusside, and nicardipine.

Acute myocardial infarction: The goal in lowering the blood pressure in these cases is to decrease cardiac work by decreasing afterload and increasing coronary perfusion pressure. The preferred medications include nitroglycerin and β-blockers.

Aortic dissection: It is critical to lower blood pressure rapidly in this condition to limit progression of the dissection. Acute aortic dissection represents **the only hypertensive emergency where rapid, aggressive blood pressure reduction is indicated.** The goal is to maintain arterial pressure as low as possible without compromising end-organ perfusion. The preferred medications include labetalol alone. If this does not adequately lower blood pressure it should be used in combination with sodium nitroprusside.

Preeclampsia/eclampsia: The most commonly used agent in the past was hydralazine. However, obstetricians are using labetalol more frequently because it has similar efficacy and fewer side effects. In addition, magnesium sulfate is generally administered for seizure prophylaxis, though it has not been shown to lower blood pressure in hypertensive pregnant patients.

COMPREHENSION QUESTIONS

17.1 A 55-year-old man presents to the ED with complaints of a severe headache, diplopia, and vomiting. His blood pressure is 210/120 mm Hg upon arrival. Which of the following is the best next step?

    A. Observe the blood pressure and recheck in 1 hour, and supportive measures for the headache and vomiting.

    B. Obtain a head CT scan, give an antihypertensive such as nicardipine, and admit to the intensive care unit.

    C. Give intravenous furosemide to decrease the blood pressure.

    D. Give lorazepam to help the patient relax.

17.2 A 54-year-old woman presents to the ED requesting medication refills on her antihypertensive medications. She has been out of her medications for 2 weeks and cannot get an appointment with her private physician until next week. She normally takes atenolol and hydrochlorothiazide. Her blood pressure is 190/100 mm Hg. The patient has no complaints. She has been waiting for 4 hours and is in a hurry to get back to work. Which of the following is the most appropriate next step?

A. Change her medications to a calcium channel blocker.

B. Admit to the intensive care unit and initiate intravenous nitroprusside.

C. Give her a prescription for her medications, instruct her to take them immediately, and have her follow-up in 48 hours.

D. Counsel the patient on the dangers of her noncompliance, admit to the hospital, and begin the patient on intravenous labetalol.

17.3 A 38-year-old man presents to the ED after a motor vehicle collision. After complete evaluation it is determined that he sustained a fractured right tibia. The patient has a history of hypertension for which he is on pharmacologic treatment. The patient is writhing on the gurney in pain. His blood pressure is 210/104 mm Hg. The patient has no complaints except for right leg pain. Which of the following is the most appropriate next step in management?

A   Pain control and monitor the patient's blood pressure.

B. Start a β-blocker and monitor the patient's blood pressure.

C. Call a social worker because of suspected drug or alcohol abuse.

D. Admit the patient to the hospital to get his blood pressure under control.

ANSWERS

17.1 **B.** This man has hypertensive encephalopathy, which is a medical emergency. He has symptomatic hypertension causing end-organ damage. A head CT scan should be obtained prior to starting treatment to rule out any intracranial pathology. The appropriate treatment is IV antihypertensive medications to decrease his mean arterial pressure by 20% to 25% over 1 hour.

17.2 **C.** This patient has hypertensive urgency. She has no symptoms related to her elevated blood pressure and no signs of end-organ damage. The patient should restart her medications and have her blood pressure reassessed in 48 hours.

17.3 **A.** Although this man has a history of hypertension, he is in excruciating pain, which could be causing his elevated blood pressure. The appropriate treatment is to control the pain, have the leg set back into place, and monitor his blood pressure. The blood pressure should decrease once his pain is controlled.

CLINICAL PEARLS

▶ Hypertensive emergency is defined as markedly elevated blood pressure in the presence of end-organ damage, whereas hypertensive urgency is markedly elevated blood pressure without end-organ effects.

▶ One of the most common reasons for hypertensive emergency is patient noncompliance with antihypertensive medication.

▶ It is critical to cautiously lower blood pressure to avoid inducing a hypoperfusion state that leads to cerebral ischemia.

▶ Patients with hypertensive emergency should be admitted to a monitored setting, preferably an intensive care unit.

REFERENCES

Amin A. Parenteral medication for hypertension with symptoms. *Annals Emerg Med.* 2008;51(3 Suppl): S10-S15. Epub 2008 Jan 11.

Blumenfeld JD, Laragh JH. Management of hypertensive crises: the scientific basis for treatment decisions. *Am J Hypertension.* 2001;14(11 Pt 1):1154-1167.

Chobanian AV, Bakris GL, Cushman WC, et al. The seventh report of the Joint National Committee on Prevention, Detection and Evaluation, and Treatment of High Blood Pressure, The JNC 7 Report. NIH Publication No. 04-5230. 2004.

Cotton DB, Gonik B, Dorman KF. Cardiovascular alterations in severe pregnancy induced hypertension: acute effects of intravenous magnesium sulfate. *Am J Obstet Gynecol.* 1984;148:162-165.

De Gaudio AR, Chelazzi C, Villa G, Cavaliere F. Acute severe arterial hypertension: therapeutic options. *Curr Drug Targets.* 2009;10(8):788-798.

Fisher ND, Williams GH. Hypertensive vascular disease. In: Kasper DL, Braunwald E, Fauci AS, Hauser SI, Longo DL, Jameson JL, eds. *Harrison's Principles of Internal Medicine.* 16th ed. New York, NY: McGraw-Hill :1463-1481.

Flanigan JS, Vitberg D. Hypertensive emergency and severe hypertension: what to treat, who to treat, and how to treat. *Med Clin North Am.* 2006;90(3):439-451.

Frakes MA, Richardson LE. Magnesium sulfate therapy in certain emergency conditions. *Am J Emerg Med.* 1997;15:182-187.

Lipstein H, Lee CC, Crupi RS. A current concept of eclampsia. *Am J Emerg Med.* 2003;21:223-226.

Marik PE, Varon J. Hypertensive crises: challenges and management. *Chest.* 2007;131(6):1949-1962.

McCoy S, Baldwin K. Pharmacotherapeutic options for the treatment of preeclampsia. *Am J Health Syst Pharm.* 2009;66(4):337-344.

Pancioli AM. Hypertension management in neurologic emergencies. *Annals Emerg Med.* 200;51(3 Suppl):S24-S27. Epub 2008 Jan.

Powers DR, Papadakos PJ, Wallin JD. Parenteral hydralazine revisited. *J Emerg Med.* 1998;16(2):191-196.

Rhoney D, Peacock WF. Intravenous therapy for hypertensive emergencies, part 1. *Am J Health Syst Pharm.* 2009;66(15):1343-1352.

Rhoney D, Peacock WF. Intravenous therapy for hypertensive emergencies, part 2. *Am J Health Syst Pharm.* 2009;66(16):1448-1457.

Sandset EC, Bath PM, Boysen G, et al; SCAST Study Group. The angiotensin-receptor blocker candesartan for treatment of acute stroke (SCAST): a randomised, placebo-controlled, double-blind trial. *Lancet.* 2011;377:741.

Selvidge R, Dart R. Emergencies in the second and third trimesters: hypertensive disorders and antepartum hemorrhage. *Emerg Med Pract.* 2004;6(12):1-20.

Sibai B, Dekker G, Kupfemine M. Preelampsia. *Lancet.* 2005;365:785-799.

Varon J. Treatment of acute severe hypertension: current and newer agents. *Drugs.* 2008;68(3):283-297.

Varon J, Marik PE. The diagnosis and management of hypertensive crises. *Chest.* 2000;118:214-227.

Vaughan CJ, Norman D. Hypertensive emergencies. *Lancet.* 2000;356:411-417.

Vidt DG. Current concepts in treatment of hypertensive emergencies. *Am Heart J.* 1986;111:220-225.

You are working in the emergency department (ED) of a 15-bed rural hospital without CT scan capabilities, and a 25-year-old, previously healthy, woman presents for evaluation of abdominal pain. The patient describes her pain as having been present for the past 3 days. The pain is described as constant, exacerbated by movements, and associated with subjective fevers and chills. She denies any recent changes in bowel habits, urinary symptoms, or menses. Her last menstrual period was 6 days ago. The physical examination reveals temperature of 38.4°C (101.1°F), pulse rate of 110 beats per minute, blood pressure of 112/70 mm Hg, and respiratory rate of 18 breaths per minute. Her skin is nonicteric. Cardiopulmonary examination is unremarkable. The abdomen is mildly distended and tender in both right and left lower quadrants. Involuntary guarding and localized rebound tenderness are noted in the right lower quadrant. The pelvic examination reveals no cervical discharge; cervical motion tenderness and right adnexal tenderness are present. The rectal examination reveals no masses or tenderness. Laboratory studies reveal white blood cell count (WBC) of 14,000 cells/mm^3, a normal hemoglobin, and a normal hematocrit. The urinalysis reveals 3 to 5 WBC/high-power field (HPF), few bacteria, and trace ketones.

► What are the most likely diagnoses?
► How can you confirm the diagnosis?

ANSWERS TO CASE 18:

Acute Abdominal Pain

Summary: A 25-year-old, previously healthy, woman presents with a 3-day history of lower abdominal pain and subjective fever. Her examination indicates the presence of fever and lower abdominal tenderness (right > left). The rectal examination is unremarkable. Her laboratory studies indicate leukocytosis.

- **Most likely diagnosis:** Likely diagnoses include complicated acute appendicitis, pelvic inflammatory disease (PID), ovarian torsion, or other pelvic pathology.

- **Confirmatory studies:** Begin with pregnancy test and pelvic ultrasonography to evaluate for possible ovarian and pelvic pathology. If these suggest pelvic source of pathology, then strong consideration should be given to perform exploratory laparoscopy or laparotomy.

ANALYSIS

Objectives

1. Learn the relationships between symptoms, findings, and pathophysiology of the various types of disease processes capable of producing acute abdominal pain.

2. Learn to develop reasonable diagnostic and treatment strategies based on clinical diagnosis, resource availability, and patient characteristics.

3. Learn the diagnosis and severity stratification for acute pancreatitis.

Considerations

This is a healthy young woman, who presents with acute pain in the lower abdomen. Based on patient age and location of pain, acute appendicitis and gynecological pathology are the most likely sources of pathology, and additional history and diagnostic studies may help to differentiate these possibilities.

Pertinent gynecological history should include history of sexual contacts, menstrual pattern, previous gynecological problems, and the probability of pregnancy. A pregnancy test should be obtained early during the evaluation process to verify the presence or absence of pregnancy, and if the history and physical examination suggest the source of pathology to have originated from the pelvic organs, a pelvic ultrasound should be obtained.

In the event that the patient is pregnant, an ultrasound should be performed to verify intrauterine gestational sac and estimate the gestational age. If an intrauterine gestational sac is not visualized by ultrasound, the possibility of ectopic pregnancy should be considered and an immediate referral should be made for a gynecologic evaluation and possible operative intervention. Whereas, if the pregnancy test is negative and pelvic pathology is strongly suspected, the initial priority would be to identify potential life-threatening and fertility-reducing processes, including tuboovarian abscesses, pelvic inflammatory diseases, and ovarian torsion.

Pelvic ultrasonography would be very valuable as the initial study to identify or rule out these processes. In the event that the pelvic ultrasound does not identify any pelvic pathology, a computed tomography (CT) scan of the abdomen and pelvis may be useful. The management approach for patient with abdominal pain varies depending on resource and expertise availability. For this patient at a 15-bed facility without CT capability, the general surgeon should be consulted early regarding the potential need for transfer to another facility or further evaluation by laparoscopy or laparotomy.

APPROACH TO:
Abdominal Pain

DEFINITIONS

ACUTE ABDOMEN: "Acute abdomen" describes the recent onset of abdominal pain. Patients with acute abdomen require urgent evaluation and not necessarily urgent operations.

FOREGUT: Foregut extends from oropharynx to mid-duodenum, including liver, biliary tract, pancreas, and spleen.

HINDGUT: Hindgut extends from distal transverse colon to rectum.

MIDGUT: Midgut extends from distal duodenum to mid-transverse colon.

REFERRED PAIN: This pain usually arises from a deep structure to a remote deep or superficial structure. The pattern of referred pain is based on the existence of shared central pathways between the afferent neurons of cutaneous dermatomes and intra-abdominal structures. Frequently, referred pain is associated with skin hyperalgesia and increased muscle tone. (Classic example of referred pain occurs with irritation of the left hemidiaphragm from ruptured spleen that causes referred pain to the left shoulder because of shared innervation by the same cervical nerves.)

SOMATIC PAIN: This pain arises from the irritation of the parietal peritoneum. This type of pain is mediated mainly by spinal nerve fibers supplying the abdominal wall and is perceived as sharp, constant, and generally localized to one of four quadrants. **Somatic pain may arise as a result of changes in pH and temperature (infection and inflammation) or pressure increase (surgical incision).**

VISCERAL PAIN: This pain is generally characterized as dull, crampy, deep, or aching. Normal embryological development of abdominal viscera results in symmetrical bilateral autonomic innervations leading to visceral pain being perceived in the midline location. Visceral stimulation can be produced by stretching and torsion, chemical stimulation, ischemia, or inflammation. Visceral pain from gastrointestinal (GI) tract structures correlate with pain location based on their embryonic origins, where foregut pain is perceived in the epigastrium, midgut pain is perceived in the periumbilical region, and hindgut pain is perceived in the hypogastrium.

CLINICAL APPROACH

Abdominal pain is a common chief complaint of patients seen in the ED, comprising approximately 5% to 8% of total visits. Overall, 18% to 25% of patients with abdominal pain evaluated in the ED have serious conditions requiring acute hospital care. In a recent series, the distribution of common diagnosis of adult ED patients with abdominal pain were listed as the following: 18% admitted, 25% undifferentiated abdominal pain (UDAP), 12% female pelvic, 12% urinary tract, and 9.3% surgical gastrointestinal. Approximately 10% of patients required urgent surgery, and most patients with UDAP were young women with epigastric symptoms who did not progress to develop significant medical problems.

Understanding of disease pathophysiology, epidemiology, clinical presentations, and the limitations of laboratory and imaging studies are important during evaluation of patients with abdominal pain in the ED. Abdominal pain can be initially categorized as "surgical" or "nonsurgical"; alternatively, pain may be approached from an organ-system approach. Overall, the surgical causes are encountered more commonly than nonsurgical causes when considering all comers with acute abdominal pain.

Surgical causes (or causes that may require surgical corrections) may be categorized by mechanism into (1) **hemorrhagic,** (2) **infectious,** (3) **perforating,** (4) **obstructive,** (5) **ischemic,** and (6) **inflammatory.** Hemorrhagic conditions causing abdominal pain include traumatic injuries to solid and hollow viscera, ruptured ectopic pregnancy, tumor rupture/hemorrhage (eg, hepatic adenomas and hepatocellular carcinomas), and leaking or ruptured aneurysms. Infectious conditions may include appendicitis, cholecystitis, diverticulitis, infectious colitis, cholangitis, pyelonephritis, cystitis, primary peritonitis, and pelvic inflammatory disease. Perforations causing abdominal pain can occur from peptic ulcers, diverticulitis, esophageal perforations, and traumatic hollow viscus injury. Obstructive processes leading to abdominal pain can occur from small intestinal obstruction, large bowel obstruction, ureteral obstruction, and biliary obstructions (see Figure 18-1 for radiograph). Ischemic causes are subcategorized as microvascular or macrovascular. Macrovascular ischemic events can occur from mechanical causes, including torsion (intestines and ovaries are most common), vascular obstruction from thrombosis, embolism, and non-occlusive low-flow states, and these can include small bowel and colonic ischemia. Microvascular ischemic events are uncommon and can occur from causes such as cocaine intoxication. Inflammatory conditions causing abdominal pain may include acute pancreatitis and Crohn disease; the mechanism of pain production associated with acute pancreatitis is not clearly known but is likely related to the local release of inflammatory mediators. Although, not all patients with abdominal pain produced by the above listed surgical causes need surgical interventions, the potential for surgical or other forms of invasive interventions are high in these patients; therefore, early surgical consultation is advisable.

Nonsurgical causes of acute abdominal pain are less common and occur most frequently in patients with history of prior endocrine, metabolic, hematologic, infectious, or substance abuse history. The endocrine and metabolic causes of abdominal pain may include diabetic ketoacidosis, Addisonian crisis, and uremia. Hematologic causes of abdominal pain include sickle cell crisis and acute leukemia.

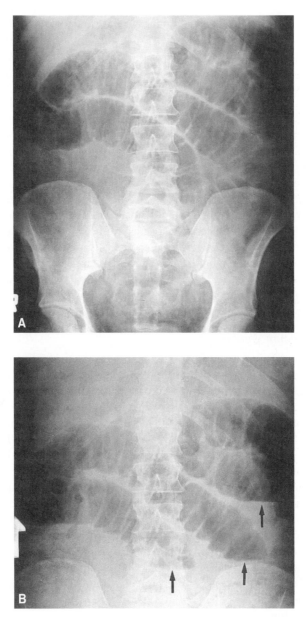

Figure 18–1. Abdominal radiographs in the supine (A) and upright (B) positions show a dilated small bowel with air-fluid levels. (Reproduced, with permission, from Kadell BM, Zimmerman P, Lu DSK. Radiology of the abdomen. In: Zinner MJ, Schwarz SI, Ellis H, et al, eds. *Maingot's Abdominal Operations.* 10th ed. New York, NY: McGraw-Hill; 1997:24.)

Systemic infectious causes of abdominal pain can include acute meningitis, TB peritonitis, acute hepatitis, and varicella zoster infections. Because the differences between surgical and nonsurgical causes of abdominal pain are often subtle, it is advisable to consult a surgical colleague for all patients with acute abdominal pain. In addition, because of the potential for complications development in some of the patients with initially nonsurgical causes of abdominal pain, surgical consultations and follow-up are essential for the management of these complex patients.

Patient evaluations should be directed toward identifying potentially serious medical conditions. Analgesia including narcotics should not be withheld in patients with pain. In the event that a diagnosis is not identified following a thorough evaluation, it may be appropriate to discharge the patient with the diagnosis of "abdominal pain of uncertain etiology." Usually, **individuals still under the effect of analgesia without a diagnosis should not be discharged.** For patients whose abdominal pain etiologies are not clearly determined, it is important to provide them with the reassurance that the pain most likely would improve and resolve; however, because of the broad overlap in the early manifestation of serious disease, the patient need to be instructed to seek early follow-up if symptoms do not resolve. Furthermore, the use of narcotic pain medications should be withheld in the individuals without clear diagnosis or follow-up.

Abdominal Pain in Women

Women make up approximately 75% of all patients evaluated in the ED with abdominal pain. Women of childbearing age represent a complex patient population from the diagnostic standpoint, because of a broader differential for pain. Acute appendicitis, biliary tract disease, urinary tract infection, and gynecological problems are the most common sources of abdominal pain in childbearing-age women. The history obtained from each patient should include details of menstrual history, sexual practices, gynecological and obstetrical history, and surgical history. For most individuals, the initial history and physical examination can help to direct the workup toward an organ system or body region. Laboratory evaluations, including CBC with differential, serum amylase, urinalysis, pregnancy test, and liver functions test, may provide additional information to help rule in or rule out certain diagnoses. When indicated, imaging such as ultrasonography and CT scans can be helpful in assessing for biliary tract and pelvic pathology, and for acute appendicitis. **Because overreliance on laboratory and/or imaging can contribute to misdiagnoses, laboratory and imaging results should always be interpreted within the proper clinical context; clinical judgment should be exercised regarding the acquisition of consultation and/or observation.**

Abdominal Pain in Elderly Patients

Elderly patients (age >65) account for approximately 15% of all ED visits, and about one-third of these visits result in inpatient admissions. In comparison to young adults, **elderly patients** with abdominal pain evaluated in the ED generally **have increased prevalence of serious diseases** causing abdominal pain, where the frequency of illnesses requiring surgical intervention has been estimated to be as high as 30%. Furthermore, the mortality rate associated with abdominal pain is increased in this population as a consequence of the increase in catastrophic illnesses (including mesenteric ischemia, leaking or ruptured aneurysm, and myocardial infarction). **Common diagnoses among elderly patients** include **biliary tract disease** (23%), **diverticular disease** (12%), **bowel obstruction** (11%), and undetermined (11%).

Due to various reasons that include atypical clinical presentations and difficulty with communications, abdominal pain in the elderly is associated with high frequency of inaccurate diagnosis (up to 60%). Inability to accurately diagnose the cause of abdominal pain contributes to delayed treatment and increased morality, as elderly patients whose abdominal pain were not accurately diagnosed in the ED have been shown to have a 2-fold increase in mortality when compared to elderly patients whose causes of abdominal pain were accurately diagnosed.

For most elderly patients, the evaluation should be broadened to help identify cardiac, pulmonary, vascular, neoplastic, and neurologic causes of abdominal pain. Often symptoms in this population are attributable to an underlying medical comorbidity. It is important to bear in mind that medications taken by many elderly patients may contribute to abdominal problems, as well as alter the clinical presentations (eg, β-blockers may blunt pulse rate response to stress). When indicated, ancillary testing should be applied to assist in establishing the diagnosis; however, it is important to remember that **the diagnostic accuracy of any test is dependent on the pretest probability, specificity, sensitivity, and disease prevalence of the test population.** Because abdominal pain in the elderly population is more frequently associated with serious pathology, appropriate consultations should be sought out and a liberal policy regarding inpatient or ED observation should be applied whenever causes cannot be clearly identified.

Patients With Acute Pancreatitis (AP)

Acute pancreatitis is an acute inflammatory condition of the pancreas that can affect adults of all ages, and in its severe forms, AP can affect all organ systems in the body. Patients are said to have severe AP when the process is associated with organ dysfunction, APACHE II scores ≥8, Ranson scores ≥3, or presence of local complications based on contrast-enhanced CT scans (eg, pancreas necrosis, pseudocysts, or peripancreatic fluid collections). Severe AP is reported in 15% to 20% of patients with AP. Mortality rates associated with mild AP is approximately 5%, whereas severe AP is associated with mortality rates up to 25%. The diagnosis of pancreatitis should be suspected when patients present with persistent abdominal or back pain associated with elevated levels of serum lipase and/or amylase. In the emergency department setting, the etiology of AP can be assessed by clinical history (these should include inquiries regarding gallstones, alcohol use, medications, infections, metabolic and autoimmune disorders, family history, and history of trauma), and laboratory studies that include liver function tests, calcium, and triglyceride levels. In approximately 80% of the patients with AP, the cause can be determined based on the clinical history and initial clinical evaluation. Identifying AP cause is generally not critical during the initial management of patients in the emergency center, but could have implications in the prevention of future disease recurrences. Severity stratification for patients is helpful during the initial evaluation, as it may help direct the triage of patients to intensive care units or specialty care facilities.

Early management of patients is directed toward the recognition and prevention of organ dysfunction in those patients with severe AP. Prompt repletion of intravascular volume is essential in the prevention of renal dysfunction. When patients do not respond appropriately to their initial fluid management, central venous pressure monitoring, pulse-oximetry monitoring, and urine-output monitoring should be considered to help direct these efforts and avoid fluid overloading patients.

Disease recurrences are common among patients with AP, especially when the cause is alcohol, metabolically-induced, or produced by anatomic abnormalities such as pancreas divisum and periampullary duodenal diverticulum. It is important to identify patients with AP that are gallstone-related, because most recurrences in these patients can be prevented by cholecystectomies.

CT scan of the abdomen is not necessary for the diagnosis or confirmation of AP. CT scans in the emergency center setting may be indicated to help confirm the diagnosis of AP when the clinical picture and/or biochemical values are not sufficient for the confirmation of diagnosis. In addition, CT scan may help identify patients with significant pancreas necrosis, which often correlates with disease severity and regional pancreatic complications (Table 18–1). CT scan with intravenous contrast performed in intravascular volume depleted patients with severe AP could contribute to acute kidney injuries and further injuries to the pancreas; therefore, these studies should be withheld until the patients' volume depletions have been corrected.

Patients with severe pancreatitis determined either by the presence of end-organ dysfunction, APACHE II >8, Ranson score >3, or CT demonstrating pancreas necrosis may benefit from close monitoring, therefore admissions to intensive care units. Over the past several years, there has been a continued trend toward the

Table 18–1 • CT SEVERITY INDEX (CTSI) FOR ACUTE PANCREATITIS	
CT Findings	Point
Pancreatic inflammation	
None	0
Focal diffuse enlargement of the pancreas	1
Pancreatic inflammation associated with inflammatory changes in the peripancreatic fat	2
Single, fluid collection or phlegmon	3
Two or more fluid collections or presence of gas in the peripancreatic region	4
Pancreatic necrosis	
No necrosis	0
≤30% necrosis	2
30%-50% necrosis	4
>50% necrosis	6
Total score (Inflammation score + necrosis score)	0-10

nonoperative or delayed-operative (>14 days) management of patients with severe AP. Critically ill patients with AP would still benefit from early consultation by a surgical specialist because other intra-abdominal processes that would require surgical interventions could mimic AP or develop as the result of severe AP.

Patients With Chronic or Recurrent Abdominal Pain

Patients with chronic or recurrent abdominal pain represent one of the most difficult diagnostic and management challenges for emergency medicine physicians. The dilemma facing ED physicians during encounters with these patients include establishing the accurate diagnosis, determining appropriate use of diagnostic studies, determining the appropriateness of analgesic medications, and follow-up.

Similar to the approach taken toward patients with acute abdominal pain, the evaluation of chronic abdominal pain should begin with a thorough history. Events and activities that trigger or alleviate the symptoms may be helpful in identifying the organ systems of pain origin. Furthermore, detail description of the patterns and location of pain are helpful for categorization of pain as visceral pain, somatic pain, or referred pain, and based on these determinations, organ system and anatomical sources of abdominal pain also may be delineated.

The physical examinations in these patients should be focused to help sort out the differential diagnosis formulated on the basis of history, and not a search for pathology. Unfortunately, the physical examination findings are sometimes difficult to interpret because of psychologic and personality changes, especially if the pain has been chronic, recurrent, and severe.

Unfortunately, no specific laboratory or imaging studies are completely sensitive or specific for the diagnosis of abdominal pain. As a general rule, diagnostic studies should be selected only if results of the studies will lead to specific additional evaluations or treatment. The CBC might be helpful in identifying leukocytosis, which may indicate an inflammatory or infectious condition, whereas the presence of anemia might help to verify the presence of ischemic colitis, GI tract malignancy, or inflammatory bowel disease. Abnormalities within the liver functions panel may help identify choledocholithiasis, stenosing papillitis, and periampullary malignancy. Serum amylase elevation is generally seen in the setting of chronic or acute pancreatitis. Elevation in erythrocyte sedimentation rate may suggest the presence of autoimmune processes or collagen vascular disorders.

Frequently, even after the completion of extensive, appropriate evaluations the patient's condition may remain unrecognized. If possible, the results of the evaluation and diagnostic studies should be discussed with the patient's primary care physician, so that the patient may be provided with additional testing and follow-up. For those patients without primary care physicians, evaluation and consultation by an appropriate primary care physician or specialist should be obtained prior to discharge from the ED.

COMPREHENSION QUESTIONS

18.1 A 30-year-old woman presents with epigastric pain that developed following dinner. The patient describes having similar pain prior to the current episode, but previous episodes were less severe. The patient was diagnosed as having gastroesophageal reflux disease by her primary care physician and prescribed a proton pump inhibitor, which has been ineffective in resolving her pain. The current pain episode has been severe and persistent for 3 hours. The patient has a temperature of 38°C (100.4°F), heart rate of 100 beats per minute, respiratory rate of 20 breaths per minute, and blood pressure of 130/90 mm Hg. The abdominal examination reveals no abdominal tenderness. The administration of 30 mL of antacids and 4 mg of morphine sulfate resulted in some relief of pain. Which of the following is the most appropriate next step?

A. Obtain CBC, amylase, liver function tests, and ultrasound of the gallbladder. Discuss with surgical consultants regarding admission to the hospital.

B. Follow up with her primary care physician in 2 weeks.

C. Admit the patient to the hospital for upper GI endoscopy.

D. Prescribe antacids and discharge the patient from the ED, with follow-up by her primary care physician.

E. Obtain an ultrasound of the gallbladder, prescribe oral antibiotics, analgesics, and arrange for an outpatient follow-up with her primary care physician.

18.2 Which of the following features best characterizes somatic pain?

A. Midline location

B. Sharp, persistent, and well-localized pain in the left lower quadrant

C. Intermittent pain

D. Pain is improved with body movement

18.3 For which of the following patients is CT of the abdomen contraindicated?

A   A 60-year-old man with persistent left lower quadrant pain, fever, and a tender mass

B. A 45-year-old alcoholic man with diffuse abdominal pain, WBC 18,000 cells/mm^3, and serum amylase of 2000

C. A nonpregnant 18-year-old woman with suprapubic and right lower quadrant pain, fever, right lower quadrant mass, and WBC of 15,000 cells/mm^3

D. A 70-year-old man with abdominal pain and distension, a 10-cm pulsatile mass in the epigastrium, and blood pressure of 70/50 mm Hg

E. A 24-year-old man with a new finding of painful, irreducible umbilical hernia who presents with 12-hour history of abdominal distension and vomiting

ANSWERS

18.1 **A.** This patient has recurrent epigastric pain, which is attributed to gastro-esophageal reflux disease. However, the fact that her symptoms have been poorly controlled with proton pump inhibitors in the past suggests that the diagnosis is probably inaccurate. Her recurrent symptoms are likely caused by biliary tract disease, and her current presentation is highly suspicious for complicated biliary tract disease such as acute cholecystitis. Choice A represents testing for the evaluation of biliary tract disease, which is appropriate in this setting. Because of her fever, outpatient management approach described in choice E is inappropriate.

18.2 **B.** Somatic pain is generally associated with irritation of the parietal perito-neum, resulting in localized, persistent, and sharp pain. This type of pain is aggravated by movement and can produce spasm in the overlying abdominal wall musculature, which is manifested as involuntary guarding.

18.3 **D.** The patient in "D" is hemodynamically unstable and possesses signs and symptoms suggestive of ruptured abdominal aneurysm. A CT scan would likely delay his care and is contraindicated in this situation. The patient described in choice A likely has diverticulitis, where CT may be appropriate for severity staging. The patient described in choice B likely has acute pancreatitis, where CT is helpful for the stratification of disease severity. The patient described in choice C may have complicated appendicitis or some other complicated GI or gynecological process, where CT can be useful for differentiation. The patient described in choice E has an incarcerated umbilical hernia with signs and symptoms of intestinal obstruction related to this finding. Surgical inter-vention is indicated based on his presentation alone.

CLINICAL PEARLS

▶ Most patients with the diagnosis of "undifferentiated abdominal pain" determined after thorough ED evaluation will have spontaneous resolu-tion of pain.

▶ Narcotic medications will affect the characteristics and intensity of all abdominal pain, regardless of etiology.

▶ Up to one-third of elderly patients with abdominal pain evaluated in the ED have conditions that may require surgical intervention.

REFERENCES

Delrue LJ, De Waele JJ, Duyck PO. Acute pancreatitis: radiologic scores in predicting severity and outcome. *Abdom Imaging.* 2009;35:349-361.

Gravante G, Garcea G, Ong SL, et al. Prediction of mortality in acute pancreatitis: a systematic review of the published evidence. *Pancreatology.* 2009;9:601-614.

McNamara R, Dean AJ. Approach to acute abdominal pain. *Emerg Med Clin N Am.* 2011;29:159-173.

Pezzeilli R, Zerbi A, DiCarlo V, et al. Practice guidelines for acute pancreatitis. *Pancreatology.* 2010;10:523-535.

Privette Jr TW, Carlisle MC, Palma JK. Emergencies of the liver, gallbladder, and pancreas. *Emerg Med Clin N Am.* 2011;29:293-317.

A two-year-old boy is brought to the emergency department (ED) because of an episode of "choking." The patient was playing with marbles when his mother left the room for a few minutes. She ran back in when she heard the patient gagging and coughing. She denies any recent fever, cough, or other upper respiratory infectious symptoms. When asked, she denies her son turning blue, having difficulty breathing or vomiting. The patient was a term baby without any significant past medical history. He is not taking any medications, and his immunizations are all up-to-date. He attends day care and has no recent sick contacts.

On examination, his temperature is 37.7°C (99.9°F), blood pressure is 93/55 mm Hg, heart rate is 105 beats per minute, respiratory rate is 24 breaths per minute, and the O_2 saturation is 98% on room air. The patient is playful and alert. His examination is unremarkable except for intermittent gagging. He has no intercostal retractions or accessory muscle use.

▶ What are the potential complications in this patient?
▶ What is the most appropriate next step?

ANSWERS TO CASE 19:
Swallowed Foreign Body

Summary: This is a two-year-old boy with probable ingestion of a foreign body (marble).

- **Potential complications:** Esophageal stricture, perforation, mediastinitis or peritonitis, paraesophageal abscess, cardiac tamponade, and aortotracheoesophageal fistula.

- **Most appropriate next step:** Because the child is stable, x-ray to localize the foreign body.

ANALYSIS

Objectives

1. Recognize the clinical scenario, signs, and symptoms of swallowed foreign bodies.
2. Learn the diagnostic and therapeutic approach to the various types of swallowed foreign bodies.

Considerations

Patients with swallowed foreign bodies may be asymptomatic or may present in extremis. Although most objects will pass through the gastrointestinal tract without problems, it is important to recognize which patients require observation and which will need intervention (Table 19–1).

APPROACH TO:
Swallowed Foreign Body

CLINICAL APPROACH

Although children 18 to 48 months account for nearly 80% of cases, edentulous adults, psychiatric patients, and prisoners also commonly swallow foreign objects. Children most commonly ingest things they can pick up and place in their mouths, such as coins, buttons, toys, and crayons. Adults are more likely to have trouble swallowing meat and bones. Although objects can be located anywhere throughout the alimentary tract, there are several areas where they lodge more frequently. In the pediatric patient, most obstructions occur in the proximal esophagus at one of 5 areas: the cricopharyngeal narrowing (most common), thoracic inlet, aortic arch, tracheal bifurcation, and hiatal narrowing. In contrast, most adult patients have distal esophageal obstructions caused by a structural or motor abnormality (eg, stricture, malignancy, scleroderma, achalasia).

Most adult patients will be able to relate a history of ingesting a foreign object or of feeling food becoming lodged. They may complain of anxiety, foreign body sensation, chest or epigastric pain, retching, vomiting, wheezing, or difficulty swallowing.

Table 19–1 • SPECIAL TYPES OF SWALLOWED FOREIGN BODIES

Foreign Body	Comments	Treatment
Food impaction	Avoid proteolytic enzymes because of risk of esophageal perforation. Avoid gas-forming agents if perforation suspected. Barium swallow after treatment to confirm clearance of the impaction and to rule out esophageal pathology.	Expectant management if handling secretions and impacted <12 h. Otherwise endoscopy preferred. Alternatives: intravenous glucagon, sublingual nifedipine, sublingual nitroglycerin, oral gas-forming agents.
Coin	Often asymptomatic. X-ray to confirm location (esophageal coins lie with flat side showing on anteroposterior x-ray).	Endoscopy preferred if at the level of the cricopharyngeus muscle. Alternative: Foley catheter removal under fluoroscopy if lodged <24 h, bougienage (pushing object into stomach). Expectant management may be considered if impacted <24 h
Button battery	High risk of mucosal burns and esophageal perforation if lodged in esophagus. X-ray to confirm location.	Surgical consult for endoscopy if in esophagus and has not passed through the pylorus or patient symptomatic. Expectant management if past the esophagus and no symptoms. Repeat radiographs until battery cleared.
Sharp or pointed objects	X-ray to confirm location.	If foreign body proximal to or in duodenum, endoscopic removal recommended given risk of intestinal perforation. If symptomatic, impacted, or foreign body past duodenum, surgical consult for endoscopy or laparotomy. Otherwise expectant management with serial radiographs.
Body packing	Ingestion of packets of drugs (most commonly cocaine or heroin). Rupture of packet may be fatal (especially with cocaine). May cause symptoms because of drug effect or gastrointestinal obstruction. Avoid endoscopy because of risk of rupture.	If packet intact, may observe and use whole bowel irrigation with polyethylene glycol to hasten passage of packets through gastrointestinal tract. Otherwise surgery to remove packets.

Data from Tintinalli J, Judith E, and J S. Stapczynski. Tintinalli's Emergency Medicine: A Comprehensive Study Guide. *New York, NY: McGraw-Hill; 2011.*

In children, the history may be less clear. Parents may have seen the child with an object in his or her mouth and suspect ingestion. Children can present with vomiting, gagging, choking, refusal to eat, or neck or chest pain. Increased salivation, drooling, or an inability to swallow suggests a complete obstruction. Patients with airway foreign bodies tend to present with more respiratory symptoms (Table 19–2).

Table 19–2 • SWALLOWED VS ASPIRATED FOREIGN BODIES		
	Swallowed Foreign Body	**Aspirated Foreign Body**
Most Common Objects	Children: coins, toys, crayons. Adults: meat, bones	Children: grapes, nuts, hot dogs, candy Adults: nonfood items more common than in children
Most Common Location	Children: cricopharyngeal narrowing Adults: distal esophagus	Children: bronchial tree Adults: proximal airway
Clinical Presentation	Anxiety, pain (neck, retrosternal, epigastric), foreign body sensation, choking, vomiting, dysphagia, inability to swallow, drooling. Air hunger and dyspnea generally less common.	Choking, coughing, hoarse voice, dyspnea, stridor, wheezing, respiratory distress (retractions, accessory muscle use, hypoxia, cyanosis). May present in delayed fashion with infectious complications (eg, recurrent pneumonia)
Treatment	Depends on symptomatology, location, type of foreign body. May include expectant management or removal of foreign body	Removal of foreign body

The physical examination should focus on identifying patients with airway compromise, inability to tolerate fluids, or active bleeding. It should include a careful evaluation of the oropharynx, neck, chest, and abdomen. Findings such as fever, subcutaneous air, or peritoneal signs suggest perforation. In patients with a suspected oropharyngeal foreign body, direct or indirect laryngoscopy can be useful. Plain x-rays may help locate radiopaque foreign bodies throughout the gastrointestinal (GI) tract and be used to follow their progression (if repeated every 2-4 hours). Many foreign bodies are not radiopaque, including chicken and fish bones.

If plain films do not reveal the object, an esophagogram, computed tomography (CT), or endoscopy are other options. If perforation is suspected, the esophagogram should be performed with a water-soluble contrast agent. If aspiration is a concern, barium is the preferred contrast agent; however, barium can obscure the visual field if endoscopy is subsequently performed. CT can be useful to identify the location and orientation of swallowed foreign bodies as well as the presence of any complications such as perforations or fistulae. Endoscopy is usually the study of choice because the object may be removed once it is visualized. Some success has been reported using metal detectors to locate and follow metallic objects.

Eighty to ninety percent of patients with normal gastrointestinal anatomy will pass swallowed foreign bodies without complications. Thus most patients are treated expectantly at first. If symptomatic, in-hospital observation should be considered for serial examinations. In general, once a foreign object passes the pylorus, it will continue through the GI tract without incident. However, if it cannot pass the esophagus or pylorus, it must be removed. Again, endoscopy is usually the method of choice. However, surgery may be necessary if there is evidence of obstruction or perforation, if the object is too big to pass safely, or if it contains toxins.

There are several special considerations when dealing with certain types of swallowed foreign bodies such as button batteries, which generally need to be removed because of their toxic effects on mucosa (see Table 19–1).

COMPREHENSION QUESTIONS

19.1 The ED director embarks on a study to see the type of patient most likely to experience foreign-body ingestion. Which of the following groups of individuals is most likely to have foreign-body ingestion?

A. Children

B. Edentulous adults

C. Prisoners

D. Psychiatric patients

19.2 A 21-year-old woman accidentally swallowed a penny. At which of the following locations is the coin most likely to be lodged?

A. Aortic arch

B. Cricopharyngeal narrowing

C. Lower esophageal sphincter

D. Thoracic inlet

19.3 A 3-year-old girl accidentally swallowed a button battery from her mother's camera. She does not appear to be in respiratory distress. She has normal vital signs and is afebrile. Plain x-ray shows the battery in the esophagus. Which of the following is the best management for this patient?

A. Avoidance of citrus drinks

B. Avoidance of magnets

C. Endoscopy

D. Expectant management

19.4 An 8-year-old girl presents to the ED having swallowed a penny as part of a bet with a friend. The abdominal radiograph reveals that the penny is in the stomach. Thirty-six hours later, it is still in the stomach. Which of the following is the best next step?

A. Endoscopy

B. Laparotomy

C. Lithotripsy

D. Observation

E. Rigid bronchoscopy

ANSWERS

19.1 **A.** Foreign-body ingestion is most common in children.

19.2 **C.** In adults, a swallowed object will most commonly lodge in the esophagus at the lower esophageal sphincter. In children, the most common location is the proximal esophagus at the cricopharyngeal narrowing.

19.3 **C.** Button battery ingestion is a true emergency with the potential for mucosal burns within 4 hours and esophageal perforation within 6 hours of ingestion. A button battery in the esophagus must be removed as soon as possible.

19.4 **A.** In general, the preferred method of swallowed foreign body removal is endoscopy (except in body packers due to the risk of packet rupture).

CLINICAL PEARLS

▶ Children account for the vast majority of cases of swallowed foreign bodies.

▶ In the pediatric patient, objects most commonly lodge in the proximal esophagus, whereas most adult patients have distal esophageal obstructions.

▶ Findings such as fever, subcutaneous air, or peritoneal signs suggest perforation and necessitate an emergent surgical consult.

▶ Button batteries in the esophagus as well as sharp, pointed objects in the stomach must be removed as soon as possible. In general, the preferred method of swallowed foreign body removal is endoscopy (except in body packers because of the risk of packet rupture).

REFERENCES

Aghababian, R. *Essentials of Emergency Medicine.* 2nd ed. Sudbury, Mass: Jones and Bartlett Publishers; 2011.

Harrigan R, and Ufberg JW , Tripp ML. *Emergency Medicine Review: Preparing for the Boards.* St. Louis, MO: Saunders/Elsevier; 2010.

Marx J A, Hockberger RS, Walls RM, et al. *Rosen's Emergency Medicine: Concepts and Clinical Practice.* 7th ed. Philadelphia, PA: Mosby/Elsevier; 2010.

Tintinalli Judith E, and Stapczynski JS. *Tintinalli's Emergency Medicine: A Comprehensive Study Guide.* New York, NY: McGraw-Hill; 2011:Chapter 80.

A 55-year-old man presents to the emergency department (ED) complaining of abdominal pain. The patient relates that he has been having intermittent pain throughout the abdomen for the past 12 hours, and since the onset of pain, he has vomited twice. His past medical history is significant for hypertension and colon cancer for which he underwent laparoscopic right colectomy 8 months ago. The patient indicates that he has not had any recent abdominal complaints. His last bowel movement was 1 day ago, and he denies any weight loss and hematochezia. On physical examination, the patient is afebrile. The pulse rate is 98 beats per minute, blood pressure is 132/84 mm Hg, and respiratory rate is 22 breaths per minute. His cardiopulmonary examination is unremarkable. His abdomen is obese, mildly distended, with well-healed surgical scars. No tenderness, guarding, or hernias are noted. His bowel sounds are diminished, with occasional high-pitched sounds. The rectal examination reveals normal tone, empty rectal vault, and hemoccult-negative stool.

▶ What is the most likely cause of this patient's problems?
▶ What are the next steps in this patient's evaluation?

ANSWERS TO CASE 20:

Intestinal Obstruction

Summary: A 55-year-old man with history of previous laparoscopic surgery for the resection of right colon carcinoma presents with intermittent abdominal pain and vomiting. The physical examination reveals no abdominal wall or groin hernias, no tenderness, and high-pitched bowel sounds.

- **Most likely diagnosis:** Bowel obstruction. It is unclear whether the intestinal obstruction is involving the large or small bowel, or whether it is complete or partial obstruction.

- **Next steps in evaluation:** Diagnostic radiography, which can be either plain x-rays or computed tomography (CT).

ANALYSIS

Objectives

1. Learn to recognize the clinical presentations of intestinal obstruction (small bowel and colon).
2. Learn the common causes of bowel obstructions.
3. Learn the approach in the selection of imaging modalities for the evaluation of patients with possible bowel obstruction.
4. Learn to recognize clinical and radiographic signs of complicated obstruction and the urgency associated with its management.

Considerations

In this patient scenario, the differential diagnosis for obstruction includes intestinal ileus, adhesions, ischemia, and obstruction from recurrence of metastatic colon carcinoma. For this individual, the probability of ileus as the cause of his abdominal symptoms is unlikely, because he has a history of crampy abdominal pain and findings of high-pitched bowel sounds, which are clinical features compatible with mechanical obstruction and not functional obstruction. **The first imaging study to consider can be an abdominal series or CT scan.** The radiographic studies will help to distinguish partial obstruction from high grade, complete obstruction. The abdominal series may delineate the level of obstruction. **The presence of stool or air in the rectal vault may suggest a partial obstruction,** whereas the presence of air and fluid levels in the small intestine, with the absence of stool and air throughout the colon, indicate a high-grade, small-bowel obstruction. His past history of colon cancer points to the possibility that recurrent cancer may be the cause of his bowel obstruction; thus, a computed tomography (CT) scan of the abdomen may be helpful in identifying any obstructing tumor masses. In addition, CT scan can help identify a transition point in the GI tract where the luminal diameter of the bowel changes, thus differentiate a mechanical obstruction from a functional obstruction.

APPROACH TO:
Bowel Obstruction

DEFINITIONS

CLOSED-LOOP OBSTRUCTION: Blockage occurs both proximal and distal to the dilated segment preventing decompression. Examples include an isolated loop of small bowel caught in a tight hernia defect, a twisting of the bowel on itself causing a volvulus, or a complete large-bowel obstruction in a patient with a competent ileocecal valve. These obstructions are unlikely to resolve with nonoperative therapy.

COMPLICATIONS OF BOWEL OBSTRUCTION: Ischemia, necrosis, or perforation as a result of obstruction.

CT SCAN OF THE ABDOMEN: This modality is increasingly used in the evaluation of patients with bowel obstruction. CT can help to differentiate functional obstruction from mechanical obstruction. It is also useful in the evaluation of patients with previous abdominal malignancy to help determine if the obstruction is related to tumor recurrence. In addition, there are a number of CT characteristics that will identify high-grade, complicated obstructions, and differentiate these from uncomplicated obstructions. Disadvantages of CT in comparison to plain abdominal radiographs include intravenous contrast exposure that has the potential of causing acute kidney injury in a patient who is hypovolemic, and excessive exposure to ionizing radiation that could have significant late carcinogenic effects.

FUNCTIONAL OR NEUROGENIC OBSTRUCTION: Luminal contents cannot pass because of bowel motility disturbances preventing peristasis. Etiologies include neurogenic dysfunction, medication-related or metabolic problems, bowel wall infiltrative processes such as collagen vascular diseases, or extraluminal infiltrative processes such as peritonitis or malignancy. Surgery generally does not improve the above conditions; however, complications related to the above conditions may require operative intervention.

MECHANICAL OBSTRUCTION: Luminal contents cannot pass through the gastrointestinal (GI) tract because of a mechanical obstruction. The treatment can be operative or nonoperative depending on the cause, severity, and duration of the obstructive process.

OPEN-LOOP OBSTRUCTION: Intestinal blockage is distal, allowing proximal bowel decompression of obstruction via nasogastric (NG) suction or emesis.

SIMPLE (UNCOMPLICATED) BOWEL OBSTRUCTION: Partial or complete obstruction of the bowel lumen without compromise to the intestinal blood flow.

UPPER GI–SMALL-BOWEL FOLLOW THROUGH: This is contrast radiography done following the administration of oral contrast. The study accurately localizes obstruction site and caliber in the small bowel. The administration of contrast may be associated with worsening of obstruction and aspiration. This study is rarely indicated in the ED setting.

CLINICAL APPROACH

The causes of bowel obstruction in young children (<5 years of age) are quite different than those found in the adult population. The following discussion is limited to adult patients. **Adhesions** represent the most common cause of **small-bowel obstruction** whereas **colorectal carcinoma** is the most common cause of **large-bowel obstruction in developed countries.** Table 20–1 lists the distribution and clinical features associated with obstructive causes.

Pathophysiology

With mechanical obstruction, **air and fluid accumulate in the bowel lumen.** The net result is an **increase in the intestinal intraluminal pressure,** which inhibits fluid absorption and stimulates the influx of water and electrolytes into the lumen. Eighty percent of air found inside the bowel lumen is swallowed air (see Figure 18–1). Because of this, NG tube decompression may be useful in preventing progression of bowel distension. Initially following the onset of mechanical obstruction, there is an increase in peristaltic activity. However, as the obstructive process progresses (usually >24 hours), coordinated peristaltic activity diminishes along with the contractile function of obstructed bowel, giving rise to dilated and atonic bowel proximal to the point of obstruction. With this progression, the patient may actually appear to improve clinically with less frequent and less intense crampy abdominal pain. The effects of mechanical obstruction on intestinal blood flow include an initial increase in blood flow. **With unrelieved obstruction, blood flow diminishes leading to a breakdown of mucosal barriers and an increased susceptibility to bacterial invasion and ischemia.**

Table 20–1 • SMALL- VS LARGE-BOWEL OBSTRUCTION	
Small-Bowel Obstruction	**Large-Bowel Obstruction**
Causes • Adhesions (70%-75%) • Malignancy (8%-10%) • Hernia (8%-10%) • Volvulus (3%) • Inflammatory bowel disease (1%) • Intussusception, gallstone ileus, radiation enteritis, intra-abdominal abscess, bezoar (all <1%)	**Causes** • Carcinoma (65%) • Volvulus (15%) • Diverticular disease (10%) • Hernias, peritoneal carcinomatosis, fecal impaction, ischemic colitis, foreign body, inflammatory bowel disease (total 10%)
Symptoms • Vomiting (more common with proximal obstruction) • Cramping pain (common, early) • Distension (variable, with greater distension seen with distal obstruction)	**Symptoms** • Distension (common and usually significant) • Postprandial cramps and bloating (very common) • Vomiting (unusual) • Bowel habit changes (common)

Clinical Presentation

The **common clinical manifestations of bowel obstruction are pain, emesis, constipation,** obstipation, distension, tenderness, visible peristalsis, and/or shock. The presence or absence of these signs and symptoms are dependent on the severity of the obstruction. Pain associated with bowel obstruction is generally severe at the onset and is characterized as intermittent and poorly localized. With the progression of small-bowel obstruction, spastic pain decreases in intensity and frequency. However, continuous pain may develop as the result of ischemia or peritonitis. Patients with **large-bowel obstruction, pain frequently present with postprandial crampy pain,** and some patients with chronic large-bowel obstruction may describe the symptoms as indigestion. Continuous pain may also develop with the progression of marked distension, ischemia, or perforation.

Emesis is a symptom found commonly in patients with intestinal obstruction. In general, patients with proximal obstruction of the small bowel report the most dramatic episodes, whereas patients with distal obstructions may not experience as much emesis. The quality of the material vomited may help indicate the level of obstruction, as obstruction in the distal small bowel may produce feculent vomitus. Contrary to common beliefs, **obstruction of the large bowel often is not associated with vomiting,** because the presence of a competent ileocecal valve (found in 50%-60% of individuals) frequently contributes to a closed-loop obstruction.

Absence of bowel movements and flatus are suggestive of a high-grade or complete obstruction. With the stimulation of peristalsis at the initiation of an obstructive episode, it is not unusual for a patient to describe having bowel movements. The presence of a recent bowel movement does not rule out the diagnosis of a bowel obstruction. The classic description of decreased stool caliber is infrequently reported by patients with large-bowel obstruction, and when reported, this finding is not specific for colonic obstruction. On the other hand, diarrhea is frequently reported by patients with progressive large-bowel obstruction. Presumably, with high-grade narrowing of the bowel lumen, passage of the solid and semisolid contents are blocked, therefore the stools become more liquid in character. Distension to some degree is generally observed in most patients with intestinal obstruction; however, this finding may be absent in patients with obstruction of the proximal small bowel; therefore, the absence of distension does not eliminate the possibility of intestinal obstruction.

Patients with uncomplicated obstruction usually have mild, ill-defined, nonlocalized abdominal tenderness. The tenderness results from distension of the bowel wall leading to the aggravation of visceral pain. In the case of open-loop obstruction, decompression by emesis or NG tube frequently results in the improvement or resolution of abdominal tenderness. **Localized tenderness is a finding that is infrequently encountered in patients with uncomplicated bowel obstruction,** and the presence of localized tenderness **is suggestive of complications involving an isolated bowel segment.** The presence of this finding should raise the suspicion for a closed-loop obstruction, bowel necrosis or perforation, and in patients without obvious need for urgent operative treatment, further evaluation with CT scan may be beneficial.

CT Finding	Clinical Implications Associated With Finding
Dilated small bowel (>2.5 cm) with transition to normal-sized bowel	Mechanical small bowel obstruction (SBO)
>50% diameter difference between proximal dilated small bowel and distal small bowel	High-grade SBO
Small-bowel feces	Moderate- to high-grade obstruction
Intraperitoneal free fluid	This finding in the setting of SBO suggests high-grade SBO
Thickened small bowel wall	High-grade obstruction
Target sign	Intussusception
Swirl sign	Internal hernia or volvulus
Reduced bowel wall enhancement	Ischemic bowel wall
Pneumatosis intestinalis	Ischemic bowel wall/necrosis

MANAGEMENT OF SMALL-BOWEL OBSTRUCTION

When identified early, patients with uncomplicated small-bowel obstruction should be managed by NPO, intravenous hydration, and NG tube decompression. This therapy is directed at correcting the fluid and electrolyte deficits and reversing the cycle of inflammatory and metabolic events associated with increased intestinal luminal pressures. Many patients with early, partial small-bowel obstruction can be successfully managed without further problems. Patients with suspected small-bowel obstruction should undergo CT imaging, which may help differentiate uncomplicated small-bowel obstructions from complicated obstructions and help identify patients at risk of developing complicated obstructions.

Typically, **patients who present late in the course of obstruction are less** likely **to resolve with nonoperative management.** Furthermore, in these patients with prolonged obstruction, the probability of **bowel ischemia and necrosis** is increased. The development of complicated small-bowel obstruction is associated with increase morbidity and mortality; therefore, every effort should be made to identify and initiate early treatment in these patients. No clinical, laboratory, and radiographic criteria will reliably predict and identify patients with small-bowel obstruction who will go on to develop bowel necrosis. **The presence of fever, tachycardia, persistent abdominal pain, abdominal tenderness, leukocytosis, and high-grade obstruction are associated with the increased likelihood of bowel necrosis. These findings should prompt early referral to a surgeon, and patients with these findings are more likely to benefit from early surgical interventions.**

The nonoperative approach does not address the source of the small-bowel obstruction. Therefore, prolonged nonoperative therapy would be considered inappropriate for patients with surgically correctable causes such as abdominal wall and groin hernias and obstructing neoplasms. Similarly, patients with no previous abdominal operations and no defined causes for intra-abdominal adhesions should undergo resuscitation and prompt evaluation to identify a possibly treatable source of obstruction (eg, Crohn disease, tumors, volvulus, and internal hernias).

MANAGEMENT OF LARGE-BOWEL OBSTRUCTION

Patients with **large-bowel obstruction are often older and more severely dehydrated** and should be managed with **nasogastric suction, intravenous fluid hydration, and close monitoring for their responses to fluid** resuscitation. Patients with inappropriate response to fluid resuscitation may require admissions to an intensive care unit where invasive monitoring may be used to guide the resuscitation efforts; alternatively, poor response to initial fluid resuscitation could indicate complications such as perforations and/or bowel necrosis, therefore early surgical interventions may be needed.

The major diagnostic dilemma in patients with suspected large-bowel obstruction is differentiating mechanical obstruction from functional obstruction (dysmotility). In most patients, a **CT scan** will help make the differentiation. When mechanical and functional obstruction cannot be differentiated by CT imaging, a contrast enema without bowel preparation may be obtained.

Colorectal carcinoma is by far the most common cause of mechanical large-bowel obstruction. The site of obstruction of colon carcinoma correlates to the luminal diameter of the large bowel, rather than with the frequency of distribution of carcinoma. The generally reported frequency of distribution of obstructing colorectal carcinoma is **splenic flexure (40%), hepatic flexure (25%), descending and sigmoid colon (25%), transverse colon (10%), and ascending colon and cecum (10%).** Less commonly, sigmoid volvulus, and diverticular disease may cause large-bowel obstruction, in these settings the plain radiographs generally will identify the sigmoid volvulus. When identified, the volvulus may be evaluated and resolved by proctosigmoidoscopy performed without bowel preparation. Because nearly all patients with large-bowel obstruction will require operative treatment, surgical consultations should be obtained early in these patients.

One of the most devastating complications associated with large-bowel obstruction is colonic perforation, which generally occurs in the cecum or right colon. **The risk for developing colonic perforation is increased among patients with severely dilated colon (>10 cm cecal diameter).** These patients may or may not present with frank peritonitis; however, most patient will have severe volume contraction as a consequence of the ongoing inflammatory changes. The diagnosis of colonic perforation should be entertained when patients fail to improve with aggressive fluid management.

COMPREHENSION QUESTIONS

20.1 A 44-year-old woman with a past history of appendicitis that was treated by appendectomy 2 years ago presents with abdominal pain of 4-day duration. Her temperature is 38.5°C (101.3°F), pulse rate is 120 beats per minute, and blood pressure is 100/84 mm Hg. Her abdomen is distended and diffusely tender, with guarding. An occasional, high-pitched bowel sound is present. A kidneys, ureters, bladder (KUB) x-ray reveals a markedly dilated small bowel without air or stool in the colon. Which of the following is the most appropriate course of management?

A. Place IV, NG tube, and Foley catheter, initiate broad-spectrum antibiotics, and obtain CT of abdomen.

B. Place IV, NG tube, and Foley catheter, initiate broad-spectrum antibiotics, and prepare patient for operation.

C. Place IV, NG tube, and Foley catheter, initiate broad-spectrum antibiotics, and attempt nonoperative treatment.

D. Place IV, NG tube, and Foley catheter, initiate broad-spectrum antibiotics, obtain CT scan of abdomen, and prepare patient for an operation.

E. Place IV, NG tube, and Foley catheter. Admit the patient to the ICU for monitoring.

20.2 Which of the following is the most likely cause of small-bowel obstruction in 25-year-old woman with no previous abdominal operations?

A. Adhesions

B. Hernia

C. Crohn disease

D. Adenocarcinoma of the small bowel

E. Endometriosis

20.3 A third-year medical student has been given an assignment to assess the relative value of methods to differentiate between functional intestinal obstruction and mechanical obstruction. The patient scenario is that of a 90-year-old woman with Alzheimer disease, urinary tract infection, and abdominal distension. Which of the following statements is most accurate for this clinical learning issue?

A. The history and physical examination is the most important test in differentiating between the two disorders.

B. The history and physical examination while often unhelpful is better than imaging tests in differentiating between the two disorders.

C. The history and physical examination is typically unhelpful in differentiating between the two disorders.

D. Imaging tests are rarely helpful, may exacerbate the condition and worsen the prognosis.

E. CT scan is helpful in differentiating between the two pathological conditions in this patient.

ANSWERS

20.1 **B.** This patient presents with signs and symptoms of high-grade small-bowel obstruction. The physical examination is highly suspicious for presence of intra-abdominal complications associated with the obstruction; therefore, CT scan is unlikely to contribute further in the diagnosis, and nonoperative therapy is inappropriate for a patient who is already exhibiting signs and symptoms of complicated small-bowel obstruction.

20.2 **B.** Statistically speaking, a hernia would be the most likely cause of small-bowel obstruction in a patient without previous abdominal operations or other causes of adhesions.

20.3 **E.** History and physical examination is often inadequate in differentiating mechanical large-bowel obstruction from functional large-bowel obstruction, and this would be especially true in a patient with Alzheimer disease and possible cause for functional large-bowel obstruction. CT scan of the abdomen, barium enema and/or 4-view radiographs of the abdomen are some of the imaging tests used in this setting.

CLINICAL PEARLS

▶ Persistent pain in a patient with small-bowel obstruction is usually suggestive of bowel ischemia or impending bowel necrosis.

▶ Localized tenderness in a patient with small-bowel obstruction may indicate an isolated segment of closed-loop obstruction, localized ischemic injury, or localized perforation.

▶ Because the symptoms and physical findings associated with large-bowel obstruction are nonspecific, they can be easily overlooked by both the patient and the physician.

▶ **Adhesions** represent the most common cause of **small-bowel obstruction**, whereas **colorectal carcinoma** is the most common cause of **large-bowel obstruction.**

REFERENCES

Arnaoutakis GJ, Eckhauser FE. Small bowel obstruction. In: Cameron JL, Cameron AM, eds. *Current Surgical Therapy.* 10th ed. Philadelphia, PA: Mosby Elsevier; 2011:93-96.

Tavakkolizadeh A, Whang EE, Ashley SW, Zinner MJ. Small intestine. In Brunicardi FC, Andersen DK, Billiar TR, Dunn DL, Hunter JG, Mathews JB, Pollock RE, eds. *Schwartz's Principle of Surgery.* 9th ed. New York, NY: McGraw-Hill; 2011:979-1012.

Webb ALB, Fink AS. Large bowel obstruction. In: Cameron JL, Cameron AM, eds. *Current Surgical Therapy.* 10th ed. Philadelphia, PA: Mosby Elsevier; 2011:154-157.

A 19-year-old woman is brought into the emergency department (ED) complaining of abdominal pain and diarrhea of 3-day duration. She has also been nauseous and has not been able to drink much liquid. Five days ago she returned from a camping trip in New Mexico, but did not drink from natural streams. She denies fever, but states that she has had some chills. Her stools have been watery, brown, and profuse. The patient denies health problems. On examination, the patient is thin and pale. Her mucous membranes are dry. Her temperature is 37.2°C (99°F), heart rate 110 beats per minute, and blood pressure 90/60 mm Hg. The skin has no lesions. Her heart and lung examinations are unremarkable except tachycardia. The abdominal examination reveals hyperactive bowel sounds and no masses. There is diffuse mild tenderness but no guarding or rebound. Rectal examination demonstrates no tenderness or masses, and is Hemoccult negative. The complete blood count reveals a leukocyte count of 16,000 cells/mm³. The pregnancy test is negative.

► What is the most likely diagnosis?
► What is the next diagnostic step?
► What is the next step in therapy?

ANSWERS TO CASE 21:

Acute Diarrhea

Summary: A 19-year-old healthy woman presents to the ED with a 3-day history of abdominal pain, nausea, and non-bloody, watery, profuse diarrhea. Five days ago, she was on a camping trip in New Mexico but did not drink from natural streams. Her mucous membranes are dry. Her temperature is 37.2°C (99°F), heart rate 110 beats per minute, and blood pressure 90/60 mm Hg. The abdominal examination reveals hyperactive bowel sounds, no masses, and diffuse mild tenderness without peritoneal signs. Rectal examination is occult blood negative. The leukocyte count is 16,000 cells/μL. The pregnancy test is negative.

- **Most likely diagnosis:** Acute volume depletion and possible electrolyte abnormalities

- **Next diagnostic step:** Stool for fecal leukocytes

- **Next step in therapy:** Intravenous fluid hydration

ANALYSIS

Objectives

1. Know a diagnostic approach to acute diarrhea including the role of fecal leukocytes and assessment for occult blood in the stools.

2. Understand that volume replacement and correction of electrolyte abnormalities are the first priorities in treatment of diarrhea.

3. Be familiar with a rational workup for acute diarrhea, and know the common etiologies of diarrhea, including *Escherichia coli*, *Shigella*, *Salmonella*, *Giardia*, and amebiasis.

Considerations

This 19-year-old woman developed severe diarrhea, and nausea. Her most immediate problem is volume depletion as evidenced by her dry mucous membranes, tachycardia, and hypotension. The **first priority** should be for **acute replacement of intravascular volume,** usually with **intravenous normal saline.** The electrolytes should be assessed, and abnormalities, such as hypokalemia, should be corrected. After volume repletion, the next priority is to determine the etiology of the diarrhea. **Up to 90% of acute diarrhea is infectious in etiology.** This patient does not have a history consistent with inflammatory bowel disease or prior abdominal surgeries. She had been camping in New Mexico recently, which predisposes her to several pathogens: *E coli*, *Campylobacter*, *Shigella*, *Salmonella*, and *Giardia*. She does not have grossly bloody stools which would usually mandate an evaluation, and suggests invasive bacterial infections such as hemorrhagic or enteroinvasive

E coli species, *Yersinia* species, *Shigella*, and *Entamoeba histolytica*. Additionally, the stool for occult blood is negative. Fetal leukocyte is an inexpensive and good test to differentiate between the various types of infectious diarrhea. If the fecal leukocytes are present in the stool, the ED physician may have a higher suspicion for *Salmonella*, *Shigella*, *Campylobacter*, *Clostridium difficile*, *Yersinia*, enterohemorrhagic and enteroinvasive *E coli*, and *E histolytica*. Stool cultures are helpful. In general, ova and parasite evaluation is unhelpful unless the history strongly points toward a parasitic source, or the diarrhea is prolonged. Most diarrheas are self-limited, and do not need evaluation. Table 21–1 summarizes the danger signs. Because of the severity of this patient's symptoms, empiric antibiotic therapy such as with ciprofloxacin might be indicated.

Table 21–1 • ETIOLOGIES OF DIARRHEA

Etiologic Agent	Incubation Time	Diarrhea	Emesis	Abdominal Pain	Fever	Comments
Staphylococcus aureus, Clostridium perfringens	4-12 h	Watery, profuse	Pronounced	Mild	Absent	Preformed toxin, may be in foods
Vibrio cholerae, enterotoxigenic Escherichia coli	8-72 h	Watery, profuse	Moderate	Mild	Absent	Enterotoxin produced
E Coli, Giardia	2-7 d	Variable, watery	Mild	Moderate	Variable	Enteroadherent or enteropathogenic
Hemorrhagic E coli, Clostridium difficile	1-3 d	Variable, often bloody	Mild	Severe	Mild	Cytotoxin producing, causing cell necrosis and inflammation
Salmonella, Campylobacter, Shigella, enteroinvasive E coli, Entamoeba histolytica	1-4 d	Often bloody	Mild	Severe	Moderate to high	Invasive organisms leading to inflammation, abdominal pain, and fever

Data from Ahlquist DA, Camilleri M. Diarrhea and constipation. In: Braunwald E, Faucis AS, Kaspar DL, et al, eds. Harrison's Principles of Internal Medicine. 15th ed. New York, NY: McGraw Hill; 2001.

APPROACH TO:
Acute Diarrhea

DEFINITIONS

ACUTE DIARRHEA: Present for less than 2-week duration.

CHRONIC DIARRHEA: Diarrhea present for greater than 4-week duration.

DIARRHEA: Passage of abnormally liquid or poorly formed stool in increased frequency.

SUBACUTE (PERSISTENT) DIARRHEA: Present for 2- to 4-week duration.

CLINICAL APPROACH

Etiologies

Approximately 90% cases of acute diarrhea are caused by infectious etiologies, and the remainder is caused by medications, ischemia, or toxins. Infectious etiologies often depend on the patient population. For instance, **travelers to Mexico or Asia will frequently contract enterotoxigenic E coli as a causative agent.** Those traveling to Russia and campers and backpackers will often be affected by *Giardia*. *Campylobacter*, *Shigella*, and *Salmonella* are also common causative agents.

Consumption of foods is also frequently a culprit. **Salmonella or Shigella** can be found in **undercooked chicken, enterohemorrhagic E coli in undercooked hamburger,** and **Staphylococcus aureus or Salmonella in mayonnaise.** Raw seafood may harbor *Vibrio*, *Salmonella*, or hepatitis A, B, or C. Sometimes the timing of the diarrhea following food ingestion is helpful.

For example, illness within **6 hours of eating a salad** (mayonnaise) suggests **S aureus, 8-12 hours post-ingestion suggests Clostridium perfringens, and 12 to 14 hours post-ingestion suggests E coli** (see Table 21–1).

Day-care settings are particularly common locales for *Shigella*, *Giardia*, and rotavirus transmission. Patients in nursing homes and who were recently in the hospital may develop C *difficile* colitis from antibiotic use. In addition, immunecompromised patients with prior history of C *difficile* infections may remain colonized and recurrent clinical infections despite appropriate treatment.

Clinical Presentation

Most patients with acute diarrhea have self-limited processes, and do not require much workup. Exceptions to this rule include **profuse diarrhea, dehydration, fever exceeding 38.5°C (101.3°F), grossly bloody diarrhea, an elderly patient, severe abdominal pain, duration exceeding 48 hours without improvement, and an immunocompromised patient.** Mortalities related to diarrheal illnesses are generally due to the inadequate recognition and treatment of dehydration, electrolyte disturbances, and acidosis.

The history should be meticulous about trying to identify prior history of GI complaints, exposure history including medications, foods, travel history, and contacts with individuals with similar symptoms. A history of recent viral illness may provide clue to the etiology. Occupational history may help identify infectious sources.

The clinician should determine what the patient can tolerate orally; in other words, if the patient is both vomiting and having profuse diarrhea, severe dehydration is likely. The amount and character of the stools may be helpful to determine etiology, as well as direct therapy.

The physical examination should focus on the vital signs, clinical impression of the patient's hydration status, indicators of sepsis, mental status, and abdominal examination. The patient's hydration status is determined by observing whether the mucous membranes are moist or dry, skin has good turgor or is tenting, jugular venous distention, and capillary refill. The principal laboratory test is the stool for microscopic and microbiological examination. Stool culture results generally require several days to become finalized and are not useful in the ED setting; however, these results may be helpful for follow-up evaluations and for patients who do not improve with initial management. Ova and parasite evaluation is generally unhelpful except in selected circumstances of very high suspicion. Stool for **C *difficile* toxin** may yield the etiology in patients who develop symptoms after **antibiotic use,** and in most instances, the enzyme immunoassay results may be available in as little as two hours. Although pseudomembranous colitis was classically associated with clindamycin usage, fluoroquinolones are reported recently as the most common antibiotics contributing to the condition. *C difficile* infections are also being increasingly reported in patients with inflammatory bowel disease (IBD), where the symptoms may be difficult to differentiate from an exacerbation of IBD. A complete blood count, electrolytes, and renal function tests are sometimes indicated.

Traveler's diarrhea most often presents as watery diarrhea occurring a few days after traveling to Mexico, South America, Africa, or South Asia. This type of diarrhea is most often caused by enterotoxigenic *E coli*, which can produce diarrhea from the generation of toxin leading to cholera-like symptoms; infections by enteroinvasive strains of *E coli* causing a shigella-like illness that is manifested by bloody mucous-producing diarrhea; and chronic infections related to *E coli* overgrowth. Fluids and electrolyte replacements are the mainstay of treatment for traveler's diarrhea. A number of agents are helpful in reducing stool frequency, and these agents include bismuth subsalicylate and loperamide.

Antibiotic therapy may be indicated when symptoms do not resolve with supportive care and stool-reducing agents. For travelers returning from the non-coastal regions of Mexico, double-strength trimethoprin-sulfamethoxazole twice a day is recommended. For other patients, ciprofloxacin (750 mg), levofloxacin (500 mg), norfloxacin (800 mg), or azithromycin (1000 mg) are recommended. For immune compromised patients and elderly patients with comorbidities, prophylaxis with trimethoprim-sulfamethoxazole or a fluoroquinolone can be prescribed.

If the etiology is still unclear and the patient is not improving while off oral intake, hospital admission and consultation with a gastroenterologist may be indicated. Radiological studies or endoscopy may be needed to determine the cause. Diseases such as inflammatory bowel disease or ischemic bowel disease must be considered.

Treatment

Fluid and electrolyte replacement are fundamental to the treatment of acute diarrhea. For mildly dehydrated individuals who can tolerate oral fluids, **sports**

drinks such as Gatorade orally are often all that is needed. In developing countries, the oral rehydration solution (ORS) introduced by the World Health Organization (WHO) has been shown to be well tolerated by patients and well received by care givers. For those with more serious volume deficits, or elderly patients or infants, hospitalization and intravenous hydration may be necessary. **Bismuth subsalicylate** may be used to alleviate the gastrointestinal symptoms, but should not be used in an immune-compromised individual because of the risk of bismuth encephalopathy. Many physicians choose to treat patients with moderately ill or severely ill appearance empirically with ciprofloxacin 500 mg twice daily for 5 days. Antimicrobial treatment may not alter the course of the disease.

Traveler's Prophylaxis

The best method in preventing traveler's diarrhea, which is principally caused by enterotoxigenic *E coli*, is avoidance of food and water in areas of high risk. Travelers should be advised to drink only bottled water, and avoid eating foods from street vendors or unhygienic locations. "*Boil it, cook it, peel it, or forget it*" remains a sound advice for individuals traveling to Latin America, the Caribbean, Africa, and South Asia. The CDC endorses **bismuth subsalicylate, two 262-mg tablets chewed well four times a day** (with meals and at bedtime), but does not advocate the use of antimicrobial agents because a false sense of security or antibiotic resistance may result. Nevertheless, many practitioners prescribe **ciprofloxacin 500 mg once a day. Medical prophylaxis (either bismuth subsalicylate or antibiotic) should not be used for longer than 3 weeks.**

COMPREHENSION QUESTIONS

Match the following etiologies (A to F) to the clinical situations in Questions 21.1 to 21.4:

    A. *E coli*

    B. *Giardia*

    C. Rotavirus

    D. *S aureus*

    E. *Vibrio*

    F. *Cryptosporidium*

21.1 During the winter, a 24-year-old woman who works at a day care develops profuse watery diarrhea.

21.2 A 22-year-old college student takes a trip during spring break to Cozumel and develops diarrhea.

21.3 Several workers develop watery diarrhea and significant emesis within 4 hours after eating food at a potluck dinner.

21.4 A 45-year-old man eats raw oysters and 2 days later develops abdominal cramping, fever to 38.3°C (101°F), and watery diarrhea.

ANSWERS

21.1 **C.** Rotavirus usually causes a watery diarrhea, and is especially common in the winter.

21.2 **A.** *E coli* is the most common etiology for diarrhea in travelers visiting Mexico.

21.3 **D.** *S aureus* usually causes prominent vomiting and diarrhea within a few hours of food ingestion as a consequence of the toxin produced.

21.4 **E.** Raw seafood may harbor *Vibrio* spec; thus, the history of eating raw oysters makes Vibrio-related infection likely.

CLINICAL PEARLS

▶ The vast majority of acute diarrhea is caused by an infectious etiology.

▶ Most acute diarrheas are self-limited.

▶ One should be cautious when assessing acute diarrhea in immunosuppressed patients, very young, or elderly patients.

▶ Significant dehydration, grossly bloody diarrhea, high fever, and nonresponse after 48 hours are warning signs of possible complicated diarrhea.

▶ In general, acute uncomplicated diarrhea can be treated with oral electrolyte-fluid solution with or without empiric ciprofloxacin.

REFERENCES

Faris B, Blackmore A, Haboubi N. Review of medical and surgical management of *Clostridium difficile* infection. *Tech Coloproctol.* 2010:DOI 10.1007/s10151-010-0574-3.

Hill Dr, Beeching NJ. Travelers' diarrhea. *Curr Opin Infect Dis.* 2010;23:481-487.

House HR, Ehlers JP. Travel-related infections. *Emerg Med Clin N Am.* 2008;26:499-516.

Pigott DC. Foodborne illness. *Emerg Med Clin N Am.* 2008;26:475-497.

A 30-year-old white man presents to the emergency department (ED) complaining of sudden onset of abdominal bloating and back pain. Patient states he was sleeping comfortably but the sudden onset of severe, constant pain that radiates from his back to his abdomen and down toward his scrotum caused him to awaken. He is unable to find a comfortable position and feels best when ambulating. He admits to having had occasional hematuria but denies ever having this type of pain before. He has no other significant medical problems. On physical examination the patient is diaphoretic and in moderate distress. His blood pressure is 128/76 mm Hg, heart rate is 90 beats per minute, temperature is 37.4°C (99.4°F), and his respiratory rate is 28 breaths per minute. His cardiovascular examination reveals tachycardia without murmurs. Lung examination is clear to auscultation. Abdominal examination demonstrates good bowel sounds, and no abdominal distension and costovertebral angle tenderness. A midstream voided urine specimen demonstrates gross hematuria.

► What is the most likely diagnosis?
► How would you confirm the diagnosis?
► What is the next step in treatment?

ANSWERS TO CASE 22:

Nephrolithiasis

Summary: A 30-year-old healthy man complains of the acute onset of severe back pain and a history of gross hematuria. He appears to be in moderate distress and has not previously experienced these symptoms.

- **Most likely diagnosis**: Nephrolithiasis.

- **Confirmation of the diagnosis:** Perform a urinalysis, complete blood count (CBC), serum chemistries, kidneys, ureters, bladder (KUB) radiograph, and intravenous pyelogram or computed tomography (CT) scan of the abdomen.

- **Next steps in treatment:** Start IV fluids and provide adequate pain management for the patient before sending him for the appropriate imaging study. Strain all urine once the diagnosis of nephrolithiasis is suspected and perform stone analysis on any stone passed.

ANALYSIS

Objectives

1. Recognize the history and typical presentation of a patient with nephrolithiasis.

2. Learn to order the appropriate laboratory and radiographic studies to diagnose nephrolithiasis.

3. Learn to treat and manage nephrolithiasis in an acute situation.

Considerations

This patient has a very typical presentation for nephrolithiasis; male (three times more common in men than in women) and the history of the sudden onset of pain that radiates from his back toward his abdomen. The emergency department physician must be careful to rule out other acute abdominal etiologies that may mimic the same presentation (Table 22–1 lists the differential diagnosis). Patients with nephrolithiasis often have difficulty in finding a comfortable position. Patients with an acute abdomen often feel better when they remain supine without moving or with their knees bent toward their chest. The pain can be described as constant, colicky, or as waxing and waning. A history of dark-brown-tinged urine may represent old blood in the urine (ie, from a stone high in the calyx), while a complaint of bright red blood in the urine may be more consistent with a lower urinary tract stone. A family history of nephrolithiasis or a personal history of stones within the urinary tract may make the diagnosis easier. On physical examination, the patients are usually normotensive, afebrile, but tachycardic. The presence of fever would suggest urinary tract infection such as pyelonephritis or some other disease process (appendicitis). The increase in heart rate is most likely related to his pain. Furthermore, costovertebral angle tenderness and hematuria on urinalysis are highly suggestive of a urinary tract process.

Table 22–1 • DIFFERENTIAL DIAGNOSIS OF NEPHROLITHIASIS
Appendicitis
Ectopic pregnancy
Salpingitis
Diverticulitis
Bowel obstruction
Renal artery embolism
Biliary stones
Ovarian torsion
Peptic ulcer disease
Abdominal aortic aneurysm
Gastroenteritis

APPROACH TO:

Nephrolithiasis

DEFINITIONS

CALCIUM OXALATE: It is the most common type of renal stone and is radio-dense.

EXTRACORPOREAL SHOCK WAVE LITHOTRIPSY (ESWL): Fluoroscopically focused shockwaves result in disintegration of the stone into fragments that are usually small enough to pass in the urine.

NEPHROLITHIASIS: A condition in which stone formation has occurred within the urinary tract system.

STONE COMPOSITION ANALYSIS: This is helpful in conjunction with metabolic workup to determine the underlying cause for stone formation when the history and physical examination does not identify risk factors for stone formation.

CLINICAL APPROACH

Epidemiology

Urinary calculus disease is a common condition that affects up to 10% of the US population. Nephrolithiasis is caused by urinary supersaturation; therefore, increases in urinary ion excretion and/or decrease in urinary volume are common factors that contribute to the process. The incidence of stone formation depends on a multitude of extrinsic and intrinsic risk factors, including socioeconomic status, diet, occupation, climate, medications, sex, and age (Table 22–2). **Nephrolithiasis is more common in men** than in women (3:1) and has its peak incidence between the ages of 30 and 50 years. Individuals exposed to high temperature either by geographic location or through occupational exposures are at increased risk of dehydration, which contributes to the risk of stone formation. Individuals with excessive sun exposure have

Table 22–2 • RISK FACTORS	
Metabolic factors	**Environmental factors**
• Hypercalciuria	• Hot, dry, increased sunlight
• Hyperuricosuria	**Drugs**
• Hypocitraturia	• Loop diuretics
• Hyperoxaluria	• Antacids
Primary hyperparathyroidism	• Acetazolamide
• Renal tubular acidosis	• Glucocorticoids
Age	• Theophylline
• 30-50 y	• Allopurinol
Sex	• Probenecid
• Male 3:1	• Triamterene
Diet	• Acyclovir
• Increased intake of calcium,	• Indinavir
• protein and oxalate	• Vitamins D and C
Socioeconomic status	

increased calcium absorption due to the increased production of vitamin D, therefore experience an increased risk of urinary calculus formation. Medications can also predispose individuals to stone formation (see Table 22–2). **Calcium-based (calcium oxalate and/or calcium phosphate) stones are the most common types of stones and account for more than 75% of urinary stones.** Other types of stone include magnesium ammonium phosphate, uric, and cystine stones. Uric acid stones tend to occur in patients with low urine pH (<6.0) and with hyperuricosuria. Cystine stones occur in the setting of cystinuria, which is a relatively common autosomal-recessive condition causing defects in the gastrointestinal and renal transport of cystine, ornithine, arginine, and lysine. **Magnesium ammonium phosphate (struvite) stones are more common in women and are usually associated with urinary infections with urease-producing organisms (*Proteus, Pseudomonas,* and *Klebsiella*).**

Clinical Presentation

The vast majority of patients with renal stones will present to the emergency department complaining of **acute onset of colicky or non-colicky renal pain.** Non-colicky pain is most likely caused by an upper urinary tract stone, whereas colicky pain is more likely caused by the stretching caused by the stone in the ureter. In addition, the presenting symptoms may include tachycardia, tachypnea, and hypertension, which are produced in response to pain. **Fever, pyuria, and severe costovertebral angle tenderness usually indicate a medical emergency, because pyelonephritis caused by obstruction often leads** to sepsis and rapid clinical deterioration. Persistent nausea and vomiting due to stimulation of the celiac ganglion may require the patient to be hospitalized.

A dipstick and microscopic examination of the voided midstream urine is very helpful, but the **amount of hematuria does not correlate with the degree of obstruction.** Although microscopic hematuria is present in 90% of cases of nephrolithiasis,

Table 22–3 • RISK FACTORS FOR NEPHROTOXICITY WITH CONTRAST DYE
Age >60 y
Dehydration
Hypotension
Multiple myeloma
Hyperuricemia
History of intravenous contrast within 72 h
Debilitated condition
Known cardiovascular disease, especially on a diuretic
Asthma
Renal insufficiency
Diabetes mellitus

a complete ureteral obstruction may present without hematuria. A careful analysis of urine sediment for crystals by an experienced individual should be performed promptly. In addition to the microscopic evaluation, a culture and sensitivity should be performed.

A KUB radiograph is sometimes helpful in identifying a urinary tract stone (90% are radiopaque). Traditionally, the intravenous pyelogram (IVP) has been the gold standard in evaluating a renal stone because it gives information about degree of obstruction as well as renal function. In many institutions, **newer-generation helical CT imaging without contrast is the preferred imaging method of choice for the evaluation of acute renal colic;** its sensitivity and specificity are greater than that of IVP, but renal function is not assessed. CT imaging also has the advantage of assessing the appendix, aorta, and diverticulitis. Regardless of test, the clinician should interpret the clinical picture in conjunction with the imaging results. Before an IVP, the patient should be questioned about allergy to contrast dye or shellfish, the possibility of pregnancy, and preexisting renal disease. Pregnant women and children generally should have ultrasound imaging first to avoid the radiation exposure. Table 22–3 lists the risk factors of nephrotoxicity associated with contrast dye.

Management

The critical issues surrounding nephrolithiasis are pain control, degree of obstruction, and presence of infection. Adequate analgesia is critical in treating a patient with nephrolithiasis, and analgesic administration should not be delayed pending test results. Depending on the severity of the pain, intravenous opiates, acetaminophen with codeine, meperidine, nonsteroidal anti-inflammatory drugs (NSAIDs), or morphine may be necessary. **NSAIDs should be used with caution in patients with renal insufficiency, in older patients, and in those with diabetes mellitus.** Evaluation of the patient's volume status will determine how much and what kind of intravenous fluids are necessary. Excessive hydration to dislodge a stone is not therapeutic and should not be attempted. Because definitive therapy is guided by the type of stones that are being formed, recovery of any passed stones and straining all urine is important for long-term management.

Conservative management, including analgesics, hydration, and antibiotics if urinary tract infection is suspected, may be all the patient needs. Most small stones (<6 mm) in diameter will produce symptoms but will typically pass without the need for interventions. **Indications for urgent urologic consultation are inadequate oral pain control, persistent nausea and vomiting, associated pyelonephritis, large stone (>7 mm), solitary kidney, or complete obstruction.** If the patient is being managed expectantly, the patient should be instructed to increase fluid intake and strain the urine until the stone is passed. Medical therapy including calcium channel blocker or α-blocker is being increasingly applied to facilitate stone passage and has been shown to be associated with a 65% increased in the likelihood of stone passage. Surgery is indicated in patients with stones larger than 5 to 8 mm, persistent pain, or failure to pass the stone despite conservative management. Stones located in the lower urinary tract system may be removed using a ureteroscope; upper urinary tract stones can be treated by ESWL.

COMPREHENSION QUESTIONS

22.1 After passing a kidney stone, a 38-year-old woman is told by her primary care physician that she had passed a magnesium ammonium phosphate stone. She is most likely to have had a urinary infection caused by which of the following organisms?

A. *Proteus*

B. *Escherichia coli*

C. *Enterococcus* species

D. Group B *Streptococcus*

E. *Staphylococcus aureus*

22.2 A 55-year-old man presents to the emergency department complaining of right flank pain for the past 2 weeks. He has noted some gross hematuria and has been unable to eat anything secondary to nausea and vomiting. Which of the following is an indication for hospitalization?

A. Gross hematuria

B. Right flank pain

C. Nausea and vomiting despite antiemetics

D. Age greater than 50 years

E. Presence of a 6-mm stone

22.3 A 39-year-old man complains of the sudden onset of severe left flank pain after running a marathon. He describes the pain as constant with radiation to his left groin area. A urinalysis shows microscopic hematuria and the presence of cystine crystals. Where is the stone most likely to be located?

A. Renal pelvis

B. Proximal ureter

C. Distal ureter

D. Uretero-vesicular junction

E. Bladder

22.4 A 33-year-old woman is pregnant at 12 weeks' gestation and presents with right flank pain and gross hematuria. She is afebrile. Which of the following imaging tests is most appropriate for this patient?

A. Ultrasonography

B. KUB

C. IVP

D. Retrograde pyelography

E. Helical CT without contrast

ANSWERS

22.1 **A.** This woman has a magnesium ammonium phosphate stone, which are common in women and are associated with urease-producing organisms. *Proteus, Pseudomonas,* and *Klebsiella* are all urease-producing organisms.

22.2 **C.** Hospitalization is required if the patient is unable to tolerate anything by mouth. Gross hematuria and flank pain are expected with nephrolithiasis. Appropriate analgesics should be prescribed for patients if they will not be hospitalized. Stones 6 mm or less will generally pass spontaneously without interventions.

22.3 **A.** Constant pain is most likely to be located in the kidney. Colicky pain is most likely to be located in the ureter and is caused by the stretching caused by the stone and inflammatory processes in the lumen of the ureter. Most stones in the renal pelvis or bladder are asymptomatic.

22.4 **A.** Because the patient is pregnant during the first trimester, the initial imaging test should be sonography to avoid the radiation-related teratogenic/mutagenic effects on the fetus.

CLINICAL PEARLS

▶ The acute presentation of nephrolithiasis resembles other pathologies; the correct studies and appropriate interpretation of laboratory data will help to establish the diagnosis.

▶ Any patient with severe nausea, vomiting, fever, or signs of infection should be hospitalized.

▶ Adequate pain control for patients with suspected nephrolithiasis is a priority even before all test results return.

▶ All urine should be strained to confirm the diagnosis and for the stone composition to be discerned.

▶ The absence of pain does not mean follow-up is unnecessary. Identifying the etiology of stone formation is important to prevent recurrence.

REFERENCES

Brener ZZ, Winchester JF, Salman H, Bergman M. Nephrolithiasis: evaluation and management. *Southern Med J.* 2011;104:133-139.

Hollingsworth JM, Rogers MA, Kaufman SR, et al. Medical therapy to facilitate urinary stone passage: a meta-analysis. *Lancet.* 2006;368:1171-1179.

Kahler J, Harwood-Nuss AL. Selected urologic problems. In: Marx JA, Hockberger RS, Walls RM, eds. *Rosen's Emergency Medicine. Concepts and Clinical Practice.* 6th ed. Philadelphia, PA: Mosby-Elsevier; 2006:1572-1606.

A 64-year-old man presents to the emergency department (ED) because of an inability to urinate for the past 24 hours. In addition, he complains of an unintentional weight loss of 20 lb over the past 6 months, night sweats, and generalized fatigue. On examination, he is thin and in moderate distress. His blood pressure is 168/92 mm Hg, heart rate is 102 beats per minute, temperature is 37.7°C (98.8°F), and respiratory rate is 22 breaths per minute. The abdominal examination reveals a tender mass in the suprapubic area. On rectal examination, the prostate is firm, nontender, and somewhat irregular.

▶ What is the most likely diagnosis?
▶ How would you confirm the diagnosis?
▶ What is the next step in treatment?

ANSWERS TO CASE 23:

Acute Urinary Retention

Summary: A 64-year-old man presents with an inability to void for the past 24 hours and a tender mass in the lower abdomen. The patient has signs and symptoms suggestive of prostate cancer, including unintentional weight loss, night sweats, a decrease in energy, and an enlarged irregular firm prostate gland.

- **Most likely diagnosis:** Acute urinary retention likely due to prostate cancer.

- **Confirming the diagnosis:** Thorough history and physical examination including a rectal examination, urinalysis, electrolytes and renal function tests, along with bedside ultrasound, if available. Prostate-specific antigen may help in the diagnosis of neoplastic disease if results will be available in the ED.

- **Next steps in treatment:** Draining the bladder by inserting a urethral catheter should relieve the patient's pain; if not, a suprapubic catheter can be placed. Treatment of the underlying disease process is also necessary.

ANALYSIS

Objectives

1. Recognize the typical signs and symptoms of acute urinary retention.

2. Know how to treat and manage acute urinary retention in the emergency department.

3. Identify when patients with acute urinary retention require hospitalization.

Considerations

Many disease processes, trauma, and medications can result in acute urinary retention (Table 23–1). In elderly men, the most common cause is prostatic hypertrophy. As with this patient, a thorough history and physical examination can help elucidate the etiology of the urinary retention. Passage of a urethral catheter to alleviate the obstruction will bring about significant pain relief. Assessment of renal function is important, as is obtaining a urinalysis to rule out concomitant urinary tract infection. Imaging studies in the ED are rarely necessary for these patients, although bedside ultrasound may help identify bladder distention or a clot in the bladder. Depending on this patient's renal function and physical status after drainage of his bladder, he may require admission.

Table 23–1 • CAUSES OF ACUTE URINARY RETENTION	
Cause	**Specific Examples**
Obstruction at the penis	Phimosis or paraphimosis Foreign body Stenosis at the meatus
Urethral obstruction	Stenosis at the meatus Calculus, tumor, foreign body, hematoma, trauma Urethral irritation Stricture
Prostate pathology	Benign prostatic hypertrophy (most common for men) Neoplasm Infarction Severe prostatitis
Neurologic diseases	Spinal cord syndromes, neurogenic bladder Tabes dorsalis, CVA Diabetes Multiple sclerosis
Medications	Anticholinergics (including antihistamines and cyclic antidepressants) Antispasmodics Spinal anesthesia Ephedrine derivatives, amphetamines

APPROACH TO:

Acute Urinary Retention

DEFINITIONS

ACUTE URINARY RETENTION: Sudden, complete inability to void accompanied by abdominal discomfort, with a palpable or percussible distended bladder containing greater than 150 mL of urine.

AZOTEMIA: Presence of nitrogenous bodies, especially urea, in the blood that develops in urinary tract obstruction when overall excretion function is impaired.

BENIGN PROSTATIC HYPERPLASIA: Overgrowth and proliferation of the epithelium and fibromuscular tissue of the prostate.

HYDRONEPHROSIS: Dilation of the renal pyelocalyceal system because of obstruction of the urinary tract system.

CLINICAL APPROACH

Because untreated urinary obstruction may lead to chronic renal failure, relieving the blockage is critical. Loss of urinary concentrating ability, azotemia, renal

Table 23–2 • TYPES OF RENAL TUBULAR ACIDOSIS (RTA)

Type	Mechanism	Laboratory Findings	Etiologies	Treatment
I (distal RTA)	Abnormality in distal hydrogen secretion	Hypokalemic hyperchloremic metabolic acidosis, urine pH >5.5	Autoimmune and genetic disorders, amphotericin, toluene, nephrocalcinosis, tubulointerstitial diseases	Oral sodium bicarbonate, potassium supplementation
II (proximal RTA)	Decreased proximal resorption of bicarbonate	Hypokalemic hyperchloremic metabolic acidosis, urine pH <5.5	Primary hyperparathyroidism, multiple myeloma, Fanconi syndrome, acetazolamide	Oral sodium bicarbonate, potassium supplementation
III[a]	Glomerular insufficiency; impaired ability to generate NH3	Normokalemic hyperchloremic metabolic acidosis, urine pH <5.5		
IV	Antagonism or deficiency of aldosterone → decreased distal acidification and sodium resorption	Hyperkalemic hyperchloremic metabolic acidosis, urine pH <5.5	Urinary obstruction, diabetes, sickle cell disease, Addison disease	Sodium bicarbonate for significant acidosis; furosemide for hyperkalemia

[a]Type III RTA is often not considered a distinct clinical entity. Thus many texts only describe Types I, II, and IV RTAs.

tubular acidosis (Table 23–2), hyperkalemia, and renal salt wasting may occur. Hypertension is common in acute urinary retention because of the increased release of renin by the involved kidneys. The most common presenting symptoms are urinary hesitancy, decreased force, terminal dribbling, nocturia, and typically overflow incontinence. Other symptoms include urinary urgency, hesitancy, and frequency, straining to void, and a sensation of incomplete bladder emptying. Pain due to bladder distention is the symptom that usually provokes the need for ED evaluation. A detailed history and physical examination will often help to identify the cause of the obstruction. History of previous instrumentation of the urinary tract, trauma, neurologic disease, prostatectomy, urologic malignancy, or chronic systemic illness may aid in the proper diagnosis and treatment. Evaluation of medications taken may help in identifying pharmacologic agents that may contribute to urinary retention (Table 23–3).

On physical examination, a palpable mass above the symphysis pubis that disappears after insertion of a urethral catheter is highly suggestive of a distended bladder (acute urinary retention). The meatus should be inspected for evidence of stenosis

Table 23–3 • MEDICATIONS THAT MAY CONTRIBUTE TO URINARY RETENTION	
Class of Medication	**Examples**
Anticholinergics	Atropine, benztropine, antihistamines, phenothiazines, cyclic antidepressants, ipratropium
β-Agonists	Isoproterenol, terbutaline
Detrusor muscle relaxants	Nifedipine, dicyclomine, hyoscyamine, oxybutynin, diazepam, NSAIDs, estrogen
Narcotics	Morphine, hydromorphone

and the penis palpated for fistulae or masses. Digital rectal examination may reveal prostatic nodules, asymmetry, tenderness, bogginess, or the typical stony hard enlargement of prostate cancer. A benign prostate on examination does not eliminate it as a cause of obstruction. Testing rectal sphincter tone, perianal sensation, and the bulbocavernosus reflex can be important in cases of suspected neurogenic bladder. In females, a pelvic examination should be performed to rule out inflammation, lesions, or an adnexal mass. Patient may also present febrile, tachypneic, or hypotensive suggesting an infection or sepsis.

Electrolytes and blood urea nitrogen (BUN)/creatinine levels should be obtained to assess renal function. The BUN may be elevated due to significant resorption secondary to the obstruction. A urinalysis is helpful to rule out concomitant infection, which would require antibiotics. Nephrolithiasis, neoplasm, or infection may cause hematuria. Imaging studies are rarely necessary in the ED, although a bedside ultrasound may help identify bladder distention or a clot in the bladder.

Management

Any patient with acute urinary retention requires relief of the obstruction as soon as possible in order to prevent progressive renal dysfunction. Initial efforts should be attempted with a standard urethral catheter. Lidocaine gel should be inserted into the urethra to anesthetize and lubricate the urethra before inserting a 16- or 18-F Foley catheter. If the ED physician is unable to pass the catheter because of an enlarged prostate, a 14- or 18-F coudé catheter may help. Occasionally a catheter may not pass secondary to urethral strictures. A urethral catheter should never be forced because urethral trauma and false passages may be created. In these situations, a urologist should be consulted. If consultation is not available, a suprapubic catheter may be placed or percutaneous bladder aspiration can be performed. These procedures may be performed with bedside ultrasound guidance.

After successful bladder drainage, complications may occur, including transient hematuria, hypotension, and postobstructive diuresis. Postobstructive diuresis can cause electrolyte abnormalities, profound fluid loss, and hypotension. Patients with this condition require monitoring of their urine output and fluid replacement. Risk factors for postobstructive diuresis include chronic bladder obstruction, fluid overload, and chronic renal disease.

Many patients with acute urinary retention can be discharged home with an indwelling urethral catheter and outpatient urologic follow-up. Admission should be considered for patients with renal dysfunction, a serious infection, or volume overload and for those who are unable to care for themselves.

COMPREHENSION QUESTIONS

23.1 An 88-year-old woman is seen in the ED complaining of significant lower abdominal pain and inability to void. She is noted to have a very full bladder. After a urethral catheter is placed, 1400 mL of urine is drained. She is afebrile with a blood pressure of 130/64 mm Hg, pulse of 74 beats per minute, and respiratory rate of 20 breaths per minute. Her laboratory results are remarkable for a BUN of 65 mg/dL and a urinalysis with moderate leukocyte esterase and many bacteria. Which of the following is the most appropriate management for this patient?

A. Discharge home with oral hydration and recheck the BUN in 48 hours.

B. Discharge home with home health nurse visits.

C. Place the patient on oral antibiotic therapy and arrange follow-up in 1 week.

D. Admit to the hospital for further therapy.

23.2 A 65-year-old man presents to the ED with progressive inability to void, suprapubic pain, and a lower abdominal mass. He has never experienced this type of pain before and is in moderate discomfort. Which of the following is your next step in management?

A. Rectal examination

B. Decompression of bladder with a urethral catheter

C. Computed tomography of the abdomen

D. Percutaneous bladder aspiration

23.3 A 35-year-old woman without any previous medical problems presents with acute urinary retention. She reports a history of increased fatigue with exertion and intermittent paresthesias but denies any history of diabetes, hypertension, or recurrent urinary infections. One year ago, she had some difficulty with double vision that had resolved spontaneously. Which of the following is the most likely diagnosis?

A. Drug abuse

B. Multiple sclerosis

C. Ovarian cancer

D. Spastic bladder

23.4 A 22-year-old woman complains of acute urinary retention, associated with vulvar burning and tingling. A urethral catheter is placed and the bladder decompressed. Which of the following is the best therapy for this patient?

A. Acyclovir

B. Azithromycin

C. Ceftriaxone

D. Doxycycline

ANSWERS

23.1 **D.** This patient needs to be hospitalized because of a concomitant urinary tract infection and renal dysfunction. At 88 years of age, she may also have difficulty caring for herself.

23.2 **B.** Decompression of the bladder with a urethral catheter should be performed before examination of the prostate. Percutaneous bladder aspiration is not indicated unless other attempts to decompress the bladder have failed.

23.3 **B.** Acute urinary retention may be the presenting symptom of multiple sclerosis (MS) in a young healthy female with no previous medical problems. MS is characterized by chronic waxing and waning of neurologic symptoms.

23.4 **A.** This is likely caused by herpes simplex virus with associated urethral irritation and urinary retention. The best treatment is acyclovir.

CLINICAL PEARLS

▶ A thorough history and physical examination will often help to identify the cause of acute urinary retention.

▶ Bladder decompression should be performed as quickly as possible to prevent further damage to the urinary system.

▶ Consultation with a urologist may be necessary if urethral catheterization cannot be accomplished with a Foley or coudé catheter.

▶ Admission should be considered for patients with renal dysfunction, a serious infection, or volume overload and for those who are unable to care for themselves.

REFERENCES

Ferri FF. *Ferri's Clinical Advisor*. Philadelphia, PA: Mosby Elsevier; 2011.

Kahler J, Harwood-Nuss AL. Selected urologic problems. In: Marx JA, Hockberger RS, Walls RM, eds. *Rosen's Emergency Medicine: Concepts and Clinical Practice*. 6th ed. Philadelphia, PA: Mosby Elsevier; 2010.

Karafin L, Schwartz GR. Renal calculi (kidney stones) In: *Principles and Practice of Emergency Medicine*. 4th ed. Williams; & Wilkins; 2001:762-763.

McCuskey CF. Chapter 37. Genitourinary emergencies. In: Stone CK, Humphries RL, eds. *Current Diagnosis & Treatment: Emergency Medicine*. 6th ed. Available at: http://www.accessmedicine.com/content.aspx?aID=3109311. Accessed March 31, 2012.

Nicks BA, Manthey DE. Male genital problems. In: Tintinalli JE, Kelen GD, Stapczynski JS, eds. *Emergency Medicine: A Comprehensive Study Guide*. 6th ed. New York, NY: McGraw-Hill; 2011: Chapter 96.

Severyn FA. Urinary-related Complaints. In: Mahadevan SV, Garmel GM, eds. *An Introduction to Clinical Emergency Medicine*. New York, NY: Cambridge University Press; 2005:543-554.

Yen DH, Lee C. Acute urinary retention. In: Tintinalli JE, Kelen GD, Stapczynski JS, eds. *Emergency Medicine: A Comprehensive Study Guide*. 6th ed. New York, NY: McGraw-Hill; 2011: Chapter 95.

An 18-year-old adolescent woman presents to the emergency department (ED) complaining of a 1-week history of abdominal pain. She tells you that she and her friends recently returned from spring break vacation in Mexico, and she has noticed a constant ache that is worse on her right side. The patient's mother is worried because her daughter has been unable to eat or drink anything for 2 days and thinks she may have become sick from drinking the water while on vacation. After asking the mother to step out of the room while you examine the patient, she tells you that she has had five sexual partners, occasionally uses condom for birth control, and has never been pregnant. Her last menstrual period was 2 weeks ago and was heavier than normal. On physical examination, her blood pressure was 100/70, pulse 110 beats per minute, respirations 22 breaths per minute, and temperature 38.9°C (102.1°F). Her heart has a regular rate and rhythm without murmurs. Lungs are clear to auscultation bilaterally. The abdominal examination reveals a diffusely tender lower abdomen, greater on the right than left and the patient exhibits voluntary guarding. Examination of the pelvis reveals a greenish, foul-smelling discharge with a red, friable-appearing cervix. Bimanual examination reveals an exquisitely tender cervix with fullness and pain in the right adnexal area. DNA assays for gonorrhea and *Chlamydia* are collected. The wet prep of the discharge shows many white blood cells (WBCs), no clue cells, no trichomonas, and no *Candida*. A urine pregnancy test is negative.

► What is the most likely diagnosis?
► What is the next diagnostic step?
► What is the next step in your treatment?

ANSWERS TO CASE 24:
Acute Pelvic Inflammatory Disease

Summary: An 18-year-old nulliparous adolescent woman complains of severe abdominal pain, vaginal discharge, fever, nausea, and vomiting. She displays cervical motion tenderness and her right adnexa appear to have some fullness and tenderness on examination.

- **Most likely diagnosis:** Pelvic inflammatory disease.

- **Next step:** Transvaginal ultrasound to rule out tubo-ovarian abscess, complete blood count (CBC), and screen for sexually transmitted infections (STIs).

- **Next treatment step:** Admit the patient and start IV antibiotic therapy.

ANALYSIS

Objectives

1. Understand the diagnosis and workup of pelvic inflammatory disease.

2. Describe the lack of clinical signs of tubo-ovarian abscess.

3. Know the criteria and treatments for both outpatient and inpatient pelvic inflammatory disease.

4. Know the common differential diagnoses for lower abdominal pain and be able to consult the appropriate specialties based on the physical examination and laboratory studies.

Considerations

This nulliparous adolescent woman has lower abdominal pain, fever, abnormal vaginal discharge, adnexal tenderness/fullness, and cervical motion tenderness. Although these symptoms may occur with other diagnoses such as appendicitis, ovarian torsion, ectopic pregnancy, or inflammatory bowel disease, the clinical symptoms are most consistent with pelvic inflammatory disease (PID). **PID is defined as an ascending infection from the vagina or cervix to the upper genital tract,** such as the endometrium, fallopian tubes, or ovaries. Although the etiology may be **polymicrobial,** sexually transmitted organisms such as **Neisseria gonorrhoeae or Chlamydia trachomatis are implicated in many cases.** Because the disease may mimic other common conditions, meticulous physical examination, clinical examination, and use of transvaginal ultrasound must be performed in conjunction to correctly diagnose a gynecologic disease from that of a general surgery process. This patient is admitted to the hospital due to inability to tolerate oral medication (nausea and vomiting) and also height of the temperature (37.8°C [102°F]).

> # APPROACH TO:
> ## Pelvic Inflammatory Disease

DEFINITIONS

CERVICAL MOTION TENDERNESS: Also referred to as a "chandelier sign." Motion of the cervix during bimanual examination elicits extreme tenderness, so as to cause the patient to jump off the bed and hit the chandelier.

PELVIC INFLAMMATORY DISEASE (PID): An ascending infection of microorganisms from the lower genital tract to the upper genital tract that is polymicrobial, but is commonly caused by *N gonorrhoeae* or *C trachomatis*. PID may also be termed salpingitis.

TUBO-OVARIAN ABSCESS (TOA): A collection of purulent material encompassing the fallopian tube and ovary comprised of predominantly anaerobic organisms. TOAs are an important complication of pelvic inflammatory disease.

CLINICAL APPROACH

Pelvic inflammatory disease is an ascending infection from the lower genital tract to the upper genital tract that may be difficult to diagnose due to the variety and severity of presenting symptoms. Risk factors for the development of PID are young age, recent menstruation, multiple sexual partners, no use of barrier contraception, and lower socioeconomic status. The clinical diagnosis of PID is fairly accurate but a broad differential diagnosis should be kept in mind in the evaluation of abdominal pain in a woman. Criteria for diagnosis include **lower abdominal tenderness, adnexal tenderness, and cervical motion tenderness.** The presence of purulent vaginal discharge, fever more than 101°F, elevated serum leukocyte count, and presence of gonorrhea or *Chlamydia* in the endocervix are supportive findings. Thus, all women who are suspected of having PID should have testing for *N gonorrhoeae* and *C trachomatis* as well as HIV.

The clinical presentation of tubo-ovarian abscess can be subtle. The majority of these patients have little or low-grade fever, slightly elevated white blood cell count, and may not have a palpable adnexal mass on pelvic examination. For this reason, those patients who are diagnosed with PID should have imaging of the pelvis to assess for TOA, since this diagnosis requires in-patient therapy.

Ultrasound imaging or computed tomography (CT) imaging of the abdomen and pelvis may be helpful to assess for other conditions. The differential diagnosis of acute PID includes appendicitis, ectopic pregnancy, endometriosis, ovarian torsion, hemorrhagic corpus luteum cyst, benign ovarian tumor, and inflammatory bowel disease. CT imaging is more helpful in assessing appendicitis. Finally, laparoscopy is considered the "gold standard" in establishing the diagnosis, by visualizing purulent discharge from the tube, and is generally considered when a patient has acute symptoms, sepsis, or is not improving on therapy.

The etiology of PID is polymicrobial as many different bacteria are harbored in the vagina. Most commonly, *N gonorrhoeae* and *C trachomatis* are isolated from a cervical culture, but other organisms, such as *Bacteroides fragilis, Escherichia coli, Peptostreptococci* sp, *Haemophilus influenzae*, and aerobic streptococci, have been isolated from acute cases of PID. Thus, organisms may be classified as either sexually transmitted organisms or endogenous.

The pathogenesis of PID may include many mechanisms. First, for ascension of infection to develop from the vagina, through the cervical canal, to the endometrium of the uterus, through the fallopian tubes and to the ovaries or peritoneum, there must be a breakdown of the natural host defense system. For instance, hormonal changes unique to a woman's cycle may play a role in the ascending infection. During a normal menstrual cycle, the cervical mucus changes based on the predominate hormone, either estrogen or progesterone. At midcycle, when estrogen predominates and progesterone is low, cervical mucus is thin and may facilitate easy ascension of bacteria. Whereas after ovulation, when progesterone is low, the cervical mucous is thick and more difficult for bacteria to penetrate. For this reason, progestin-containing contraception via the oral contraceptive or depot medroxyprogesterone acetate (depo provera) decreases the incidence of PID. Menses is another time when woman are at greater risk for developing PID because the cervical mucous plug is lost due to outward menstrual flow and organisms may also ascend to the upper genital tract. Retrograde menstrual flow has also been attributed to the risk of bacteria ascending from the uterus into the fallopian tubes, ovaries, or peritoneal cavity.

Treatment of PID varies widely depending on the clinical presentation of the patient. Treatment should provide broad-spectrum coverage of the suspected pathogens, and should be initiated as soon as a presumptive diagnosis has been made in order to prevent long-term sequelae or complications from acute PID, such as tubal damage leading to infertility, chronic pain, or ectopic pregnancies. **Of note, postinfectious tubal infertility is the second most common reason for female infertility in the United States.**

Uncomplicated PID in a compliant patient may be treated as an outpatient. However, **certain criteria for hospitalization** exist for the management of complicated PID (Table 24–1). Although IV antibiotics are used to treat the symptoms of PID, laparoscopy is useful in cases with an uncertain diagnosis, suspicion of a ruptured TOA, or when a patient fails to respond to IV antibiotics. A ruptured TOA

Table 24–1 • CRITERIA FOR HOSPITALIZATION
Surgical emergencies (eg, appendicitis) cannot be excluded
Pregnancy
Lack of response clinically to oral antimicrobial therapy
Patient is unable to follow or tolerate an outpatient oral regimen
Severe illness, nausea, and vomiting, or high fever
Tubo-ovarian abscess
Adolescent, nulliparous, or questionable compliance
Presence of an intrauterine device

Table 24–2 • THERAPY FOR PELVIC INFLAMMATORY DISEASE
Outpatient therapy: • Ceftriaxone 250 mg IM in a single dose *plus* doxycycline 100 mg PO bid for 14 d *with or without* metronidazole 500 mg PO bid for 14 d   • Cefoxitin 2 g IM in a single dose and probenecid, 1 g PO administered concurrently in a single dose *plus* doxycycline 100 mg PO bid for 14 d *with or without* metronidazole 500 mg PO bid for 14 d   • Other parenteral third-generation cephalosporin (eg, ceftizoxime or cefotaxime) *plus* doxycycline 100 mg PO bid for 14 d *with or without* metronidazole 500 mg PO bid for 14 d
Inpatient therapy: The first two bullet points are the same: • Cefotetan 2 g IV q12h or cefoxitin 2 g IV q6h and doxycycline 100 mg PO or IV q12h   • Clindamycin 900 mg IV q8h and gentamycin 2 mg/kg IV loading dose followed by 1.5 mg/kg q8h   • Ofloxacin was not mentioned on the CDC website, but the last half of the bullet point was: ○ Ampicillin/sulbactam 3 g IV q6h and doxycycline 100 mg PO or IV q12h

Data from Centers for Disease Control and Prevention. 2010 Guidelines for treatment of sexually transmitted diseases. MMWR. 2010;59(RR-12):1.

presents as shock, and is a surgical emergency. Thus, the patient who is brought into the emergency department with hypotension, significant abdominal pain, and a signs of infection should receive fluid resuscitation and arrangements for rapid surgical management.

Treatment options can be divided into **oral treatment and parenteral treatment.** Fluoroquinolone-resistant gonorrhea has rendered quinolone therapy as a secondary regimen. Outpatient management includes **intramuscular ceftriaxone and oral doxycycline 100 mg twice daily for 14 days with or without metronidazole** (Table 24–2). Patients should ideally be seen back in 48 hours to assess for improvement. A common inpatient management is intravenous cefotetan 2 g every 12 hours and oral or IV doxycycline 100 mg every 12 hours. Improvement should occur after 24 to 48 hours of therapy. When a tubo-ovarian abscess is suspected, clindamycin or metronidazole is used in the place of doxycycline since anaerobic bacteria are the main concern. TOAs are an exception to the rule that "abscesses require drainage"—the majority of TOAs can be treated with antibiotic therapy and followed with imaging for resolution. Approximately one-third of TOAs will need surgical therapy.

After clinical improvement on intravenous therapy, the patient is changed to oral antibiotic therapy for 10 days. If there is no improvement after 72 hours of therapy (decreased fever, improvement in abdominal pain, reduction in uterine/adnexal tenderness), a more in-depth workup is needed. **Follow-up and treatment of a known sexual partner** is essential for decreasing the incidence of recurrence of PID. Known **complications are infertility, pelvic adhesions leading to chronic pelvic pain, risk of ectopic surgery, Fitz-Hugh-Curtis syndrome, and chronic PID.**

COMPREHENSION QUESTIONS

24.1 A 22-year-old woman is noted to have lower abdominal pain associated with some dysuria and abnormal menses. Her appetite has decreased recently. The pregnancy test is negative. Which of the following findings would most likely suggest pelvic inflammatory disease?

A. Endometrial biopsy showing atypical cells

B. Vaginal wet mount demonstrating clue cells

C. Cervical motion tenderness on physical examination

D. Pain on rectal examination

24.2 A 32-year-old woman is noted to have a 2-day history of low-grade fever and lower abdominal tenderness. The examination reveals cervical motion tenderness and adnexal tenderness. Which of the following is best in assessing for possible tubo-ovarian abscess?

A. Degree of temperature

B. Elevation of leukocyte count

C. Pelvic examination revealing adnexal mass

D. Ultrasound of the pelvis

E. Rebound tenderness of the abdominal examination

Match the following diseases (A to F) to the clinical situations in Questions 24.3 to 24.6:

A. Ectopic pregnancy

B. Appendicitis

C. Gastroesophageal reflux disease (GERD)

D. Crohn disease

E. Cholelithiasis

F. Pancreatitis

G. Ovarian torsion

24.3 A 21-year-old woman experiences crampy abdominal pain that begins near the umbilicus and moves to the lower right quadrant. The pain has progressed over days, and is intermittent and crampy. The patient is afebrile and complains of some nausea.

24.4 A 41-year-old woman complains of pain in the upper abdomen especially after eating. The pain seems to travel to her right shoulder. She has bloating at times.

24.5 A 35-year-old man complains of epigastric abdominal pain which seems to "bore straight to the back." He has nausea and vomiting.

24.6 A 22-year-old woman complains of intermittent severe abdominal pain with diarrhea. She also has some joint pain.

ANSWERS

24.1 **C.** Although cervical motional tenderness is not specific for acute salpingitis, and can be seen with other acute inflammatory conditions of the lower abdomen such as diverticulitis and appendicitis, it is a classic finding of pelvic inflammatory disease.

24.2. **D.** Imaging is the best way to assess for TOA. Tubo-ovarian abscess is often subtle in its presentation and may not be associated with fever or elevated WBC. Most TOAs can be treated medically with antibiotics rather than requiring surgical therapy.

24.3 **G.** The intermittent crampy abdominal pain is classic for ovarian torsion. Although this patient's pain moves from the umbilicus to the lower quadrant area, it has lasted longer than 24 hours, without fever.

24.4 **E.** The right upper quadrant abdominal pain following meals (especially fatty meals) is very typical of cholelithiasis. The pain often radiates to the right scapula. If she had fever, cholecystitis would be suspected.

24.5 **F.** Pancreatitis usually presents with midepigastric pain that penetrates straight to the back, is constant in nature, and is associated with nausea and vomiting. Common etiologies include alcohol abuse and gall stones.

24.6 **D.** Inflammatory bowel disease (Crohn disease or ulcerative colitis) often affects individuals in their teens or twenties, with abdominal pain, diarrhea (often bloody), and extraintestinal manifestations such as joint pain or eye findings.

CLINICAL PEARLS

▶ The classic triad of symptoms for diagnosing PID include lower abdominal tenderness, adnexal tenderness, and cervical motion tenderness.

▶ Laparoscopy remains the gold standard for diagnosing PID.

▶ TOAs often present in a subtle or indolent fashion and require imaging for diagnois. TOAs require hospital antibiotic therapy and the majority can be treated medically.

▶ Patients with a ruptured TOA present in shock. This is a surgical emergency.

▶ Long-term sequelae of PID include infertility, pelvic adhesions, chronic pelvic pain, risk of ectopic pregnancy, and Fitz-Hugh-Curtis syndrome.

▶ Disseminated gonococcal infection, although uncommon, is a serious complication of untreated gonorrhea, which is a very common infection.

▶ Persons found to have a positive gonorrhea culture should also be treated for *Chlamydia* because concomitant infection is found in as many as 40% of patients. In any person presenting with asymmetric polyarthritis, tenosynovitis, and pustular skin lesions, disseminated gonococcal infection should be considered in the differential diagnosis.

REFERENCES

Centers for Disease Control and Prevention. 2010 guidelines for treatment of sexually transmitted diseases. *MMWR.* 2010;59(RR-12):1.

Cohen CR. Pelvic inflammatory disease. In: Klausner JD, Hook III EW, eds. *Current Diagnosis & Treatment of Sexually Transmitted Diseases.* New York, NY: McGraw-Hill; 2007.

Hemsell DM. Gynecologic infection. In: Schorge J, Schaffer J, Halvorson L, Hoffman B, Bradshaw K, Cunningham F, eds. *Williams Gynecology.* New York, NY: McGraw-Hill; 2008: 73-76.

Sweet RL, Gibbs RS. *Infectious Diseases of the Female Genital Tract.* 5th ed. Baltimore, MD: Lippincott Williams & Wilkins; 2009.

A 27-year-old woman notice that since 1 day ago, she has noticed that her mouth has been drooping in the right corner, and it is difficult for her to drink water without drooling. She cannot close her right eye completely, and her right eye is red and irritated. She denies having headaches, visual disturbances, nausea, or vomiting. She does not have any history of trauma. Her past medical history is unremarkable. She is not taking any medications. Her mother had a stroke when she was 60 years old. The patient states that she is from Michigan and has not been traveling recently. On physical examination, the right corner of her mouth droops, and the right nasolabial fold is absent. The right lower eyelid is sagging, and the patient cannot completely close her right eye. On attempts to close the right eye, the eye rolls upward. The patient also cannot wrinkle her forehead. The other cranial nerves seem to be normal, and the neurologic examination reveals no deficits other than as stated.

▶ What is your diagnosis?
▶ How will you manage this condition?

ANSWERS TO CASE 25:

Bell Palsy (Idiopathic Facial Paralysis)

Summary: A 27-year-old woman has acute onset of right facial weakness and right eye irritation. She denies trauma and has no other cranial nerve or neurological problems.

- **Most Likely Diagnosis:** Facial nerve palsy most likely idiopathic (Bell palsy)

- **Management of condition:** Protection of the eye and a course of prednisone

ANALYSIS

Objectives

1. Differentiate an upper motor neuron process from a lower motor neuron process and review the differential diagnoses for each.

2. Understand the clinical presentation of Bell palsy.

3. Learn the management of Bell palsy.

Considerations

This 27-year-old woman is affected by the abrupt onset of right facial weakness. Notably, her upper facial muscles are affected, which is consistent with a peripheral neuropathy. She has none of the findings suggestive of a more complicated process (Table 25–1). Her symptoms are likely caused by paralysis of the seventh cranial nerve, which is mainly a motor nerve supplying all the ipsilateral muscles of facial expression. The drooping of the right corner of the mouth represents paralysis of the orbicularis oris muscle. Tearing of the right eye (epiphora) occurs because paralysis of the orbicularis oculi muscle prevents closure of the eyelids and causes the lacrimal duct opening to sag away from the conjunctiva. The inability to wrinkle the forehead is a result of paralysis of the frontalis muscle. Affected individuals will often have the Bell phenomenon upon attempted closure of the eyelids, the eye on the paralyzed side rolls upward.

Table 25–1 • RED FLAGS FOR SUSPECTED FACIAL NERVE PALSY
Cranial nerve involvement other than VII
Bilateral facial weakness
Weakness, numbness of arms or legs
Unaffected upper facial muscles (forehead)
Headache, visual deficits, nausea or vomiting
History of travel through woods, tick bite
Recurrent unilateral facial paralysis
Slow progression of symptoms
Ulceration or blisters near ear

APPROACH TO:
Facial Paralysis

Approach to Bell Palsy

The seventh cranial nerve exits the cranium through the stylomastoid foramen and supplies all the muscles concerned with facial expression. It also has a small sensory component which conveys taste sensation from the anterior two-thirds of the tongue and cutaneous impulses from the anterior wall of the external auditory meatus. A complete interruption of the facial nerve at the stylomastoid foramen paralyzes all the muscles of the face on the affected side. Taste sensation is intact because the lesion is beyond the site where the chorda tympani has separated from the main trunk of the facial nerve. If the nerve to the stapedius muscle is involved, there is often hyperacusis. If the geniculate ganglion or the motor root proximal to it is involved, lacrimation and salivation may be reduced.

Although the most common cause of facial paralysis is Bell palsy, this is a diagnosis of exclusion. In other words, the emergency department (ED) physician should be careful of presuming a facial palsy is Bell palsy without considering other possible etiologies. Other causes of nuclear or peripheral facial nerve palsy include Lyme disease, tumors of the temporal bone (carotid body, cholesteatoma, dermoid), Ramsey Hunt syndrome (herpes zoster of the geniculate ganglion), and acoustic neuromas. Malignant otitis externa, stroke, Guillain-Barré disease, polio, sarcoid, and human immunodeficiency virus (HIV) infection are other processes that must be considered.

All forms of peripheral facial nerve palsy must be distinguished from the supranuclear type. In the latter, the frontalis and orbicularis oculi muscles are spared because the innervation of the upper facial muscles is bilateral and that of the lower facial muscles is mainly contralateral. In other words, **if the patient has drooping of the mouth but is able to wrinkle his or her forehead normally, an intracranial process should be suspected.** With supranuclear lesions, there may also be a dissociation of emotional and voluntary facial movements. Because Bell palsy is a diagnosis of exclusion, a very careful history and physical examination are critical to detect any other neurological abnormalities.

The onset of Bell palsy is abrupt, and symptoms can progress from weakness to complete paralysis over a week. Over half of the patients with Bell palsy will recall a preceding viral prodrome. Associated symptoms may include pain behind the ear, ipsilateral loss of taste sensation, decreased or overflow tearing, and hyperacusis. The patient may complain of heaviness and numbness on the affected side of the face; however, no sensory loss is demonstrable. Eighty percent of patients recover within weeks to a few months. The presence of incomplete paralysis in the first week is the most favorable prognostic sign. If the presentation is atypical or there is no improvement at 6 months, laboratory studies, imaging studies (eg, computed tomography, magnetic resonance imaging), or motor-nerve conduction studies should be considered.

Treatment

The patient should use an eye patch while sleeping to protect the eye and prevent corneal drying and abrasions. While awake, he or she should apply artificial tears to the affected eye every hour. Massaging of the weakened muscles may improve muscle tone and aid in recovery.

Medical therapy should be started as soon as possible but can be considered for up to 1 week after the onset of symptoms. Although treatment regimens are controversial, most experts recommend the use of corticosteroids. Corticosteroids are hypothesized to decrease facial nerve edema. Thus prednisone 1 mg/kg/d can be given orally for 7 to 10 days (with or without a taper). Because some studies implicated herpes simplex virus as a causative agent of Bell palsy, antivirals were routinely incorporated into the treatment regimen. However, further studies have shown conflicting results regarding the efficacy of antiviral therapy. If physicians choose to prescribe antiviral agents, valacyclovir and famciclovir are favored due to their less frequent dosing and greater bioavailability. These agents do cost substantially more than acyclovir, which requires more frequent dosing. If medical therapy is unsuccessful, patients may benefit from surgical decompression of the facial nerve.

COMPREHENSION QUESTIONS

25.1 A 32-year-old woman complains of facial weakness for several weeks that has gradually worsened. The upper face and lower face are both affected. She does not have weakness of the arms or legs. Which of the following would suggest a diagnosis other than Bell palsy?

A. Absence of symptoms in arms

B. Absence of symptoms in legs

C. Gradual onset over several weeks

D. Upper facial weakness

25.2 A 55-year-old woman complains of weakness of her right facial muscles along with numbness of her right cheek region. Which of the following is the next step?

A. Obtain magnetic resonance imaging of the brain.

B. Obtain a rapid plasma reagin (RPR) serology.

C. Perform a lumbar puncture.

D. Recommend eye protection and observation.

Match the following mechanisms (A to E) to the clinical scenarios presented in Questions 25.3 to 25.5:

    A. Pressure on the cerebellopontine nucleus

    B. Edema of the nerve at the stylomastoid foramen

    C. Immunoglobulins against the acetylcholine receptor

    D. Multifocal myelin destruction in the central nervous system

    E. Autoimmune attack on myelinated motor nerves particularly of the lower extremities

25.3 A 22-year-old woman is on the ventilator because of inability to breathe. This condition began 3 weeks ago when she had weakness of both legs following a bout of gastroenteritis. Her deep tendon reflexes are absent.

25.4 A 32-year-old woman has a 5-year history of progressive weakness during the day. She cannot look upward for long periods of time because of fatigue.

25.5 A 35-year-old man had eye weakness 2 years ago with full resolution. Now he has difficulty with his right handgrip. His deep tendon reflexes are normal to increased.

ANSWERS

25.1 **C.** The onset of Bell palsy is abrupt with maximum weakness occurring within 1 week. Facial nerve palsy due to tumors of the temporal bone is insidious, and the symptoms gradually progress.

25.2 **A.** The numbness over the cheek is concerning and inconsistent with Bell palsy. The facial nerve supplies all the muscles of the face. Injury to this nerve produces paralysis of the facial muscles. Drooping of the corner of the mouth is one of the findings. The tongue is supplied by the hypoglossal nerve. Middle ear lesions producing facial palsy will cause loss of taste over the anterior two-thirds of the tongue, but alteration of taste sensation does not occur. The sensory component of the facial nerve is limited to the anterior wall of the external auditory meatus. Further evaluation with magnetic resonance imaging (MRI) may be warranted.

25.3 **E.** This presentation of ascending paralysis is classic for Guillain-Barré syndrome, and typically the deep tendon reflexes are absent.

25.4 **C.** Myasthenia gravis is characterized by progressive weakness throughout the day, particularly involving the eye muscles. These symptoms are due to immunoglobulin G antibodies against the acetylcholine receptors.

25.5 **D.** Multiple sclerosis typically affects young individuals with waxing and waning weakness and full recovery between exacerbations. The mechanism is multifocal destruction of the myelin in the central nervous system.

CLINICAL PEARLS

▶ Bell palsy is an idiopathic seventh cranial nerve peripheral neuropathy, leading to both upper and lower facial weakness.

▶ The diagnosis of Bell palsy is one of exclusion.

▶ The most important assessment in a patient who presents with possible Bell palsy is to rule out serious disorders such as intracranial tumors and strokes.

▶ Protection of the eye to prevent corneal drying and abrasions is accomplished with an eye patch during sleep and lubricants to the affected eye.

▶ The prognosis of Bell palsy is usually favorable, but persistent weakness, the appearance of other neurologic deficits, or blisters that appear on the ear are indications for referral.

REFERENCES

Axelsson S, Lindberg S, Stjernquist-Desatnik A. Outcome of treatment with valacyclovir and prednisone in patients with Bell's palsy. *Ann Otol Rhinol Laryngol.* 2003;112:197.

Baringer JR. Herpes simplex virus and Bell's palsy. *Ann Intern Med.* 1996;124:63.

Benatar M, Edlow J. The spectrum of cranial neuropathy in patients with Bell's palsy. *Arch Intern Med.* 2004;164:23-83.

Brodal A. The cranial nerves. In: *Neurological Anatomy in Relation to Clinical Medicine.* 3rd ed. New York, NY: Oxford;1980:448-577.

Engstrom M, Berg T, Stjernquist-Desatnik A, et al. Prednisolone and valaciclovir in Bell's palsy: a randomised, double-blind, placebo-controlled, multicentre trial. *Lancet Neurol.* 2008;7:993-1000.

Gilden DH, Tyler KL. Bell's palsy—is glucocorticoid treatment enough? *N Engl J Med.* 2007;357:1653.

Hato N, Yamada H, Kohno H, et al. Valacyclovir and prednisolone treatment for Bell's palsy: a multicenter, randomized, placebo-controlled study. *Otol Neurotol.* 2007;28:408.

Hauser WA, Karnes WE, Annis J, Kurland LT. Incidence and prognosis of Bell's palsy in the population of Rochester, Minnesota. *Mayo Clin Proc.* 1971;46:258.

Karnes WE. Diseases of the seventh cranial nerve. In: Dyck PJ, Thomas PK, Lambert EH, et al, eds. *Peripheral Neuropathy.* 2nd ed. Philadelphia, PA: WB Saunders; 1984:1266-1299.

Marx, John A, Robert S. Hockberger, Ron M. Walls, James Adams, and Peter Rosen. *Rosen's Emergency Medicine: Concepts and Clinical Practice.* Philadelphia, PA: Mosby/Elsevier; 2010.

Sullivan FM, Swan IR, Donnan PT, et al Early treatment with prednisolone or acyclovir in Bell's palsy. *N Engl J Med.* 2007;357(16):1598-1607.

Worster A, Keim SM, Sahsi R, Pancioli AM; Best Evidence in Emergency Medicine (BEEM) Group: do either corticosteroids or antiviral agents reduce the risk of long-term facial paresis in patients with new-onset Bell's palsy? *J Emerg Med.* 2010;38(4):518-523. Epub 2009 Oct 21 (Review).

A 26-year-old woman presents to the emergency department (ED) with a 6-hour history of worsening abdominal pain. She states the pain initially was a dull pain near her umbilicus but has since moved to her lower right side. She rates the pain as 8 on a scale of 10 and crampy in nature. The patient states that she noted some vaginal spotting this morning, but denies any passage of clots or tissue. The patient ate breakfast that morning, but states she has not eaten since because she feels nauseous. She denies any fever or chills or any change in her bowel habits. Upon further questioning, the patient states her last menstrual period was 2 months ago, but her periods are irregular. She also states that she was told that she had a vaginal infection a year ago but does not recall having been treated for the illness. On physical examination, her blood pressure is 120/76 mm Hg, heart rate is 105 beats per minute, and she is afebrile. In general, she is in mild distress. The abdomen reveals tenderness to palpation in her right lower quadrant that is greater than that in the left lower quadrant. The examination reveals some minimal voluntary guarding, but no rebound tenderness is appreciated. On pelvic examination, the uterus appears mildly enlarged without cervical motion tenderness. There are no masses or tenderness in the adnexal region. Her complete blood count (CBC) reveals a mildly elevated white blood cell count with a left shift. A beta–human chorionic gonadotropin (β-hCG) was 4658 mIU/mL. A transvaginal sonogram reveals an empty uterus but no adnexal masses or free fluid is noted.

▶ What is the most likely diagnosis?
▶ What is the next step?
▶ What is the initial treatment?

ANSWERS TO CASE 26:

Ectopic Pregnancy

Summary: A 26-year-old woman complains of severe abdominal pain, nausea, and vaginal spotting. She has a positive pregnancy test, a quantitative β-hCG level of 4658 mIU/mL, and a transvaginal sonogram showing no intrauterine pregnancy.

- **Most likely diagnosis:** Ectopic pregnancy.

- **Next step:** Diagnostic versus operative laparoscopy.

- **Initial treatment:** Establish an IV line and stabilize the patient in preparation for surgery.

ANALYSIS

Objectives

1. Understand the diagnosis and workup of ectopic pregnancy.

2. Know the different sonographic appearances of ectopic pregnancy.

3. Know the common differential diagnoses for lower abdominal pain and be able to consult the appropriate specialties based on the physical examination.

Considerations

This patient presents to the emergency department with complaints of vaginal bleeding, abdominal pain, and a positive pregnancy examination. Her quantitative hCG level is above the threshold of 1200 to 1500 mIU/mL, and no intrauterine pregnancy is seen on transvaginal sonography; thus, her risk for an ectopic pregnancy approaches 85%. Other diagnoses should be considered, such as threatened abortion, incomplete abortion, pelvic inflammatory disease, or appendicitis. Ectopic pregnancy is defined as a pregnancy that develops after implantation of the blastocyst anywhere other than in the lining of the uterine cavity.

APPROACH TO:
Ectopic Pregnancy

DEFINITIONS

ECTOPIC PREGNANCY: Pregnancy that develops after implantation anywhere other than the lining of the uterus.

RUPTURED ECTOPIC PREGNANCY: Ectopic pregnancy that has eroded through the tissue in which it has implanted, producing hemorrhage from exposed vessels.

SALPINGECTOMY: Surgical excision and removal of the oviduct and ectopic pregnancy.

SALPINGOSTOMY: Surgical excision of the ectopic pregnancy with preservation of the tube. The tube remains opened to heal by secondary intention.

CLINICAL APPROACH

Ectopic pregnancy is defined as a pregnancy outside the lining of the uterus, most commonly occurring in the oviduct, but it may also be found in the abdomen, ovary, or cervix. The incidence of the ectopic pregnancy has increased in the United States for three reasons: (1) the increased incidence of salpingitis caused by increased infection with *Chlamydia trachomatis* or other sexually transmitted diseases, (2) improved diagnostic techniques, and (3) the increase in assisted reproductive technology pregnancies. Other risk factors include prior tubal surgery, previous ectopic pregnancy, use of exogenous progesterone, and a history of infertility agents. The most common presenting symptoms are abdominal pain, absence of menses, and irregular vaginal bleeding. Other symptoms found on physical examination may include a palpable adnexal tenderness, uterine enlargement, tachycardia, hypotension, syncope, peritoneal signs, and fever.

Approximately half of the episodes of ectopic pregnancy are linked to previous salpingitis, although these episodes may be asymptomatic. Prior infections are likely to lead to anatomic tubal pathology that prevents the normal passage of an embryo into the uterus. In the remaining incidences of ectopic pregnancy, an identifying factor cannot be determined and may be linked to a physiologic disorder. Increased levels of estrogen and progesterone interfere with tubal motility and increase the chance of ectopic pregnancy.

Approximately 97% of ectopic pregnancies occur in the oviduct, specifically in the ampullary region. The remainder of ectopic pregnancies implant in the abdomen, cervix, or ovary. Pathogenesis of ectopic pregnancy begins as the embryo invades the lumen of the tube and its peritoneal covering. As the embryo continues to grow, surrounding vessels may bleed into the peritoneal cavity, resulting in a hemoperitoneum. The stretching of the tube results in abdominal pain until necrosis ensues and results in rupture of the ectopic pregnancy.

The differential diagnosis of ectopic pregnancy includes many other gynecologic and surgical illnesses. Most common are salpingitis, threatened or incomplete abortion, ruptured corpus luteum, adnexal torsion, and appendicitis. The diagnosis of ectopic pregnancy must be considered in any woman of reproductive age with abnormal vaginal bleeding and abdominal pain.

Diagnosis of ectopic pregnancy may be aided with the use of transvaginal ultrasound. Visualization of the pelvic organs may reveal the absence of an intrauterine pregnancy, the presence of a complex adnexal mass, or the presence of an embryo in the adnexa. It is important to note that with higher resolution ultrasound, **the hCG discriminatory zone is closer to 1200 to 1500 mIU/mL than the traditionally quoted figure of 1500 to 2000 mIU/mL, in which an intrauterine pregnancy is almost always seen on transvaginal sonography.** Lack of visualization of an intrauterine gestational sac on transvaginal sonography confers up to an 85% risk of an ectopic pregnancy. At times, sonography can visualize an ectopic pregnancy even with hCG levels lower than this threshold; the **level of hCG does not reliably correlate with the size of the ectopic pregnancy.** When hCG levels are lower than the above threshold, the ED physician should rely on the clinical impression to diagnose an ectopic pregnancy.

In a reliable and asymptomatic patient whose initial hCG level is below the threshold, a repeat hCG level can be obtained in 48 hours. The **hCG should increase by at least 66% over 48 hours;** lack of normal rise strongly implies an abnormal pregnancy, although the test does not indicate the location of the pregnancy (ectopic or miscarriage). A definitive diagnosis of ectopic pregnancy can most always be made by direct visualization of the pelvic organs using laparoscopy if the diagnosis remains uncertain.

More pregnancies are associated with in vitro fertilization, which carries a higher risk of ectopic pregnancy, and multiple gestation. Notably, in women who have IVF pregnancies, a proven intrauterine pregnancy may not rule out ectopic pregnancy, since these patients can have heterotopic pregnancies (concomitant intrauterine and ectopic pregnancies).

Treatment options include both medical and surgical therapy. Medical treatment consists of using intramuscular **methotrexate,** a folinic acid antagonist that interferes with deoxyribonucleic acid (DNA) synthesis, repair, and cellular replication. Actively dividing tissue, such as fetal cell growth is susceptible to methotrexate and may be used for treatment of ectopic pregnancy under specific conditions (Figure 26–1). Methotrexate is found to be more successful if the hCG is less than 5000 mIU/mL, if the fetus is smaller than 3.5 cm, and if there is no detectable fetal cardiac activity. It is important to note that each individual patient may present with different complaints and different levels of hCG, and at times medical management involves multiple doses of methotrexate.

Potential problems associated with medical management of ectopic pregnancy include drug side effects and treatment failure. Some patients treated with methotrexate will develop acute abdominal pain due to the process of "tubal abortion." In these individuals, pelvic sonography is useful- if the vital signs are stable, and the ultrasound does not show much intra-abdominal fluid, the patient may be observed in the hospital to assess for resolution of the pain. However, those

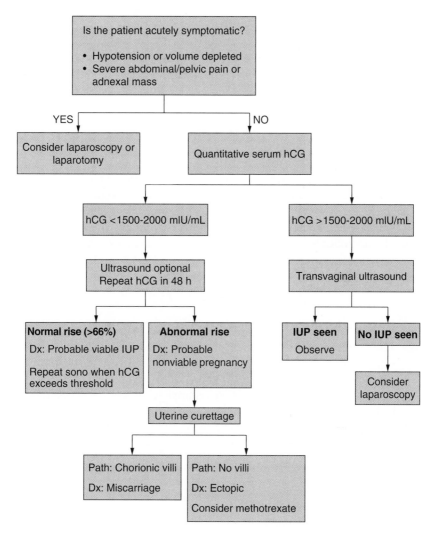

Figure 26–1. Algorithm for the management of suspected ectopic pregnancy.

patients who have hypotension or evidence of intra-abdominal bleeding should go to the operating room.

If medical therapy fails, surgical intervention is necessary. Surgical management commonly consists of laparoscopy and/or laparotomy. A few common surgical techniques used for treatment of ectopic pregnancy include salpingotomy, salpingostomy, and partial salpingectomy. These techniques can be used to treat the majority of unruptured ectopic pregnancy, whereas exploratory laparotomy may be used in cases of ruptured ectopic pregnancy.

COMPREHENSION QUESTIONS

26.1 A 22-year-old woman complains of lower abdominal pain and vaginal spotting. Which of the following tests is the first priority?

   A. Pelvic ultrasound

   B. KUB (kidneys, ureters, bladder) radiograph

   C. hCG level

   D. *Chlamydia* antigen test of the cervix

26.2 A 22-year-old woman underwent methotrexate treatment for an ectopic pregnancy 1 week ago and complains of lower abdominal cramping. She denies vaginal bleeding, dizziness, or vomiting. On examination, her blood pressure is 120/80 mm Hg and her heart rate is 80 beats per minute. The abdomen reveals mild tenderness. Which of the following is the best management?

   A. Observation

   B. Surgical management of the ectopic pregnancy

   C. Administration of folinic acid

   D. Transfusion of 2 units of red blood cells

26.3 A 42-year-old woman complains of an acute onset of significant abdominal pain of 6 hours duration. She states that she underwent in vitro fertilization and is currently 8 weeks pregnant. Her blood pressure is 90/60 mm Hg and her heart rate is 110 beats per minute. Her quantitative hCG level is 22,800 mIU/mL. Transvaginal sonography reveals a singleton intrauterine gestation with cardiac activity, and a moderate amount of free fluid in the cul de sac. Which of the following is the most likely diagnosis?

   A. Heterotopic pregnancy

   B. Ruptured corpus luteum

   C. Cirrhosis with ascites

   D. Urinary tract infection

26.4 A 33-year-old woman complains of vaginal bleeding and abdominal cramping. She passed some blood clots. Her last menstrual period was 6 weeks previously. On examination her cervical os is open to 1 cm. Her quantitative hCG level is 2000 mIU/mL. Which of the following is the most likely diagnosis?

   A. Ectopic pregnancy

   B. Incomplete abortion

   C. Completed abortion

   D. Incompetent cervix

26.5 A 28-year-old woman complains of lower abdominal cramping pain for about 3 hours, and passed what was described as "liver-like" tissue, after which her pain resolved. In the ED, her blood pressure is 120/70 mm Hg and heart rate is 80 beats per minute. Her uterus is firm and the cervix is closed. The hCG level is 2000 mIU/mL. Transvaginal sonography reveals no intrauterine pregnancy. Which of the following is the next step?

A. Laparoscopy

B. Methotrexate therapy

C. Progesterone level

D. Repeat hCG level in 48 hours

ANSWERS

26.1 **C.** In general, any woman in the childbearing age group with abdominal pain or abnormal vaginal bleeding should have a pregnancy test. If pregnant, then ectopic pregnancy should be ruled out.

26.2 **A.** A large number of women who undergo methotrexate treatment of ectopic pregnancy will have some abdominal discomfort. As long as there are no signs of rupture such as hypotension, severe pain, or free fluid on ultrasound, expectant management may be practiced.

26.3 **A.** In vitro fertilization with embryo transfer produces a rate of coexisting intrauterine pregnancy and ectopic pregnancy of up to 3% (markedly higher than the spontaneous rate of 1:10,000). Thus, a woman who has undergone in vitro fertilization who presents with abdominal fluid and hypotension must be suspected as having an ectopic pregnancy, even when an intrauterine pregnancy has been visualized on sonography.

26.4 **B.** The presence of uterine cramping, vaginal bleeding, passage of tissue, and an open cervical os in a pregnant woman is consistent with an incomplete abortion. Uterine curettage would be the therapy.

26.5 **D.** This patient likely has a completed abortion with the resolution of symptoms following passage of tissue and now with a small uterus and closed cervical os. Nevertheless, there is still a possibility of ectopic pregnancy and perhaps the "tissue" passed was only blood clot. The tissue should be sent for pathologic analysis. Also, a repeat hCG level should be performed to ensure that all tissue has passed. The hCG level should fall by about 50% in 48 hours if all tissue has passed. A plateau in the hCG level may indicate incomplete abortion or ectopic pregnancy. Dilation and curettage would generally be performed, and if chorionic villi found the diagnosis is miscarriage; absence of chorionic villi establishes the diagnosis of ectopic pregnancy which may be treated by surgery or methotrexate.

CLINICAL PEARLS

▶ In any woman of childbearing age, consider pregnancy. If the pregnancy test is positive, consider an ectopic pregnancy.

▶ Consider pregnancy even when a woman has had a tubal ligation or is using contraception.

▶ When the serum quantitative hCG level is above 1500 to 2000 mIU/mL and transvaginal ultrasound does not reveal an intrauterine pregnancy, the risk of ectopic pregnancy is high.

▶ Surgery, not methotrexate, is the best treatment for the patient who is hemodynamically unstable or with significant abdominal pain.

▶ Laparoscopy remains the gold standard for ectopic pregnancy.

REFERENCES

Cunningham FG, Leveno KJ, Bloom SL, et al. Ectopic pregnancy. In: Cunningham FG, Leveno KJ, Bloom SL, Hauth JC, Rouse DJ, Spong CY, eds. *Williams Obstetrics*. 23rd ed. New York, NY: McGraw-Hill; 2010: Chapter 10.

Hoover KW, Tao G, Kent KC. Trends in the diagnosis and treatment of ectopic pregnancy in the United States. ACOG. March 2010;115(3):495-502.

Silva C, Sammel MD, Zhou L, et al. Human chorionic gonadotropin profile for women with ectopic pregnancy. ACOG. March 2006;107(3):605-610.

A 25-year-old G1P0 woman at 11 weeks' gestation is noted to be lethargic by her husband. The patient was noted to have numerous episodes of nausea and vomiting over the past 1 1/2 months, which has persisted despite antiemetic therapy and adjustments in her diet. The patient had been admitted to the hospital 2 weeks ago due to emesis. She was brought in by EMS when her husband arrived after work to find her unarousable. On examination, the patient is lethargic but will respond to painful stimuli and open her eyes. Her blood pressure is 92/44 mm Hg and heart rate 130 beats per minute. Her respiratory rate is 14 breaths per minute. O_2 saturation is 99% on room air. The patient's mucous membranes are dry. She otherwise has a normal examination. The fetal heart tones are 150 beats per minute. The urinalysis shows a dipstick of specific gravity 1.027 and 3+ ketones.

▶ What is the most likely diagnosis?
▶ What is your next step in management?
▶ What is the differential diagnosis?

ANSWERS TO CASE 27:

Hyperemesis Gravidarum and OB Emergencies Less than 26 Weeks' Gestation

Summary: A 25-year-old G1P0 woman at 11 weeks' gestation has a 6-week history of persistent emesis. She is found to be lethargic and noted to be hypovolemic with blood pressure of 92/44 mm Hg and heart rate of 130 beats per minute. Her respiratory rate is 14 breaths per minute. The fetal heart tones are 150 beats per minute. The urinalysis shows a dipstick of specific gravity 1.027 and 3+ ketones.

- **Most likely diagnosis:** Hyperemsis gravidarum, severe

- **Next step in management:** Immediate isotonic fluid replacement, and also assess for electrolyte abnormalities and correction of these problems

- **Differential diagnosis:** Acute pancreatitis, molar pregnancy or twin pregnancy, peptic ulcer disease, hyperthyroidism, and cholelithiasis

ANALYSIS

Objectives

1. Know the common complications in pregnant women less than 26 weeks' gestation.

2. Understand the diagnostic strategy and management of those complications.

3. Know the physiologic changes in pregnancy and their impact on common diseases in pregnancy.

Considerations

This patient described in the scenario above is significantly ill and needs aggressive fluid replacement, electrolyte replacement, and correction of metabolic abnormalities. Replacement with 2 L of normal saline quickly is warranted. Assessment of comprehensive metabolic panel, electrolytes, amylase, lipase, urinalysis for leukocytes, calcium, magnesium, and CBC with differential should be performed. She has complicated hyperemesis gravidarum, and needs a diagnostic workup such as pelvic ultrasound if not previously performed, right upper quadrant ultrasound, and thyroid function tests. The patient should be admitted to the hospital. Antiemetic therapy, and fluid replacement and nothing by mouth should be initiated. The patient should be followed carefully once discharged to ensure that she doesn't become so volume depleted.

APPROACH TO:

Medical Complications in Pregnancies Before 26 Weeks

INTRODUCTION

There are numerous emergencies or urgencies that bring a pregnant woman into the emergency department. For this chapter, the discussion will be focused on: hyperemesis gravidarum, spontaneous abortion, asthma exacerbation, hyperthyroidism/thyroid storm, preterm premature rupture of membranes, and pyelonephritis.

Hyperemesis Gravidarum

Nausea and vomiting in pregnancy is very common, affecting up to 75% of pregnant women. However, hyperemesis gravidarum, which is defined as intractable emesis with volume depletion and metabolic/electrolyte alterations is less common, with prevalence of about 2% of pregnancies. Typically it occurs in women in the first trimester, and is diagnosis of exclusion. The emergency physician should not be lulled into complacency because nausea and vomiting is so common in pregnant women. The evaluation should include addressing the degree of volume depletion and exploring the possibility of metabolic issues such as electrolyte abnormalities, renal or liver function abnormalities, and the possibility of other etiologies. A urinalysis should also be performed. Hyperemesis gravidarum is a diagnosis of exclusion.

Pregnant women are typically young and healthy, and significant hypovolemia with compensation without appearing ill. A careful history should be taken regarding the amount of oral intake, medications taken if any, and the presence of other possible causes of emesis. The differential diagnosis includes pancreatitis, gall stones, peptic ulcer disease, appendicitis, ovarian torsion, pyelonephritis, and gastroenteritis. Additionally, high hCG level as associated with molar pregnancies or multiple gestation is seen with hyperemesis. Thus an ultrasound should be performed to assess for adnexal masses and to define the type of pregnancy.

Treatment depends on the severity of the patient's condition. Patients with mild volume depletion can be given IV hydration or a trial of oral fluids, and prescribed antiemetic medications. Pyridoxine (vitamin B_6) has efficacy as a first-line agent. Ondansetron (Zofran), while pregnancy Class B, has become the most common parenteral and oral antiemetic used in US emergency departments due to its efficacy, and it has become the first choice in hyperemesis in the last several years. As an adjunctive agent, corticosteroids have also been used. For patients who have failed outpatient therapy, or who have moderate to severe volume depletion should be hospitalized for more intensive therapy and monitoring. Rarely, patients will be so severely affected that total parenteral nutrition is required.

Spontaneous Abortion

Patients who present with vaginal bleeding during pregnancy are said to have a threatened abortion. In this circumstance, approximately 10% of cases will involve ectopic pregnancy (see Case 26), 40% will result in a spontaneous abortion, and 50% will result in a normal pregnancy carried to term. When the patient presents to the emergency department, a careful history and physical examination should be performed including assessing for cramping, passage of tissue, risk factors for ectopic pregnancy, and hemodynamic alterations. The physical examination should be focused on assessing volume status, abdominal tenderness, pelvic examination for the state of the cervix, and the presence of adnexal masses or tenderness. The hCG level and transvaginal ultrasound usually help to determine the type of pregnancy. For instance, if the hCG level is above the threshold of 1500 mIU/mL and nothing is seen in the uterus indicating an intrauterine pregnancy, in the absence of history indicative of tissue passing, this is consistent with an ectopic pregnancy. Women with threatened abortion should be instructed to bring in any passed tissue for histologic analysis.

An inevitable abortion must be differentiated from an incompetent cervix. With an inevitable abortion, the uterine contractions (cramping) lead to the cervical dilation. With an incompetent cervix, the cervix opens spontaneously without uterine contractions and, therefore, affected women present with painless cervical dilation. This disorder is treated with a surgical ligature at the level of the internal cervical os (cerclage). Hence, one of the main features used to distinguish between an incompetent cervix and an inevitable abortion is the presence or absence of uterine contractions.

The treatment of an **incomplete abortion,** characterized by the **passage of tissue and an open cervical os,** is dilatation and curettage of the uterus. The primary complications of persistently retained tissue are bleeding and infection. A completed abortion is suspected by the history of having passed tissue and experiencing cramping abdominal pain, now resolved. The cervix is closed. Serum hCG levels are still followed to confirm that no further chorionic villi are contained in the uterus.

Asthma Exacerbation

Asthma is one of the most common medical conditions complicating pregnancy, with an incidence of 4% to 9%. The clinical course of asthma in pregnancy is relatively unpredictable; however, there is evidence to suggest that worsening of asthma may be related to baseline asthma severity. Approximately one-third of pregnant asthmatics experience worsening of symptoms while one-third improve and one-third remain the same. Exacerbations are more common in the second and third trimester and are less frequent in the last 4 weeks of pregnancy. Asthma typically follows a similar clinical course with successive pregnancies. As such, this patient would be expected to do relatively well given that her symptoms were well controlled prior to this pregnancy and in previous pregnancies.

Asthma symptoms correlate poorly with objective measures of pulmonary function. Therefore, the next step in the evaluation of this patient is to perform an objective measure of airway obstruction. The single best measure is the **forced expiratory volume (FEV$_1$),** which is the volume of gas exhaled in 1 second by a forced exhalation after a full inspiration. This value, however, can only be obtained by spirometry, thus limiting its clinical use. The **peak expiratory flow rate (PEFR)** correlates well with FEV$_1$ and can be measured with inexpensive, disposable portable peak flow meters. Both the FEV$_1$ and PEFR remain unchanged throughout pregnancy and may be used as measures of asthma control and severity.

Treatment of an acute exacerbation during pregnancy is **similar** to that of non-pregnant asthmatics. In other words, a rule of thumb is that pregnant women should be treated similarly to nonpregnant asthmatics. Patients should be taught how to recognize the signs and symptoms of early exacerbations so that they may begin treatment at home promptly. **Initial treatment consists of a short-acting inhaled beta-2-agonist** (albuterol), up to three treatments of 2 to 4 puffs by MDI (metered-dose inhaler) at 20 minute intervals for up to three treatments, or single nebulizer treatment for up to 1 hour. A good response is characterized by PEFR greater than 80% of personal best and resolution of symptoms sustained for 4 hours. Patients may be continued on beta-2-agonists every 3 to 4 hours for 24 to 48 hours. Inhaled corticosteroids (ICS) should be initiated or if already taking ICS, the dose should be doubled. Follow-up appointment with their physician should be made as soon as possible. Inadequate response to initial therapy (PEFR <80%) or decreased fetal activity warrants immediate medical attention.

Prevention of hypoxia is the ultimate goal for the pregnant woman who presents to the hospital during an acute asthma attack. Initial assessment should include a brief history and physical examination to assess the severity of asthma and possible trigger factors such as a respiratory infection. Patients with imminent respiratory arrest include those who are drowsy or confused, have paradoxical thoracoabdominal movement, bradycardia, pulsus paradoxus, and decreased air movement (no wheezing). Intubation and mechanical ventilation with 100% oxygen should be performed in these circumstances and the patient should be admitted to the intensive care unit. Because of the changes in the respiratory physiology in pregnancy (ie, a respiratory alkylosis with partially metabolic compensation), different thresholds for action exist (Table 27–1). A $Paco_2$ greater than 35 mm Hg, with a pH less than 7.35 in the presence of a falling Pao_2 is a sign of impending respiratory failure in a pregnant asthmatic. Intubation is warranted when the $Paco_2$ is 45 mm Hg or more and rising.

Premature Rupture of Membranes

Premature rupture of membranes (PROM) is defined as the ROM prior to the onset of labor. Preterm PROM (PPROM) is the ROM that occurs prior to 37 completed weeks. Approximately 3% of all pregnancies are complicated by PPROM and is the underlying etiology of one-third of preterm births. Normal fetal membranes are biologically very strong in preterm pregnancies. The weakening mechanism is likely multifactorial. Studies have shown PPROM to be associated with intrinsic (intrauterine stretch/strain from polyhydramnios and multifetal pregnancies, cervical incompetence) and

Table 27–1 • ARTERIAL BLOOD GAS FINDINGS IN PREGNANCY			
Parameter	Nonpregnant	Pregnancy	Mechanism
pH	7.40	7.45	Respiratory alkylosis
Po_2	80-100 mm Hg	90-110 mm Hg	Increased minute ventilation
Pco_2	40 mm Hg	28 mm Hg	Respiratory alkylosis
HCO_3	24 mEq/L	18 mEq/L	Partial metabolic acidosis compensation

extrinsic factors (ascending bacterial infections). There is evidence demonstrating an association between ascending infection from the lower genital tract and PPROM. This section will be restricted to gestational age less than 26 weeks.

PPROM is associated with significant maternal and fetal morbidity and mortality. The time from rupture of membranes to delivery is known as "latency." The latency period is inversely proportional to the gestational age at PPROM. Latency period of 1 week or less is present in 50% to 60% of PPROM patients. During this period amnionitis occurs in 13% to 60%, and abruptio placentae occurs in 4% to 12%. Maternal and fetal complications decrease with increasing gestational age at the time of PPROM. Multiple complications have been associated with PPROM.

The primary maternal morbidity is chorioamnionitis. Incidence varies with population and gestational age at PPROM, with reported frequency from 15% to 40%. Chorioamnionitis typically precedes fetal infection but this is not always the case, and therefore close clinical monitoring is required. Fetal morbidity and mortality varies with gestational age and complications, particularly infection. The most common complication is respiratory distress syndrome (RDS). Other serious fetal complications include necrotizing enterocolitis, intraventricular hemorrhage, and sepsis. The three causes of neonatal death associated with PPROM are prematurity, sepsis, and pulmonary hypoplasia. Preterm infants born with sepsis have a mortality rate four times higher than those without sepsis.

Management of PPROM starts with initial evaluation and diagnosis of rupture of membranes. The primary patient complaint is experiencing a "gush" of fluid but some patients will report persistent leakage of fluid. This patient history of rupture of membranes is accurate in 90% of cases. Diagnosis is established on sterile speculum evaluation. Confirmatory findings include pooling of amniotic fluid in posterior fornix and/or leakage of fluid on Valsalva; positive nitrazine test of fluid (vaginal pH 4.5-6.0, amniotic fluid pH 7.1-7.3, nitrazine turns dark blue above 6.0-6.5); amniotic fluid *ferning* on microscopy. Should the initial tests be ambiguous or negative, in the face of continued clinical suspicion other diagnostic modalities can be utilized. The ultrasound finding of oligohydramnios is usually confirmatory.

At the time of the initial evaluation, the patient's cervical os should be **visually** assessed for dilatation and possible prolapse of umbilical cord or fetal limb. In general, a digital examination of the cervix should be avoided since bacterial may be theoretically inoculated with an examination. Ultrasound evaluation of the gestational age, fetal weight, fetal presentation, placental location, and assessment of amniotic fluid index (AFI) are vital for treatment planning. A low AFI (<5.0 cm) and low maximum vertical fluid pocket (<2.0 cm) at the time of initial assessment is associated with shorter latency, increased RDS, and increased composite morbidity.

Management

Patients diagnosed with PPROM would benefit from an admission to the hospital in all likelihood until delivery. Once PPROM is verified, the treatment plan must balance the maternal, fetal, neonatal risks/benefits of prolonged pregnancy or expeditious delivery and possible inclusion of medical intervention. For those gestations that are previable, observation in the hospital or careful follow-up with an obstetrician is advisable.

In the absence of clinical signs of labor, abruption, or maternal or fetal signs of infection most patients in this gestational age will benefit from an expectant management with daily assessment of the maternal and fetal well-being.

Maternal and fetal assessment

1. **Maternal:** The criteria for the diagnosis of clinical chorioamnionitis include maternal pyrexia, tachycardia, leukocytosis, uterine tenderness, malodorous vaginal discharge, and fetal tachycardia. During inpatient observation, the woman should be regularly examined for such signs of intrauterine infection and an abnormal parameter or a combination of them may indicate intrauterine infection. The frequency of maternal and fetal assessments (temperature, pulse, and fetal heart rate auscultation) should be between 4 and 8 hours.

2. **Fetal:** Electronic fetal heart rate tracing is useful when the gestation is considered viable, because fetal tachycardia may represent a sign of fetal infection and is frequently used in the clinical definition of chorioamnionitis in some studies. Fetal tachycardia is often the earliest sign of infection. However, checking intermittent fetal heart activity for previable gestation is preferable.

Use of steroids: A meta-analysis of 15 randomized controlled trials involving more than 1400 women with preterm rupture of the membranes demonstrated that antenatal corticosteroids reduced the risks of respiratory distress syndrome. This is generally administered at 24 weeks or beyond in the absence of clinical infection.

Use of antibiotics: The use of antibiotics following PPROM was associated with a statistically significant reduction in chorioamnionitis. There was a significant reduction in the numbers of babies born within 48 hours and 7 days. Neonatal infection was significantly reduced in the babies whose mothers received antibiotics.

PPROM under 23 weeks: There are insufficient data to make recommendations in the setting of PPROM under 23 to 24 weeks including the possibility of home, day-care, and outpatient monitoring. It would be considered reasonable to maintain the woman in hospital for at least 48 hours before a decision is made to allow her to go home. The management of these cases should be individualized and outpatient monitoring restricted to certain groups of women after careful consideration of other risk factors and the access to the hospital.

Hyperthyroidism

Hyperthyroidism in pregnancy is more difficult to recognize due to the hyperdynamic physiologic changes in pregnancy. However, unintended weight loss, nervousness, palpitations, tachycardia, or tremor are clinical manifestations that bear evaluation. The diagnosis is made clinical suspicion and thyroid function tests, such as thyroid-stimulating hormone (TSH) and free T4 levels. The immediate treatment includes β-blocking agents and thioamides.

The patient who presents acutely to the emergency department should be started on β-blockers urgently to relieve the adrenergic symptoms of tachycardia, tremor, anxiety, and heat sensitivity by decreasing the maternal heart rate, cardiac output, and myocardial oxygen consumption. Longer-acting agents, such as atenolol and metoprolol 50 to 200 mg/d, are recommended. β-Blockers are contraindicated in patients with asthma and congestive heart failure and should not be used at the time of delivery due to possible neonatal bradycardia and hypoglycemia.

Thioamides inhibit thyroid hormone synthesis by reduction of iodine organification and iodotyrosine coupling. Both propylthiouracil (PTU) and methimazole have been used during pregnancy, but PTU has been traditionally preferred because of concern regarding reduced transplacental transfer of PTU compared to methimazole. However, recent studies do not confirm this finding. Teratogenic patterns associated with methimazole include aplasia cutis and choanal/esophageal atresia; however, these anomalies do not occur at a higher rate in women on thioamides compared to the general population.

Side effects of thioamides include transient leukopenia (10%); agranulocytosis (0.1%-0.4%); thrombocytopenia, hepatitis, and vasculitis (<1%) as well as rash, nausea, arthritis, anorexia, fever, and loss of taste or smell (5%). Agranulocytosis usually presents with a fever and sore throat. If a CBC indicates agranulocytosis, the medication should be discontinued. Treatment with another thioamide carries a significant risk of cross-reaction as well.

Initiation of thioamides in a patient with a new diagnosis during pregnancy requires a dose of PTU 100 to 150 mg three times daily or methimazole 10 to 20 mg twice daily. Free T4 levels are used to monitor response to therapy in hyperthyroid patients and should be checked in 4 to 6 weeks. The PTU or methimazole can be adjusted in 50 mg or 10 mg increments, respectively, with a therapeutic range for free T4 of 1.2 to 1.8 ng/dL. The goal of treatment is to maintain the free T4 in the upper normal range using the lowest possible dose in order to protect the fetus from hypothyroidism. The required dose of thioamide during pregnancy can increase up to 50% for patients with a history of hyperthyroidism prior to conception. The patient's TSH should be checked at the initial prenatal visit and every trimester. Medication adjustments, testing intervals, and therapeutic goals for the free T4 are the same as for patients with new-onset disease.

The most common cause of hyperthyroidism is Graves disease, which occurs in 95% of all cases at all ages. The diagnosis of Graves disease is usually made by the presence of elevated free T4 level or free thyroid index with a suppressed TSH in the absence of a nodular goiter or thyroid mass. The differential diagnosis of hyperthyroidism, in the order of decreasing frequency, includes subacute thyroiditis, painless (silent or postpartum) thyroiditis, toxic multinodular goiter, toxic adenoma (solitary autonomous hot nodule), iodine-induced (iodinated contrast or amiodarone), iatrogenic overreplacement of thyroid hormone, factitious thyrotoxicosis, *struma ovarii* (ovarian teratoma), and gestational trophoblastic disease. The general symptoms of hyperthyroidism include palpitations, weight loss with increased appetite, nervousness, heat intolerance, oligomenorrhea, eye irritation or edema, and frequent stools. The general signs include diffuse goiter, tachycardia, tremor, warm, moist skin, and new-onset atrial fibrillation. Diagnosis during pregnancy is even more difficult because the signs and symptoms of hyperthyroidism may overlap with the hypermetabolic symptoms of pregnancy. Discrete findings with Graves disease include a diffuse, toxic goiter (common in most young women), ophthalmopathy (periorbital edema, proptosis, and lid retraction in only 30%), dermopathy (pretibial myxedema in <1%), and acropachy (digital clubbing).

The pathogenesis of Graves disease is characterized by an autoimmune process with production of thyroid-stimulating immunoglobulins (TSIs) and TSH-binding inhibitory immunoglobulins (TBIIs) that act on the TSH receptor on the thyroid gland to mediate thyroid stimulation or inhibition, respectively. These antibodies, in effect, act as TSH agonists or antagonists, to stimulate or inhibit thyroid growth, iodine trapping, and T4/T3 synthesis. Maternal Graves disease complicates 1 out of every 500 to 1000 pregnancies. The frequency of poor outcomes depends on the severity of maternal thyrotoxicosis with a risk of preterm delivery of 88%, stillbirth of 50%, and risk of congestive heart failure of over 60% in untreated mothers.

Thyroid Storm

Maternal thyroid storm is a medical emergency characterized by a hypermetabolic state in a woman with uncontrolled hyperthyroidism. Thyroid storm occurs in less than 1% of pregnancies but has a high risk of maternal heart failure. Usually, there is an inciting event, such as infection, cesarean delivery, or labor, which leads to acute onset of fever, tachycardia, altered mental status (restlessness, nervousness, confusion), seizures, nausea, vomiting, diarrhea, and cardiac arrhythmias. Shock, stupor, and coma can ensue without prompt intervention, which includes OB-ICU admission, supportive measures, and acute medical management. Therapy includes a standard series of drugs, each of which has a specific role in suppression of thyroid function: PTU or methimazole blocks additional synthesis of thyroid hormone, and PTU also blocks peripheral conversion of T4 to T3. Saturated solutions of potassium iodide or sodium iodide block the release of T4 and T3 from the gland. Dexamethasone decreases thyroid hormone release and peripheral conversion of T4 to T3. Propranolol inhibits the adrenergic effects of excessive thyroid hormone. Phenobarbital can reduce extreme agitation or restlessness and may increase catabolism of thyroid hormone. Fetal surveillance is performed throughout, but intervention for fetal indications should not occur until the mother is stabilized.

Pyelonephritis

A pregnant woman is at greater risk for pyelonephritis and its complications such as sepsis and acute respiratory distress syndrome (ARDS). Most cases of pyelonephritis in pregnancy are caused by infection with gram-negative aerobic bacteria, but an increasing number are due to group B *Streptococcus*. Approximately 7% of affected women will develop pulmonary insufficiency due to ARDS (see Figure 27–1), presumably related to release of endotoxin. For these reasons, a pregnant patient with pyelonephritis should be admitted to the hospital. The diagnosis is established with the classic triad of fever, costovertebral angle (CVA) tenderness, and pyuria.

The patient should be placed on IV hydration, antibiotics aimed at the most common etiology, *E Coli*, and monitored for complications. Bacteria and/or their component toxins can produce a sepsis syndrome that, unchecked, will develop into septic shock. The cornerstone of management is early diagnosis, but often that is not easy. A program of early goal-directed therapy has been shown to reduce mortality from septic shock. However, not all patients with septic shock require the same treatment interventions. The woman in our case scenario, for example, requires aggressive fluid resuscitation and transfer to an intensive care unit. Per hour 1 to 2 L

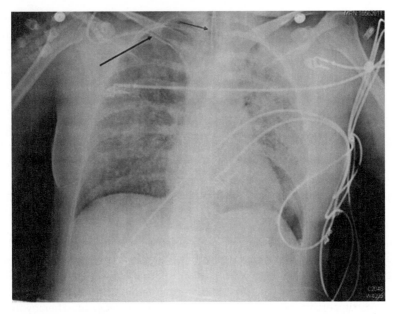

Figure 27–1. CXR showing diffuse bilateral alveolar opacities consistent with ARDS. (Reproduced, with permission, from Longo DL, Fauci As, Kasper DL, et al. *Harrison's Principles of Internal Medicine.* 18th ed. New York, NY: McGraw-Hill; 2010. Figure 27-1.

(not the 125 cc/h she was receiving) would be appropriate. The total volume needed should be determined by monitoring central venous pressure. An arterial catheter should be placed to monitor blood pressure and obtain timely pH and blood gas measurements. If adequate fluid resuscitation has not elevated the mean arterial pressure above 65 mm Hg, then vasopressors would be indicated. Adequate oxygenation should be maintained, with endotracheal intubation and mechanical ventilation, if necessary. The ceftriaxone she was receiving likely does not need to be changed, but some authorities prefer ampicillin and gentamicin for the treatment of pyelonephritis in pregnancy. Surgical intervention is seldom necessary for septic shock secondary to pyelonephritis, but prolonged hypotension and ischemia can lead to gangrene of the extremities and amputation in severe cases. When septic shock results from necrotizing fasciitis, extensive debridement of necrotic tissue is an essential component of management. Antibiotic therapy should include vancomycin for methicillin-resistant *Staphylococcus* and clindamycin for *Streptococcus*; there is evidence that clindamycin may directly inhibit synthesis of group A streptococcal toxins.

COMPREHENSION QUESTIONS

27.1 A 35-year-old woman G2P1 at 24 weeks' gestation comes into the emergency department with fever of 102°F, dysuria, and costovertebral angle tenderness. The urinalysis shows numerous bacteria and leukocytes. The patient asks whether she can be treated as an outpatient. Which of the following is the best response?

A. Outpatient therapy with oral cephalexin is acceptable.

B. Outpatient therapy with an initial dose of ceftriaxone IM and then oral nitrofurantoin is acceptable.

C. Outpatient therapy is acceptable if this is the patient's first episode of pyelonephritis.

D. In-patient therapy is preferred in this patient.

27.2 The patient in Question 27.1 is treated with antibiotic therapy for 2 days, and develops acute shortness of breath and is noted to have an O_2 sat of 89% on room air. Which of the following is the most likely cause of her hypoxemia?

A. Pulmonary embolism

B. Pneumonia

C. ARDS

D. Aspiration

27.3 A 28-year-old G1P0 woman is noted to be at 7 weeks' gestation by dates. She comes into the ED with vaginal bleeding. The physical examination is otherwise unremarkable. There are no adnexal masses or tenderness and the uterus is nontender and the cervix is closed. The hCG level is 2000 mIU/mL, and the transvaginal ultrasound shows no intrauterine gestation, no adnexal masses, and no free fluid. Which of the following is the most likely diagnosis?

A. Ectopic pregnancy

B. Completed abortion

C. Incomplete abortion

D. Molar pregnancy

27.4 A 31-year-old woman G3P2 woman at 19 weeks' gestation complains of jitteriness, weight loss, and palpitations. She has a history of Graves disease and had been taking PTU and propranolol until she stopped 2 weeks ago due to concern about the medications' effect on her pregnancy. The patient is noted to have a temp of 102°F, BP 160/100 mm Hg, heart rate 130, and she is confused and disoriented. Which of the following is the most likely diagnosis?

A. Acute β-blocker withdrawal syndrome

B. Sepsis due to PTU-induced neutropenia

C. Thyroid storm

D. Hyperparathyroidism

27.5 A 27-year-old G1P0 woman at 18 weeks' gestation complains of significant nausea and vomiting throughout her pregnancy, and has not been able to keep any foods or liquids down. She has been admitted to the hospital numerous times. Her BP is 100/60 mm Hg and heart rate 110, and urinalysis shows negative nitrates, negative leukoesterase, and ketones is 2 +/4. Which of the following statements is most accurate about this patient?

A. The presence of ketones in the urine in consistent with significant volume depletion.

B. The patient's gestational age of 18 weeks is expected for hyperemesis gravidarum.

C. Vitamin B_1 is useful for this patient's condition.

D. The patient may be expected to have hyperkalemia.

27.6 A 31-year-old G2P1 woman is noted to be at 20 weeks' gestation. She presents to the ED with a history of leakage of fluid per vagina earlier in the day. On speculum examination, there is no fluid in the vagina. The fern and nitrazine tests are negative. Which of the following is the best next step for this patient?

A. Inform the patient that she does not have rupture of membranes.

B. Hospitalize the patient and assume that she has rupture of membranes.

C. Treat with an oral antibiotic for presumed UTI.

D. Perform an ultrasound examination.

ANSWERS

27.1 **D.** Pregnant women with pyelonephritis should be admitted to the hospital in general because of the complications such as sepsis, preterm labor, miscarriage, or ARDS. Endotoxin-induced pulmonary injury is a well-documented complication of pyelophritis and occurs more commonly in pregnant women.

27.2 **C.** A patient who develops acute shorness of breath and hypoxemia after treatment for pyelonephritis should be assumed to have endotoxin-mediated pulmonary injury, or ARDS. A chest x-ray will usually reveal patchy bilateral infiltrates in the lung fields. The treatment is supplemental oxygen and supportive therapy.

27.3 **A.** When the hCG level exceeds the threshold of 1500 and no gestational sac is seen on TV ultrasound, the likelihood of an ectopic pregnancy is high (in the range of 85%). These patients usually go to laparoscopy to confirm the diagnosis. When the hCG level is below the threshold, then the next step is generally to repeat the hCG level in 48 hours to assess for a normal rise (>66% rise) which would indicate a normal intrauterine pregnancy, versus an abnormal rise (<66%) which would be either an ectopic pregnancy or a miscarriage.

27.4 **C.** Thyroid storm is present with hyperthyroidism in conjunction with CNS dysfunction (seizures, confusion, lethargy), and/or autonomic instability (fever). Thyroid storm carries a worse prognosis and usually requires immediate admission to the ICU and aggressive therapy consisting of PTU, β-blockers, and steroids. A common precursor to thyroid storm is a patient who has stopped taking medications and a stressor such as infection or surgery.

27.5 **A.** With hyperemesis gravidarum, the presence of moderate to significant ketones is associated with significant volume depletion. The patient is typically hypokalemic. The usual gestational age for hyperemesis is the first trimester, although less commonly, women can persist later and ever rarer, throughout the pregnancy. Vitamin B$_6$ is a useful adjunctive treatment.

27.6 **D.** When the history suggests PROM, but the speculum examination is negative, ultrasound to assess for amniotic fluid volume is helpful. If oligohydramnios is diagnosed, the patient is assumed to have ROM, and should be admitted to the hospital.

CLINICAL PEARLS

▶ Nausea and vomiting in pregnancy is common, so that significant volume or metabolic derangements in these patients can be minimized.

▶ Hyperemesis is a diagnosis of exclusion.

▶ The physiologic changes of pregnancy should be considered when interpreting ABGs. For instance when the P$_{CO_2}$ exceeds 40 mm Hg in a pregnant asthmatic, severe hypercarbia is present and intubation should be considered.

▶ Dyspnea and hypoxemia after treatment for pyelonephritis is usually caused by endotoxin-related pulmonary injury, ARDS.

▶ Hyperthyroidism is typically treated with methimazole or PTU, and a β-blocker.

▶ When the hCG level exceeds the threshold of 1200 to 1500 mIU/mL and no gestational sac is seen in the uterus on transvaginal ultrasound, then an ectopic pregnancy is highly likely.

▶ The history for a gush of fluid followed by constant leakage is 90% accurate for rupture of membranes.

▶ In there is strong clinical suspicion, and the speculum examination is negative for ROM, an ultrasound assessment for amniotic fluid volume is helpful.

REFERENCES

American College of Obstetricians and Gynecologists. Diagnosis and treatment of gestational tropho-blastic disease. ACOG *Practice Bulletin 53*. Washington, DC: 2004.

American College of Obstetricians and Gynecologists. Medical management of abortion. *ACOG Practice Bulletin 67*. Washington, DC: 2005.

Andrews JI, Shamshirsaz AA, Diekema DJ. Nonmenstrual toxic shock syndrome due to methicillin-resistant *staphylococcus aureus*. *Obstet Gynecol*. 2008;112:933-938.

Casey BM, Leveno KJ. Thyroid disease in pregnancy. Clinical expert series. *Obstet Gynecol*. 2006;108:1238-1292.

Katz VL. Recurrent and spontaneous abortion. In: Katz VL, Lentz GM, Lobo RA, Gersenson DM, eds. *Comprehensive Gynecology*. 5th ed. St. Louis, MO: Mosby-Year Book; 2007:359-388.

Lu MC, Hobel CJ. Antepartum care: preconception and prenatal care, genetic evaluation and teratology, and antenatal fetal assessment. In: Hacker NF, Moore JG, Gambone JC, eds. *Essentials of Obstetrics and Gynecology*. 4th ed. Philadelphia, PA: Saunders; 2004:83-103.

Martin SR, Foley MR. Intensive care in obstetrics: an evidence-based review. *Am J Obstet Gynecol*. 2006;195:673-689.

Neal DM, Cootauco AC, Burrow G. Thyroid disease in pregnancy. *Clin Perinatol*. 2007;34:543-557.

Parillo JE. Septic shock—vasopressin, norepinephrine, and urgency. *N Engl J Med*. 2008;358:954-956.

A 10-week-old infant is brought to the emergency department (ED) by his mother for 1 day of fever. The mother tells you that her son was delivered vaginally at full term and was the product of an uncomplicated pregnancy. He has had regular well-baby checks and has been gaining weight appropriately. He has met his normal developmental milestones and vaccinations are up-to-date. He has had no prior illnesses. This morning his mother noticed he felt warm to the touch and discovered an axillary temperature of 101°F. No other signs or symptoms of infection including runny nose, cough, difficulty breathing, rash, nuchal rigidity, seizure activity, abdominal distension, vomiting, or diarrhea. She states her son has been breast-feeding less than normal, but overall has had a normal number of wet diapers. She is very concerned because this is her first child and he has never had a fever before.

On examination, the child is found to have a heart rate of 180 beats per minute, a blood pressure of 90/50 mm Hg, a respiratory rate of 40 breaths per minute, an oxygen saturation of 99% on room air, and a rectal temperature of 102.7°F. He is overall well appearing and has an unremarkable physical examination. Although he cries when you perform the examination, his mother is able to console him easily.

▶ What is the most likely diagnosis?
▶ What is the next step in management?
▶ What is the best therapy?

ANSWERS TO CASE 28:

Fever Without a Source in the 1- to 3-Month-Old Infant

Summary: A previously healthy 10-week-old infant is brought in by his mother for fever The cause of the fever is not clearly identified by the history or physical examination. His vital signs in the emergency department are significant for fever and tachycardia. His examination is unremarkable.

- **Most likely diagnosis:** Fever without a source (FWS).

- **Next step**: Order CBC, blood cultures, urinalysis, urine culture. You may also order stool studies, a chest x-ray, and perform a lumbar puncture depending on the clinical presentation.

- **Best therapy:** It is up to physician discretion to decide which well-appearing infants with fever without a source should receive antibiotics. If antibiotics are given, the best drug is ceftriaxone, either IV or IM.

ANALYSIS

Objectives

1. Understand the appropriate workup for fever without a source in the well-appearing 1- to 3-month-old infant.

2. Appreciate the controversy regarding the management of fever without a source in this age group.

3. Learn the treatment options for fever without a source in a 1- to 3-month-old infant.

Considerations

This 10-week-old infant presented with fever without any other signs or symptoms of infection including runny nose, cough, difficulty breathing, rash, nuchal rigidity, seizure activity, abdominal distension, vomiting, or diarrhea. Importantly, the emergency physician must be aware that the 1- to 3-month-old infant will not manifest the same signs of infection as an older child. For this reason, the workup of fever in this age group must remain broad and one must have a low threshold for both further testing and treatment with antibiotics.

APPROACH TO:
Fever Without a Source in the 1- to 3-Month-Old Infant

DEFINITIONS

FEVER WITHOUT A SOURCE: Fever without a source is an acute febrile illness in which the etiology of the fever is not apparent after a careful history and physical examination. A rectal temperature greater than 38°C (100.4°F) is defined as a fever.

SERIOUS BACTERIAL ILLNESS (SBI): Illnesses including bacteremia, pneumonia, urinary tract infection, skin and soft tissue infections, bone and joint infections, enteritis, or meningitis due to a bacterial pathogen.

CLINICAL APPROACH

Diagnosis of Potential Fever in the 1- to 3-Month-Old Infant

While many parents will bring in their infants for a chief complaint of fever, not all parents will have actually taken their child's temperature with a thermometer. If an infant has had a rectal temperature more than 38°C at home but is afebrile and well appearing in the emergency department, this infant still requires full workup for fever. If the parent only reports a tactile fever and the infant is afebrile and well appearing in the emergency department, no laboratory testing for fever workup is required. Temperature must be measured with a rectal thermometer in order to rule out a fever. Axillary and tympanic membrane thermometers are not adequate to evaluate for fever in an infant. If an infant is brought in bundled and has a mildly elevated temperature, it is worthwhile to recheck a rectal temperature 15 minutes after unbundling the infant. However, a temperature more than 38.5°C should never be attributed to bundling.

Evaluation of Fever Without a Source in the 1- to 3-Month-Old Infant

The evaluation of fever in this age group has changed dramatically in the last 30 years in the wake of vaccines targeting haemophilus influenzae type b and *Streptococcus pneumoniae*. These vaccines have dramatically decreased the burden of SBI in this age group. Prior to the development of these vaccines, the majority of febrile infants in this age group were hospitalized and often started on empiric antibiotic therapy. Morbidity and mortality for SBI was high and early clinical identification was very difficult.

Given the controversy and difficulties identifying infants with SBI several decision rules have been developed. These are the Rochester, Boston, and Philadelphia criteria, each using a combination of factors including history, physical examination, and laboratory parameters to identify low-risk infants. Although all these criteria use slightly different testing strategies, all of the criteria support the use of CBC, blood cultures, urinalysis, and urine culture to identify infants at low risk for SBI. Test results suggestive of high risk for SBI include WBC greater than or equal to $15,000/mm^3$ or less than or equal to $5000/mm^3$, a band-to-neutrophil ratio of greater than or equal to 0.2, a urine dipstick test positive for nitrite or leukocyte esterase, or a finding of greater than or equal to 5 WBCs/hpf or organisms seen on Gram stain.

Routinely obtaining chest x-rays and lumbar punctures in this age group are somewhat more controversial. Although there is disagreement between the decision rules, one meta-analysis of a combined group of 361 febrile infants found that infants which have tachypnea >50 breaths per minute, rales, ronchi, retractions, wheezing, coryza, grunting, stridor, nasal flaring, or cough should have a chest x-ray.

Similar to chest x-ray, routine lumbar puncture is another area of controversy among the decision rules. Several observational studies suggest that infants can be identified as low risk for SBI without performing a lumbar puncture. However, other physicians feel that the significant morbidity and mortality associated with bacterial meningitis outweighs the low incidence of the disease, and thus argue in support of routine lumbar puncture in the workup of fever without a source. Cerebrospinal fluid (CSF) with greater than or equal to 8 WBC/mm^3 or organisms on Gram stain is considered high risk for SBI. Additionally, sending stool for WBCs and culture is recommended for infants in this age group with diarrhea. Greater than 5 WBC/hpf in the stool specimen is considered high risk for SBI.

While this case has focused on the well-appearing 1- to 3-month-old infant with fever without a source, it is worthwhile to note that ill-appearing infants in this age group have a much higher risk of SBI, and all of these infants should be treated with empiric antibiotics and admitted to the hospital. Up to 45% of these infants will test positive for SBI.

Pathogens

Routine vaccinations with *Haemophilus influenzae* type b vaccine (Hib) and heptavalent pneumococcal conjugate vaccine (PCV7) have dramatically decreased the rates of SBI infants. After the introduction of the Hib vaccine, the majority (90%) of infections were due to pneumococcus. The PCV7 vaccine further changed the landscape of SBI, decreasing the incidence of invasive pneumococcal disease 65% to 80% in children younger than 3 years of age. Although much less common, other pathogens are emerging as prominent causes of SBI in this age group, including *E Coli*, *Staphylococcus aureus*, *Neisseria meningitides*, *Salmonella* species, and *Streptococcus pyogenes*. Furthermore, non-vaccine serotypes of *S Pneumoniae* are noted to be increasingly prevalent in this age group.

Treatment

Antibiotics must be considered for all 1- to 3-month-old infants with fever without a source. The empiric antibiotic of choice is c eftriaxone, which may be given IV or IM. The regular dose is 50 mg/kg; however, if meningitis is suspected, the dose should be increased to 100 mg/kg. If lumbar puncture is not performed, antibiotics should be withheld because giving empiric antibiotics in this situation could mask the presentation of bacterial meningitis on follow-up examination. For ill-appearing infants in this age group, consideration should be given to augmenting empiric ceftriaxone by adding vancomycin to cover for methicillin-resistant *Staphylococcus aureus* (MRSA) and *Streptococcus pneumonia* resistant to ceftriaxone. Ampicillin should also be considered for the ill-appearing infant to cover for possible *Listeria monocytogenes*.

COMPREHENSION QUESTIONS

28.1. An 8-week-old previously healthy infant, product of a full-term pregnancy, is brought by his older sister to the emergency department for a fever up to 101.2°F. The sister, who is 17 years old, states that she is the primary caretaker for her brother because the only adult at home is her mother who is struggling with cocaine and alcohol abuse. The sister states that although her brother has not been eating well, he is taking in a normal amount of formula and has not had cough, runny nose, altered behavior, vomiting, or diarrhea. Overall, the patient is well appearing. You perform an appropriate workup for this infant with FWS and find a WBC count of 10,000/mm^3, and a UA with 2 WBCs/hpf. You also elect to do an LP and the CSF shows 1 WBC/mm^3 and no organisms on Gram stain. What is the most appropriate disposition for this patient?

A. Discharge the patient home after giving a dose of IV Ceftriaxone.

B. Discharge the patient home but do not give any antibiotics.

C. Give a dose of IV ceftriaxone and admit the patient to the hospital.

D. Order a chest x-ray, stool WBCs and culture, and then admit the patient to the hospital.

28.2. An 11-week-old male infant is brought in by his mother for 4 days of fever (Tmax 100.8°F) associated with cough and runny nose. The child was the product of a full-term healthy pregnancy and his vaccines are up-to-date. He is overall well appearing and has normal vital signs. A chest x-ray demonstrates no evidence of pneumonia. A rapid respiratory syncytial virus (RSV) test comes back positive. Which of the following statements most accurately describes the risk of SBI in the RSV positive infant?

A. SBI is just as common in RSV-positive infants as in RSV-negative infants.

B. SBI is less common in RSV-positive infants as in RSV-negative infants.

C. SBI is equally as common in RSV-positive infants as in RSV-negative infants.

D. There is no risk of SBI in the febrile infant with a positive RSV test.

28.3. A 9-week-old well-appearing female infant is brought in to the emergency department with a chief complaint of a fever up to 102°F at home. The infant has not had any vomiting or cough and the examination is unremarkable including a thorough skin examination. In the ED, the infant is afebrile but had been given ibuprofen by mom 2 hours prior to arrival. A catheter urinalysis comes back positive for 20 WBCs/hpf. What is the best management for this patient?

A. Send urine cultures, give her IV antibiotics, and admit her to the pediatric service.

B. Send urine cultures, give her PO antibiotics, and discharge her home.

C. Give her an IM shot of ceftriaxone and send her home with PO antibiotics.

D. Send urine cultures, give IV or IM antibiotics, and evaluate the social situation.

28.4. A 6-week-old male infant is brought in by his parents for evaluation of fever of 39°C. The infant is ill appearing and lethargic and does not want to breast-feed. His parents also reported that his cry sounds different. The patient is given antipyretics, a bolus of 20 cc/kg IV fluids and labs are sent. A thorough examination including skin does not reveal any source of infection, and urinalysis, chest x-ray, and CSF are all normal and cultures are sent. What is the best management of this patient?

A. Give him an IM shot of ceftriaxone and discharge home with close follow-up.

B. Give him IV ceftriaxone and admit to the pediatric service.

C. Give him IV ceftriaxone, vancomycin, and ampicillin and admit to the pediatric service.

D. Do not give any antibiotics at this time and admit to the pediatric service for observation.

ANSWERS

28.1 **C.** This case demonstrates the importance of good follow-up and an adequate social situation when considering discharging the well-appearing infant with FWS. In order to discharge a well-appearing infant with FWS, one must ensure follow-up within 24 hours. There must also be adequate social support to ensure the patient can be brought back to the hospital if his condition worsens. In general, this means that the patient's family should have access to a telephone and transportation. In this case, the social situation is less than ideal as a minor is primarily caring for the patient and the only adult in the family is incapacitated by polysubstance abuse to the point that she has not even come to the hospital with her ill infant. There is no indication for a chest x-ray or stool studies in this patient as he has no respiratory symptoms and no diarrhea.

28.2 **B.** A positive RSV test in a 1- to 3-month-old infant with a fever decreases the risk of SBI, but does not completely eliminate this risk. Most studies demonstrate that the risk of SBI in the RSV-positive population is decreased by approximately 50%. The most common SBI in the RSV-positive patient is a urinary tract infection. There are no studies at this time which have been powered enough to detect difference in rates of bacteremia and meningitis in RSV-positive and RSV-negative patients as both bacteremia and meningitis in this age group is relatively uncommon. Thus, RSV-positive infants in this age group with fever should at least receive a urinalysis and urine culture. It remains unclear whether or not clinicians can safely forgo blood and spinal fluid testing in these same infants.

28.3 **D.** Urinary tract infection is the most common cause of SBI in infants with fever without a source and the prevalence has not changed with the PCV7 vaccine. A positive urine is defined as greater than10 WBCs per high power field. A negative urine dipstick or urinalysis does not exclude UTI as pyuria is absent on initial urinalysis in up to 20% febrile infants with pyelonephritis. Thus, a urine culture must be obtained on all patients. Additionally, catheter samples should always be obtained as bag specimens are often contaminated. Infants younger than 8 weeks of age should be admitted to the hospital. Well-appearing infants greater than 8 weeks may be discharged home if the parents are reliable and follow-up within 24 hours is possible. Infants younger than 3 months of age should be given parenteral antibiotics (ceftriaxone 50 mg/kg) with admission or discharge and may need additional parenteral doses even if discharged home.

28.4 **C.** Infants who have an abnormal cry and temperature greater than 38.5°C or are ill appearing have an increased risk of SBI. Up to 45% of ill-appearing young infants may have SBI and, thus, require extensive workup including blood, urine, CSF, and CXR. Ill-appearing infants in this age group should receive parenteral antibiotic therapy to cover the likely pathogens in this age group regardless of initial laboratory results (*S pneumoniae, S aureus, N meningitides, H influenza* type b) and should be admitted to the hospital. Of note, vancomycin should be administered to infants with soft tissue infection or CSF pleocytosis. In infants 29 to 60 days of age, ampicillin should also be given to cover *Listeria monocytogenes*.

REFERENCES

Anbar RD, Richardson-de Corral V, O'Malley PJ. Difficulties in universal application of criteria identifying infants at low risk for serious bacterial infection. *J Pediatr.* 1986;109(3):483.

Bramson RT, Meyer TL, Silbiger ML et al. The futility of the chest radiograph in the febrile infant without respiratory symptoms. *Pediatrics.* 1993;92(4):524-526.

Cheng TL, Partridge JC. Effect of bundling and high environmental temperature on neonatal body temperature. *Pediatrics.* 1993;92(2):238.

Hoberman A, Wald ER, Reynolds EA et al. Is urine culture necessary to rule out urinary tract infection in young febrile children? *Pediatr Infect Dis J.* 1996;15(4):304.

Ishimine P. The evolving approach to the young child who has fever and no obvious source. *Emerg Med Clin North Am.* Nov 2007;25(4):1087-1115,vii.

Jaskiewicz JA, McCarthy CA, Richardson AC, et al; Febrile Infant Collaborative Study Group. Febrile infants at low risk for serious bacterial infection—an appraisal of the Rochester criteria and implications for management. *Pediatrics.* 1994;94(3):390.

Rudinsky SL, Carstairs KL, Reardon JM, et al. Serious bacterial infections in febrile infants in the post-pneumococcal conjugate vaccine era. *Acad Emerg Med.* Jul 2009;16(7):585-590.

Yiannis L, Katsogridakis MD, MPH, Kristine L, Cieslak MD. Empiric antibiotics for the complex febrile child: when, why, and what to use. *Clin Pediatr Emerg Med.* 2008;9:258-263.

A 60-year-old woman with hypertension and diabetes presents to the emergency department (ED) with severe left eye pain, redness, and blurred vision for 3 hours. She reports that her symptoms began while watching a movie in the local cinema. She initially thought that she had eyestrain, but then her eye began to progressively ache. She denies any symptoms in her right eye. The patient denies preceding trauma, photophobia, ocular discharge, increased tearing, or prior eye surgery. She occasionally wears nonprescription reading glasses because she is farsighted. There are no prior similar events. She also reports seeing colored halos around the light fixtures in the ED, and having a headache over her left brow, some nausea, and one episode of vomiting. She denies dizziness, weakness, imbalance, abdominal pain, or chest pain. She is fully compliant with her medications, She also and reports having taken an over-the-counter cold medicine for nasal congestion for the past 2 days.

On examination, her blood pressure is 155/88 mm Hg, pulse is 88 beats per minute, respirations are 18 breaths per minute, and temperature is 36.8°C (98°F). She is alert, but in obvious discomfort, although able to tolerate ambient light. She has no periorbital signs of trauma. The left conjunctiva has **ciliary flush** (circumferential reddish ring around the cornea), but no discharge or visible foreign body. Visual acuity is 20/30 in the right eye; but only finger counting in the left eye. Visual fields are grossly intact. Gentle palpation of the closed left eye reveals that it is much firmer than the right. Her left pupil is 5 mm, fixed, and unreactive. Her right eye appears normal; the pupil is 3 mm and briskly reactive. She does not experience pain in the left eye when direct light is applied to the right eye (absent consensual photophobia). Extraocular movements are intact and non-painful. The left cornea is slightly cloudy, which makes fundoscopy difficult. The right fundus appears normal. Her temporal arteries are pulsatile and nontender. The rest of the physical examination, including the remainder of the neurological examination, is normal.

▶ What is your next diagnostic step?
▶ What is the most likely diagnosis?
▶ What is your next therapeutic step?

ANSWERS TO CASE 29:

Red Eye

Summary: This is a 60-year-old woman with acute onset of left eye redness, pain, and markedly decreased visual acuity. The left eye feels firmer to palpation than the right eye. The left cornea is edematous with a fixed and dilated pupil.

- **Next diagnostic step:** Slit-lamp examination should be performed and intra-ocular pressures must be measured in both eyes. The intraocular pressures, measured using a Tono-Pen are 18 mm Hg and 52 mm Hg in the right and left eye, respectively. Slit-lamp examination reveals bilateral narrow anterior chambers. Cell and flare (inflammatory changes) are absent. There is no evidence of hyphema (blood) or hypopyon (white cells) in the anterior chamber. Fluorescein staining is unremarkable.

- **Most likely diagnosis:** Acute angle-closure glaucoma.

- **Next step:** Lowering the intraocular pressure (IOP) should be initiated as quickly as possible to preserve vision.

ANALYSIS

Objectives

1. Become familiar with the vision-threatening causes of a painful red eye.

2. Understand the basic treatment modalities and disposition options for vision-threatening causes of a painful red eye.

3. Recognize the clinical settings, signs, and symptoms, as well as complications, of acute angle-closure glaucoma.

4. Understand the key treatment modalities for angle-closure glaucoma.

Considerations

This 60-year-old woman complains of non-traumatic acute onset of left eye pain, redness, and vision loss with a significant increase in IOP noted on examination. This case is an example of acute angle-closure glaucoma (AACG), a true ophthalmologic emergency characterized by rapidly elevated intraocular pressure, which compromises blood flow to the optic nerve **and can result in permanent vision loss.** It is likely that her underlying narrow ant chamber angle, plus the combination being in dim lighting and taking an over the counter decongestant (usually a sympathomimetic or anticholinergic), limited outflow of aqueous humor, as the cornea and iris apposed one another.

APPROACH TO:

Red Eye

ACUTE ANGLE-CLOSURE GLAUCOMA

The **mechanism of AACG or primary angle-closure glaucoma is pupillary block** of the trabecular meshwork outflow pathway. Normally, aqueous humor is produced by the ciliary body in the posterior chamber, and diffuses through the pupil into the anterior chamber where it is drained via the trabecular meshwork. A balance exists between aqueous humor production and outflow to maintain a normal IOP. However, some individuals are predisposed to acute angle closure glaucoma from aqueous humor outflow obstruction secondary to anatomical and environmental factors. Many other forms of glaucoma have a far more insidious, benign presentation, with an inexorable loss of vision. **Delay in diagnosis and treatment of AACG results in permanent loss of vision,** as the increased IOP causes optic nerve ischemia. The provider must always consider this diagnosis because it is possible to get sidetracked evaluating the associated symptoms of headache, nausea, vomiting or abdominal pain, by looking for neurologic or gastrointestinal etiologies. Risk factors for a narrow angle closure include age-related lens thickening and hyperopia (farsightedness), which results in a shortened eyeball, and a relatively shallow anterior chamber. There is a 75% risk of a similar attack in the fellow eye if left untreated. Medications which cause pupil dilatation can also trigger AACG, including anticholinergics, tricyclic antidepressants, adrenergic agonists, and topical mydriatics.

The incidence of narrow angles in the United States is 2% in white patients, and the rate of AACG is 0.1% in these individuals. Globally, the highest prevalence rates of AACG occur in certain Asian groups, for example, Mongolians and Inuits. African Americans have much higher rates of chronic angle-closure glaucoma (CACG) but lower rates of AACG. Persons between ages of 55 and 65 years have the highest incidence of AACG. The incidence in women is three to four times the rate in men. AACG is likely to occur in 33% to 50% of a patient's first-degree relatives, so the patient should inform their family members.

Acute angle-closure glaucoma can occur with stress, fatigue, dim lighting, or sustained work at close range. The patient may present with mild unilateral eye ache or intense pain, blurring, nausea, vomiting, abdominal pain, diaphoresis, and frontal headache. The **hallmarks of the physical examination** include a **fixed, dilated, midposition** pupil, diffuse conjunctival injection, **corneal edema** (clouding), and a shallow anterior chamber (Figure 29–1). Slit-lamp examination may reveal mild cell and flare, but no hyphema or hypopyon. The IOP will be elevated (normal is 9-21 mm Hg); pressures can reach 80 mm Hg in AACG. The other eye must always be examined for anterior chamber depth (the angle is usually narrow) and IOP.

Management

The therapeutic goal of the initial management of acute angle-closure glaucoma is to decrease IOP by decreasing aqueous production and increasing outflow. The principal treatment modalities include aqueous suppressants, osmotic agents, and miotic agents.

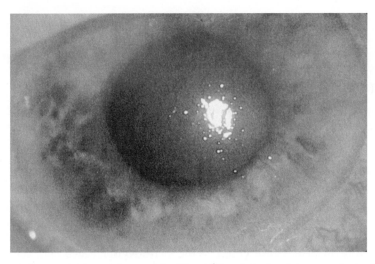

Figure 29–1. Acute angle-closure glaucoma. Pupil is mid-dilated, fixed, and the cornea is cloudy. *(Reproduced, with permission, from Tintinalli JE, Kelen GD, Stapczynski JS, eds. Emergency Medicine. 6th ed. New York, NY: McGraw-Hill;2004:1460.)*

After corneal edema subsides, **the definitive treatment is a laser peripheral iridectomy,** performed by an ophthalmologist.

Treatment to lower the intraocular pressure should be initiated in the ED in **consultation with an ophthalmologist.** Intraocular pressure is first lowered by decreasing aqueous humor production with agents such as topical **β-blockers (timolol 0.5%), an α-2-agonist (apraclonidine), and a carbonic anhydrase inhibitors (acetazolamide 500 mg orally or IV).** Patients with sulfa allergy may not tolerate acetazolamide. **Osmotic agents,** such as mannitol and glycerol, can be used instead of acetazolamide to dehydrate the vitreous humor, which decreases intraocular fluid volume, and thus lowers IOP. Mannitol may induce hypotension in patients with poor cardiac function, and glycerol should be avoided in diabetic patients. **Miotics (pilocarpine)** enhance trabecular outflow by constricting the pupil to disrupt the corneal-iris apposition. Intraocular pressure should be first lowered by the administration of topical β-blockers and acetazolamide prior to the administration of pilocarpine as the ischemic iris sphincter may be unresponsive to pilocarpine at extremely high intraocular pressures (>50 mg Hg). Pilocarpine is only used in patients with native lenses since pilocarpine will induce movement in artificial lens. Systemic concerns related to topical β-blocker administration include asthma, severe chronic obstructive pulmonary disease (COPD), bradycardia, heart block, congestive heart failure, and myasthenia gravis. Systemic absorption of topical agents can be reduced up to 70% by instructing the patient to close his or her eyes while occluding the lower tear ducts at the root of the nose after applying the drops. Punctal occlusion decreases drug absorption by the nasal mucosa. The patient should also receive analgesic and antiemetic medications.

Table 29–1 • DIFFERENTIAL DIAGNOSIS OF THE RED EYE	
Processes That Usually Do Not Impair Vision	**Processes That Can Impair Vision**
• Viral conjunctivitis/allergic conjunctivitis • Nongonococcal or nonchlamydial conjunctivitis • Subconjunctival hemorrhage • Dacrocystitis • Blepharitis • Episcleritis • Peripheral corneal pterygium • Preseptal cellulitis	• Corneal infection (gonococcal infection/ chlamydia/herpes simplex virus/herpes zoster virus) • Keratitis • Corneal ulcer • Anterior uveitis • Scleritis • Pterygium (encroaching on the paracentral cornea) • Orbital cellulitis • Endophthalmitis

Differential Diagnosis of the Red Eye

Other vision-threatening and painful causes of a red eye include severe conjunctivitis, keratitis, corneal ulcer, anterior uveitis, endophthalmitis, orbital cellulitis, scleritis, and temporal arteritis (Table 29–1). Causes of acute vision loss are outlined in Table 29–2.

In this case, the absence of any discharge makes the possibility of **conjunctivitis** highly unlikely, but discharge can be scant. However, gonococcal conjunctivitis (the most serious form of bacterial conjunctivitis) produces a copious purulent discharge with an intensely red eye, and may potentially perforate the cornea. With chlamydial conjunctivitis the clinical course is more chronic; although the conjunctivae are very red, there is scant discharge. The incidence of sexually transmitted chlamydial conjunctivitis is increasing.

Corneal inflammation, or **keratitis,** may be due to viral, bacterial, or protozoal infection, contact lenses, trauma, or ultraviolet light. Severe keratitis can progress to a **corneal ulcer,** which may be visible to the unaided eye as a white defect. Distinguishing an **ulcer** from a corneal abrasion is clinically significant and can

Table 29-2 • DIFFERENTIAL DIAGNOSIS OF ACUTE VISION LOSS	
Painful Vision Loss	**Painless Vision Loss**
AACG	Retinal detachment
Corneal ulcer	Vitreous hemorrhage
Anterior uveitis	Posterior vitreous detachment
Scleritis	Central retinal artery occlusion
Endophthalmitis	Central retinal vein occlusion
Optic neuritis	
Temporal arteritis	

be challenging. Examination with the slit lamp is required. The major distinction is the hazy/cloudy stroma that lies beneath the ulcer in contrast to the clear stroma deep to most abrasions. A slit-lamp examination is a necessary part of the evaluation of all patients with a red eye. Fluorescein staining should be included in every examination and may be the only way to identify the classic dendrite with terminal bulb markings found in herpes simplex keratitis. Herpes zoster dendrites taper at their ends and are typically associated with periorbital dermatomal vesicular eruptions, or lesions at the tip of the nose (Hutchinson sign of nasociliary involvement). Patients with HIV are at risk for complications of herpes zoster virus (HZV), and must undergo careful corneal and retinal evaluation to prevent vision loss.

Anterior uveitis (iritis) is associated with pain, blurred vision, photophobia (direct and consensual), circumcorneal redness, and anterior chamber cells and flare. A hypopyon (layer of white cells) may be visible along the inferior rim of the anterior chamber. The affected pupil is smaller, irregular, and minimally reactive. IOP can be elevated. Etiologies include idiopathic, infectious (tuberculosis, syphilis, herpes simplex/zoster, toxoplasmosis, cytomegalovirus [CMV]), autoimmune (sarcoidosis, collagen-vascular diseases, human leukocyte antigen [HLA] B27-associated), and post-traumatic. Uveitis due to herpes simplex virus (HSV) and HZV is common in HIV positive patients. Because treatment involves topical corticosteroids with their attendant risk of glaucoma, cataracts, or reactivation of herpes simplex infections, patients should be referred to an ophthalmologist. An immune recovery uveitis occurs in 15.5% of HIV-positive patients with CMV retinitis.

Endophthalmitis is inflammation of the vitreous humor and can be endogenous, secondary to hematogenous spread from a distant site, or exogenous from inoculation after penetrating trauma. Traumatic endophthalmitis usually develops within three days of penetrating injury, retained foreign body, or ocular surgery. Hallmarks include decreased vision, eye pain, hypopyon, anterior chamber cells and flare, an absent red reflex, and a hazy vitreous. Varying degrees of eyelid swelling, chemosis (conjunctival swelling), and severe conjunctival injection will also be present. Causative organisms include Bacillus cereus, coagulase-negative *Staphylococcus*, *Streptococcus*, gram-negative rods, and fungi. Any patient with a hypopyon requires an emergent ophthalmology consult. Orbital CT or ultrasound B-scan microscopy (UBM) may help diagnose a foreign body. Systemic and intravitreal antibiotics will be necessary to preserve any remainder of vision.

Orbital cellulitis, defined as infection deep to the orbital septum, is usually associated with blurred vision, diplopia, conjunctival injection, lid swelling, proptosis, fever, toxicity, and limited or painful ocular motility. An orbital computed tomography (CT) (axial and coronal cuts) is diagnostic, and will often reveal sinusitis (often ethmoid). Admission and parenteral antibiotics are indicated, because of the infection can potentially spread into the brain. Preseptal or periorbital cellulitis is a superficial and far less serious entity but it can be difficult to distinguish from orbital cellulitis. In general, these patients are less toxic appearing, with less pain. Most of these patients can be discharged on oral antibiotics with close follow-up to make sure they didn't have an early presentation of the more serious orbital cellulitis.

Subconjunctival hemorrhages should be **painless and not affect vision.** These hemorrhages are often spontaneous or may be associated with minor trauma including coughing and sneezing. In the setting of blunt trauma, continue evaluating for hyphema, globe rupture, or retrobulbar hemorrhage if the patient complains of pain or vision changes. Patients should be informed that the redness (bruise) might take weeks to spontaneously resolve.

Blunt trauma to the eye may result in a **hyphema** (blood in the anterior chamber) and painful, blurred vision. Blood may be visible to the unaided eye if it layers, or it may only be seen with the slit-lamp in the anterior chamber (microhyphema) on maximum magnification. Initial treatment includes elevating the head 30 degrees, an eye shield to prevent additional trauma, mydriatics to paralyze the ciliary body allowing the iris to rest, pain medication, antiemetics, and consultation. Complications include staining of the cornea by the red cells producing a partially opaque cornea, elevated IOP secondary to red blood cells occluding the trabecular outflow tract, and rebleeding.

Scleritis symptoms include severe eye pain, redness, and decreased vision. An underlying systemic disorder, such as a connective tissue disease, autoimmune disorder, herpes simplex virus (HSV), herpes zoster, HIV, Lyme disease or syphilis, is frequently the cause. Rheumatoid arthritis is the most common systemic cause of scleritis. HZV is the most common infectious cause of scleritis. The conjunctival, episcleral, and scleral vessels are inflamed, either diffusely or focally. Unlike episcleral vessels, which blanch with topical vasoconstrictors and move under cotton swabs, scleral vessels do not. Additionally, the entire sclera may have a bluish or violaceous hue and may be very tender upon palpation. Treatment of the underlying disorder may involve systemic corticosteroids, immunosuppressive therapy, and nonsteroidal anti-inflammatory drugs (NSAIDs).

Temporal arteritis is associated with an ischemic optic neuropathy causes **vision loss.** These patients often present with **temporal artery tenderness, temporal headache, or jaw claudication.** Patients are usually **older than age 50 years,** and will have an **elevated erythrocyte sedimentation rate (ESR)** and an afferent pupillary defect (contracts to indirect light but not to direct light). A temporal artery biopsy showing giant cells is required for definitive diagnosis. Timely treatment with systemic steroids may prevent blindness in the other eye.

Optic neuritis is caused by demyelinating inflammation of the optic nerve that is highly associated with multiple sclerosis and typically occurs within the third decade of life. These patients complain of subacute eye pain (worse with extraocular movements), vision loss, and decreased color perception (more prominent with red). On examination the eye may appear grossly normal but there will be an afferent pupillary defect (absent papillary response to direct light) and edema of the optic nerve disc on fundoscopy in the affected eye. MRI is useful for confirming optic nerve inflammation and screening for underlying lesions suggestive of multiple sclerosis. Treatment involves hospital admission for intravenous steroids.

Other causes of non-traumatic acute vision loss are listed in Table 29–2 and focus on posterior chamber pathology that present with **acute painless vision loss:** these including retinal detachment, central retinal artery occlusion, central retinal vein occlusion, vitreous hemorrhage, and posterior vitreous detachment.

COMPREHENSION QUESTIONS

29.1 A 40-year-old man complains of the acute onset of left eye redness with circumcorneal injection (ciliary flush) and pain with bright lights. On examination, his pupil is small and minimally reactive with cell and flare noted on slit lamp examination. He also has pain in the affected eye when light is directed in the unaffected eye (consensual photophobia). Which of the following is the most likely diagnosis?

A. Acute angle-closure glaucoma

B. Anterior uveitis

C. Herpes simplex virus infection

D. Corneal abrasion

29.2 A 50-year-old woman is diagnosed with acute angle-closure glaucoma. She has acutely decreased visual acuity. Which of the following is the most likely mechanism for this condition?

A. Increased IOP caused by increased aqueous humor production

B. Nonreactive pupil leading to increased intraocular pressure

C. Decreased outflow of the aqueous humor

D. Separation of the retina leading to decreased visual acuity

29.3 A 50-year-old woman with redness, severe pain, a bluish scleral tinge, and decreased vision in her right eye is noted to have scleritis. Which of the following is the most common condition associated with scleritis?

A. Systemic lupus erythematosis

B. Rheumatoid arthritis

C. Inflammatory bowel disease

D. Syphilis

29.4 A 36-year-old woman has been diagnosed with glaucoma. She also has asthma which has been well controlled. After using the drops prescribed for her glaucoma, she develops an exacerbation of her asthma. Which of the following medications is most likely responsible for her asthmatic exacerbation?

A. Anticholinergic agent

B. β-blocker agent

C. Alpha-agonist agent

D. Beta-agonist agent

ANSWERS

29.1 **B.** Anterior uveitis usually presents as photophobia, red eye with pain, and cell with flare are noted on slit-lamp examination.

29.2 **C.** In acute angle-closure glaucoma the sudden rise in IOP is a consequence of blocked outflow, usually due to a pupillary block, and not increased production of aqueous humor.

29.3 **B.** Rheumatoid arthritis is the most common systemic disease associated with scleritis.

29.4 **B.** Bronchospasm is associated with the use of topical β-blockers which can be systematically absorbed.

CLINICAL PEARLS

▶ A useful working differential diagnosis for vision-threatening causes of red eye includes acute angle-closure glaucoma, anterior uveitis, endophthalmitis, corneal ulcer, corneal infection, chlamydial/gonococcal conjunctivitis, orbital cellulitis, hyphema, retrobulbar hemorrhage, and scleritis.

▶ Subconjunctival hemorrhages should be painless and does not affect vision. In the setting of blunt trauma, continue evaluating for hyphema, hypopyon, globe rupture, endophthalmitis, or retrobulbar hemorrhage if the patient complains of pain or vision changes and emergently consult an ophthalmologist.

▶ Slit-lamp examination, fluorescein staining, and measurement of intraocular pressure are essential elements of a thorough evaluation of the red eye.

▶ Beware of systemic complications from topical ophthalmologic medications. Allergic reactions and complications such as bronchospasm from topical β-blockers are common.

REFERENCES

Allingham RR, Damji K, Freedman S, et al, eds. *Shields' Textbook of Glaucoma.* 5th ed. Philadelphia, PA: Lippincott William & Wilkins; 2005.

Choplin NT, Lundy DC, eds. *Atlas of Glaucoma.* 2nd ed. London: Informa UK Ltd.; 2007.

Dargin JM, Lowenstein RA. The Painful Eye. *Emerg Med Clin N Am.* 2008;26:199-216.

Ehlers JP, Shah CP, eds. *The Wills Eye Manual.* 5th ed. Philadelphia, PA: Lippincott Williams & Wilkins; 2008.

Friedman NJ, Kaiser PK, Trattler WB, eds. *Review of Ophthalmology.* Philadelphia,PA: Elsevier, Inc.; 2005.

Galor A, Jeng BH. Red eye for the internist: When to treat, when to refer. *Cleveland Clin J Med.* 2008; 75(2):137-144.

Leibowitz HM. The red eye. *N Engl J Med.* 2000;343:345-351 (Classic).

Mahmood AR, Narang AT. Diagnosis and management of the acute red eye. *Emerg Med Clin N Am.* 2008;26:35-55.

Moayedi S. Head, neck and ophthalmologic manifestations of HIV in the emergency department. *Emerg Med Clin N Am.* 2010;28:265-271.

Muftuoglu O, Hosal BM, Karel F, Zilelioglu G. Drug-induced intraocular lens movement and near visual acuity after intraocular lens implantation. *Cataract Refract Surg.* 2005;31(7):1298-1305.

Riordan-Eva P, Whitcher JP, eds. *Vaughan & Asbury's General Ophthalmology.* 16th ed. New York, NY: Lange Medical Books/McGraw-Hill; 2004.

Roy H. The red eye. *Compr Ther.* 2006;32(1):43-46.

Shingleton BJ, O'Donoghue MW. Blurred vision. *N Engl J Med.* 2000;343:556-562.

Swadron SP. Pitfalls in the management of headache in the emergency department. *Emerg Med Clin N Am.* 2010;28:127-147.

An otherwise healthy 19-year-old man is brought to the emergency department (ED) by his roommate who states that he has "not been acting right" for the past 24 hours. Per the roommate, the patient had complained of a headache 2 days prior to arrival, and has been progressively somnolent and confused since then. The patient has no past medical history and does not take any medications. His roommate states that the patient is a college student who does not use any illegal drugs and occasionally drinks alcohol. Review of systems is positive for headache and altered mental status as stated above as well as a tactile fever for the past 2 days. Additional review of systems is unobtainable as the patient is unable to answer any questions. On physical examination the patient is noted to be febrile to 38.5°C (101°F) orally, with a heart rate of 120 beats per minute, blood pressure of 114/69, and a respiratory rate of 20 breaths per minute. His oxygen saturation is 98% on room air. The head and neck examination are significant for dry mucous membranes and nuchal rigidity. His cardiopulmonary examination is within normal limits with the exception of tachycardia. The abdomen is soft and nontender. His skin is noted to be warm and well perfused without any rash. The neurologic examination is significant for an altered mental status with a Glasgow coma score (GCS) of 10 (eyes open to voice [3], patient moans to painful stimuli [2], and localizes painful stimuli [5]). The motor examination is symmetric, and the patient appears to be sensate in all extremities. His reflexes are 2+ bilaterally throughout the upper and lower extremities with downgoing toes. Laboratory studies reveal a leukocytosis of 24,000/mm^3 with a left shift, and are otherwise unremarkable. A CT scan is completed which shows no mass, shift, bleed, or edema.

▶ What is the most likely diagnosis?
▶ What is the next diagnostic study of choice?
▶ What is the most appropriate treatment of this condition?

ANSWERS TO CASE 30:

Bacterial Meningitis

Summary: This is a 19-year-old man who presents with the classic triad for bacterial meningitis—fever, neck stiffness, and altered mental status.

- **Most likely diagnosis:** Bacterial meningitis
- **Next diagnostic study:** Lumbar puncture
- **Appropriate treatment:** Intravenous antibiotics ± steroids

ANALYSIS

Objectives

1. Understand the diagnostic and therapeutic approach to bacterial meningitis including when to obtain neuroimaging, when to perform a lumbar puncture, and what empiric therapies to initiate.

2. Recognize the clinical presentation of acute bacterial meningitis.

Considerations

Bacterial meningitis is an inflammation of the leptomeninges (pia/arachnoid/dura-maters) from infection of the arachnoid space, characteristically accompanied by white blood cells in the cerebrospinal fluid. It is one of the ten most common potentially devastating infections and can affect both adults and children. Mortality rates have been reported as high as 50% in some series, yet most cohorts appear to have mortality between 10% and 30%. Of patients who survive, approximately 25% will go on to have a permanent neurologic deficit. It is incumbent upon the emergency physician to consider this diagnosis in patients presenting with any combination of the following signs and symptoms: fever, altered mental status, nuchal rigidity and headache. Although the classic triad includes fever, altered mental status, and nuchal rigidity, only 44% to 50% of patients will present with all three features. Almost all patients (99%-100% in the largest study published) have headache plus at least one of these three clinical signs. Fever is present in 79% to 95% of patients at presentation and another 4% will develop fever within 24 hours of presentation. Altered mental status (typically confusion or lethargy) is present in 78% to 83% of patients with 16% to 22% responsive to only painful stimuli and 6% unresponsive to all stimuli. Nuchal rigidity is present in 83% to 94% of patients on initial examination, and often persists for more than one week after treatment and resolution of infection.

Altered mental status (AMS) in an otherwise healthy individual can be caused by a number of serious illnesses including infectious, metabolic, toxicologic, and neurologic etiologies. As with any seriously ill emergency department patient, the initial priorities include managing the ABCs (airway, breathing, and circulation), including airway protection, as needed for a depressed level of consciousness.

This patient presents with a GCS of 10, yet appears to be protecting his airway on initial examination.

Immediately reversible causes of altered mental status, such as hypoglycemia, hypoxia, and drug intoxication should be recognized and treated during the initial examination. If a reversible cause of AMS is not identified, and bacterial meningitis is suspected, prompt diagnosis and treatment is critical.

Additional findings that may raise ones concerns for the diagnosis of meningitis include seizures, focal neurologic deficits, rash, septic arthritis, papilledema and photophobia. Seizures have been described in 15% to 30% of patients and are most commonly associated with infections due to *Streptococcus pneumoniae*. Focal neurological deficits are seen in 10% to 35% of patients with *Listeria monocytogenes* as part of a rhombencephalitis syndrome including ataxia with or without nystagmus, and cranial nerve palsies. *Neisseria meningitidis* may cause palpable purpura in 11% to 64% of patients, and concomitant septic arthritis in 7% to 11%. Papilledema and/or photophobia are rarely present, having been described in less than 5% of cases.

APPROACH TO:
Suspected Bacterial Meningitis

CLINICAL APPROACH

The approach to suspected bacterial meningitis involves appropriate use of diagnostic studies and therapeutic interventions in a timely manner. Although no randomized controlled trial exists to prove it, the best experimental and observational data suggest that time to antibiotics has a profound effect on clinical outcomes. Therefore, our goal in the emergency department is to maintain a high index of suspicion and **not** delay treatment while diagnostic studies are being completed.

Diagnosis

The cornerstone of the diagnosis of meningitis is analysis of the cerebrospinal fluid (CSF), which is obtained by lumbar puncture (LP). LP can confirm the presence of inflammatory cells in the CSF, identify the causative organism by Gram stain and culture, and help in ruling out other potential causes of the patient's symptoms (idiopathic intracranial hypertension or pseudotumor cerebri, subarachnoid hemorrhage, autoimmune disease, etc). When it is expected that there will be a significant delay in obtaining the LP, it is recommended to obtain blood cultures and then initiate treatment with antibiotics with or without dexamethasone, prior to obtaining the CSF (see the section Treatment). A common cause for delay of diagnosis is the time it takes to obtain a computed tomography (CT) scan of the head. The goal of CT scanning prior to performing an LP is to identify those patients that may be at risk of brain herniation during the procedure. Current Infectious Diseases Society of America (IDSA) guidelines for CT before LP include patients who present with altered mental status or a depressed level of consciousness, focal findings on neurologic examination, or a handful of other specific risk factors (Table 30–1). All other patients can safely have an LP performed without an antecedent CT scan.

Table 30–1 • INDICATIONS FOR HEAD CT PRIOR TO LP
Altered level of consciousness
Altered mental status
Focal neurologic deficit
Immunocompromised state[a]
History of CNS disease[b]
New-onset seizure (less than 1 week prior to presentation)
Papilledema
History of evidence of head trauma

[a]Including HIV, AIDS, post-transplant, on immunosuppressant medications.
[b]Including mass lesions, strokes, focal infection, surgery.

Administration of antibiotics has minimal effect on chemistry and cytology of CSF, but can reduce the yield of Gram stain and culture. In fact, administration of antibiotics can result in sterile CSF cultures within an hour in patients suffering from meningococcal infections. Pneumococcal infections, however, will typically remain culture positive up to 4 to 10 hours after administration of parenteral antibiotics. Importantly, Gram stains can positively identify an organism in 10% to 15% of patients who have sterile cultures after antibiotic administration.

Identification of the causative organism allows clinicians to safely narrow the spectrum of antimicrobial therapy. However, in the emergency department we are often unable to know with certainty what organism will eventually be identified, and are therefore required to initiate empiric therapy on the basis of epidemiologic data and local resistance patterns. Gram stain of the CSF is successful in identifying the microorganism in approximately 80% of cases. As Gram stain results are typically available 1 to 2 days before culture results, it is helpful to know the Gram-stain pattern of the most common organisms. The presence of gram-positive diplococci suggests *Streptococcus pneumoniae* infection, while gram-negative diplococci suggest *Neisseria meningitidis* infection. Small pleomorphic gram-negative coccobacilli suggests *Haemophilus influenzae*, while gram-positive rods and coccobacilli suggest *Listeria monocytogenes* infection. Additional cases will be identified by culture of the CSF and blood; yet this information is rarely available during the initial emergency department presentation. Additional analyses of the CSF should include opening pressure (which can be the only abnormality present in cases of cryptococcal meningitis), CSF protein, CSF glucose, cell count with differential, and CSF lactate. Unfortunately, despite all of these tests it can still be quite difficult to distinguish between the possible causes of meningitis (bacterial, viral, tubercular, neoplasms, autoimmune, etc) (Table 30–2). Therefore, most patients with CSF pleocytosis (presence of an elevated number of WBCs) should be admitted to the hospital and treated for meningitis while awaiting the results of CSF culture.

Treatment

The most important element of treatment after stabilization of the ABCs is initiation of appropriate antimicrobial therapy. The most common organisms to cause

Table 30–2 • ANALYSIS OF THE CEREBROSPINAL FLUID

Test	Normal Value	Significance of Abnormality
Opening pressure	<200 mm H$_2$O	Higher pressures indicate the presence of elevated intracranial pressure (39% are ≥350 mm H$_2$0, 9% are ≤140 mm H$_2$0)
CSF appearance	Clear	Cloudy CSF indicates the presence of WBCs, RBCs, bacteria, and protein
Cell count	<5 WBC/mm^3	All types of meningitis have an elevated WBC count. ≥2000/microL or PMN ≥1180/microL is 99% predictive. 13% are ≤100/microL
	<1 PMN/mm^3	Increased PMNs suggest a bacterial etiology[a]
Gram stain	No organisms	Identifies organisms in 80% of bacterial meningitis; 60% if the patient is pretreated
Protein	14-45 mg/dL	Elevated in acute bacterial/fungal meningitis ≥220 mg/dL is 99% predictive
Glucose	50-80 mg/dL	≤40 mg/dL in 50%-60% of patients with bacterial meningitis (eg, 40%-50% are ≥40 mg/dL), a ratio of CSF/serum glucose ≤0.4 is 80% sensitive for bacterial meningitis. ≤34 mg/dL is ≥99% predictive
India ink	Negative	Positive in 33% of cryptococcal meningitis
Cryptococcal Ag	Negative	90% accuracy for cryptococcal disease
Acid-fast stain	Negative	Positive in 80% of tuberculous meningitis
CSF Lactate	<35 mg/dL	CSF lactate is rarely normal in cases of bacterial meningitis

Abbreviations: CSF = cerebrospinal fluid; PMN = Polymorphonuclear leukocyte; WBC = white blood cells; Ag = antigen.
[a]Viral meningitis typically has a lymphocyte predominance; however, in the first 48 hours PMNs may predominate.

bacterial meningitis in adult patients are *Neisseria meningitidis* and *Streptococcus pneumoniae*. Initial therapy should include a third generation cephalosporin in a sufficient dose to achieve adequate CSF concentration. Ceftriaxone or cefotaxime at a dose of 2 g is typically recommended in the United States. As a result of an increasing worldwide prevalence of drug resistant *Streptococcus pneumoniae*, most authorities now recommend a dose of vancomycin along with the third-generation cephalosporin until a resistance profile can be obtained.

Patients who are older than 50 years of age, alcoholic, or immunocompromised are at higher risk for additional organisms including *Listeria monocytogenes, Haemophilus influenzae*, and aerobic gram-negative bacilli, and should therefore have ampicillin added to the empiric antibiotic regimen. Patients less than 1 month of age are at risk for infection with *Streptococcus agalactiae, Klebsiella* sp, *E coli*, and *L monocytogenes* and require yet another empiric regimen (Table 30–3).

In addition to adequate antimicrobial therapy, a number of recent studies have shown improved outcomes with adjunctive dexamethasone either before or with the first dose of antibiotics. The theory is that meningitis leads to significant morbidity and mortality as a result of the inflammatory response in the CSF. This response can be heightened when antimicrobials are administered, which will lead to bacterial

Table 30–3 • EMPIRIC ANTIMICROBIAL THERAPY BASED ON PATIENT AGE		
Patient Age	Common Pathogens	Empiric Antibiotics
<1 month	Streptococcus agalactiae, Escherichia coli, Listeria monocytogenes, Klebsiella species	Ampicillin plus cefotaxime or ampicillin plus an aminoglycoside
1-23 months	Streptococcus pneumoniae, Neisseria meningitidis, S agalactiae, Haemophilus influenzae, E coli	Vancomycin plus a third-generation cephalosporin[a]
2-50 years	N meningitidis, S pneumoniae	Vancomycin plus a third-generation cephalosporin[a]
>50 years	S pneumoniae, N meningitidis, L monocytogenes, aerobic gram-negative bacilli	Vancomycin plus a third-generation cephalosporin[a] plus ampicillin

[a]Ceftriaxone or cefotaxime.
Data from Tunkel A, Hartman B, Kaplan S, et al. Practice guidelines for the management of bacterial meningitis. Clin Infect Dis. 2004;39:1267-1284.

lysis and release of additional inflammatory mediators. Administering a dose of corticosteroids (dexamethasone 0.15mg/kg IV every 6h) with or before the first dose of antibiotics may attenuate the inflammatory response. If antibiotics have already been initiated as an outpatient or before steroid administration, the subsequent addition of dexamethasone has no demonstrated efficacy and may cause harm.

The evidence supporting the use of dexamethasone is based largely on a single randomized double-blinded placebo-controlled trial that compared dexamethasone 10 mg IV q6h × 4 d versus placebo in 301 adults with bacterial meningitis (suspected disease plus either cloudy CSF, a positive Gram stain, or >1000 WBC/mm^3). In this trial, the number needed to treat (NNT) to prevent an unfavorable outcome was 10 and the NNT to prevent death was 12.5. There was, however, some heterogeneity in the results, with the greatest benefit found in those patients with an intermediate GCS of 8 to 11 and those with disease ultimately found to be due to *Streptococcus pnuemoniae*. For most patients, a single dose of dexamethasone is unlikely to be harmful, and in general most authorities recommend that if you are giving antibiotics for suspected bacterial meningitis, it should be preceded or accompanied by a dose of dexamethasone.

Once a patient is diagnosed with bacterial meningitis, family members and close contacts (such as this patient's roommate) are often concerned about whether they should receive antibiotic prophylaxis to prevent them from developing a similar infection. Current CDC guidelines recommend antibiotic prophylaxis (typically with a fluoroquinolone or rifampin) for close contacts (anyone in the same household or day-care center or anyone in direct contact with the patient's oral secretions) of patients with meningitis due to *Neisseria meningitidis*. Antibiotics for close contacts of patients with meningitis due to *Haemophilus influenzae* are no longer recommended if all contacts 4 years of age or younger are fully vaccinated against Hib disease. Given the high morbidity and mortality of meningococcal infections, vaccination against N meningitidis is recommended for freshmen college students who live in dormitories, as they are at moderately increased risk of contracting this disease.

COMPREHENSION QUESTIONS

30.1 A 30-year-old man presents with altered mental status, fever, and nuchal rigidity. You suspect bacterial meningitis. Which of the following is the appropriate order of your actions?

A. Head CT, lumbar puncture, blood cultures, steroids, antibiotics

B. Blood cultures, head CT, lumbar puncture, steroids, antibiotics

C. Blood cultures, steroids, antibiotics, head CT, lumbar puncture

D. Lumbar puncture, blood cultures, steroids, antibiotics, head CT

E. Head CT, blood cultures, steroids, antibiotics, lumbar puncture

30.2 Which of the following are the appropriate empiric antibiotics to administer to a 65-year-old man with suspected bacterial meningitis?

A. Vancomycin alone

B. Vancomycin and ceftriaxone

C. Vancomycin and ceftriaxone and amoxicillin

D. Vancomycin and ceftriaxone and ampicillin

30.3 Approximately what percentage of patients with bacterial meningitis present with the classic triad of fever, neck stiffness, and altered mental status?

A. <50%

B. Between 51%-75%

C. Between 76%-99%

D. >99%

ANSWERS

30.1 **C.** Neuroimaging is indicated in this patient prior to lumbar puncture given his altered mental status. Given the high suspicion for bacterial meningitis, antibiotic administration should not be delayed for the head CT. It is expected that one would obtain blood cultures and administer dexamethasone prior to the antibiotics in this case.

30.2 **D.** All adults with suspected bacterial meningitis get a third-generation cephalosporin and most institutions advocate for vancomycin to cover drug-resistant *Streptococcus pneumoniae*. Ampicillin is added because this patient is older than the age of 50.

30.3 **A.** Although the triad in the question is considered classic, studies have found that it is only present in less than half of the cases. If headache is added to the other 3, then at least 2 of the 4 symptoms are present in approximately 95% of patients.

CLINICAL PEARLS

▶ The classic triad of fever, neck stiffness, and a change in mental status is present in less than 50% of patients with bacterial meningitis.

▶ Younger patients that are otherwise healthy do not require neuroimaging prior to LP if they have a normal neurologic examination including mental status.

▶ Initial antimicrobial therapy in adults should include a third-generation cephalosporin and vancomycin to cover drug-resistant *S pneumoniae*.

▶ Patients older than 50 years, alcoholics, and immunocompromised patients should have ampicillin added to the empiric antimicrobial therapy to cover *L monocytogenes*.

▶ Dexamethasone prior to or with the first dose of antibiotics has been shown to decrease neurologic sequelae as well as mortality among adults with bacterial meningitis.

REFERENCES

Aronin SI, Peduzzi P, Quagliarello VJ. Community-acquired bacterial meningitis: risk stratification for adverse clinical outcome and effect of antibiotic timing. *Ann Intern Med.* 1998;129:862.

Attia J, Hatala R, Cook DJ, Wong JG. The rational clinical examination. Does this adult patient have acute meningitis? *JAMA.* 1999;282:175.

de Gans J, van de Beek D. Dexamethasone in adults with bacterial meningitis. *N Eng J Med.* 2002;347(20):1549-1556.

Durand ML, Calderwood SB, Weber DJ, et al. Acute bacterial meningitis in adults. A review of 493 episodes. *N Eng J Med.* 1993;328:21.

Geiseler PJ, Nelson KE, Levin S, et al. Community-acquired purulent meningitis: a review of 1,316 cases during the antibiotic era, 1954-1976. *Rev Infect Dis.* 1980;2:725.

Hasbun R, Abrahams J, Jekel J, et al. Computed Tomography of the head before lumbar puncture in adults with suspected meningitis. *N Eng J Med.* 2001;345(24):1727-1733.

Kanegaye JT, Soliemanzadeh P, Bradley JS. Lumbar puncture in pediatric bacterial meningitis: defining the time interval for recovery of cerebrospinal fluid pathogens after parenteral antibiotic pretreatment. *Pediatrics.* 2001;108:1169.

Talan DA, Hoffman JR, Yoshikawa TT, Overtuft GD. Role of empiric parenteral antibiotics prior to lumbar puncture in suspected bacterial meningitis: state of the art. *Rev Infect Dis.* 1988;10:365.

Tunkel A, Hartman B, Kaplan S, et al. Practice guidelines for the management of bacterial meningitis. *Clin Infect Dis.* 2004;39:1267-1284.

van de Beek D, de Gans J, Spanjaard L, et al. Clinical features and prognostic factors in adults with bacterial meningitis. *N Eng J Med.* 2004;351(18):1849-1859.

van de Beek D, de Gans J, Tunkel A, et al. Community-acquired bacterial meningitis in adults. *N Eng J Med.* 2006;354(1):44-53.

Whitney C, Farley M, Hadler J, et al. Increasing prevalence of multidrug-resistant *Streptococcus pneumoniae* in the United States. *N Eng J Med.* 2000;343(26):1917-1924.

A 37-year-old man, known to be an insulin-dependent diabetic (IDDM), is brought into the emergency department (ED) by ambulance after a motor vehicle accident. Per EMS, he was the restrained driver of a vehicle when he apparently lost control of the car and drove into the center divide at highway speeds. Witnesses reported that the vehicle rolled over multiple times and the air bag did not deploy. There is severe damage to the front of the vehicle. Vital signs taken in the field showed a blood pressure of 110/85 mm Hg, heart rate 140 beats per minute, respiration rate 24 breaths per minute, oxygen saturation 98% on 15 L of oxygen via nonrebreather mask. During transport to the ED, the patient begins to seize. Paramedics describe tonic-clonic movements of all four extremities. He is given lorazepam 2-mg IV push with almost immediate resolution of the seizure. In the ED, on examination (once the seizure has stopped), his airway is patent, breath sounds are equal bilaterally, and pulses are bounding throughout. His Glasgow coma scale (GCS) is 8. His blood glucose is 75. It is noted that his right pupil is 5 mm and nonreactive, his left pupil is 3 mm and reactive. His tone is normal in all four extremities. His reflexes are 2+ throughout. His toes are downgoing bilaterally. His cardiovascular, respiratory, and abdominal examination are unremarkable. He is not wearing a medic-alert bracelet. His CT scan of the head reveals a large right-frontal intraparenchymal hemorrhage.

▶ What is the most likely diagnosis?
▶ What is your next step?

ANSWERS TO CASE 31:

Seizure Induced by Traumatic Brain Injury

Summary: A 37-year-old man, unrestrained driver in motor vehicle accident, seizing en route to the ED and found to have right-sided blown pupil, GCS 8, and no known history (hx) of seizures.

- **Most likely diagnosis:** Seizure likely secondary to acute intraparenchymal bleed from a traumatic brain injury.

- **Next step:** Aggressive management of ABCs (airway, breathing, and circulation) with rapid sequence intubation to protect the airway, management of ICP, and anticonvulsant treatment to prevent reoccurrence of seizures.

ANALYSIS

Objectives

1. Develop a methodological approach to the assessment of the patient who presents to the emergency department with first-time seizure and status epilepticus.

2. Understand the diagnostic and therapeutic approach to the patient presenting to the emergency department with first-time seizure and status epilepticus.

Considerations

This 37-year-old man with IDDM presents with a seizure after being involved in a motor vehicle accident. It is important to consider the order of events in traumas such as this, especially when the history is limited. This patient may have had a seizure while driving secondary to hypoglycemia, and then crashed his car. He may also have a past medical history of epilepsy and be subtherapeutic on his anticonvulsant medications. He may have lost control of the car for some unknown reason, and then crashed the car causing traumatic brain injury, intraparenchymal bleeding, and subsequent seizure.

APPROACH TO:

Seizure Disorders

DEFINITIONS

SEIZURE: A **seizure** is any event involving an abnormal firing of neurons that causes a sudden change in behavior characterized by changes in sensory perception or motor activity. It can sometimes occur in the presence of precipitating factors (provoked seizure).

EPILEPSY: The term **epilepsy** is applied when 2 or more unprovoked seizures occur more than 24 hours apart.

STATUS EPILEPTICUS: Status epilepticus is historically defined as more than 30 minutes of continuous seizure activity or two or more sequential seizures without return to normal mental baseline.

CLINICAL APPROACH

Classifications

Seizures can be divided into two major classifications based on their origin. *Neurogenic* seizures represent the majority of seizures seen in the ED and result from excessive discharge of cortical neurons. *Psychogenic*, or nonepileptic, seizures (NES) are increasingly common and may be extremely difficult to distinguish from true seizures. Unlike neurogenic seizures, these *pseudoseizures* are not the result of abnormal cortical discharge, and are often associated with major stress or emotional trauma. *Unclassified* seizures are difficult to fit into a single class and are considered when there is inadequate data.

Neurogenic seizures can be broken down into 2 main subgroups depending on their manifestation. *Generalized seizures* involve abnormal neuronal activity in both hemispheres of the brain and are accompanied by a loss of consciousness. They can be further characterized based on the pattern of motor activity, such as tonic (rigid trunk and extremities), clonic (symmetrical rhythmic jerking of the trunk and extremities), tonic-clonic (tonic phase followed by clonic phase), atonic (sudden loss of postural tone), and myoclonic (brief, shock-like muscular contractions). *Partial (focal) seizures* involve neuronal discharge in a localized area of one cerebral hemisphere and are subclassified into simple (consciousness is maintained) and complex (impaired level of consciousness).

Status epilepticus (SE) is present when patients have more than 30 minutes of continuous seizure activity or have 2 or more sequential seizures without full recovery of consciousness in between. SE is the initial presentation of a seizure disorder in approximately one-third of cases. The most common cause of SE is discontinuation of anticonvulsant medications. The catecholamine surge that accompanies SE can cause tachycardia, hypertension, hypotension, cardiac arrhythmias, respiratory failure, hyperglycemia, acidosis, and rhabdomyolysis. Nonconvulsive SE can also occur and must be ruled out in any patient who does not regain consciousness within 20 to 30 minutes of cessation of a single generalized seizure and should be considered in any patient with unexplained confusion or coma.

Etiology

It is important to consider the etiology of a patient's seizure as it may influence the clinical approach. Primary, unprovoked seizures in a patient with a known history of epilepsy are usually managed pharmacologically with the goal of restoring normal neuronal function. However, seizures can also present as secondary manifestations of other primary diseases.

Common etiologies of secondary seizures include head trauma, intracranial masses or hemorrhages, infections such as meningitis or encephalitis, metabolic disturbances (ie, glucose or electrolyte abnormalities), and drugs or toxins. Additional common conditions that may present as seizures include hypertensive encephalopathy and anoxic-ischemic injury secondary to cardiac arrest or severe hypoxemia. Eclampsia must also be considered in pregnant women as a potential etiology of seizures.

Diagnosis

History: History is essential in the evaluation of a seizure patient, especially in a first-time seizure. It is important to ask the patient and/or witnesses the circumstances leading up to the seizure, including a description of the ictal movements and the postictal period. Any symptoms associated with the seizure should also be addressed to help direct work-up and management. For example, a headache prior to the seizure is concerning for intracranial hemorrhage, while a fever and/or general malaise in a patient who presents with a seizure is worrisome for infectious causes. Patients with a known seizure disorder should be questioned about the type and frequency of their seizures as well as medication compliance. Past medical history, medications, and social history including drug and alcohol use and HIV risk factors are also important to consider.

Examination: Patients presenting to the ED with seizure require a thorough physical examination. A detailed neurologic examination is the key component of the evaluation. Focal deficits may be a critical clue to the ultimate diagnosis or may represent a common transient postictal neurologic insult referred to as a Todd paralysis. The head and neck examination should include the tongue to look for lacerations, head or facial trauma, and signs of meningismus. Cardiopulmonary examination should include auscultation for heart murmurs or an irregular rhythm suggesting an embolic or syncopal event. Although rare, extremity fractures or dislocations are commonly missed when they do occur and should be ruled out by a thorough musculoskeletal examination.

Diagnostic Workup: Appropriate laboratory studies in patients with first-time seizures include glucose, serum electrolytes such as sodium, calcium, and magnesium, assessment of renal function, hematology studies such as a complete blood cell count, and drug or toxicology screen. Women of childbearing age also require a pregnancy test.

Neuroimaging studies should be performed when a clear etiology to the seizure is not identified or whenever an acute intracranial process is suspected. American College of Emergency Physicians (ACEP) guidelines recommend a head CT be performed in patients with a history of recent head trauma, persistent altered mental status or headache, fever, malignancy, immunocompromised status, anticoagulation, or in patients who have a new focal deficit, are over 40, or have a partial-onset seizure.

A lumbar puncture is an essential part of the workup if clinical presentation is suggestive of an infectious process. Use of the EEG is uncommon in the ED evaluation of first-time seizure except in the assessment of nonconvulsive status epilepticus, or to establish status epilepticus in a patient who has been given long-acting paralytic agents.

MANAGEMENT

Initial stabilization of the patient requires (a) **ABCs,** (b) bedside **glucose** analysis, (c) **pulse oximetry,** (d) **cardiac monitoring,** and (d) **anticonvulsant** therapy if seizure activity continues at time of evaluation.

Aggressive airway protection is critical as seizure patients have decreased gag reflexes and are at risk for aspiration. Positioning the patient on their side with frequent suctioning, if necessary, will lower the risk for aspiration. Patients who continue to seize despite therapy or those unable to protect their airway with conservative measures require intubation.

Pharmacologic Therapy

Parenteral **benzodiazepines** are first-line therapy for active seizures (including SE) and are effective in terminating seizures in 75% to 90% of patients. They suppress seizure activity by directly enhancing GABA (gamma-aminobutyric acid)-related neuronal inhibition. **Lorazepam** is generally preferred up to a dose of 0.1 mg/kg given at 2 mg/min. **Lorazepam** and **diazepam** (0.2 mg/kg IV given at 5 mg/min) are equally effective at terminating the initial seizure, while lorazepam is superior for preventing recurrence of the seizure. IV **midazolam** has been less studied but has shown a trend toward superior efficacy and decreased incidence of adverse outcomes compared to lorazepam and diazepam. Options for patients without intravenous access include IM midazolam or lorazepam (midazolam is probably the best option) in addition to rectal diazepam.

If a benzodiazepine does not terminate seizure activity, second-line agents for abortive therapy include **phenytoin** or **fosphenytoin.** Phenytoin does not directly suppress electrical activity at the seizure focus but rather slows recovery of voltage-activated sodium channels and thus suppresses neuronal recruitment. Thus, concurrent benzodiazepine administration is necessary when treating active seizures. The total oral dose of phenytoin is about 20 mg/kg with a maximum of 400 mg every 2 hours. It can also be given via slow IV administration up to 18 mg/kg. The rate can be no greater than 50 mg/min to avoid **hypotension** and **cardiac dysrhythmias** associated with its propylene glycol diluent. **Fosphenytoin** is the prodrug of phenytoin, is **water soluble,** and can be administered at 150 mg/min without significant toxicity. Cerebellar findings, such as nystagmus and ataxia, are the most common neurological side effects associated with phenytoin. While parenteral loading is most common, oral loading is appropriate in patients who report medication noncompliance or are found to have a subtherapeutic phenytoin level.

Phenobarbital is a CNS depressant that directly suppresses cortical electrical activity and is often used after benzodiazepines and phenytoin have failed. The onset of intravenous phenobarbital is 15 to 30 minutes with a long duration of action of up to 48 to 96 hours. Adverse effects of phenobarbital include profound **respiratory depression** and **hypotension,** limiting its use as abortive seizure therapy to third-line therapy.

Parenteral **valproic acid** has shown some recent promise as abortive seizure therapy, and is considered an alternative in cases where benzodiazepine or phenytoin use is limited by hypotension or hypersensitivity. Although similar to phenytoin in mechanism of action, it is generally well tolerated with mild side effects. Recommended loading dose for valproic acid is 15 to 20 mg/kg at a rate of 3 to 6 mg/kg/min, although more rapid bolus infusions have been safely administered.

Additional agents to be considered for abortive seizure therapy include **propofol, barbiturates** (other than phenobarbital), and inhaled anesthetics such as **isoflurane. Propofol** acts as a direct GABA agonist and global CNS depressant. While studies are limited showing its efficacy in SE, it has been shown to provide almost immediate suppression of seizure activity after a bolus infusion. Barbiturates (**pentobarbital** and **thiopental**) directly enhance GABA-mediated neuronal inhibition while suppressing all other brainstem functions and thus can also induce respiratory arrest, myocardial depression, and hypotension. **Isoflurane anesthesia** suppresses electrical seizure foci and is the treatment of last resort for the patient in SE, as these are patients who will have required intubation and ventilatory support.

Levetiracetam is a relatively new antiepileptic drugs (AEDs) with a mechanism of action that is atypical compared to other AEDs. Clinical studies suggest that it might have a significant effect in generalized seizures and was recently approved by the FDA as adjunctive treatment for primary generalized tonic-clonic seizures in adults and children aged 6 years and older. It is not yet recommended for abortive seizure therapy.

Patients in SE who require intubation are ideally induced with a benzodiazepine, serving to both sedate and to abate the seizure. If the patient requires paralysis for management purposes, it cannot be assumed that the patient's seizure has been terminated. In this situation, anticonvulsant therapy should be continued and **EEG monitoring** of the patient should be arranged.

SPECIAL CASES

Drug-Induced Seizures

Therapy for drug-induced seizures is guided by general seizure management principles. There are no clear evidence-based guidelines for the management of drug-related seizures and usually require therapy that is specific to the etiological agent. **Cocaine is one of the most frequent causes of drug-induced seizures.** Approximately 15% of cocaine users will experience a drug-induced seizure. Seizures caused by cocaine are a result of a combination of a lowered seizure threshold and hypersympathetic state. They are often associated with hyperthermia and high lactate levels. These seizures are usually self-limited, but in cases **of status epilepticus, should be treated with high doses of benzodiazepines.**

Tricyclic antidepressants cause seizures as a consequence of their anticholinergic properties. In addition to standard seizure therapy, patients with status epilepticus secondary to tricyclic overdose should be treated with sodium bicarbonate in an effort to obtain a blood pH of approximately 7.5. This will decrease the free form of the drug in the patient's CNS as well as mitigate the drug's sodium channel–blocking effect on the heart.

Isoniazid-induced seizures are associated with a high mortality rate and typically occur within 120 minutes of an acute overdose. Isoniazid binds pyridoxine, the active form of vitamin B_6, a cofactor for glutamic acid decarboxylase, and gamma-aminobutyric acid (GABA) transaminase. INH toxicity and depleted **vitamin B_6 lead to a reduction in** levels of CNS inhibitory transmitter GABA and ultimately can result in status epilepticus. Treatment of seizures secondary to isoniazid toxicity is often refractory to standard measures and **should be treated with IV pyridoxine.** The dose of pyridoxine is based upon the amount of drug ingested.

Alcohol Withdrawal Seizures

Alcohol withdrawal seizures (AWS) are a leading cause of seizures in adults. These seizures often occur as part of a constellation of early withdrawal symptoms **typically within 6 to 48 hours after the last drink.** Other withdrawal symptoms including sweating, anxiety, tremor, auditory/visual hallucinations, agitation, nausea/vomiting, headache, and disorientation often occur prior to the onset of seizures. The more serious withdrawal syndrome of delirium tremens can be associated with seizures that may occur as long as 7 days post alcohol cessation. The more common and classic early AWS often occur in bunches of up to 4 to 6 seizures. However, these almost always cluster over a fairly brief period of time and they rarely persist past twelve hours from onset. Recent evidence recommends the use of benzodiazepines to reduce the incidence of seizures and delirium. Phenytoin does not have a role in managing either AWS or controlling recurrent alcohol-related seizures in the ED; however it may play a role in alcoholics who have underlying seizure disorders. The data for use of other anticonvulsants like carbamazepine in alcohol withdrawal seizures are limited.

CT imaging of the head has a high diagnostic yield in patients with their first alcohol-related seizure as these patients have a high incidence of structural intracranial lesions, such as subdural hematomas or other intracranial hemorrhages. Alcoholism is also a common cause of hypoglycemia and other metabolic abnormalities, thus electrolytes should be checked. IV fluid hydration with a glucose-containing solution in addition to thiamine, magnesium, potassium, and multivitamins is also indicated.

Neurocysticercosis

Neurocysticercosis (NCC) is an infection of the brain with larvae of *Taenia solium* (pork tapeworm) and is the most common cause of adult onset seizures in the developing countries of Latin America, sub-Saharan Africa, and Southeast Asia. It is also becoming increasingly prevalent in nonendemic countries with large immigrant populations. Seizures can vary from simple partial seizures to generalized tonic clonic. Diagnosis is confirmed via neuroimaging with visualization of active or calcified cysts in the brain. Treatment is usually initiated by a neurologist and consists of an antihelminth medication such as albendazole, combined with an antiepileptic medication.

Pseudoseizures

Pseudoseizures, also known as **psychogenic seizures,** are often the result of major stress or emotional trauma. These psychogenic nonepileptic seizures are often difficult to distinguish from physiologic seizures. Patients with **psychogenic seizures tend to have multiple seizure patterns,** which are usually **not followed by a**

postictal period. Urinary incontinence and injury such as tongue biting has been reported in up to 20% of patients with psychogenic seizure. Unlike in physiologic seizures, noxious stimuli such as ammonia capsules may elicit responses from patients having psychogenic seizures. The observation of purposeful movement during a psychogenic seizure also is typical. Management of pseudoseizures involves reassurance and patient education with psychiatric consultation often recommended.

Patient Disposition

Disposition of patients will likely depend on the etiology of their seizure (if known), the known seizure history, and the availability of adequate outpatient follow-up. All patients need to be provided detailed **seizure precautions,** and locally mandated reporting requirements must be noted in the patient's chart. Currently, the law in 6 states (California, Delaware, Nevada, New Jersey, Oregon, and Pennsylvania) requires physicians to report patients with seizures. They should also be warned about limiting activities when and where sudden loss of consciousness would be especially dangerous such as operating heavy equipment, swimming alone, cooking with hot water or even bathing.

In patients with known epilepsy who present with a single seizure, it is acceptable to send laboratory test results for anticonvulsant levels (if appropriate), give a loading dose of the appropriate anticonvulsant, and then discharge them with the appropriate follow-up. Subtherapeutic levels of antiseizure medication can be a result of medical noncompliance or increased metabolism, often caused by concurrent medication intake. Any history or physical examination findings consistent with a new seizure pattern should be addressed, as would be the case in a first-time seizure patient (Tables 31–1 and 31–2). Patients should also be thoroughly educated regarding the risks and benefits of noncompliance with antiepileptic medications.

In patients without a history of epilepsy who present with a single unprovoked seizure, a more thorough workup is indicated. If this initial workup is unremarkable, it is acceptable to discharge the patient home with follow up neuroimaging and an appointment with a neurologist. They will not necessarily need to be discharged on new antiepileptic medications but they will need education about restrictions in patients with seizures.

Patients without a history of seizure who do not return to baseline and remain postictal should be admitted to the hospital until they return to their baseline mental status and the underlying etiology of their seizures is determined. Patients in status epilepticus are usually admitted to the ICU for management and evaluation.

Table 31–1 • COMMON CAUSES OF REACTIVE SEIZURES
Metabolic encephalopathies: Hypomagnesemia, hyponatremia, hypocalcemia, hypoglycemia, hepatic or renal failure
Infectious encephalopathies: Central nervous system abscess, meningitis, encephalitis
Central nervous system lesions: Neoplasm, arteriovenous malformations, vasculitis, acute hydrocephalus, intracerebral hematomas, cerebrovascular accident, posttraumatic seizures, migraine/vascular headache, degenerative disease (multiple sclerosis)
Intoxications: Medications (tricyclic antidepressants, isoniazid, theophylline), recreational drugs (cocaine), alcohol and drug withdrawal, lead, strychnine, camphor, eclampsia

Table 31–2 • ACUTE SEIZURE MANAGEMENT: DRUG THERAPY

Drug	Adult Dose	Pediatric Dose	Duration of Action	Comments
First-line therapy				
Lorazepam	0.1 mg/kg IV at 1-2 mg/min up to 10 mg	0.05-0.1 mg/kg IV	2-8 h	Rapid acting; longer duration of action than diazepam; prolonged CNS depression possible
Diazepam	0.2 mg/kg IV at 2 mg/min up to 20 mg	0.2-0.5 mg/kg IV up to 20 mg	5-15 minutes	Rapid acting; short effective half-life
Midazolam	2.5-15 mg IV 0.2 mg/kg IM	0.15 mg/kg IV then 2-10 µg/kg/min	1-15 minutes	Significant amnestic effect
Second-line therapy				
Phenytoin	20 mg/kg IV at <50 mg/min	20 mg/kg IV at 1 mg/kg/min	24 h	Hypotension and arrhythmias at high infusion rates; cardiac monitoring required
Phenobarbital	20 mg/kg IV at 60-100 mg/min		1-3 d	Long lasting; may be given as IM loading dose
Third-line therapy				
Pentobarbital	5 mg/kg IV at 25 mg/min, then titrate to EEG		Minutes	Intubation, ventilation, and pressor support required; respiratory arrest, hypotension, and myocardial depression common
Isoflurane	Via general endotracheal anesthesia		Minutes	Monitor with EEG

COMPREHENSION QUESTIONS

31.1 A 34-year-old man is brought into the ED with a seizure of new onset. It is determined that it was likely to be metabolic in etiology. Which of the following is the most likely diagnosis?

A. Hyperthyroidism

B. Hypocalcemia

C. Hypoglycemia

D. Hypomagnesemia

31.2 A 28-year-old woman is brought into the ED by paramedics because of seizure activity that has persisted for 40 minutes despite intravenous valium at the house and en route. Which of the following is the most likely reason for this patient's condition?

A. Meningitis

B. Noncompliance with seizure medications

C. Cocaine

D. Benzodiazepine allergy

31.3 A 21-year-old man is brought into the ED for a seizure which was witnessed. It was described as tonic clonic and lasting for 3 minutes. Currently, the patient appears alert, oriented, and with normal vital signs. He has no nuchal rigidity. He admits to being diagnosed with HIV disease, but otherwise has no medical problems. He denies head trauma, or alcohol or illicit drug use. He denies headache. Which of the following is the best next step?

A. Emergent CT or MRI imaging of the brain

B. Begin fosphenytoin for seizure disorder

C. Observation because this is his first seizure

D. Stat EEG

ANSWERS

31.1 **C.** New-onset seizure in the ED caused by metabolic abnormalities is rare. Hypoglycemia is considered the most common metabolic cause of seizure. Symptomatic hypoglycemia occurs most commonly as a complication of insulin or oral hypoglycemic therapy in diabetics. Hyperglycemia, hypocalcemia, and hypomagnesemia are other, less-common metabolic causes of seizure.

31.2 **B.** A patient who experiences 30 minutes of continuous seizure activity or a series of seizures without return to full consciousness between seizures is considered to be in status epilepticus. The most common cause of status epilepticus is discontinuation of anticonvulsant medications.

31.3 **A.** Diagnostic imaging with head CT or MRI is recommended for seizure patients with suspicion of head trauma, elevated intracranial pressure, intracranial mass, persistently abnormal mental status, focal neurologic abnormality, or HIV disease.

CLINICAL PEARLS

▶ Identifying the patient within one of the following subgroups facilitates the evaluation and management of the seizure patient in the emergency department: (a) new-onset (first-time) seizure, (b) recurrent seizures in patients with epilepsy, (c) febrile seizures, (d) post-traumatic seizures, and (e) alcohol- and drug-related seizures.

▶ The possibility of reactive seizures should be considered in all seizure patients who present to the ED, including patients with a history of epilepsy. Failure to treat the underlying cause of reactive seizure is a major pitfall.

▶ Seizures may be confused with other nonictal states such as syncope, hyperventilation, and breath-holding spells in children, migraines, transient global amnesia, cerebral vascular disease, narcolepsy, and psychogenic seizures.

▶ Prolonged altered mental status following a seizure should not be attributed to an uncomplicated postictal state.

REFERENCES

Armon K, Stephenson T, MacFaul R, et al. An evidence and consensus based guideline for the management of a child after a seizure. *Emerg Med J*. 2003;20(1):13-20.

Beghi E. Treating epilepsy across its different stages. *Ther Adv Neurol Disord*. 2010;3(2):85-92.

Botero D, Tanowitz HB, Weiss LM, Wittner M. Taeniasis and cysticercosis. *Infect Dis Clin North Am*. 1993;7:683.

Harden CL, Huff JS, Schwartz TH, et al. Reassessment: neuroimaging in the emergency patient presenting with seizure (an evidence-based review): report of the Therapeutics and Technology Assessment Subcommittee of the American Academy of Neurology. *Neurology*. 2007;69:1772.

Krumholz A, Wiebe S, Gronseth G, et al. Practice parameter: evaluating an apparent unprovoked first seizure in adults (an evidence-based review): report of the Quality Standards Subcommittee of the American Academy of Neurology and the American epilepsy Society. *Neurology*. 2007;69:1996.

Matthaiou DK, Panos G, Adamidi ES, Falagas ME. Albendazole versus praziquantel in the treatment of neurocysticercosis: a meta-analysis of comparative trials. *PLoS Negl Trop Dis*. Mar 12, 2008;2(3):e194.

Pollack CV, Pollack ES. Seizures. In: Marx JA, Hockberger RM, Walls JA, eds. *Emergency Medicine: Concepts and Clinical Practice*. 5th ed. St Louis, MO: Mosby-Year Book; 2002.

Prasad K, Al-Roomi K, Krishnan PR, Sequeira R. Anticonvulsant therapy for status epilepticus. *The Cochrane Database of Systematic Reviews 2005*, Issue 4. Art. No: CD003723.

Scheuer ML, Pedley TA. The evaluation and treatment of seizures. *N Engl J Med*. 1990;323(21):1468-1474.

Seamans CM, Slovis CM. Seizures: classification and diagnosis, patient stabilization and pharmacologic interventions. In: *EMR textbook*. 2002. Available at: http://www.emronline.com/articles/textbook/44. Access date

Shearer P, Park D. Seizures and status epilepticus: diagnosis and management in the emergency department. emergency medicine practice. 2006;8(8).

Turnbull TL, Vanden Hoek TL, Howes DS. Utility of laboratory studies in the emergency department patient with a new-onset seizure. *Ann Emerg Med*. 1990;19(4):373-377.

A 76-year-old nursing home patient is transferred to the emergency department (ED) for reported altered mental status. The patient is confused and unable to provide any relevant information about his condition. According to EMS, the patient has been in the nursing home since he fractured his tibia 4 weeks prior. The patient has a past medical history of hypertension, diabetes, and chronic obstructive pulmonary disease (COPD).

His vital signs are BP 150/90 mm Hg, HR 110 beats per minute, RR 20 breaths per minute, T 36.7°C, and oxygen saturation of 92% on 4-L nasal cannula. On physical examination, the patient appears sleepy but is arousable. He has a difficult time following directions and appears confused. His pupils are 4 mm, equal and reactive. His mucous membranes appear dry. He is tachycardic and his lung sounds are clear and equal bilaterally. His abdomen is soft and nontender. There is a cast on his left lower extremity. The capillary refill on his toes is less then 2 seconds, he has strong femoral pulses. His skin reveals poor turgor and there is tenting. His motor and sensory examinations are normal.

Laboratory results reveal a WBC 12 cells/mm^3 and hemoglobin 10 mg/dL. His sodium is 110 mEq/L, potassium 4.1 mEq/L, BUN 52 mg/dL, creatinine 1.0 mg/dL, magnesium 1.7 mEq/L, and glucose 125 mg/dL. His urine drug screen is positive for opiates and benzodiazepines. His urinalysis is negative for infection.

▶ What is the most likely diagnosis?
▶ What is the best management?

ANSWERS TO CASE 32:
Altered Mental Status

Summary: This is a 76-year-old man from a nursing home with a history of hypertension, diabetes, and COPD. He presents to the ED with altered mental status (AMS). He has limited mobility due to a cast on his left lower leg secondary to a tibia fracture. His examination reveals dehydration and lab tests are consistent with significant hyponatremia and prerenal azotemia.

- **Most likely diagnosis:** Electrolyte abnormality (hyponatremia) secondary to deconditioning and dehydration.

- **Next step in management:** Intravenous fluid hydration and consider hypertonic saline.

ANALYSIS

Objectives

1. Recognize the diversity in presentation of patients with altered mental status and understand the diagnostic approach to the workup.

2. Be able to order the appropriate workup for patients and learn the initial management.

Considerations

This is a 76-year-old man who presents to the ED from a nursing home. The presentation of altered mental status in a nursing home patient should elicit concerns for underlying **infection** (eg, sepsis, meningitis, UTI), **electrolyte and metabolic abnormalities** (eg, hypo- or hyperglycemia, hyponatremia), **delirium,** and **hypoxia.** In the younger population, it is important to keep in mind other common causes of altered mental status such as **intoxications** and **withdrawal syndromes.**

Once the patient's airway, breathing, and circulation (ABCs) are addressed, the first step in management is to **obtain a capillary blood glucose to rule out hypoglycemia.** The patient appears dehydrated and an electrolyte panel should immediately be sent to the lab and intravenous fluid started for resuscitation.

APPROACH TO:
Altered Mental Status

DEFINITIONS

CONFUSION: Reversible disturbance of consciousness, attention, cognition, and perception that occurs within a short period of time

DELIRIUM: Global disturbance in consciousness and cognition, with an inability to relate to environment and process sensory input that is not better explained by preexisting or evolving dementia

DEMENTIA: Progressive, irreversible decline in mental function affecting judgment, memory, reasoning, comprehension

AGITATION: Excessive restlessness with increased mental and physical activity

COMA: Severe alteration of consciousness where one cannot be aroused

STUPOR: Level of decreased responsiveness where an individual requires aggressive or unpleasant stimulation

OBTUNDED: Level of diminished arousal or awareness frequently from extraneous causes (infection, intoxication, metabolic states)

CLINICAL APPROACH

The phrase "altered mental status" generally refers to a change from an individual's "normal" mental state. This may reflect a change in behavior, speech, comprehension level, judgment, mood, or level of consciousness (awareness or arousal state). Changes in mental status should be thought of in terms of organic, functional or psychiatric, or as a mixed disorder. Organic causes have a pathological basis primarily with a systemic or metabolic root, however structural lesions must also be considered. Functional or psychiatric diseases do not have a clearly defined physiologic foundation.

The reticular activating system (RAS) is physiologically responsible for our level of arousal. Signals from the RAS run through the pons in the brainstem, through the thalami, then project to both cerebral hemispheres. Any disruption in this pathway will lead to a decreased level of arousal. Examples of this may be through chemical depression via endogenous or exogenous agents or via structural abnormalities such as decreased blood flow resulting in ischemia.

Altered mental status and confusion are estimated to occur in 2% of all ED patients, 10% of hospitalized patients, and 50% of elderly hospitalized patients.

The evaluation of a patient with altered mental status can be a diagnostic challenge and a **complete history** and **physical examination** (Table 32–1) is imperative to the workup. Because the patient often cannot provide a reliable history, it is important **to obtain information from all available sources** such as family, friends, bystanders, and nursing home staff. The severity of illness must be quickly assessed and any life-threatening issues must be rapidly addressed (See Table 32-2).

Assessing the patient's ABCs, and quickly recognizing and managing reversible causes of AMS, such as hypoglycemia or hypoxia, are critical steps in

Table 32–1 • PHYSICAL EXAMINATION FINDINGS SUGGESTING MEDICAL CONCERNS FOR ALTERED MENTAL STATUS

Blood pressure	Neurologic (motor/sensory) findings
• *Significant hypertension* Hypertensive encephalopathy, increased intracranial pressure, thyrotoxicosis, intracranial hemorrhage, pregnancy-induced hypertension, toxicologic (eg, sympathomimetics, serotonin syndrome) • *Significant hypotension* Septic shock, cardiogenic shock, neurogenic shock, medication reaction, myocardial infarction	• *Focal motor or sensory deficit:* Stroke, space-occupying lesion, hypoglycemia, Todd paralysis (postictal), Wernicke encephalopathy • *Asterixis:* Hepatic failure, uremia, other metabolic derangements • *Rigidity:* Neuroleptic malignant syndrome • *New asymmetry or fixed pupils:* Stroke, space-occupying lesions • *Bilaterally pinpoint pupils:* Toxicologic etiology (eg, opioids, clonidine, organophosphates), pontine stroke • *Bilaterally dilated pupils:* Toxicologic etiology (eg, sympathomimetics, anticholinergics, hallucinogens) • *Breath odor:* Acetone—ketoacidosis, toxic ingestion; Fetor hepaticus—hepatic encephalopathy; ethanol—ethanol or other volatile intoxication
Pulse	**Funduscopic examination**
• *Bradycardia* Toxicologic (eg, β-blockers, calcium channel blockers), increased intracranial pressure, hypothyroidism • *Tachycardia* Toxicologic (eg, cyclic antidepressants, sympathomimetics, anticholinergics), sepsis, thyrotoxicosis, decreased cardiac output, withdrawal syndromes, hypoxia, hypoglycemia	• *Papilledema or retinal hemorrhage:* Space-occupying lesion, hypertensive encephalopathy, subarachnoid hemorrhage
Respiration	**Neck**
• *Hypoventilation* Toxicologic (eg, opioids, barbiturates), stroke, increased intracranial pressure, COPD, CO_2 retention • *Hyperventilation* Thyrotoxicosis, ASA overdose, acidosis, sepsis, CHF, COPD	• *Nuchal rigidity or other meningeal signs with or without fever:* CNS infection, subarachnoid hemorrhage

(Continued)

Table 32–1 • PHYSICAL EXAMINATION FINDINGS SUGGESTING MEDICAL CONCERNS FOR ALTERED MENTAL STATUS (CONTINUED)

Temperature	Abdominal
• *Fever/hyperpyrexia:* CNS infections, urinary tract infections, skin infections/sepsis, neuroleptic malignant syndrome, serotonin syndrome, toxicologic (eg, anticholinergics, salicylates, sympathomimetics), stroke, heat stroke, thyrotoxicosis, withdrawal syndromes • *Hypothermia:* Sepsis, toxicologic (eg, alcohol, barbiturates), hypothyroidism, hypoglycemia	• *Ascites/hepatomegaly:* Hepatic encephalopathy, spontaneous bacterial peritonitis, HIV, hepatitis
General appearance	**Skin**
• *Signs of head trauma or occult hematoma:* Intracranial hemorrhage (can include occult signs like hemotympanum, retinal hemorrhage, CSF rhinorrhea)	• *Needle marks:* Parenteral substance abuse, CNS infection • *Petechiae/purpura:* Intracranial hemorrhage, Rocky Mountain spotted fever, CNS infection/sepsis

Data from Karas S. Behavioral emergencies: differentiating medical from psychiatric disease. Emerg Med Prac.*2002;4(3):7-8.*

early management. A systematic approach guided by your history and physical and gathering understanding as to how mentation is altered (see Definition list) should be undertaken. The mini-mental state examination (MMSE) or Quick Confusion Scale (QCS) can be used and these ask are 4 to 7 questions that can be used in reassessment to monitor change in mental status.

If altered patient is unable to provide a history, then gathering as much information as possible from EMS, nursing home staff, family or bystanders is critical. EMS may be able to provide clues by describing the scene from where they transported the patient. Was there an empty pill vial? Did the patient verbalize any recent complaints? When was the patient last seen normal? What is the baseline mental status? Was the change in mental status abrupt or gradual? Has the condition changed since first recognized?

Special consideration must be given to pediatric and geriatric populations. Seizures with prolonged postictal states, head injuries, and accidental ingestions are common causes for altered mental status in the pediatric population. In the geriatric population a change in mental status may occur concomitant with existing dementia. Electrolyte abnormalities and dehydration are common causes in addition to hypo and hyperglycemia and thyroid hormone abnormalities. The elderly are more prone to subdural hematomas due to age-related cerebral atrophy; increasing the vulnerability of the bridging veins to tearing. Polypharmacy and unintentional overdoses also commonly cause an alteration in mental status.

Many mnemonics are used to aid in the clinical workup for altered mental status. One popular pneumonic is AEIOU TIPS (see Table 32–3). In elderly patients who are confused and forgetful, understanding the differences between dementia and delirium is critical (Table 32–4).

Table 32–2 • CRITICAL AND EMERGENT DIAGNOSES OF CONFUSION

Critical
- Hypoxia/diffuse cerebral ischemia
  - Respiratory failure, CHF, MI
- Systemic
  - Hypoglycemia
- CNS infections
- Hypertensive encephalopathy
- Increased intracranial pressure

Emergent
- Hypoxia/diffuse cerebral ischemia
  - Severe anemia
- Systemic disease
  - Electrolyte/fluid disturbances
  - Endocrine disease (thyroid/adrenal)
  - Hepatic failure
  - Nutrition/Wernicke's encephalopathy
  - Sepsis/infection
- Intoxication and withdrawal
  - CNS sedatives
  - Ethanol
  - Medication side effects, anticholinergics
- CNS disease
  - Trauma
  - Infections
  - Stroke
  - Subarachnoid hemorrhage
  - Epilepsy/seizures
    - Postictal state
    - Nonconvulsive status epilepticus
    - Complex partial status epilepticus
- Neoplasm

Table 32–3 • AEIOU TIPS—MNEMONIC FOR TREATABLE CAUSES OF ALTERED MENTAL STATUS

A	Alcohol (intoxication/withdrawal)
E	Epilepsy, electrolytes, encephalopathy (hepatic, hypertensive, Wernicke), endocrine (thyroid/adrenal)
I	Insulin (hypoglycemia/hyperglycemia), intussusception
O	Opioids, oxygen (hypoxia)
U	Urea (metabolic)
T	Trauma, temperature (hypothermia, hyperthermia)
I	Infection (systemic, CNS), ingestion (drugs/toxins)
P	Psychiatric, porphyria
S	Shock, subarachnoid hemorrhage, stroke, seizure, space-occupying lesion, snake bite

Table 32–4 • CHARACTERISTICS OF DELIRIUM AND DEMENTIA

Delirium	Dementia
Abrupt onset—days to weeks	Gradual onset—usually progressive
Early disorientation	Late disorientation
Moment to moment variability	Often more stable
Altered level of consciousness	Level of conscious most often normal
Short attention span	Attention span is reduced

Data from Smith J, Seirafi J. Delirium and dementia. In: Rosen P, Barkin R, eds. Emergency Medicine, Concepts and Clinical Practice. *7th ed. Philadelphia, PA: Mosby; 2009: 1372.*

Glasgow Coma Scale

The Glasgow coma scale (Table 32–5) was created as an assessment tool to quantify the degree of depression in the level of consciousness in patients with head trauma. Its purpose was to track the progress of patients' neurologic status. Its use has widened to include patients with undifferentiated change in mental status. The scoring scale utilizes assessments of eye opening, and motor and verbal function to provide a rapid indication on any alteration of function. A higher score corresponds to a higher level of consciousness.

Management

Stabilization of Life Threats Always start by addressing the ABCs and treat any immediate threats to life. Opening the airway and providing a jaw thrust and

Table 32–5 • GLASGOW COMA SCALE

Eye Opening		
	Spontaneous eye opening	4
	Opens to verbal commands	3
	Opens to painful stimuli	2
	No response	1
Verbal Response		
	Oriented	5
	Disoriented	4
	Inappropriate words	3
	Incomprehensible sounds	2
	No response	1
Motor Response		
	Obeys commands	6
	Localizes to pain	5
	Withdraws to pain	4
	Abnormal flexion	3
	Abnormal extension	2
	No response	1

supplemental oxygen are the first steps in treating hypoxic causes of AMS. Subsequently begin bag-valve-mask ventilation. If the underlying cause of apnea or hypoventilation cannot immediately be corrected (eg, naloxone for opiate overdose), then the patient will require endotracheal or nasotracheal intubation and mechanical ventilation.

Assess circulation by feeling for pulses, placing the patient on a cardiac monitor, assess skin perfusion, and check blood pressure. The only way to fix a hypoperfused brain is to restore circulation. Begin CPR if the patient is pulseless or a nonperfusing rhythm (v-fib, pulseless v-tach) is seen on the monitor and prepare for defibrillation or cardioversion. If there is a pulse, but signs of shock are present (mottled skin, cool extremities), you need to assure adequate volume (IV fluids), hemoglobin (transfusion), and peripheral vascular resistance (pressors).

As soon as adequate airway, breathing and circulatory support has been established then make a global assessment of neurologic functioning. Assess the GCS scale. Check for pupil size and reactivity. Look for any spontaneous movement, especially noting seizure-like activity or lack of movement on one side suggesting a stroke or below a certain level (spinal cord injury). Any suspicion of cord injury requires placement of a cervical collar and immobilization. Undress the patient and onto his or her side to look for any signs of trauma, drug patches or infection sources.

Infectious Fever, recent history of infection, or any signs of infection on physical examination need to be addressed immediately. Any patient who is altered with a fever should always raise the suspicion for meningitis. It is prudent to empirically treat (ceftriaxone and vancomycin and pretreat with steroids) these patients while you proceed with the diagnostic workup (lumbar puncture). If the history and physical suggests any other sources of infection (pneumonia, UTI), appropriate antibiotics and cultures should be started right away. Indwelling lines need to be removed or changed and any fluid collections must be drained.

Metabolic Hypoglycemia is a common cause of altered mental status. If you cannot quickly determine blood glucose go ahead and give an amp of D50 (25 g of dextrose). In addition to unconsciousness, hypoglycemia can cause seizures and the patient may have a prolonged postictal phase. If the patient is unconscious and intravenous access is difficult, you can consider administering intramuscular glucagon, which acts as a counterregulatory hormone to increase serum glucose levels.

Hypo- and hypernatremia are primarily problems of water metabolism and are frequently associated with volume overload or dehydration states. Hyponatremia can cause altered mental status, focal neurologic abnormalities, and seizures. This should be treated with hypertonic (3%) saline. Hypernatremia should respond to appropriate rehydration. These patients typically require admission to the intensive care unit.

Hypo- and hypercalcemia can result from several metabolic abnormalities or paraneoplastic syndromes. Hypocalcemia should be treated with calcium, whereas the initial treatment for hypercalcemia is intravenous fluid hydration.

Primary CNS Seizure is a common cause for AMS. Always rule out hypoglycemia first. Benzodiazepines are the first-line therapy. Send blood for levels if the patient is on anticonvulsants with measurable levels or metabolites. Load subtheraputic patients where appropriate.

Tumors can present as altered mental status. Any previous cancer history, focal neurologic findings, headache, or papilledema should prompt a head CT scan. IV contrast enhances the ability of plain CT to identify tumors. If there is evidence of edema or mass-effect, then consider administering steroids to help reduce vasogenic edema. Obtain an emergent neurosurgic consultation. These patients typically require admission to the intensive care unit.

Brain abscesses can be identified with a contrast-enhanced head CT scan. These patients should immediately be placed on antibiotics and be seen by a neurosurgeon.

Drugs and Toxins Many overdoses can lead to altered mental status. Look for signs of a toxidrome (sedative/hypnotic, sympathomimetic, anticholinergic, cholinergic, and opiate/opioid). Most toxidromes can be treated with supportive measures, however specific antidotes exist for each (see Case 40).

Ethanol intoxication is a common ingestion for ED patients. These patients need to be thoroughly evaluated to exclude other causes of their change in mental status (stroke, hypoglycemia, Wernicke encephalopathy, intracranial bleed, toxic alcohol). Once serious causes are ruled out, these patients require supportive care until they can be discharged.

Withdrawal states can lead to altered mental status. Patients with ethanol and benzodiazepine withdrawal are typically hyperadrenergic, agitated, and confused. These patients require administration of benzodiazepines, supportive care, and inpatient admission.

Trauma A CT scan should be performed immediately in patients with evidence of head trauma and altered mental status. It is important to rule out an intracranial injury such as acute bleeding, skull fracture, and evidence of increased intracranial pressure. The trauma or neurosurgical service should be contacted for any positive findings.

Disposition Unless the patient with altered mental status presents to the ED with an identifiable reversible cause for his or her change in mental status (heroin overdose), the majority of patients who present to the ED with altered mental status will require admission for further inpatient workup.

COMPREHENSION QUESTIONS

32.1 A 77-year-old women is brought to the ED by her daughter. The daughter provides the history that her mother is usually alert and oriented and performs all of her activities of daily life (ADLs) by herself. Over the past week, the patient has been eating and drinking less and tells her daughter that she is not hungry. Yesterday she had an episode of incontinence and this morning she woke up confused, unable to follow commands and kept asking where her husband was (he's been deceased for over 5 years). The patient is tachycardic with a HR in the 130s, appears dehydrated, has a low-grade fever, and smells of urine. The most likely cause of her altered mental status is?

   A. Alzheimer dementia

   B. Alcohol Intoxication

   C. Overmedication

   D. Urinary tract infection

32.2 A 45-year-old man who runs his own business has been struggling with his finances since undergoing three surgeries to fix his right shoulder. He has been visiting multiple doctors to help control his pain. EMS was called to his office after an employee found the patient on his office floor with a bottle of vodka and a prescription medication bottle lying next to him. Which of the following should be the first course of action in the ED?

   A. Administer naloxone as he likely overdosed on pain medications.

   B. Give thiamine to prevent Wernicke-Korsakoff syndrome.

   C. Obtain a capillary blood glucose check.

   D. Disrobe the patient, place on a monitor, and obtain vital signs.

32.3 A 68-year-old woman was brought to the ED after her friends noticed that during lunch the patient began slurring her speech and started acting confused. They were about to take her home when she developed jerking movements of the extremities and become unresponsive. When EMS arrived she was conscious, hypertensive at 160/90 mm Hg, with otherwise normal vital signs. She was not talking or following commands. After addressing the ABCs, what is the most appropriate next step in the management of this patient?

   A. Administer lorazepam as she likely had a seizure.

   B. Administer glucose as she likely is having a hypoglycemic episode.

   C. Obtain a head CT scan as she may be having a stroke or intracranial hemorrhage.

   D. Treat her blood pressure emergently as she is having a hypertensive emergency.

ANSWERS

32.1 **D.** Infection is a common cause of altered mental status especially in the elderly population. The history suggests a urinary tract infection concomitant with dehydration. This is the most likely cause of this patient's altered mental status. Alzheimer's does not develop rapidly, but rather gradually over time. The history is not suggestive of alcohol abuse and additional history and physical examination signs should be present to suggest a medication overuse.

32.2 **D.** In all patients the ABCs take priority. The patient should be assessed and the physical examination performed before administering any medications. In this patient with altered mental status of unknown etiology, the "coma cocktail" will likely be administered, but should be guided by the physical examination and history.

32.3 **C.** This presentation is concerning for a stroke. The history obtained from friends in this case is critical to making a diagnosis for this patient. She did have a seizure and may be in a postictal state. However, the history of slurred speech and confusion raise suspicion for stroke and as soon as the patient is stable, she should undergo a CT scan. It is important to first establish the type of stroke before altering the blood pressure as it can be detrimental if the blood pressure is lowered too much and too rapidly in patients with ischemic stroke.

CLINICAL PEARLS

▶ Be sure to talk with family, EMS, nursing home care providers and review medical records for important pieces of historical information, new medications, and baseline behavior and functional status.

▶ Check vitals signs frequently, making sure to get accurate readings on pulse oximetry, temperature, and blood pressure.

▶ A glucose level should be checked immediately in all patients with altered mental status.

▶ Be careful not to classify a confused elderly patient as demented without first ruling out organic causes of their confusion.

REFERENCES

Cooke JL. Depressed consciousness and coma. In: Rosen P, Barkin R, eds. *Emergency Medicine, Concepts and Clinical Practice*. 7th ed. Philadelphia, PA: Mosby; 2009:106-112.

Huff, JS. Confusion. In: Rosen P, Barkin R, eds. *Emergency Medicine, Concepts and Clinical Practice*. 7th ed. Philadelphia, PA: Mosby; 2009:101-105.

Karas, S. Behavioral emergencies: differentiating medical from psychiatric disease. *Emerg Med Prac.* 2002;4(3):1-20.

Nassisi D, Okuda Y. ED management of delirium and agitation. *Emerg Med Prac.* 2007;9(1):1-20.

Smith J, Seirafi J. Delirium and dementia. In: Rosen P, Barkin R, eds. *Emergency Medicine, Concepts and Clinical Practice.* 7th ed. Philadelphia, PA: Mosby; 2009:1365-1378.

A 6-year-old boy presents to the emergency department (ED) with his parents complaining of a limp for 3 days. The limp began following a fall from a playground structure, and has worsened to the point that the child is no longer willing to walk. The patient was treated two weeks ago for an acute otitis media with Augmentin, and he currently has a runny nose attributed to allergies. There have been no fevers, emesis, cough, abdominal pain, recent travel or insect bites.

His blood pressure is 95/68 mm Hg, pulse is 102 beats per minute, respirations are 20 breaths per minute, and temperature is 37.5°C (99.5°F). On physical examination, he is well appearing and his right hip is noted to be flexed with slight abduction and external rotation. The joint is warm to touch, and he resists passive range of motion testing. The right knee is normal, and there are no other findings on physical examination.

▶ What is your next step?
▶ What is the most likely diagnosis?
▶ What is the best treatment for this problem?

ANSWERS TO CASE 33:

Transient Synovitis

Summary: The patient is a 6-year-old boy with right hip pain who is refusing to ambulate. He appears well with normal vital signs; his examination reveals decreased passive range of motion of the right hip.

- **Next step:** Perform an ultrasound to evaluate for hip effusion, consider an arthrocentesis to evaluate synovial fluid.

- **Most likely diagnosis:** While it is essential to consider the serious etiologies of pediatric hip pain, this child most likely has transient synovitis (TS).

- **Best treatment for this problem:** After excluding septic arthritis, osteomyelitis and other non-benign etiologies, treat for transient synovitis with NSAIDs and bed rest for 7 to 10 days.

ANALYSIS

Objectives

1. Recognize the clinical presentation of transient synovitis, and appreciate the similarities of its presentation to septic arthritis and other serious pathologies of limp.

2. Learn about the diagnosis and treatment of suspected septic arthritis.

3. Be familiar with the other etiologies of limp in a child.

Considerations

Transient synovitis is the most common cause of acute hip pain in children aged 3 to 10 years old. The arthralgia is caused by a temporary inflammation of the synovium, the soft tissue that lines the non-cartilaginous surfaces of the hip joint. While the etiology is not clearly understood, the disease is suspected to be secondary to an infection as up to 50% of patients report a recent upper respiratory tract infection. Fever typically is absent but may occur. Most patients will complain of unilateral hip pain, and up to 5% will have bilateral pain. There is a male-to-female predominance of slightly more than 2:1.

While this case is a typical example of transient synovitis, the diagnosis not to miss is **septic arthritis,** an infection that can lead to rapid destruction of the articular joint cartilage. This disease can lead to long-term morbidity if not diagnosed early, and joints of the lower extremity are affected in more than 90% of the cases.

In general, children with septic arthritis will have a history of fever, malaise and/or anorexia within the week prior to presentation. Occasionally, the presentation is more subtle, and the symptoms may be attenuated by recent antibiotic use. Neonates and infants with septic arthritis may present with irritability, poor feeding, and pseudoparalysis of the affected limb

On physical examination, the position of comfort will be with the hip flexed, abducted, and externally rotated. Passive range of motion exercises will be resisted and painful. Appropriate initial laboratory studies include complete blood count (CBC), blood cultures, erythrocyte sedimentation rate (ESR), and C-reactive protein (CRP). Plain radiographs are key to rule out obvious alternative diagnoses, and bedside ED ultrasound may identify a hip effusion. The definitive diagnosis of septic arthritis is made by examination of synovial fluid obtained by arthrocentesis.

Approximately 3% of children who present to the emergency department for limp will have septic arthritis. Causative bacterial organisms vary with age group, but *Staphylococcus aureus* is the most common organism, followed by Group A *Streptococcus* (*S pyogenes*) and *S pneumoniae*. *Kingella kingae* has recently become a common pathogen in children younger than 3, and *Neisseria gonorrhoeae* should be considered in neonates and sexually active adolescents. Empiric antibiotic coverage should include an antistaphylococcal agent with gram-negative coverage added when age appropriate. Definitive treatment is by immediate surgical drainage and washout in addition to antibiotics.

APPROACH TO:
Child With a Limp

DEFINITION

LIMP: A limp is an uneven, jerky or laborious gait, usually caused by pain, weakness, or deformity.

CLINICAL APPROACH

The differential diagnosis of the pediatric limp is broad, and the emergency physician must use a systemic approach to identify or exclude the conditions that require emergent treatment. The cause of limp can often be determined through careful history taking and physical examination. Laboratory tests, imaging and diagnostic testing can then be applied to confirm clinical suspicions.

Obtaining a History

History taking is challenging in a young child who may be unable to communicate verbally, or have difficulty localizing the site of the pain. Obtaining the following information will help to narrow the differential.

1. Age (age specific diagnoses)

2. Onset of pain (acute versus chronic)

3. Duration of pain (intermittent, constant, or worse at particular times of day)

4. Location of pain (bone, joint, soft tissue, neurologic or intra-abdominal)

5. Preceding events (history of trauma, recent viral illness or antibiotic use)

6. Constitutional symptoms (fever, malaise, weight loss)

Table 33–1 • COMMON CAUSES OF LIMP BY AGE					
Age (y)	Infectious	Trauma	Inflammatory	Developmental	Neoplasia
Toddler (1-3)	Septic arthritis	Toddler fracture	Transient synovitis	Developmental dysplasia of the hip	Leukemia
	Osteomyelitis	Child abuse	Juvenile rheumatoid arthritis	Clubfoot	
Juvenile (4-10)	Septic arthritis	Fracture	Transient synovitis	Developmental dysplasia of the hip	Ewing sarcoma
	Osteomyelitis	Legg-Calve-Perthes disease	Juvenile rheumatoid arthritis		Osteoid osteoma
Adolescent (11-17)	Septic or gonococcal arthritis	Fracture	Juvenile rheumatoid arthritis	Osteochondritis dessicans	Osteosarcoma
	Osteomyelitis	Slipped capital femoral epiphysis	Osgood-Schlatter		Ewing sarcoma
					Osteoid osteoma

There is overlap among age groups, but knowing which diseases are common in each age group is a good place to start when making a list of potential diagnoses (Table 33–1).

Limps that are acute in onset are more likely to be due to trauma or infection. Chronic limps are suggestive of systemic illness, **Legg-Calve-Perthes disease (LCP) (avascular necrosis),** or **slipped capital femoral epiphysis (SCFE).** Pain that is worse at night is more typical of a malignancy, and morning stiffness is commonly associated with **juvenile rheumatoid arthritis.** The location of the pain may be typical of a musculoskeletal etiology, but referred pain and alternative diagnoses such as appendicitis, and testicular or ovarian torsion should be entertained. A history of trauma can suggest fracture or contusion, while a recent illness or constitutional symptoms may direct the physician to consider **osteomyelitis,** septic arthritis, or transient synovitis.

Physical Examination

First, the gait should be observed if the child is ambulatory. The child should be fully undressed, vital signs reviewed, and the general appearance of "sick or not sick" considered. The extremities should be inspected for skin erythema, rash, tenderness, deformity, muscle atrophy and abnormal range of motion. The **log roll test** is particularly useful in evaluating hip rotation. To perform the log roll test, the leg is straightened, and the foot is manipulated medially (internal rotation of the hip) and laterally (external rotation of the hip). Pain with this maneuver suggests inflammation, infection, or trauma.

The presence or absence of a fever has not been found to be helpful in making a definitive diagnosis. In a series of 95 children with septic arthritis, most had a low-grade fever, but one-third were afebrile at presentation. Absence of fever should not sway the clinician from the diagnosis.

Lastly, if there are any inconsistencies between the history and physical examination, the possibility of non-accidental trauma, or child abuse, must be explored.

Laboratory Studies

Laboratory studies are not routinely indicated in a child who has normal vital signs, appears well, and has a history consistent with an immediate preceding trauma. However, a complete blood count (CBC), erythrocyte sedimentation rate (ESR), C-reactive protein (CRP), and blood cultures are useful if entities such as osteomyelitis, neoplasm, septic arthritis, and transient synovitis remain on the differential.

Synovial fluid analysis, which includes cell count, Gram stain, culture and sensitivity testing, may be required to distinguish between septic arthritis and transient synovitis. A synovial fluid white blood cell count of >50,000 cells/μL with a predominance (>90%) of polymorphonuclear (PMN) leukocytes suggests septic arthritis. The Gram stain may rapidly identify the organism, and the culture and sensitivity results will allow the antibiotic regimen to be narrowed. Notably, synovial fluid has bacteriostatic effects, and organisms may not grow in the routine culture. The likelihood of identifying the organism can be improved by placing a synovial fluid sample in a blood culture medium. Finally, neonates and adolescents with a suspected septic arthritis should be tested for gonorrhea.

Imaging Studies

In contrast to laboratory studies, most children with a limp require radiographic evaluation. Plain films should be ordered with a minimum of two views and the joints above and below the area of concern should be included. If possible, weight-bearing views should be obtained, and if the hip is involved, the contralateral hip should be filmed for comparison. Radiographs can identify fracture, late avascular necrosis, soft tissue swelling, and destructive bony lesions.

A bone scan uses IV technetium 99m-labeled methylene diphosphate to identify areas of increased cellular activity and blood flow. This test can be useful to detect early Legg-Calve-Perthes disease, osteomyelitis, stress fractures, and osteoid osteomas. Magnetic resonance imaging (MRI) can be helpful in detecting osteomyelitis, early avascular necrosis, and bone malignancies. Computed tomography (CT) is rarely indicated for musculoskeletal complaints; however the test may be necessary when intra-abdominal entities, such as appendicitis, or pelvic etiologies are in the differential.

Ultrasound (US) is perhaps the most useful imaging study after plain films in the evaluation of the pediatric limp. Recent studies have demonstrated that the use of bedside ED ultrasound can reliably detect a joint effusion (Figure 33–1). In one series of 96 children who underwent hip US for possible septic arthritis, none of the 40 patients who had normal US findings were later discharged with the diagnosis of septic arthritis. Early detection of a joint effusion and ultrasound guidance of arthrocentesis can decrease the time to definitive diagnosis and treatment

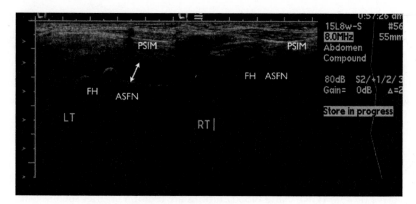

Figure 33–1. Ultrasound demonstrating a left hip effusion. The right hip is normal. The echogenic linear focus which courses along the left femoral neck is felt to represent periosteal new bone. An effusion is diagnosed when the distance between the anterior surface of the femoral neck and the posterior surface of the iliopsoas muscle is greater than 5 mm, or there is a greater than 2 mm difference from the contralateral hip. FH, femoral head; ASFN, anterior surface femoral head; PSIM, posterior surface iliopsoas muscle.

of septic arthritis. Additionally, the detection of bilateral hip effusions raises the clinical suspicion for rheumatologic conditions and transient synovitis. One study showed that up to 25% of patients with transient synovitis have bilateral effusions.

Alternate Etiologies of Pediatric Limp

Septic Arthritis is most common in children <3 years old. The male-to-female ratio is 2:1. The hip is the most common site (80%) with the most common organism being *S aureus*. Others: group A beta-hemolytic *Streptococcus*, *S pneumoniae*, *Haemophilus influenzae* type B, *Kingella kingae* (after URI), *Salmonella* (sickle cell patients), *Pseudomonas aeruginosa*, *Neisseria meningitidis*, *N gonorrhoeae*, gram-negative bacilli. Pain in the affected joint, fever, edema, swelling, inability to bear weight, anorexia, irritability, pseudoparalysis may be presenting symptoms. There are no published clinical decision rules but a recent study notes that infection is indicated by: (1) inability to bear weight, (2) fever, (3) ESR >40 mm/h, (4) WBC >12,000/mm^3. Though the incidence is low, when present, IV antibiotics and surgical irrigation and debridement must be implemented immediately as disability due to destruction of joint tissue may ensue.

Osteomyelitis of the femur or pelvis can present as hip pain. The proximal femur is the most common site of bone infection in children, and may also involve the joint given the intracapular location (Figure 33–2). On examination, there may be focal erythema, swelling, and warmth near the location of the metaphysis. Similar to septic arthritis, the presentation may be attenuated by the recent antibiotic use. Plain films may not show bony changes until 10 to 20 days after symptoms began. MRI is the ideal study with a sensitivity of 92% to 100%. The most common organisms are the same as those that cause septic arthritis, and patients with osteomyelitis require empiric antibiotic therapy and emergent orthopedic consultation for bone aspiration.

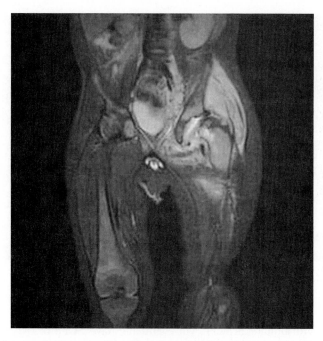

Figure 33–2. An example of osteomyelitis of the left proximal femur, ischia, and iliac bones with associated left hip septic arthritis. There is also extensive myositis surrounding the left hip. There is possible pus under pressure or necrotic changes may be present in the left proximal femur.

Legg-Calve-Perthes disease (vascular necrosis of the femoral head) develops when an insufficient blood supply to the femoral head leads to necrosis. It is commonly found in boys aged 4 to 10 years, and its cause is unknown. The child usually presents with a limp and may complain of hip or knee pain. On physical examination, the child will have decreased range of motion at the affected hip. X-rays may show fragmentation and then healing of the femoral head (Figure 33–3), and a bone scan will show decreased blood perfusion to the femoral head. Ten to twenty percent of patients will have bilateral disease, and the aim of treatment is to keep the femoral head within the acetabulum to allow healing to occur. A brace, cast, or splint may be required to immobilize the hip's position. Patients should be referred to an orthopedist for possible surgical management.

Slipped Capital Femoral Epiphysis (SCFE) remains one of the most common disorders affecting the hip in adolescence. SCFE is characterized by the posterior displacement of the capital femoral epiphysis from the femoral neck through the growth plate. It is most common in obese boys aged 11 to 15 years. Children who grow rapidly and who have hormonal imbalances such as hypothyroidism and acromegaly are also at risk. In addition to a limp, patients will complain of hip and/or knee pain. On examination, patients will have impaired internal rotation and passive hip flexion may be associated with compensatory external rotation. Plain films of the hip or pelvis will often show displacement of the femoral head, commonly described as "fallen ice cream from the cone". Approximately 30% to 60%

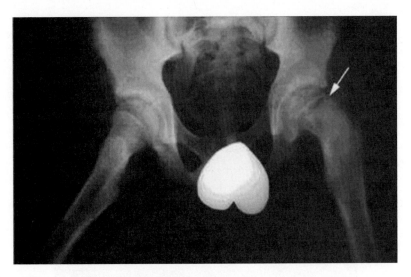

Figure 33–3. Avascular Necrosis of the Femoral Head

of patients with unilateral SCFE will eventually have SCFE of the contralateral hip. Once the diagnosis is suspected, weight-bearing should be avoided and most patients will require surgery to reattach the femoral head to the femur.

Toddler's fracture is a nondisplaced fracture of the distal tibial shaft that occurs most commonly in a child younger than 2 years who is learning to walk. Frequently, there is no definite history of a traumatic event, and the child is brought to the office due to reluctance to bear weight on the leg. On physical examination, maximal tenderness can usually be elicited over the fracture site. On plain film, the typical findings are a nondisplaced hairline spiral fracture of the tibia and no fibular fracture. It is not uncommon for initial radiographs to be normal and the diagnosis of this fracture made several days after the injury when follow-up radiographs show a lucent line or periosteal reaction.

Osgood-Schlatter syndrome is caused by a reaction of the bone and cartilage of the tibial tubercle to repetitive stress (eg, jumping) and is believed to represent tiny stress fractures in the apophysis. The condition is also associated with rapid growth spurts. Physical examination reveals tenderness and swelling over the tibial tubercle. Running, jumping, and kneeling worsen the symptoms. The condition is managed with ice, anti-inflammatory medication, and a decrease in activity. Daily stretching of the quadriceps and hamstrings is also beneficial. Patients with severe pain may require immobilization using crutches or a knee immobilizer. Individual regulation of activity is usually effective; pain may recur until the tubercle matures (ie, ossifies completely).

COMPREHENSION QUESTIONS

33.1 A 2-year-old girl presents with refusal bear weight on the left leg and a fever to 38.7°C (101.6°F) for 2 days. She has significant guarding when you attempt to range her left hip. In consideration of the differential diagnosis, which of the following diagnostic tests would be most useful?

A. Radiograph of both hips

B. Complete blood count

C. Blood culture

D. Ultrasound examination of the hip

33.2 The mother of an 8-year-old boy is told that her son's limping and knee pain is caused by Legg-Calve-Perthes disease. Which of the following best explains the condition of the femoral head?

A. Dislocation

B. Subluxation

C. Avascular necrosis

D. Dysplasia

33.3 A 5-year-old girl is brought into the emergency center due to significant hip pain. There is no history of trauma or fall. She has had a recent respiratory infection. Which of the following is the most likely diagnosis?

A. Subacute osteomyelitis

B. Transient synovitis

C. Developmental dysplasia of the hip

D. Malignant degeneration of the hip

E. Slipped capital femoral epiphysis

33.4 A 13-year-old overweight adolescent boy presents to his pediatrician's office with chronic left hip pain for 2 months. He has a Trendelenburg gait and has decreased range of motion of the left hip. Which of the following is the most likely diagnosis for this patient?

A.   Slipped capital femoral epiphysis

B.   Transient synovitis

C.   Osgood-Schlatter

D.   Legg-Calve-Perthes disease

33.5 A12-month-old male infant presents with his concerned mother after rolling off the bed in the night. X-ray reveals a femoral shaft fracture, and you note that this child has had three other visits to the emergency department for injury. What is your next step in management of this patient?

A.   Urgent orthopedic consultation

B.   Order a skeletal survey

C.   Report your concerns to the appropriate child protection services

D.   All of the above

ANSWERS

33.1 **D.** Osteomyelitis, septic arthritis, and transient synovitis should be considered in the differential of this child. Osteomyelitis and a septic arthritis are orthopedic emergencies, which require prompt intervention. Transient synovitis is often hard to distinguish clinically from the prior two entities. To make a definite diagnosis, an ultrasound should be performed to evaluate for an effusion and guide arthrocentesis. The synovial fluid of a septic joint will have a marked neutrophilia.

33.2 **C.** Legg-Calve-Perthes disease is commonly found in boys aged 4 to 8 years. It results in avascular necrosis of the femoral head.

33.3 **B.** Transient synovitis is the most common cause of hip pain in children aged 3 to 10 years. Though a benign process, it is often hard to distinguish from a septic joint or osteomyelitis. The child can be safely treated with bed rest and anti-inflammatories.

33.4 **A.** SCFE is commonly found among overweight pubertal children. A Trendelenburg gait is described as the pelvis tilting downward on the unaffected side when a patient steps on the affected side. There is also an accompanying subtle shift of the torso. Legg-Calve-Perthes is in the differential but more common among children aged 4 to 8. Transient synovitis presents more acutely. Osgood-Schlatter usually presents in athletic kids who have reproducible tibial tubercle tenderness.

33.5 **D.** Child abuse should be suspected as this is likely to be a non-ambulatory child. The mechanism sounds suspicious, was not witnessed, and there may have been delay in seeking medical care. Treating the injury, alerting the appropriate authorities of your concerns, and obtaining a skeletal survey is essential for the safety of the child. A typical skeletal survey includes skull, chest, pelvis, and entire limb x-rays.

CLINICAL PEARLS

▶ Always order an ultrasound and perform arthrocentesis in a child with fever who refuses to move a joint. Transient synovitis should be a diagnosis of exclusion.

▶ Consider Legg-Calve-Perthes disease in boys aged 4 to 8 who present with a limp as it requires a high index of suspicion.

▶ SCFE treatment is operative and 30% to 60% will eventually have bilateral disease. To prevent delay in diagnosis of the second slip, all patients should be followed closely by an orthopedist until the child has finished growing.

▶ Perform a thorough history (with and without the parent) and physical on children who present with fractures to evaluate for possible child abuse.

REFERENCES

Clark MC: Approach to the child with a limp. Available at: www.uptodate.com. Accessed: June 8, 2010.

Frank G, Mahoney HM, Eppes SC. Musculoskeletal infections in children. *Pediatr Clin North Am.* 2005;52:1083.

Kiang KM, Ogunmodede F, Juni BA, et al. Outbreak of osteomyelitis/septic arthritis caused by kigella kingae among child care center attendees. *Pediatrics.* 2005;116:e206.

Kienstra AJ; Macias CG: Slipped capital femoral epiphysis. Available at: www.uptodate.com. Accessed: May 9, 2012.

Kocher MS. Validation of a clinical prediction rule for the differentiation between septic arthritis and transient synovitis of the hip in children. *J Bone Joint Surg Am.* 2004;86A:1629.

Krogstad P: Bacterial arthritis: Clinical features and diagnosis in infants and children. Available at: www.uptodate.com.

Nelson JD. Skeletal infections in children. *Adv Pediatr Infect Dis.* 1991;6:59.

Nigrovic PA: Overview of hip pain in childhood. Available at: www.uptodate.com. Accessed: April 16, 2012.

Shetty AK, Gedalia A. Septic arthritis in children. *Rheum Dis Clin North Am.* 1998;24:287.

Sonnen GM, Henry NK. Pediatric bone and joint infections: Diagnosis and antimicrobial management. *Pediatr Clin North Am.* 1996;43:933-947.

Viera RL, Levy JA. Bedside ultrasonography to identify hip effusions in pediatric patients. *Ann Emerg Med.* 2010;55:284.

A 16-month-old child is brought in by EMS after a witnessed tonic-clonic event at home by his mother. The mother, a 33-year-old G2 woman, reports that he was born vaginally at term after an uneventful pregnancy. His birth weight was 3700 g, and he was discharged on the second hospital day. The mother noted that the child has been well appearing, is not taking any medications and there had been no recent travel. He had been active for the past week with no apparent complaints. The mother thinks the seizure lasted about 5 minutes but it ceased by the time EMS arrived at the home. The vital signs on the chart include a temperature of 38.4°C (101.1°F) (rectal), a heart rate of 130 beats per minute, a respiratory rate of 24 breaths per minute, and a systolic blood pressure of 100 mm Hg. On initial evaluation, the child is well appearing, well-perfused, and in no respiratory distress. His mental status is back to baseline per the mother, and on further evaluation, the child has no rashes or murmurs but is noted to have a bulging erythematous tympanic membrane. Acetaminophen is ordered and the child is observed and reevaluated several times over the next couple of hours. No laboratory studies are ordered initially.

▶ What is the most likely diagnosis?
▶ What is the next step in management of this patient?

ANSWERS TO CASE 34:

Febrile Seizure

Summary: This is a 16-month-old child with a febrile seizure and acute otitis media. The combination of a relatively brief seizure in a febrile child in this age group who awakens back to baseline is consistent with a diagnosis of febrile seizure. Uncomplicated presentations require a thorough history and physical examination but rarely any additional testing. The presence of a focal infection like otitis media is common but not essential for the diagnosis. Providing the child returns to a baseline playful state, admission to the hospital is not necessary.

- **Most likely diagnosis:** Simple febrile seizure and acute otitis media

- **Next step in management:** Medication to reduce the fever followed by a period of observation and reevaluation

ANALYSIS

Objectives

1. Learn the specific definition of a simple febrile seizure

2. Understand current standards for an age-based approach to the evaluation of a simple febrile seizure in the pediatric patient.

3. In cases of concurrent infection, specifically otitis media (OM), determine the need for further evaluation and/or testing in a simple febrile seizure.

Considerations

This infant has experienced a witnessed seizure at home and is noted to be febrile but well appearing and back at his baseline in the emergency department, and without neurologic deficits. As with all sick emergency department patients the evaluation begins with assessment of airway, breathing, and circulation. After the initial assessment, resuscitation and stabilization, etiology for the seizure must be investigated. This subject can be complex considering the large number of potential causes. The greatest immediate threat and concern is the possibility of CNS infection. Infectious causes must be addressed before less acute etiologies are considered.

APPROACH TO:
Febrile Seizures

DEFINITIONS

SIMPLE FEBRILE SEIZURE: The definition for a simple febrile seizure is very specific: age between 6 months and 60 months, generalized tonic-clonic convulsions, spontaneous cessation of convulsion within 15 minutes, return to alert mental status after convulsion, documentation of fever (>38.0°C), one convulsion with a 24-hour period, and absence of neurologic abnormality on examination.

COMPLEX FEBRILE SEIZURE: This heterogeneous group is beyond the scope of this chapter. The causes, presentations, assessments, and treatments are broad and complex. A standard treatment recommendation **does not exist** and the clinician must evaluate and treat the child with a complex febrile seizure on a case-by-case manner.

WELL-APPEARING INFANT: An infant who appears to both caretaker and health care practitioner to interact appropriately for age, has no increased work of breathing, has normal skin color, and no evidence of dehydration on the clinical examination.

ACUTE OTITIS MEDIA: Bacterial (suppurative) infection of middle ear fluid indicated by acute onset of signs and symptoms accompanied by a middle ear effusion.

CLINICAL APPROACH

A simple febrile seizure is a traumatic event for the caregiver, and in almost all cases, the child will be brought in by ambulance, with the emergency medicine physician evaluating the patient after the tonic clonic activity has ceased. If the child does not appear toxic, distressed, or hemodynamically unstable, a period of observation is recommended. During this period (usually under 1 hour), the clinician should have a discussion with the caregiver and EMS regarding the duration of the event, recent illnesses, and new medications. Additional useful history includes any possible exposures to chemicals or medications in the household and if there exists a family history of seizure disorders. Also, documentation of a fever greater than 38.0°C should be obtained, and antipyretic medications can be administered (oral or rectal based on the infants mental status).

A thorough physical examination should be performed, looking specifically for any source of infection and clinical signs that are worrisome for bacterial meningitis (petechial rash, nuchal rigidity, failure to fully engage or to return to baseline level of awareness, etc). The child's entire body should be examined for any signs of trauma or abuse such as old ecchymoses, scratches, or scars. The provider should observe the interaction between the child and care giver to raise or lowers ones suspicion for possible abuse.

For infants that meet the strict definition of a simple febrile seizure, further testing (serum electrolytes, glucose, lumbar puncture, and neuroimaging) is not warranted. Multiple retrospective studies have demonstrated the extremely low incidence of bacterial meningitis in children with a simple febrile seizure and no clinical signs of meningitis. Unfortunately, since the clinical presentation of bacterial meningitis can be more subtle in children younger than 12 months of age, some experts recommend lumbar puncture even for simple febrile seizures in this population (6 months to 12 months).

Infants with concurrent infections (bacterial enteritis, urinary tract infection, or otitis media) with a simple febrile seizure should be treated for the underlying illness, not changing the standard management. This child was found to have a case of acute otitis media (AOM).

Acute Otitis Media

The diagnosis of AOM requires a middle ear effusion and signs of middle ear inflammation. The disease exists on a spectrum with otitis media with effusion, which lacks a bacterial infection or inflammation. Diagnosis of a middle ear effusion can be confirmed on otoscopy by finding bubbles or an air-fluid level and a tympanic membrane that is abnormally colored (not translucent), opaque, and/or not mobile with pneumatic pressure. Acute inflammation can either be confirmed by a history of fever and ear pain (or tugging) or direct visualization of a bulging and red tympanic membrane.

Streptococcus pneumoniae, nontypeable *Haemophilus influenzae*, and *Moraxella catarrhalis* are thought to cause over 90% of cases of AOM; however, current vaccine patterns may alter future etiologies. Complications of AOM are rare, but include hearing loss, tympanic membrane perforation, and mastoiditis. Of most concern in this case would be the rare complication of intracranial extension causing meningitis, brain abscess, or central venous thrombosis. These complications must be entertained if AOM is encountered in the setting of a seizure, especially if the child experienced a complex febrile seizure.

There exists much controversy over when to treat AOM with antibiotics. Most professional guidelines recommend any child younger than the age of 2 be treated with antibiotics and children older than the age of 2 may be treated with a "watchful waiting" approach if they have mild or moderate symptoms. Amoxicillin remains the drug of choice. The widespread use of antibiotics in the developed world is widely thought to be responsible for the low incidence of severe complications of AOM seen in the ED.

Risk of Seizure Recurrence

One-third of children who have a simple febrile seizure will experience another by the age of 6 years old. Children who experience a simple febrile seizure have a small increase in their likelihood of developing epilepsy, but the risk is still only 1% in children that have had a simple febrile seizure.

Prevention and Treatment

Antibiotic and/or antipyretic therapy has not been shown to decrease the recurrence rates of simple febrile seizures. Caretakers can often feel overwhelmed in an effort to reduce the fever to prevent another seizure and must be reassured that such measures have not been shown to reduce recurrence.

Continuous antiepileptic medications (eg, valproic acid, phenobarbital, etc.) are not recommended for first-time febrile seizures.

Case Resolution

The toddler discussed above is observed in the emergency department for 1 hour. He is noted to be playful, active, and in no distress. After a careful physical examination, the child is discharged home with his mother to follow-up with his pediatrician. Parents should be instructed to return to the emergency department immediately for repeat seizure, change in behavior, vomiting, etc. An expectation should be shared that the AOM should improve within 72 hours of antibiotic treatment, and if not, they should return to their pediatrician or the emergency department. As with any pediatric patient, an attempt should be made to contact the patient's primary pediatrician prior to leaving the ED.

COMPREHENSIVE QUESTIONS

34.1 A 2-year-old toddler is brought in by her family after a seizure episode today. The family states that the child was in her normal state of health when they noticed her entire body jerking rhythmically for several minutes, during which she did not respond to their voice. After 1 hour, the child remained somnolent and minimally responsive at home and was brought to the ED for evaluation. The mother states the infant was coughing and having clear nasal discharge for the past 24 hours, but otherwise well. The mother, a 26-year-old G4 woman, reports that the toddler was born vaginally at term after an uneventful pregnancy. His birth weight was 3100 g, and he was discharged on the second day. The mother states the child received his 2-month vaccinations and has been feeding well today. The vital signs on the chart include a temperature of 39.0°C (102.2°F) (rectal), a heart rate of 140 beats per minute, a respiratory rate of 30 per minute, and a systolic blood pressure of 80 mm Hg. On the initial evaluation (about 30 minutes after the child is brought to the emergency department), the child is somnolent and not at baseline mental status per the mother. Further evaluation finds no physical examination abnormalities other than mild clear nasal discharge. The child has a normal cardiac, lung and skin examination. Which of the following criteria indicates this was a complex febrile seizure?

A.   Age of the child involved

B.   Height of the fever

C.   Generalized tonic-clonic nature of the seizure

D.   Lack of return to baseline mental status after convulsion

E.   Preceding upper respiratory infection symptoms

34.2 A 16-month-old child is brought in by EMS after an episode of shaking visualized by mother that lasted 3 minutes. On arrival to the ED, the child is back to baseline mental status as per mother. The mother states the infant was coughing for the past 24 hours, but otherwise well. The mother, a 22-year-old G1 woman, reports that he was born vaginally at term after an uneventful pregnancy. The mother states the child received his 2-month vaccinations and has been playful and active but was noted to have a mild nonproductive cough for 2 days. The vital signs on the chart include a temperature of 39.3°C (102.7°F) (rectal), a heart rate of 150 beats per minute, a respiratory rate of 34 breaths per minute, and a systolic blood pressure of 80 mm Hg. On the initial evaluation, the child is well appearing, well perfused, and in no respiratory distress. The child has a normal cardiac, pulmonary, and has no rashes. Discharge instructions to the parent of the above toddler should include:

A. Recommended use of around-the-clock antipyretic therapy

B. Recommend beginning continuous anticonvulsive medications to prevent development of epilepsy.

C. Outpatient neurologic testing including electroencephalography

D. Rectal diazepam if the child becomes febrile again to prevent further seizures

E. Appropriate follow-up with the toddler's pediatrician and reassurance

34.3 A 36-month-old toddler is brought in by EMS after an episode of shaking visualized by mother that lasted 12 minutes. On arrival to the ED, the child is resting comfortable in the bed with his mother. The mother states the toddler was tugging at his left ear and coughing for the past 2 days, but otherwise well. The mother, a 31-year-old G4 woman, reports that he was born vaginally at term after an uneventful pregnancy. The toddler has received all of his vaccinations and never had a seizure in the past. The vital signs on the chart include a temperature of 38.4°C (101.1°F) (rectal), a heart rate of 140 beats per minute, a respiratory rate of 22 per minute, and a systolic blood pressure of 110 mm Hg. On the initial evaluation, the child is well appearing, well perfused, and in no respiratory distress. The oropharynx is injected with injected pharyngeal tonsils. The left tympanic membrane is erythematous and nonmobile during air insufflation. The child has a normal cardiac, pulmonary, and has no rashes. What is the most appropriate management of the toddler?

A. Obtain laboratory testing (CBC) to determine the presence of an underlying infection

B. Neuroimaging to determine the presence of an underlying CNS infection

C. Treatment of the otitis media (OM) with conservative therapy (NSAIDs) and instructions to follow up with the child pediatrician in 24 hours

D. Lumbar puncture to determine a meningeal infection

E. Inpatient admission for ENT consultation

ANSWER

34.1 **D.** A simple febrile seizure is characterized by strict criteria. If the child does not return to their baseline mental status shortly after convulsion, even in the setting of fever, it is considered a complex febrile seizure, and alternative causes must be explored.

34.2 **E.** Research has shown that a simple febrile seizure cannot be prevented by antipyretics or antiepileptics. After a first occurrence, the risk of future epilepsy is low, and no action need be taken initially as long as the symptoms fit the strict criteria for simple febrile seizure.

34.3 **C.** This patient had a simple febrile seizure so there is a very low suspicion for a direct extension of the acute otitis media into the intracranial space. The AOM is the cause of the fever and likely related seizure. Given the patient is over 2 years old, expert recommendations endorse a watchful waiting approach to treatment. An alternative acceptable approach would be to provide antibiotics from the ED, but still ensure close follow-up with the patient's pediatrician.

REFERENCES

American Academy of Pediatrics Subcommittee on Management of Acute Otitis Media. Diagnosis and management of acute otitis media. *Pediatrics*. 2004;113:1451.

Febrile seizures: clinical practice guideline for the long-term management of the child with simple febrile seizures. *Pediatrics*. Jun 2008;121(6):1281-1286.

Fetveit A. Assessment of febrile seizures in children. *Eur J Pediatr*. Jan 2008;167(1):17-27.

Hampers LC, Spina LA. Evaluation and management of pediatric febrile seizures in the emergency department. *Emerg Med Clin North Am*. Feb 2011;29(1):83-93.

A 57-year-old man presents to the emergency department (ED) with a 1-month history of worsening low back pain. The pain radiates down the back of both legs and suddenly increased yesterday. For the past 2 days, the patient has been having difficulty voiding and has had "to force the urine out." He has also noticed that the skin around his anus feels numb when he wipes with toilet tissue. He has worked in a warehouse for 30 years but has been on light duty for the past month due to his back pain. He denies prior trauma to or surgery on his back.

▶ What is the most likely diagnosis?
▶ What is the next diagnostic step?

ANSWERS TO CASE 35:

Low Back Pain

Summary: A 57-year-old warehouse worker has a 1-month history of worsening low back pain with radiation bilaterally to his legs. The pain increased suddenly and is now associated with perianal numbness and difficulty voiding. He denies trauma to his back or prior surgery.

- **Most likely diagnosis:** Cauda equine syndrome (CES)

- **Next diagnostic step:** Magnetic resonance imaging (MRI) of the lumbar and sacral spine

ANALYSIS

Objectives

1. Review the possible etiologies of low back pain.

2. Learn how to evaluate a patient with low back pain.

3. Identify the "red flags" associated with serious causes of low back pain.

Considerations

Low back pain is a common complaint and can be caused by a multitude of disease processes. Although benign mechanical causes are most common, the ED physician must consider the "cannot miss" diagnoses: cauda equina syndrome, spinal fracture, spinal infection (epidural abscess or spondylitis), and malignancy. A careful history and physical examination are important to identify "red flags" that may herald the presence of serious disease (Table 35–1). Most patients with back pain do not

Table 35–1 • "RED FLAG" SIGNS AND SYMPTOMS OF LOW BACK PAIN
Patients younger than 18 years old or older than 50 years
Significant trauma (or mild trauma in patients older than 50 years)
Chronic steroid use
Osteoporosis
History of cancer
Recent infection
Immunocompromise
History of intravenous drug use
Pain worse at night, lasting longer than 6 weeks, or refractory to analgesics and rest
Associated systemic symptoms (fever, unexplained weight loss, malaise, night sweats, diaphoresis, nausea, syncope)
Acute onset
Use of anticoagulants or coagulopathy
Abnormal vital signs (including unequal blood pressures or pulse deficits)
Neurologic deficits (including extremity weakness, numbness, paresthesias, loss of rectal sphincter tone, urinary retention)

require any diagnostic studies in the ED. However, if a serious etiology is suspected, laboratory studies and imaging may be necessary. In general, pain control is a high priority for these patients. If the patient is critically ill, stabilization of the ABCs and surgical consultation may be needed.

APPROACH TO:
Low Back Pain

CLINICAL APPROACH

Back pain is the second most common complaint that impels people to visit their primary care physicians. Seventy to ninety percent of adults suffer from acute low back pain during their lifetime. The differential diagnosis of low back pain is extensive. Common causes include muscle strain, ligamentous injury, osteoarthritis, disk herniation, spondylolisthesis, and fracture. Infectious etiologies are epidural abscess, spondylitis, diskitis, and herpes zoster. Malignancies that cause low back pain may be primary or, more commonly, metastatic. Rheumatologic diseases such as ankylosing spondylitis and Reiter syndrome are other considerations. Back pain may also be referred from various gastrointestinal, genitourinary, gynecologic, and vascular sources (most ominously from an abdominal aortic aneurysm). Miscellaneous causes include sickle cell pain crisis and functional back pain.

The history and physical examination are important to distinguish benign causes from potentially life-threatening ones. Table 35–2 describes the typical findings for patients with the "cannot miss" causes of low back pain. Important historical questions include location, duration, and onset of pain; aggravating and alleviating factors; associated symptoms; work history; history of trauma; and past medical history (including comorbidities, medications, and family history).

The ED physician should note the patient's vital signs because any abnormalities may herald a life-threatening disease process (eg, hypotension due to sepsis or a ruptured abdominal aortic aneurysm). The physical examination should screen for signs of systemic disease and possible sources of referred back pain. If possible, gait and range of motion of the back should be observed. Inspection of the back can identify bony abnormalities such as scoliosis and skin lesions that suggest infection (erythema, warmth) or trauma (swelling, ecchymosis). The back should be palpated to isolate the area of maximal tenderness. Point tenderness over the spinous processes may indicate a destructive lesion of the spine. Pain that is severe or excessive has increased suspicion of acute spinal infection or AAA. The neurologic examination should focus on identifying any focal weakness, dermatomal sensory loss, and decreased or absent deep tendon reflexes. Straight-leg raise (SLR) testing involves the examiner passively elevating the supine patient's leg (with knee extended) 30 to 70 degrees. If the SLR elicits radicular pain in the low back radiating down the leg to below the knee, it is indicative of sciatic nerve root irritation. This test is more sensitive (80%) than specific (40%). A positive crossed SLR (elevation of the unaffected leg causes radicular pain in the affected leg) is very specific (90%) but insensitive (25%). Digital rectal examination should

Table 35–2 • "CANNOT MISS" CAUSES OF LOW BACK PAIN				
Disease	Etiology	Clinical Presentation	Diagnostics	Treatment
Cauda equina syndrome	Central disk herniation multiple, bilateral nerve roots	Bilateral leg pain and weakness, urinary retention and overflow incontinence, decreased rectal tone, saddle anesthesia	CT, MRI (preferred imaging)	Intravenous dexamethasone, emergent surgical decompression
Spinal fracture	Significant blunt trauma or minimal trauma in patient with osteoporosis	Midline tenderness along spine	Plain x-ray, CT	Orthopedic consultation. May require admission
Spinal infection	Most commonly due to *Staphylococcus aureus*. Risk factors: intravenous drug use, elderly, immunocompromised, alcoholism, recent bacterial infection or back trauma	Back pain (even at rest/night), fever, midline cultures, tenderness along spine. Focal neurologic deficits as late finding	CBC, ESR, blood plain x-ray, CT, myelography, MRI (preferred imaging)	Intravenous antibiotics, surgical drainage and decompression
Malignancy	Most commonly metastatic (breast, prostate, lung common). May also be primary (eg, multiple myeloma, leukemia, lymphoma)	Pain lasting longer than 1 month, worse at night, unrelieved by rest; unexplained weight loss; mild to moderate spinal tenderness	CBC, ESR, plain x-ray, CT, MRI	May benefit from intravenous dexamethasone and radiation therapy

Abbreviations: CT = computed tomography; MRI = magnetic resonance imaging; CBC = complete blood count; ESR = erythrocyte sedimentation rate.

be performed on patients with severe pain or neurologic deficits to assess sphincter tone and perianal sensation.

Most patients who present with low back pain do not require any diagnostic tests or imaging studies in the ED. The history and physical examination can help separate the majority of patients with simple, self-limited musculoskeletal back pain from the minority with more serious underlying causes. If rheumatologic causes, malignancy, or infection are concerns, a complete blood count, erythrocyte sedimentation rate, and urinalysis may be helpful. Indications for plain x-rays include age less than 18 years or older than 50 years; recent trauma; history or suspicion of malignancy; pain lasting longer than 4 to 6 weeks; history of fever, intravenous drug use, or immunocompromised; and progressive neurologic deficits. Further imaging by computed tomography or magnetic resonance imaging may be required if a strong suspicion of fracture, spinal infection, malignancy, or cauda equina syndrome exists.

Treatment

If a patient with low back pain is hemodynamically unstable, cardiac monitoring and resuscitation with intravenous fluids is mandated. If infection is suspected, antibiotics should be administered. Stable patients benefit from pain management. Depending on the severity of the pain, intravenous narcotics such as morphine or fentanyl may be required. If the pain is less severe, oral narcotics or nonsteroidal anti-inflammatory drugs (NSAIDs) may be sufficient. Benzodiazepines may be useful adjuncts to provide some muscle relaxation and sedation.

Patients with simple musculoskeletal back pain can be treated with pain control (primarily acetaminophen and NSAIDs). Oral narcotics may be used for a short period of time if the pain is not adequately controlled by the aforementioned medications. Application of local heat or ice may provide some pain relief. Although strict bed rest was once the recommended treatment, resumption of normal daily activities has been shown to hasten recovery and resolution of pain. Strenuous exercise should be avoided until the acute pain has subsided. Nearly all patients recover with conservative management within 4 to 6 weeks.

Admission should be considered for patients with underlying etiologies that require inpatient management, those with abnormal vital signs, those requiring intravenous narcotics for pain control, and those who cannot walk.

COMPREHENSION QUESTIONS

35.1 Which of the following describes the most common location of herniated disc of the lumbar spine region?

A. L1-L2

B. L2-L3

C. L3-L4

D. L4-L5

35.2 Which of the following is the most sensitive finding for cauda equina syndrome?

A. Decreased anal sphincter tone

B. Saddle anesthesia

C. Urinary retention

D. Weakness or numbness in the low extremities

35.3 A 27-year-old woman with a 1-week history of progressive pain radiating from the lumbar spine down the back of the leg presents to the ED. Her physical examination is normal except for complaints of back pain with movement. Which of the following is the most appropriate imaging test?

A. No imaging is necessary; attempt conservative therapy.

B. Obtain plain films of the lumbar spine.

C. Perform MRI.

D. Perform CT.

ANSWERS

35.1 **D.** The L4-L5 interspace is the most commonly affected.

35.2 **C.** Urinary retention with overflow incontinence is the most sensitive finding for cauda equina syndrome (90%).

35.3 **A.** No imaging is necessary. If the patient has no risk factors in the history and physical examination for serious disease other than sciatica, treat conservatively and do not perform any diagnostic tests in the ED.

CLINICAL PEARLS

▶ Most patients with acute low back pain have resolution of symptoms within 4 to 6 weeks.

▶ Pain that interferes with sleep, significant unintentional weight loss, or fever suggests an infectious or neoplastic cause of back pain. Low back pain with associated bowel and bladder dysfunction is suspicious for cauda equina syndrome.

▶ Most patients do not require diagnostic tests or imaging studies. However, further testing may be advisable if there is a concern for rheumatologic, infectious, neoplastic processes; fracture; or cauda equina syndrome.

▶ Pain control is important in the management of patients with low back pain. Acetaminophen, NSAIDs, and narcotics are all viable options.

REFERENCES

Deyo RA, Weinstein JN. Low back pain. *N Engl J Med*. 2001;344:363-370.

Frohna WJ, Della-Giustina D. Neck and back pain. *Tintinalli's Emergency Medicine: A Comprehensive Study Guide*. 7th ed. New York, NY: McGraw-Hill; 2011; Chapter 276.

Hermance TC, Boggs LR. Chapter 19: Arthitis and back pain. Stone CK, Humphries RL: *Current Diagnosis and Treatment: Emergency Medicine*. 6th ed. Available at: http://www.accessmedicine.com/content.aspx?aID=3100883.

Jarvik JG, Deyo RA. Diagnostic evaluation of low back pain with emphasis on imaging. *Ann Intern Med*. 2002;137:586-597.

Marx JA, Hockberger RS, Walls RM, eds. *Rosen's Emergency Medicine: Concepts and Clinical Practice*. 6th ed. Philadelphia, PA: Mosby Elsevier; 2006:260-268, 701-717.

Morris EW, Di Paola M, Vallence R, Waddell G. Diagnosis and decision making in lumbar disk prolapse and nerve entrapment. *Spine*. 1986;11:436.

A 70-year-old woman is transferred from a nursing home to the emergency department (ED) due to fever and shortness of breath. Per her daughter, the patient has had a productive cough for 2 days and became more short of breath and less responsive earlier today. The patient's past medical history is significant for diabetes mellitus, hypertension, and high cholesterol. Her vital signs include temperature 38.9°C (102.1°F), heart rate 104 beats per minute, blood pressure 130/85 mm Hg, respiratory rate 28 breaths per minute, and room air oxygen saturation 91% (96% with 3-L oxygen by nasal cannula). On examination, she is awake but slow to answer questions. The daughter states that her mother is usually more alert than this. Her skin is dry and warm to touch. Her heart sounds are regular and mildly tachycardic without any S_3 or S_4. On auscultation, she has rhonchi at the right lung base. She does not have any jugular venous distention, lower extremity edema, or calf tenderness.

► What is the most likely diagnosis?
► How should this patient be managed?

ANSWERS TO CASE 36:

Bacterial Pneumonia

Summary: A 70-year-old woman is sent from a nursing home due to fever, productive cough, and shortness of breath. On examination, she is febrile, mildly tachycardic, tachypneic, and hypoxic on room air. She has rhonchi in the right lung base but does not have any signs of congestive heart failure or a peripheral deep venous thrombosis.

- **Most likely diagnosis:** Healthcare-associated pneumonia

- **Management:** Supplemental oxygen, intravenous antibiotics, blood and sputum cultures, and admission

ANALYSIS

Objectives

1. Define community-acquired versus hospital-acquired versus healthcare-associated pneumonia.

2. Describe the various clinical presentations of pneumonia.

3. Learn the management of pneumonia including the best choices for empiric antibiotic administration.

Considerations

This 70-year-old woman presents with history and physical examination findings consistent with pneumonia. **Pneumonia is the most common cause of death from infectious disease and the seventh leading cause of death overall in the United States.** Clinical presentations and common etiologic organisms vary among different patient populations. Because this patient is a nursing home resident, she is at risk for infection with multidrug-resistant bacteria. Pneumonia may be associated with significant morbidity and mortality, especially among immunocompromised and elderly patients. However, prompt initiation of therapy can result in improved patient outcomes. Treatment includes appropriate empiric antibiotics, disease assessment, and respiratory support.

APPROACH TO:
Bacterial Pneumonia

DEFINITIONS

COMMUNITY-ACQUIRED PNEUMONIA (CAP): Pneumonia that occurs in a patient living in the general population or community.

HOSPITAL-ACQUIRED PNEUMONIA (HAP): Pneumonia that arises 48 hours or more after hospital admission. HAP includes ventilator-associated pneumonia (VAP; infection which develops more than 48 to 72 hours after intubation).

HEALTHCARE-ASSOCIATED PNEUMONIA (HCAP): Pneumonia that occurs in a patient with substantial healthcare contact (intravenous antibiotics, chemotherapy, or wound care within the past 30 days; nursing home or long-term care facility resident; hospitalization for 2 or more days within the past 90 days; hemodialysis).

CLINICAL APPROACH

Pneumonia is caused by aspiration or inhalation of pathogenic organisms into the lungs or less commonly by hematogenous spread. Thus patients with impaired host defenses (mucociliary clearance or overall immune system) and those with an increased risk of bacteremia or aspiration are at higher risk for developing pneumonia. These higher-risk patients include the elderly, smokers, those with an impaired gag reflex, and HIV-positive patients. Viral respiratory infections can also lead to the development of a superimposed bacterial pneumonia.

The most common causes of CAP are *Streptococcus pneumoniae*, *Haemophilus influenzae*, *Legionella*, *Mycoplasma*, and *Chlamydia*. HAP and HCAP are most commonly due to aerobic gram-negative bacilli such as *Pseudomonas aeruginosa*, *Escherichia coli*, *Klebsiella pneumoniae*, and *Acinetobacter*. Aspiration pneumonias are often polymicrobial, including anaerobic organisms such as *Peptostreptococcus*, *Bacteroides*, and *Fusobacterium*. Immunocompromised patients are at risk for infection with uncommon bacterial, fungal, and viral pathogens (eg, *Aspergillus*, cytomegalovirus, tuberculosis, *Pneumocystis jiroveci*). Although the specific etiologic organism cannot be identified with certainty without serologic or microbiologic confirmation, historical information may help narrow the list of likely pathogens based on clinical symptomatology and risk factors for specific infections (Table 36–1).

The typical presentation of bacterial pneumonia includes fever, productive cough with purulent sputum, dyspnea, and pleuritic chest pain. However, patients at the extremes of age may have minimal or no respiratory symptoms. Infants may be brought to the ED for fever, irritability, or respiratory distress. The elderly may present with altered mental status, a decline in baseline function, or sepsis. Patients with impaired immune systems may also present atypically.

The physical examination may reveal fever, tachypnea, tachycardia, or hypoxia. Severe illness may be heralded by severe respiratory distress, marked hypoxia, cyanosis, altered mental status, or hypotension. On auscultation, wheezes, rhonchi, rales,

Table 36–1 • SPECIFIC ORGANISMS, RISK FACTORS, AND CLASSIC PRESENTATIONS		
Organism	Risk Factors	Classic Clinical Presentation
Chlamydia	Exposure to infected individuals	Mild subacute illness; fever, sore throat, nonproductive cough
Haemophilus influenzae	Diabetes, chronic obstructive pulmonary disease, malignancy, alcoholism, malnutrition, sickle cell disease, immunocompromised	Insidious worsening of chronic cough and sputum production (acute onset less common)
Klebsiella pneumoniae	Diabetes, alcoholism, chronic debilitating illness, aspiration risk	Acute onset of fever, rigors, chest pain, "currant jelly" sputum
Legionella	Smokers, transplant patients, immunocompromised, chronic lung disease	Severe illness with high fever, lethargy, cough. May have associated gastrointestinal symptoms (abdominal pain, vomiting, diarrhea), myocarditis, pancreatitis, pyelonephritis, sinusitis
Mycoplasma	Exposure to infected individuals	Subacute illness; sore throat, cough, headache, fever, malaise; may have associated bullous myringitis, rash, arthritis
Pseudomonas aeruginosa	Prolonged hospitalization, nursing home resident, high-dose steroids, structural lung disease	Severe pneumonia, cyanosis, confusion
Staphylococcus aureus	Intravenous drug abuse, recent influenza infection, chronic lung disease, immunocompromised, aspiration risk	Insidious onset of low-grade fever, dyspnea, sputum production
Streptococcus pneumoniae	Diabetes, sickle cell disease, splenectomy, malignancy, alcoholism, cardiovascular disease, immunocompromised, elderly, children <2 years	Abrupt onset of single shaking chill, pleuritic chest pain, bloody or rust-colored sputum

or bronchial breath sounds may be appreciated. Decreased breath sounds and dullness to percussion suggest the presence of a pleural effusion. Patients at the extremes of age and those who are immunosuppressed may have atypical examination findings. For example, the elderly are often afebrile (or even hypothermic). In these patients, tachypnea may be the most sensitive sign of pneumonia

A chest x-ray is an important diagnostic tool in patients with suspected pneumonia as pulmonary infiltrates will confirm the diagnosis. In some cases, a patient with an initial negative chest radiograph may have infiltrates that "blossom" after rehydration or that are visualized using other types of imaging (eg, computed tomography is more sensitive than plain x-ray). The radiographic appearance of the infiltrates may suggest (but not definitively identify) a possible etiologic organism.

For example, lobar consolidation is typical of *Streptococcus pneumoniae* or *Klebsiella*. *Staphylococcus aureus*, *Pseudomonas*, and *Haemophilus influenzae* typically cause multilobar disease. Patchy infiltrates are consistent with *Legionella*, *Mycoplasma*, and chlamydial infection. Aspiration pneumonias usually result in infiltrates in dependent areas of the lungs (posterior segment of upper lobe or superior segment of lower lobe). Cavitary lesions, pleural effusions, and pneumatoceles may also be seen with bacterial pneumonias. Immunocompromised patients are especially likely to have atypical radiographic findings (eg, more diffuse or multilobar infiltrates).

Treatment

The initial management of patients with pneumonia includes assessment and, if needed, cardiopulmonary stabilization which may require supplemental oxygen or intubation for patients with severe respiratory distress or respiratory failure.

Antibiotics should be initiated promptly in order to decrease mortality and improve patient outcome. Antibiotics are usually chosen based on the most likely pathogens as determined by assessment of risk factors, clinical presentation (including severity of symptoms and presence of sepsis), and radiographic findings. Healthy patients without any use of antimicrobials in the past 3 months with presumed CAP are best treated with a macrolide (azithromycin). Patients with comorbid diseases or recent antimicrobial use should receive a respiratory fluoroquinolone (levofloxacin) or a β-lactam (cefpodoxime) plus a macrolide as a reasonable alternative. Patients admitted to the ICU require antibiotics that cover a broader range of organisms. A β-lactam (ceftazidime) plus either azithromycin or a fluoroquinolone may be used. If *Pseudomonas* or community-acquired methicillin-resistant *Staphylococcus aureus* (MRSA) infection is suspected, additional antimicrobial coverage is required. If concern for aspiration pneumonia consider anaerobic coverage such as clindamycin.

Patients with concern for HAP or HCAP who are at a risk for multidrug-resistant pathogens should receive a 3-drug combination therapy: (1) antipseudomonal cephalosporin (cefepime, ceftazidime), antipseudomonal carbapenem (imipenem or meropenem), or piperacillin-tazobactam; (2) antipseudomonal fluoroquinolone (ciprofloxacin or levofloxacin); and (3) anti-MRSA coverage (linezolid or vancomycin).

Those without risk factors for multi-drug–resistant (MDR) organisms may be treated with a single agent: ceftriaxone, ampicillin/sulbactam, ciprofloxacin, moxifloxacin, levofloxacin, or ertapenem.

Disposition

Factors to be considered include patient's age and comorbidities, physical examination and diagnostic findings, ability to tolerate oral medications, social situation, and ability to obtain close follow-up. Obviously, any patient with unstable vital signs, respiratory distress, hypoxia, severe infection, or intractable vomiting requires a hospital stay.

COMPREHENSION QUESTIONS

36.1 A 55-year-old man with a history of alcoholism complains of a month of subjective fevers, productive cough with greenish sputum tinged with blood. Examination reveals poor dentition with halitosis, coarse breath sounds, and clubbing of his fingers. On chest x-ray, there is a 2-cm cavitary lesion with an air-fluid level in the right lower lobe. Which of the following is the most appropriate treatment?

A. Isolate the patient and initiate antituberculosis treatment.

B. Start intravenous clindamycin.

D. Schedule a bronchoscopy.

E. Discharge with oral amoxicillin-clavulanate.

36.2 A 25-year-old woman with no past medical history presents with fever and productive cough. Her vital signs include temperature 38.8°C (101.9°F), heart rate 115 beats per minute, respirations 20 breaths per minute, blood pressure 115/89 mm Hg, and pulse oximetry 97% on room air. On examination, rhonchi are present in the right lung field. Chest x-ray shows a right middle lobe infiltrate. Which of the following should her treatment include?

A. Admission for intravenous ceftriaxone and vancomycin

B. Admission for intravenous ceftriaxone and azithromycin

C. Outpatient treatment with oral azithromycin

D. Outpatient treatment with oral amoxicillin

36.3 A 65-year-old smoker with past medical history of chronic obstructive pulmonary disease and diabetes presents with productive cough, chills, and pleuritic chest pain. His vital signs include temperature 38.9°C (102.1°F), heart rate 110 beats per minute, blood pressure 140/89 mm Hg, respiratory rate 24 breaths per minute, and pulse oximetry 92% on room air. On examination, he has a barrel chest with diffuse wheezes bilaterally. His chest x-ray reveals a left-lower-lobe infiltrate and pleural effusion. Which of the following is the best treatment?

A. Outpatient treatment with azithromycin

B. Outpatient treatment with levofloxacin

C. Inpatient treatment with ceftriaxone, azithromycin, and vancomycin

D. Inpatient treatment with ceftriaxone and azithromycin

36.4 An 89-year-old was brought by ambulance from a nursing home for fever and cough. His vital signs include temperature 39.9°C (103.9°F), heart rate 120 beats per minute, blood pressure 89/69 mm Hg, respiratory rate 36 breaths per minute, and pulse oximetry 88% on a nonrebreather face mask. He is clammy and lethargic. He has coarse breath sounds bilaterally although decreased on the left. Which of the following is the most appropriate initial intervention?

A. Administer intravenous antibiotics

B. Draw blood cultures

C. Intubation

D. Obtain a chest x-ray

ANSWERS

36.1 **B.** The history of alcoholism, presence of periodontal disease, duration of illness, symptoms and signs, and radiographic findings suggest an anaerobic source. Clindamycin provides the appropriate antimicrobial coverage.

36.2 **C.** This is a healthy individual with CAP who can be treated as an outpatient with an oral macrolide. She has no risk factors for drug-resistant *Streptococcus pneumonia* nor any indications for admission.

36.3 **D.** This patient is a candidate for inpatient treatment due to his comorbidities and abnormal vital signs. However, he does not appear to require ICU admission. Thus, ceftriaxone and azithromycin are the best options of those listed.

36.4 **C.** Although these are all appropriate interventions, this patient has significant hypoxia and respiratory distress despite noninvasive supplemental oxygen administration. Thus intubation is required.

CLINICAL PEARLS

▶ Historical information may help narrow the list of likely pathogens based on clinical symptomatology and risk factors for specific infections.

▶ Patients at the extremes of age and those immunocompromised may present atypically (clinically as well as radiographically).

▶ The chest x-ray is usually the most important diagnostic study in patients with suspected pneumonia.

▶ Empiric antibiotics are chosen based on the most likely pathogens (as determined by assessment of risk factors, clinical presentation, and radiographic findings).

▶ Factors to be considered when determining need for admission include the patient's age and comorbidities, physical examination and diagnostic findings, ability to tolerate oral medications, social situation, and ability to obtain close follow-up.

REFERENCES

American Thoracic Society, Infectious Diseases Society of America. Guidelines for the management of adults with hospital-acquired, ventilator-associated, and healthcare-associated pneumonia. *Am J Respir Crit Care Med*. 2005;171:399-416.

File TM. Community-acquired pneumonia. *Lancet*. 2003;362:1991-2001.

Mandell LA, Wunderink RG, Anzueto A, et al. Infectious Diseases Society of America/American Thoracic Society consensus guidelines on the management of community-acquired pneumonia in adults. *Clin Infect Dis*. 2007;44:S27-S72.

Metlay JP, Kapoor WN, Fine MJ. Does this patient have community-acquired pneumonia? Diagnosing pneumonia by history and physical examination. *JAMA*. 1997;278:1440-1445.

Moran GJ, Talan DA. Pneumonia. In: JA Marx, RS Hockberger, RM Walls eds. *Rosen's Emergency Medicine: Concepts and Clinical Practice*. Philadelphia, PA: Mosby/Elsevier; 2010.

Niederman MS, Mandell LA, Anzueto A, et al. Guidelines for the management of adults with community-acquired pneumonia: diagnosis, assessment of severity, antimicrobial therapy, and prevention. *Am J Respir Crit Care Med*. 2001;163:1730-1754.

Read RC. Evidence-based medicine: empiric antibiotic therapy in community-acquired pneumonia. *J Infect*. 1999;39:171-178.

A 43-year-old man is brought in on an EMS (emergency medical services) stretcher after a syncopal episode. After obtaining a palpated pressure of 80 mm Hg systolic and heart rate of 120 beats per minute, EMS placed an 18-gauge IV and initiated infusing normal saline en route to the hospital. The patient relates a 3- to 4-day history of dark, tarry stools (about 3-4 times per day). Today he passed out while having a bowel movement. He is currently complaining of mild epigastric pain and lightheadedness. He denies any hematemesis, hematochezia, chest pain, shortness of breath, and any similar past episodes. He admits to drinking 1 to 2 beers each day and is not regularly under the care of a physician.

On examination, his vital signs are temperature 36.6°C (97.9°F), blood pressure 92/45 mm Hg (after 900-mL IV fluid prior to arrival), heart rate is 113 beats/minute, and respiratory rate is 24 breaths/minute. The patient is pale with dried, dark stool covering his legs. He has mild tenderness to palpation in the epigastrium but no rebound or guarding. He does not have spider angioma, gynecomastia, palmar erythema, or ascites. The rectal examination reveals grossly melanic stool.

► What is the most likely diagnosis?
► What is the best therapy?

ANSWERS TO CASE 37:
Gastrointestinal Bleeding

Summary: This 43-year-old man presents tachycardic and hypotensive after several episodes of melena.

- **Most likely diagnosis:** Upper gastrointestinal (GI) bleed with hemorrhagic shock.

- **Best therapy:** Stabilization of the ABCs, including IV access and volume resuscitation. Consider the use of blood products and proton pump inhibitors. Endoscopy is indicated for early diagnosis and treatment.

ANALYSIS

Objectives

1. Learn the differences in presentations and outcomes between upper and lower GI bleeding.

2. Understand the priorities, evaluations, and management of patients with GI hemorrhage.

Considerations

This 43-year-old man is in class III hemorrhagic shock (see Case 7), because he is hypotensive and has a heart rate of 120. These findings correlate with up 1500 to 2000 mL of acute blood loss. The most important priorities are stabilization by addressing the ABCs, including placing two large-bore intravenous lines, giving boluses of normal saline, and monitoring the blood pressure, heart rate, pulse oximetry, and urine output. Laboratory evaluations should include complete blood count (CBC), electrolytes, renal and liver function tests, coagulation studies, in addition to the typing and cross matching of blood. The main priorities are to determine whether there has been significant blood loss, maintain hemodynamic stability, and determine if the bleeding is active. After stabilization, a focused history should be taken to determine the probable etiology of the gastrointestinal bleeding. Chronic nonsteroidal anti-inflammatory drug (NSAID) or aspirin use may indicate gastritis. His history and physical examination do not reveal obvious causes or signs of portal hypertension. Although the history of tar-colored stools suggest an upper GI bleeding source and directs the initial evaluation to this source, the possibility of bleeding distal to the ligament of Treitz (lower GI bleeding) cannot be excluded at this time. An initial room-temperature water lavage via a nasogastric (NG) tube may identify gross blood or "coffee-ground" fluid, which may establish the diagnosis of upper GI bleeding, determine if the bleeding is active, and determine the rate of hemorrhage. **Upper endoscopy is likely to be the most valuable diagnostic and treatment modality of choice for this patient. Differentiation of GI bleeding patients as possessing potential upper GI bleeding sources versus lower GI bleeding sources is important early on, because patients with upper GI bleeding have significantly** greater potential for rapid and large volume hemorrhage in comparison to those with lower GI bleeding sources. Similarly, the differentiation of upper GI bleeding patients into those with variceal bleeding and those with non-variceal bleeding is helpful to begin empirical pharmacologic therapy with octreotide in those patients with suspected bleeding from a variceal source.

APPROACH TO:
GI Bleeding

CLINICAL APPROACH

GI bleeding is classified as upper or lower based on whether it arises proximal or distal to the ligament of Treitz. Common causes of upper GI bleeding include peptic ulcer disease, esophageal or gastric varices, Mallory-Weiss tear, esophagitis, and gastritis (Figure 37–1). The most common etiologies of lower GI bleeding are upper GI bleeding, hemorrhoids, diverticulosis, angiodysplasia, malignancy, inflammatory bowel disease, and infectious conditions (Figure 37–2). In children, Meckel diverticulum, polyps, volvulus, and intussusception are the common causes of GI bleeding.

GI bleeding is also classified as either overt or occult. Overt bleeding is clinically obvious bleeding that presents as hematemesis, coffee-ground emesis, melena, or hematochezia, and occult GI bleeding is when a patient presents either with clinical anemia and/or microcytic anemia from chronic GI tract blood loss. From the

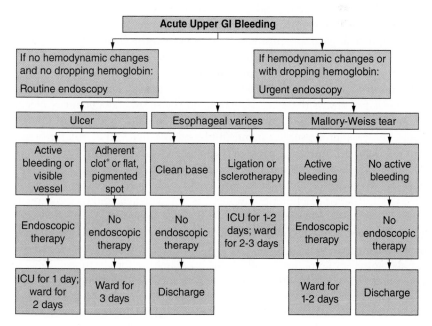

Figure 37–1. Algorithm for upper GI bleeding.

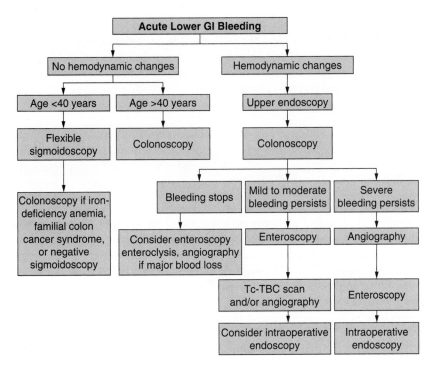

Figure 37–2. Algorithm for lower GI bleeding.

standpoint of emergency medical care, overt GI bleeding needs to be addressed on an urgent basis to resuscitate and control the bleeding source; whereas, occult GI bleeding may require treatment of symptomatic anemia and referral to a gastroenterology and/or surgical specialist to identify and treat the chronic bleeding source.

When taking a history, the clinician should focus on the nature, duration, and amount of bleeding. Classically, patients with an upper GI bleed present with hematemesis and melena, while hematochezia suggests a lower GI source. However, this is not always the case, depending on the speed and amount of bleeding. It is important to ask about syncope, weakness, chest pain, dyspnea, and confusion because these symptoms suggest significant blood loss. In addition, risk factor assessment may help determine the cause of the bleeding (Table 37–1).

During the physical examination, careful attention should be paid to the vital signs and for evidence of hypovolemic shock (tachypnea, tachycardia, hypotension). Cool, pale, or diaphoretic skin suggests hypovolemia, and pale conjunctiva, nail beds, or mucous membranes suggest anemia. If stigmata of chronic liver disease (jaundice, caput medusae, spider angiomata, palmar erythema, and gynecomastia) are present, variceal bleeding should be considered as a potential bleeding possibility. The abdominal examination should focus on searching for peritoneal signs, such as guarding and rebound, although most patients with GI bleeding do not exhibit abdominal pain.

Bedside testing includes a rectal examination to check for hemorrhoids, anal fissures, and occult blood in the stool. All patients should have a nasogastric tube with

Table 37–1 • GI BLEEDING SOURCES AND CLINICAL FEATURES/RISK FACTORS	
Etiology	**Risk Factors**
Esophageal and/or gastric varices	Alcoholism, cirrhosis
Peptic ulcer disease	*Helicobacter pylori* infection, NSAID use, alcohol use, heredity, tobacco use
Gastritis	NSAID use, alcohol use, steroids, burns, major trauma, head injury
Mallory-Weiss tear	Recent vomiting or retching, alcohol use, esophagitis
Aortoenteric fistula	History of prior abdominal aortic reconstruction
Diverticulosis	High-fat diet, older age
Colon cancer	Weight loss, change in bowel habits
Angiodysplasia	Older age, cardiovascular comorbidities

room temperature normal saline (NS) or water lavage. If blood is present (bright red or "coffee ground"), an upper GI source is more likely.

After IV access is obtained, blood should be sent for complete blood count, electrolytes, blood urea nitrogen (BUN)/creatinine, coagulation studies, and type and screen or cross-match. In patients with chest pain, dysrhythmia, or risk factors for coronary artery disease, an electrocardiogram (ECG) should be obtained.

Treatment

Treatment begins with stabilizing the ABCs. Intubation may be necessary to protect the patient's airway and in preventing aspiration. **IV access (large-bore peripherals or central) is a high priority.** Volume resuscitation should begin with 2 L of NS or lactated Ringer solution. For patients who are hemodynamically unstable after crystalloid infusion, have ongoing blood loss, or whose hemoglobin is less than 7 mg/dL, packed red blood cells (PRBCs) should be transfused. **Fresh-frozen plasma and vitamin K** may be indicated in patients with coagulopathies caused by **liver disease** or anticoagulation therapy. As a general rule, **a proton pump inhibitor should be given to patients with upper GI bleeding to decrease rebleeding rates.** Surgery is indicated for massive or refractory bleeding.

In patients with variceal bleeding, somatostatin analog such as octreotide, or vasopressin, can be helpful. However, vasopressin has fallen out of favor because of the side effects and the risk of end-organ ischemia.

In patient with massive variceal bleeding, balloon tamponade with a **Sengstaken-Blakemore tube may be useful for the temporary control of bleeding, while arrangements for definitive therapy are made.**

Various modalities exist to identify the source of bleeding. In upper GI bleeding patients, endoscopy is the study of choice because the procedure can also be therapeutic through use of lasers, electrocoagulation, sclerosant injections, clip placements, and band ligations. For lower GI bleeds, anoscopy, sigmoidoscopy, or colonoscopy are preferred for the localization of bleeding sources. Tagged red blood cell (RBC) scans are an alternative in stable patients. When lower GI bleeding that is massive or continuous, angiography can be useful to localize the bleeding, and for some cases angiography-directed embolizations can be applied to stop the bleeding.

In general, patients with lower GI bleeding rarely exhibit hemodynamic instability unless the process has gone on unrecognized. Similarly, most lower GI bleeding episodes are self-limiting. The treatments for lower GI bleeding are therefore less urgent than treatments for upper GI bleeding, and the majority of patients with lower GI bleeding can be managed outside of an ICU environment following their management in the emergency department. The number one priority following the initial the management of lower GI bleeding patient is localization of the bleeding site, so that endoscopic, interventional radiology procedure, or surgical therapy can be implemented in the unusual event that the bleeding does not stop.

COMPREHENSION QUESTIONS

37.1 Which of the following conditions is a risk factor for peptic ulcer disease?
   A. Age greater than 50
   B. Estrogen replacement therapy
   C. Acetaminophen use
   D. *Chlamydia trachomatis*
   E. *Helicobacter pylori infection*

37.2 A 43-year-old man complains of acute onset of vomiting bright red blood. He denies alcohol use and history of peptic ulcer disease. He complains of dizziness, appears anxious, and his blood pressure is 120/70 mm Hg and heart rate is 90 beats per minute. Which of the following is the best next step in managing his condition?
   A. Morphine sulfate
   B. Endoscopic examination
   C. Chest radiograph
   D. Intravenous fluid resuscitation
   E. Orotracheal intubation

37.3 In the patient described in Question 37.2, which of the following modalities is best to identify the source of bleeding?
   A. Tagged RBC scan
   B. Endoscopy
   C. Angiography
   D. Laparotomy
   E. Serial hemoglobin determination

37.4 A 58-year-old woman is brought into the ED complaining of bright red bleeding per rectum that was of acute onset. She denies abdominal pain. She is hemodynamically stable. Which of the following is the most likely etiology of her condition?

A. Varices

B. Gastritis

C. Diverticulosis

D. Mallory-Weiss tear

E. Peptic ulcer disease

ANSWERS

37.1 **E.** Risk factors for peptic ulcer disease include *H pylori* infection, NSAID use, alcohol use, heredity, and tobacco use.

37.2 **D.** Stabilization of the patient is always the first priority. The ABCs come first; assuming that his airway and breathing are stable, then circulation is next. Fluid administration very likely will be helpful, as the patient's dizziness and anxiety are signs of hypovolemic shock.

37.3 **B.** Endoscopy is the preferred modality to identify the source of bleeding in upper GI bleeding. Tagged red cell studies are more commonly used for the evaluation of lower GI bleeding.

37.4 **C.** This patient's clinical presentation is suggestive of lower GI bleeding. Common causes of lower GI bleeding are diverticulosis, upper GI bleeding, hemorrhoids, angiodysplasia, malignancy, inflammatory bowel disease, and infectious conditions. Bleeding with diverticulosis is described as painless and abrupt, "as though a water faucet was suddenly turned on." The other choices are common causes of upper GI bleeding.

CLINICAL PEARLS

▶ Although most GI bleeds resolve spontaneously, each case is potentially life threatening. The main priorities are to determine whether there has been significant blood loss and to maintain hemodynamic stability.

▶ In upper GI bleeds, endoscopy is the study of choice because it can also be used to treat. Anoscopy, sigmoidoscopy, or colonoscopy are preferred in lower GI bleeds.

▶ In general, all patients with GI bleeding are admitted. If hemodynamically unstable or actively bleeding, they should be admitted to an ICU setting.

REFERENCES

Abrkun AN, Bardou M, Kuipers EJ, et al. International consensus recommendations on the management of patients with nonvaiceal upper gastrointestinal bleeding. *Ann Intern Med.* 2010;152:101-113.

Barnert J, Messmann H. Diagnosis and management of lower gastrointestinal bleeding. *Nat Rev Gastroenterol Hepat,* 2009;6:637-646.

A 63-year-old woman arrives in the emergency department (ED) in respiratory distress. The paramedics who transported her were not able to obtain any information about her past medical history but did bring her bag of medications, which includes furosemide.

On examination, her temperature is 37.5°C (99.5°F), blood pressure 220/112 mm Hg, heart rate 130 beats per minute, respiratory rate 36 breaths per minute, and oxygen saturation 93% on high-flow oxygen. The patient's skin is cool, clammy, and diaphoretic. She is alert but can only answer yes-or-no questions because of dyspnea. She has jugular venous distension to the angle of the jaw, rales in both lung fields, and +2 pretibial edema bilaterally. Her heart sounds are regular although tachycardic with an S_3/S_4 gallop.

▶ What is the most likely diagnosis?
▶ What is the most appropriate next step?

ANSWERS TO CASE 38:

Congestive Heart Failure/Pulmonary Edema

Summary: This is a 63-year-old woman in respiratory distress with signs of pump failure and fluid overload.

- **Most likely diagnosis:** Congestive heart failure (CHF) and pulmonary edema

- **Most appropriate next step:** Management of the ABCs, preload and afterload reduction, and diuresis

ANALYSIS

Objectives

1. Recognize the clinical presentation and complications of CHF.

2. Understand the diagnostic and therapeutic approach to suspected CHF.

Considerations

This 63-year-old woman is brought into the ED with signs of severe CHF: dyspnea, tachypnea, hypoxia, hypertension, and tachycardia. Her medications include furosemide, strongly suggesting a history congestive heart failure. This clinical presentation is classic for a CHF exacerbation. Rapid assessment of the ABCs, IV access, and prompt initiation of preload and afterload reduction and diuresis are the mainstays of therapy. Supplemental oxygen should be administered. Non-invasive positive pressure ventilation (NIPPV) or endotracheal intubation may be necessary for severe cases as well as those refractory to treatment. Once the patient is stabilized, it is important to try to identify any precipitants of the exacerbation. Diagnostic tests should be directed at excluding myocardial infarction, a common cause of worsening CHF.

APPROACH TO:

Congestive Heart Failure/Pulmonary Edema

CLINICAL APPROACH

Emergency physicians must be comfortable identifying and treating patients with heart failure (HF) as this condition is the most common reason for hospitalization of patients older than 65 and is increasing in prevalence. In addition, HF is associated with a significant morbidity and mortality. Patients with HF have a 50% mortality rate at 4 years after the onset of symptoms.

The right side of the heart receives blood from the peripheral circulation and sends it to the lungs for oxygenation. The left side subsequently receives oxygenated blood from the lungs and pumps it back into the circulation. Disruption of these functions leads to loss of normal contractile ability and HF. After HF occurs,

Table 38–1 • COMMON PRESENTATIONS OF HEART FAILURE

Type of Failure	Symptoms	Examination Findings
Right sided	Peripheral edema, right upper quadrant pain, no pulmonary symptoms	Dependent edema, right-upper-quadrant tenderness, hepatomegaly, hepatojugular reflex, jugular venous distension
Left sided	Dyspnea, orthopnea, paroxysmal nocturnal dyspnea, fatigue, weakness, cough	Tachypnea, pulmonary crackles or wheezes, S_3 or S_4

the heart cannot provide enough blood to meet the body's metabolic needs or must maintain elevated ventricular filling pressures to do so. The term "congestive" refers to abnormal fluid retention resulting from this loss of contractility. There are many causes of HF, the most common of which are coronary artery disease and hypertension.

Failure of the right side of the heart results in increased systemic venous pressures while left-sided failure causes increased pulmonary venous pressures. Each has different symptoms and physical findings (Table 38–1), although the two conditions often occur concomitantly.

This condition can also be divided into HF due to systolic dysfunction (impaired contractility) versus failure resulting from diastolic dysfunction (impaired ventricular relaxation and filling). Although patients with HF commonly have both types of dysfunction, distinguishing between the two can be important because patients with diastolic dysfunction are preload dependent. As a result, they may be sensitive to reductions in diastolic filling volumes (due to aggressive diuresis or venodilation) and become hypotensive.

Clinical Evaluation

During the evaluation, the clinician must be able to distinguish patients with CHF from those with other conditions with similar clinical presentations such as pneumonia, pneumothorax, pulmonary embolus, and exacerbation of chronic obstructive pulmonary disease (COPD) (Table 38–2). In addition, the clinician must try to determine what caused the patient's condition to decompensate. The most common precipitants are cardiac causes (eg, myocardial ischemia or infarction) and noncompliance with medications or dietary restrictions. Other causes include uncontrolled hypertension, valvular dysfunction, arrhythmia, infection, volume overload, pulmonary embolism, thyrotoxicosis, and iatrogenic etiologies.

The sequence of the clinical evaluation depends on the patient's clinical status. Those with significant respiratory distress require aggressive interventions while a focused history, physical examination, and diagnostic testing are performed simultaneously. If the patient is stable, a more detailed history can be obtained. Important historical points include the onset, duration, and character of respiratory complaints; any associated symptoms (such as chest pain or fever); past medical history (including prior heart disease and cardiac workup); and current medications (including recent changes in doses and any missed doses).

Table 38–2 • DIFFERENTIAL DIAGNOSES OF HEART FAILURE
Dyspnea
• Asthma or chronic obstructive pulmonary disease exacerbation
• Pneumonia
• Pneumothorax
• Pulmonary embolus
• Pleural effusion
• Physical deconditioning or obesity
Peripheral edema
• Deep venous thrombosis
• Hypoproteinemia (liver failure, nephrotic syndrome, renal failure)
Decreased cardiac output
• Acute myocardial infarction
• Drug effect
• Pericardial tamponade
• Valvular insufficiency
• Dysrhythmia
• Tension hydro- or pneumothorax

On examination, patients with CHF may show signs of hypoperfusion: clammy skin, delayed capillary refill, and thready pulses. If the patient is hypotensive, intra-arterial blood pressure monitoring is important because noninvasive measurements are often inaccurate in vasoconstricted individuals. Patients may have crackles, rales, or wheezes on auscultation. An S_3 or S_4 is common but may be difficult to hear in a busy ED. The cardiac examination may also reveal the murmur of a ventricular septal defect or acute mitral regurgitation or the irregularly irregular rhythm of atrial fibrillation—all of which can precipitate acute pulmonary edema. The ED physician should also note any jugular venous distention or peripheral edema.

Although x-ray findings may lag behind clinical symptoms by up to 6 hours, chest radiography still provides valuable information for the clinician. In early CHF, the chest x-ray shows upper zone vascular redistribution (cephalization). As the pulmonary congestion increases, interstitial edema and Kerley B lines become prominent, followed by opacification of the air spaces with alveolar edema. Other findings may include cardiomegaly and pleural effusions. The x-ray may also help exclude other causes of dyspnea and respiratory distress (eg, pneumothorax or pneumonia).

Laboratory studies should include complete blood count, electrolytes, blood urea nitrogen/creatinine, and urinalysis. If there is a suspicion of acute coronary syndrome, cardiac enzymes should be sent. The B-type natriuretic peptide (BNP) is a hormone released from the ventricles in response to stretch. It is most useful in patients with a mixed clinical picture (eg, a patient with CHF and COPD). Levels less than 100 pg/mL make HF unlikely and those greater than 500 pg/mL make it highly likely. Levels between these two extremes are indeterminate. The BNP level also has prognostic significance and can be used to monitor response to therapy. In obese patients, BNP levels tend to be lower than expected based on the observed symptoms. Furthermore, BNP levels may lag behind the patient's clinical picture. Electrocardiograms (ECGs) are helpful in detecting evidence of cardiac ischemia or infarction and arrhythmias. Liver enzymes may be of use in patients with hepatomegaly, and lactate levels in those with suspected cardiogenic shock.

Treatment

Treatment of cardiogenic pulmonary edema consists of oxygenation, vasodilation, diuresis, and augmentation of cardiac contractility if needed. High-flow oxygen should be the first intervention. Noninvasive positive-pressure ventilation via continuous or biphasic positive airway pressure may be necessary if hypoxia continues. Ultimately, the patient may require intubation if refractory to the aforementioned interventions. Vasodilation is obtained by reducing preload. This is most effectively and rapidly achieved with nitroglycerin, which can be given via sublingual, topical, or intravenous routes. In the critically ill patient, intravenous nitroglycerin is best. Diuresis with furosemide or bumetanide effectively reduces intravascular volume and preload, thus reducing pulmonary congestion. In addition, angiotensin-converting enzyme (ACE) inhibitors may play a role in preload reduction and in the treatment of CHF. Morphine is no longer recommended as standard therapy for CHF due to an association with increased rates of intubation and ICU admission. If patients do not improve with this therapy, an inotrope, such as dobutamine, may be given to increase myocardial contractility. If the patient is hypotensive, dopamine is a useful vasopressor.

COMPREHENSION QUESTIONS

38.1 A 62-year-old woman is sent to the ED from her primary physician's office with worsening heart failure. The patient has had congestive heart failure, previously controlled with oral digoxin and furosemide. Which of the following is the most likely reason for the exacerbation of her CHF?

A. Valvular dysfunction

B. Arrhythmia

C. Myocardial ischemia and infarction

D. Thyrotoxicosis

38.2 A 55-year-old man has symptoms of worsening orthopnea, tachypnea, and rales on pulmonary examination. The liver is percussed at 6 cm at the midclavicular line. His jugular vein is at +2 cm at 45 degrees. Which of the following is the best description of this patient's disease process?

A. Right-sided heart failure

B. Left-sided heart failure

C. Biventricular heart failure

D. Acute respiratory distress syndrome

38.3 A 58-year-old man is brought into the ED by paramedics because of worsening dyspnea. He has congestive heart failure due to cardiovascular disease. On examination, his blood pressure is 150/100 mm Hg and heart rate 104 beats per minute. He has jugular venous distension and rales in both lung fields. Which of the following is the most effective and most rapid method of reducing preload in this patient?

A. Diuretics

B. Nitroglycerin

C. Dobutamine

D. Morphine

38.4 A 54-year-old man complains of acute onset of worsening fatigue and dyspnea. He has alcohol-induced cardiomyopathy and congestive heart failure. Which of the following is the best workup for his CHF exacerbation?

A. Chest x-ray, cardiac enzymes, ECG

B. Computed tomography (CT) scan of the chest, ECG, D-dimer test

C. Echocardiogram, ECG, thallium stress test

D. Arterial blood gas, cardiac enzymes, pulmonary angiography

ANSWERS

38.1 **C.** Myocardial ischemia and infarction is one of the most common precipitants of a CHF exacerbation (as well as noncompliance with medications).

38.2 **B.** Left-sided heart failure can present with dyspnea, orthopnea, paroxysmal nocturnal dyspnea, tachypnea, crackles or wheezes, and an S_3 or S_4 gallop. The lack of jugular venous distension and/or hepatomegaly suggests absence of right-sided heart failure.

38.3 **B.** Nitroglycerin is the most effective and most rapid means of reducing preload in the patient with CHF.

38.4 **A.** The workup of a CHF exacerbation includes chest x-ray, ECG, electrolytes, BUN/creatinine, and cardiac enzymes. A BNP level may also be sent.

CLINICAL PEARLS

▶ The most common causes of CHF include coronary artery disease and hypertension while the most common causes of an acute exacerbation are myocardial ischemia or infarct and noncompliance.

▶ BNP is a hormone released by the ventricles in response to stretch. It can be useful as a marker for heart failure.

▶ Treatment of CHF includes oxygenation, correction of the underlying cause, and relief of symptoms by vasodilation, diuresis, and possibly inotropic support.

REFERENCES

Collins SP, Ronan-Bentle S, Storrow AB. Diagnostic and prognostic usefulness of natriuretic peptides in emergency department patients with dyspnea. *Ann Emerg Med.* 2003;41:532-544.

Humphries RL. Chapter 32: Cardiac emergencies. Stone CK, Humphries RL. *Current Diagnosis and Treatment: Emergency Medicine.* 6th ed. Available at: http://www.accessmedicine.com/content.aspx?aID=3106633.

Kosowsky JM, Kobayashi L. Acutely decompensated heart failure: diagnostic and therapeutic strategies for the new millennium. *Emerg Med Pract.* 2002;4(2):1-28.

Maisel AS, Krishnaswamy P, Nowak RM, et al. Rapid measurement of B-type natriuretic peptide in the emergency diagnosis of heart failure. *N Engl J Med.* 2002;347:161-167.

Niemann JT. Congestive heart failure and cor pulmonale. *Harwood Nuss' Clinical Practice of Emergency Medicine,* 4th ed. 2005.

O'Brien JF, Falk JL. Heart failure. In: Marx JA, Hockberger RS, Walls RM, eds. *Rosen's Emergency Medicine: Concepts and Clinical Practice.* 7th ed. Philadelphia, PA: Mosby Elsevier; 2009: Chapter 79.

Peacock WF. Congestive heart failure and acute pulmonary edema. In: Tintinalli JE, Kelen GD, Stapczynski JS, eds. *Emergency Medicine: A Comprehensive Study Guide.* 7th ed. New York, NY: McGraw-Hill; 2011: Chapter 57.

A 25-year-old woman is brought to the emergency department (ED) by police after attempting to break into a grocery store. When they apprehended her, they noted her pupils were large and that she seemed "high." The patient states that she has been "smoking" for the past year. She notes that without her "smokes," she craves the drug, becomes very sleepy, depressed, and has a huge appetite. In the ED, she complains of chest pain. The patient has a temperature of 38°C (100.4°F), heart rate of 120 beats per minute, and blood pressure of 160/90 mm Hg. Her pupils are both 6 mm and reactive. Her thyroid is normal to palpation. The heart and lung examinations reveal tachycardia, but are otherwise normal. Neurologic examination is unremarkable.

▶ What is the most likely diagnosis?

ANSWER TO CASE 39:

Cocaine Intoxication

Summary: This 25-year-old woman was arrested while attempting to burglarize a grocery store. She lost her job because she was late and stealing, secondary to her desire to "smoke." She has required more and more of the drug to get high and has been unsuccessful in her attempts to quit "smoking." She suffers from cravings, sleepiness, depression, and hyperphagia when she is unable to "smoke." While high, the patient feels euphoric and a sense of heightened energy. Her pupils are widely dilated; she has a low-grade fever, tachycardia, and hypertension. She has unintentionally lost 30 lbs over 6 months.

- **Most likely diagnosis:** Cocaine intoxication

ANALYSIS

Objectives

1. Recognize the clinical manifestations of cocaine intoxication.

2. Know the treatment for acute cocaine intoxication.

Considerations

This patient has many of the clinical signs and symptoms of cocaine intoxication. Cocaine, a sympathomimetic with local anesthetic characteristics, has potent vasoconstrictive properties. Acute cocaine intoxication can be a medical emergency. Rapidly fatal complications include severe hypertension (with concomitant end-organ damage), hyperthermia, and dysrhythmia. The mainstays of treatment are benzodiazepines (often in large dosages) and supportive measures. β-Blockers are contraindicated due to the risk of unopposed α-adrenergic stimulation. Acute cocaine intoxication may be difficult to distinguish from other conditions such as heat stroke, sedative-hypnotic withdrawal, intoxication with other sympathomimetics/anticholinergics, thyrotoxicosis, and infections or structural lesions of the central nervous system.

APPROACH TO:
Cocaine Intoxication

CLINICAL APPROACH

Cocaine is the second most commonly used illicit drug, second only to marijuana. With such widespread use, ED visits related to cocaine intoxication and its complications have risen substantially. A recent study shows that 14% of people older than 12 years have tried cocaine. Before the mid 1980s, the main routes of administration were intranasal and intravenous injection of cocaine hydrochloride. During the 1980s, crack cocaine emerged as the form of choice. Frequently, cocaine is combined with other drugs for various effects. Examples include mixing with heroin ("speedball") or alcohol ("liquid lady").

Cocaine causes release of norepinephrine, epinephrine, serotonin, and dopamine. This leads to a general stimulatory state including vasoconstriction and increased myocardial contractility. Cocaine also acts as a local anesthetic through sodium channel blockade. This effect is also responsible for many of the dysrhythmias and conduction abnormalities associated with cocaine use.

Symptoms of cocaine intoxication include euphoria, feelings of power or aggression, agitation, anxiety, hallucinations (classically formication, a tactile sensation of insects crawling on the skin), and delusions. Physical examination may reveal mydriasis, tachycardia, hypertension, hyperthermia, diaphoresis, tremors, or seizures. Coingestants or contaminants may result in atypical presentations (eg, cocaine plus heroin: mixed sympathomimetic-opioid presentation).

Table 39–1 lists the acute complications of cocaine intoxication. The effects on the cardiovascular and neurologic systems are of major concern. Severe dysrhythmias, myocardial infarction, seizures, and subarachnoid hemorrhage may result and potentially kill the patient. Body packers, who swallow cocaine wrapped in packets to smuggle it into the country, may die precipitously if a packet ruptures. Patients with seizures, altered mental status, dysrhythmias, or hemodynamic instability are

Table 39–1 • ACUTE COMPLICATIONS OF COCAINE INTOXICATION	
Autonomic	Hyperthermia, rhabdomyolysis, hypertension, dehydration
Cardiac	Dysrhythmia, myocarditis, endocarditis, cardiomyopathy, myocardial infarction or ischemia, coronary artery dissection, aortic rupture
Central nervous system	Seizures, intracranial hemorrhage or infarction, altered mental status, spinal cord infarction, intracranial abscess, acute dystonia
Pulmonary	Pulmonary hemorrhage, barotrauma (pneumothorax, pneumomediastinum, pneumopericardium), pneumonitis, asthma, pulmonary edema
Gastrointestinal	Intestinal ischemia, bowel necrosis, splenic infarction, ischemic colitis, gastrointestinal bleeding
Renal	Renal insufficiency or failure, renal infarction
Miscellaneous	Deep venous thrombosis, nasal perforation, sinusitis, oropharyngeal burn, infection (local or systemic), placental abruption, spontaneous abortion

at increased risk of developing rhabdomyolysis, which may in turn result in renal failure. Half of those who develop acute renal failure die.

Chest pain is a frequent complaint of those who present to the ED after cocaine use. Cocaine causes coronary vasoconstriction while also increasing the myocardial oxygen demand and platelet aggregation. The ED physician must maintain a high index of suspicion for myocardial ischemia and infarction, even with an atypical history and normal initial ECG; between 0.7% and 6% of these patients will have an acute myocardial infarction. These patients are typically younger, nonwhite, cigarette smokers without other risk factors for coronary artery disease. Benzodiazepines, often in large doses, are useful in treating cocaine-induced chest pain. If acute coronary syndrome is suspected, aspirin, nitrates, and morphine are advisable. **β-blockers should *not* be used due to the risk of an unopposed α-adrenergic effect, leading to increased hypertension and coronary vasoconstriction.** Thrombolytic therapy of an acute myocardial infarction should be avoided if coronary vasospasm or dissection is suspected or severe, uncontrolled hypertension exists. Emergent coronary artery catheterization may provide the best diagnostic information.

For patient with hyperthermia or agitation, a basic metabolic panel and creatine kinase help rule out renal failure, metabolic acidosis, and rhabdomyolysis. If coronary ischemia or infarction is suspected, ECGs and cardiac enzymes should be obtained. The ECG may reveal conduction abnormalities (including widened QRS complexes), dysrhythmias, or ST-segment or T-wave abnormalities consistent with myocardial ischemia or infarction. Patients with altered mental status or seizures should have a computed tomography of the head performed.

In general, patients with acute cocaine intoxication require only supportive care including monitoring and intravenous fluids. Agitation is best controlled using benzodiazepines such as lorazepam or diazepam. Phenothiazines (such as haloperidol) should be avoided because they may lower the seizure threshold, contribute to hyperthermia, and have dysrhythmic effects. Atrial dysrhythmias may respond to benzodiazepines or other standard therapies (except β-blockers). Intravenous sodium bicarbonate administration may be useful for wide-complex tachycardias (or lidocaine if the dysrhythmia is refractory to bicarbonate). The drug of choice to treat severe hypertension is the α-antagonist phentolamine. Intravenous nitroglycerin or nitroprusside may also be used. Again, β-blocking agents should be avoided. Even labetalol (mixed α- and β-blocker) has been associated with excess morbidity and mortality in animal studies of cocaine toxicity. Seizures are treated with benzodiazepines. Hyperthermia requires continuous monitoring of core temperature and rapid cooling. Patients with rhabdomyolysis require increased fluid resuscitation in order to maintain 1 to 3 mL/kg/h of urine output.

Asymptomatic body packers may be carefully monitored and given activated charcoal and polyethylene glycol to hasten the passage of the packets of cocaine. These packets usually contain ten times the lethal dose of cocaine and are rapidly fatal if ruptured. If the patient becomes hypertensive, hyperthermic, or agitated or manifests other signs of cocaine intoxication, benzodiazepines should be given and surgery should be emergently consulted for operative removal of the packets. Endoscopy is usually avoided due to a risk of packet perforation.

The patient who responds to sedation and has no further complications may be discharged from the emergency department after a period of observation.

Patients with ongoing chest pain, ECG changes, enzyme elevations or requiring ongoing pharmacologic treatment should be admitted to a monitored bed for further observation. Body packers need to be observed until all packets have passed.

COMPREHENSION QUESTIONS

39.1 A 25-year-old man is brought to the emergency room by police because of suspected cocaine intoxication. He is noted to be very agitated (fighting against five burly policemen) and wild eyed. On examination, his blood pressure is 180/100 mm Hg and heart rate 110 beats per minute. He is noted to have rotatory nystagmus. The neurologic examination reveals no focal abnormalities. Which of the following is the most likely diagnosis?

A. Amphetamine intoxication

B. Cocaine intoxication

C. Opiate intoxication

D. Phencyclidine intoxication

39.2 A 28-year-old man is noted to have extremely elevated blood pressure (210/130 mm Hg) associated with chest pain and dyspnea. His urine drug screen is positive for cocaine metabolites. Which of the following is the best next step?

A. Albuterol intravenously

B. Ephedrine intravenously

C. Labetalol intravenously

D. Lorazepam intravenously

39.3 A 35-year-old man is brought to the ED with altered level of consciousness, drowsiness, and pinpoint pupils. Which of the following is the most appropriate initial therapy for this patient?

A. Activated charcoal

B. Bicarbonate

C. Lorazepam

D. Naloxone

ANSWERS

39.1 **D.** Phencyclidine intoxication often presents with agitation, superhuman strength, and rotatory or vertical nystagmus.

39.2 **D.** Benzodiazepines should be used as the first-line agent for nearly all cocaine toxicities. The hypertension is caused by sympathetic stimulation. β-Blockers are contraindicated because they can result in unopposed α-adrenergic stimulation and exacerbation of the chest pain and hypertension. Hypertension not responsive to benzodiazepines may require intravenous phentolamine, an α-adrenergic antagonist.

39.3 **D.** This patient likely has an opiate intoxication (drowsiness and pinpoint pupils). Cocaine intoxication usually causes agitation and dilated pupils. Naloxone counteracts the effect of opioids.

CLINICAL PEARLS

▶ The clinical manifestations of cocaine intoxication result from sympathetic overstimulation and vasoconstriction.

▶ Cocaine intoxication can cause life-threatening complications, such as dysrhythmias, hyperthermia, and hypertensive emergencies.

▶ Cocaine can cause a quinidine-like effect, prolonging the QT interval and leading to wide-complex dysrhythmias, bradycardia, and hypotension.

▶ β-Blockers are avoided in patients with cocaine intoxication because of the risk of unopposed α-adrenergic stimulation.

▶ Benzodiazepines are a mainstay of treatment for cocaine toxicity and many of its complications.

REFERENCES

Aghababian RV, Allison EJ Jr, Boyer EW, et al, eds. *Essentials of Emergency Medicine*. Sudbury, MA: Jones and Bartlett; 2006:798-807.

Marx JA, Hockberger RS, Walls RM, eds. *Rosen's Emergency Medicine: Concepts and Clinical Practice*. 7th ed. Philadelphia, PA: Mosby Elsevier; 2009.

McCord J, Jneid H, Hollander JE, et al. Management of cocaine-associated chest pain and myocardial infarction: a scientific statement from the American Heart Association Acute Cardiac Care Committee of the Council on Clinical Cardiology. *Circulation*. 2008;117;1897-1907.

Schaider J, Hayden SR, Wolfe R, Barkin R, Rosen P, eds. *Rosen and Barkin's 5-Minute Emergency Medicine Consult*. 3rd ed. Philadelphia, PA: Lippinott Williams & Wilkins; 2007:238-239.

Tintinalli JE, Kelen GD, Stapczynski JS, eds. *Emergency Medicine: A Comprehensive Study Guide*. 7th ed. New York, NY: McGraw-Hill; 2011.

An 18-year-old woman is brought by a friend to the emergency department (ED) about 30 minutes after she took "a bunch" of Tylenol. The patient states she was upset with her parents who grounded her after she came home late from a party; she swallowed half a bottle of extra-strength Tylenol in order to "make them feel sorry." She is tearful, says she was "stupid," and denies any true desire to hurt herself or anyone else. She has no other complaints and denies any past attempts to hurt herself. On examination, her blood pressure is 105/60 mm Hg, heart rate is 100 beats per minute, and respiratory rate is 24 breaths per minute (crying). Her pupils are equal and reactive bilaterally. Her sclera is clear, and her mucous membranes are moist. The lungs are clear and the heart sounds are regular. The abdominal examination is benign with normal bowel sounds. She is awake and alert without any focal neurologic deficits.

▶ What is the most appropriate next step?
▶ What are the potential complications of this ingestion?
▶ What is the mechanism of acetaminophen toxicity?

ANSWERS TO CASE 40:
Acetaminophen Toxicity

Summary: This is an 18-year-old woman with an acute acetaminophen overdose 30 minutes prior to arrival in the ED. She is alert and oriented with stable vital signs.

- **Most appropriate next step:** Obtain IV access; send appropriate laboratory studies; administer activated charcoal; evaluate need for *N*-acetylcysteine (NAC)

- **Potential complications:** Hypoglycemia, metabolic acidosis, hepatic failure, and renal failure

- **Mechanism:** Production of toxic metabolite, *N*-acetyl-*p*-benzoquinoneimine (NAPQI)

ANALYSIS

Objectives

1. Learn the general approach to the poisoned patient.

2. Recognize the clinical signs and symptoms of acetaminophen toxicity.

3. Understand the evaluation and treatment of patients with acetaminophen toxicity.

Considerations

Acetaminophen (APAP) is one of the most commonly used analgesics and antipyretics. It is available in a variety of prescription, over-the-counter, and combination medications labeled for fever, cold, cough, and pain relief. As a result, it is the most common over-the-counter agent reported in accidental and intentional overdoses, leading to more hospitalizations after overdose than any other pharmaceutical agent. A toxic exposure to APAP is suspected when more than 200 mg/kg or more than 10 g is ingested in a single dose or over the course of 24 hours. In addition, an ingestion of more than 150 mg/kg or more than 6 g per day for at least 2 consecutive days is potentially toxic. Hepatotoxicity is the most life-threatening complication, but may be indolent; thus, serum APAP level and a precise time of ingestion are important to plot on a nomogram to assess likelihood of toxicity. This patient was forthcoming about the medication used in the overdose; however, many patients will underreport or deny the use of APAP. Consequently, an APAP level should be drawn on all suspected overdose patients. Although clinical evidence of hepatotoxicity may be delayed for 24 to 72 hours, NAC therapy is most effective if started within 8 hours of ingestion. Because this patient reported the ingestion within 30 minutes, there is time for a serum APAP level, activated charcoal decontamination, and then NAC therapy. If time is an issue, NAC treatment should be initiated without delay. Emesis should not be induced because of the possible delay in therapy. After medical stabilization, assessment of suicide potential is important.

APPROACH TO:
Acetaminophen Toxicity

CLINICAL APPROACH

Although APAP is safe at therapeutic dosages, ingestions more than 200 mg/kg can lead to liver failure and death. Under normal circumstances, most APAP is metabolized in the liver and excreted by the kidneys. Of the remainder, approximately 5% is excreted unchanged in urine. Another 5% is metabolized by the hepatic cytochrome P450 system to form NAPQI. This toxic intermediate is then detoxified by conjugation with glutathione. In acute APAP overdose, glutathione depletion leads to accumulation of NAPQI which then binds to hepatocyte intracellular proteins causing toxicity. APAP toxicity can be divided into four clinical phases (Table 40–1).

Clinical Evaluation

When approaching the poisoned or overdose patient, the clinician's priorities are to perform a rapid assessment, stabilize the ABCs, decontaminate, minimize absorption, and administer any antidotes. Important historical information includes type, amount, and timing of ingestion; current symptoms; circumstances of the ingestion (accidental or intentional); and possible coingestants. The physical examination should focus on the abdomen (RUQ tenderness) and mental status (signs of encephalopathy). A complete physical examination is important to search for any concomitant toxic syndromes (toxidromes) (Table 40–2). Table 40–3 lists common antidotes. Consulting with the local poison control center is also recommended for any suspected ingestion or overdose.

Diagnostic studies include serum electrolytes, blood urea nitrogen (BUN)/creatinine, glucose, liver enzyme levels, coagulation studies, and urinalysis (as well as pregnancy test if appropriate). Because coingestion is common, a toxicology screen and salicylate level should be obtained. An ECG should be obtained to evaluate for dysrhythmias associated with other ingestants and electrolyte abnormalities.

Table 40–1 • CLINICAL PHASES OF APAP TOXICITY			
Phase 1	**Phase 2**	**Phase 3**	**Phase 4**
Preinjury period (30 min to 24 h after ingestion)	Onset of liver injury (24-72 h after ingestion)	Maximum liver injury (72-96 h after ingestion)	Recovery period (4-10 d after ingestion)
Nonspecific symptoms: anorexia, nausea, vomiting, malaise, diaphoresis, anxiety; may be asymptomatic	Nausea, vomiting, right upper quadrant and epigastric pain and tenderness, elevated liver enzymes	Anorexia, nausea, vomiting, peak liver enzyme abnormalities; fulminant liver failure (encephalopathy, coagulopathy, hypoglycemia, metabolic acidosis), renal failure, and death	Resolution of hepatic dysfunction

Table 40–2 • COMMON TOXIDROMES

Toxidrome	Clinical Findings	Common Agents
Anticholinergic	Tachycardia, hyperthermia, dry skin and mucous membranes, delirium, urinary retention, mydriasis, flushed skin, absent bowel sounds	Antihistamines, phenothiazines, tricyclic antidepressants, scopolamine, Jimson weed, belladonna
Cholinergic	Salivation, lacrimation, urination, diarrhea, miosis, bradycardia, emesis	Organophosphate insecticides, pilocarpine, betel nuts
Opioid	Coma, respiratory depression, pinpoint pupils	Codeine, heroin, morphine, meperidine, hydrocodone
Sedative-hypnotic	Decreased level of consciousness, respiratory depression, hypotension, variable pupillary changes, hypothermia, seizures	Barbiturates, benzodiazepines
Sympathomimetic	Hypertension, tachycardia, mydriasis, hyperpyrexia, arrhythmias	Cocaine, methamphetamine, ephedrine, ecstasy

If the patient's mental status is altered, a computed tomography (CT) scan of the head is also recommended. However, the single best predictor of the risk of hepatotoxicity is a serum APAP level. This should be drawn 4 hours postingestion, or immediately if the time of ingestion is unknown. Using the APAP level and the Rumack-Matthew nomogram, the clinician can then predict the severity of toxicity and determine the need for NAC therapy (Figure 40–1). The APAP level between 4 and 24 hours is plotted; if the level falls above the lower line, known as the treatment line, NAC should be initiated. This nomogram is not applicable for chronic ingestions, delayed ingestions, unknown time or duration of ingestion, extended release APAP, or coingestions.

Treatment

Initial treatment of the patient with an APAP overdose consists of stabilizing the ABCs, obtaining IV access, and placing the patient on cardiac and oxygen saturation monitors. Gastric lavage is rarely necessary due to the rapid gastrointestinal absorption of APAP. Activated charcoal can reduce gastric absorption of the drug but may also adsorb oral NAC. Thus, if activated charcoal is given, separating the first dose of NAC and activated charcoal by 1 to 2 hours may be preferable. NAC, the antidote for APAP toxicity, acts by replenishing glutathione stores and combining with NAPQI as a glutathione substitute. It is most effective when given within 8 hours of ingestion. The indications for NAC include a toxic level as determined using the Rumack-Matthew nomogram or evidence of hepatic failure. NAC can be empirically started if an APAP overdose is suspected and an APAP level will not be available within 8 hours of the ingestion; the NAC can then be discontinued if the APAP level is nontoxic and the patient is asymptomatic. Any patient who requires NAC treatment should be admitted to the hospital. Although the nomogram is not applicable for ingestions greater than 24 hours prior to ED arrival, NAC therapy may still be helpful.

Table 40–3 • COMMON ANTIDOTES: DOSES AND INDICATIONS

Antidote	Pediatric	Adult	Poison
N-acetylcysteine	140 mg/kg PO, then 70 mg/kg PO q4h for 18 total doses OR 150 mg/kg IV over 15 min-1 h, then 50 mg/kg IV over 4 h, then 100 mg/kg over 16 h		Acetaminophen
Activated charcoal	1 g/kg PO		Most ingested poisons
Crotalidae polyvalent immune Fab	4-6 vials IV initially over 1 h; may be repeated 2 vials every 6 h for 18 h		Envenomation by Crotalidae
Calcium gluconate 10% (9 mg/mL elemental calcium)	0.2-0.25 mL/kg IV	10 mL IV	Hypermagnesemia, hypocalcemia (ethylene glycol, hydrofluoric acid), calcium-channel antagonists, black widow spider venom
Calcium chloride 10% (27.2 mg/mL elemental calcium)	0.6-0.8 mL/kg IV	10-30 mL IV	
Cyanide antidote kit			
Amyl nitrate	Not typically used	1 ampule in oxygen chamber of ambu-bag 30 sec on/ 30 sec off	Cyanide poisoning
Sodium nitrite (3% solution)	0.33 mL/kg IV	10 mL	Hydrogen sulfide (use only sodium nitrite)
Thiosulfate (25% solution)	1.65 mL/kg IV	50 mL IV	
Deferoxamine	Initial dose: 20 mg/kg IM/IV (15 mg/kg/h IV); 1 g max	Initial dose: 1 g IM/IV (15 mg/kg/h IV); 6 g/d max	Iron
Dextrose	0.5 g/kg IV	1 g/kg IV	Hypoglycemia
Digoxin immune Fab	(Empiric)	(Empiric)	
Acute	10-20 vials IV	10-20 vials IV	Digoxin and cardiac glycosides
Chronic	1-2 vials IV	4-6 vials IV	
Ethanol 10% for IV administration	10 mL/kg over 30 min, then 1.2 mL/kg/h[a]		Ethylene glycol, methanol
Folic acid/leucovorin	1-2 mg/kg q4-6h IV		Methotrexate (only leucovorin)
Fomepizole	15 mg/kg IV, then 10 mg/kg q12h		Methanol, ethylene glycol, disulfiram
Flumazenil	0.01 mg/kg IV	0.2 mg IV	Benzodiazepines
Glucagon	50-150 µg/kg IV	3-10 mg IV	Calcium channel blocker, β-blocker
Hydroxycobalamin (may be used with sodium thiosulfate)	70 mg/kg IV over 30 min (5 g max)	5 g IV over 30 min	Cyanide, nitroprusside

(Continued)

Table 40–3 • COMMON ANTIDOTES: DOSES AND INDICATIONS (CONTINUED)

Antidote	Pediatric	Adult	Poison
IV lipid emulsion 20%	1.5 mL/kg IV over 1 min (may repeat × 2), then 0.25 mL/kg/min IV	100 mL IV over 1 min, then 400 mL IV over 20 min	Calcium channel blocker, β-blocker (rescue therapy)
Methylene blue	1-2 mg/kg IV Neonates: 0.3-1 mg/kg	1-2 mg/kg IV	Oxidizing chemicals (eg, nitrites, benzocaine, sulfonamides)
Octreotide	1 μg/kg SC q6h	5-100 μg SC q6h	Refractory hypoglycemia after oral hypoglycemic agent ingestion
Naloxone	As much as is needed. Typical starting dose 0.01 mg/kg IV	As much as is needed. Typical starting dose 0.4-2 mg IV	Opioid, clonidine
Physostigmine	0.02 mg/kg IV	0.5-2 mg IV	Anticholinergic substances (not cyclic antidepressants)
Pralidoxime (2-PAM)	20-40 mg/kg IV, then 20 mg/kg/h	1-2 g IV, then 500 mg/h	Cholinergic substances
Protamine	1 mg neutralizes 100 U of unfractionated heparin; administered over 15 min		Heparin
	0.6 mg/kg IV (empiric)	25-50 mg IV (empiric)	
Pyridoxine	Gram for gram of ingestion if amount of isoniazid is known		Isoniazid, Gyromitra esculenta, hydrazine
	70 mg/kg IV (5 g max)	5 g IV	
Sodium bicarbonate	1-2 mEq/kg IV bolus then 2 mEq/kg/h IV		Sodium channel blockers, alkalinization of urine or serum
Thiamine	5-10 mg IV	100 mg IV	Wernicke syndrome, "wet" beri-beri
Vitamin K$_1$	1-5 mg/d PO	20 mg/d PO	Anticoagulants (eg, warfarin)

[a]This is an approximation. Doses should be titrated to ethanol level of 100-150 mg/dL.

The standard 72-hour NAC regimen is an oral loading dose of 140 mg/kg followed by maintenance doses of 70 mg/kg every 4 hours for 17 additional doses. Because of its acrid smell and taste, oral NAC often induces nausea and vomiting. Dilution in fruit juice or a chilled drink and the administration of antiemetics can be helpful.

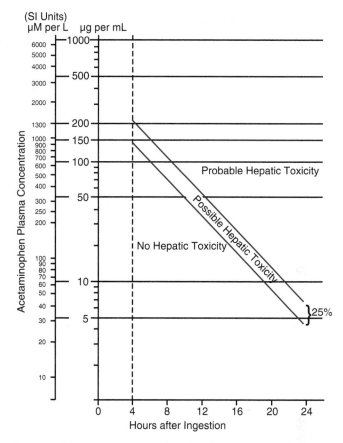

Figure 40–1. Acetaminophen toxicity nomogram based on serum acetaminophen concentration versus time after ingestion.

If the patient has intractable vomiting or fulminant hepatic failure, intravenous NAC may be indicated (150 mg/kg loading dose, followed by 50 mg/kg over 4 hours, followed by 100 mg/kg over 16 hours). Intravenous NAC should be used cautiously as rate-related anaphylactoid reactions can occur.

A small fraction of patients will develop fulminant hepatic failure, associated with a 60% to 80% mortality rate. Most deaths associated with liver failure occur 3 to 5 days postingestion, attributed to cerebral edema, sepsis, hemorrhage, multiorgan failure, or acute respiratory distress syndrome.

COMPREHENSION QUESTIONS

40.1 A 16-year-old adolescent girl is brought to the ED after taking a number of pills from her parents' medicine cabinet. The parents have brought in all the medication bottles. Which of the following is most concerning for toxicity?

A. Ampicillin

B. Diphenhydramine

C. Fluoxetine

D. Theophylline

40.2 A 34-year-old man admits taking "the whole bottle" of acetaminophen over the course of 36 hours because of a severe headache. Which of the following is the best guide to determine whether to initiate NAC therapy?

A. Initiate NAC due to potentially toxic exposure

B. Serum APAP level and liver enzymes

C. Plotting the serum APAP level on the nomogram

D. If over 24 hours have elapsed, NAC therapy is not efficacious

40.3 A 25-year-old man is brought into the ED 1 hour after a witnessed overdose of 20 to 25 pills of acetaminophen tablets. At what time would be the best time to draw the APAP level?

A. As soon as the patient arrives in the ED

B. At 2 hours postingestion

C. At 4 hours postingestion

D. At 8 hours postingestion

40.4 A 38-year-old school teacher took a "large number of Tylenol tablets" and is found to have an APAP level of 200 µg/mL. The estimated time postingestion is 8 hours. The first dose of NAC is given. Which of the following is the next step to guide therapy?

A. Check APAP level 4 hours after the first NAC dose and if below the toxicity line, no further NAC needed.

B. Check the APAP level 12 hours after the first NAC dose and if below the toxicity line, no further NAC needed.

C. Check the APAP level and liver function tests at the 8 hour after the first NAC dose and if in the normal/nontoxic range, then no further NAC needed.

D. Give the entire course of NAC and no further APAP levels are necessary.

Match the following antidotes (A to H) to the clinical situations (Questions 40.5 to 40.8):

    A. Calcium gluconate

    B. Deferoxamine

    C. Digoxin Fab

    D. Glucagon

    E. N-acetylcysteine

    F. Naloxone

    G. Physostigmine

    H. Vitamin K

40.5 A 45-year-old man takes too many of his antihypertensive pills and is noted to have a heart rate of 40 beats per minute.

40.6 A 22-year-old pregnant woman with preeclampsia receiving intravenous medication to prevent seizures develops weakness and difficulty breathing.

40.7 A 24-year-old man is brought into the ED with somnolence, pinpoint pupils, and track marks on his arm.

40.8 A 56-year-old woman taking tablets to "thin her blood" is noted to be bleeding from her gums and has multiple bruises on her arms and legs. Life-threatening bleeding can be addressed with transfusion with clotting factors.

ANSWERS

40.1 **D.** Theophylline has a very narrow therapeutic index, with toxic effects of tachycardia, nausea, vomiting, and seizures.

40.2 **A.** At 24 hours postingestion, NAC therapy may still be useful. Due to the historically toxic exposure, NAC should be started while a serum APAP level and liver enzymes are checked. If the APAP level is undetectable and the liver enzymes are normal, subsequent doses of NAC can be discontinued. The Rumack-Matthew nomogram is not applicable for ingestions more than 24 hours prior to evaluation.

40.3 **C.** A serum APAP should be drawn 4 hours postingestion; the nomogram has relevance between 4 hours and 24 hours postingestion.

40.4 **D.** Once it is determined by the nomogram that the APAP dose is potentially toxic, the entire NAC regimen is given. No further APAP levels need to be drawn.

40.5 **D.** Glucagon is effective in treating calcium-channel blocker or β-blocker overdose.

40.6 **A.** This patient is likely receiving magnesium sulfate for seizure prophylaxis, and the antidote for hypermagnesemia is calcium gluconate.

40.7 **F.** Naloxone is the treatment of choice for opiate overdose. This individual likely is a heroin abuser.

40.8 **H.** This patient likely has warfarin overdose, which is treated by vitamin K.

CLINICAL PEARLS

▶ Because the devastating effects of APAP toxicity may be delayed for 24 to 72 hours and antidotal therapy is most effective if started within 8 hours of ingestion, the clinician must have a high level of suspicion of APAP toxicity in any poisoned patient.

▶ APAP toxicity is caused by the formation of a toxic metabolite, N-acetyl-p-benzoquinoneimine (NAPQI).

▶ N-acetylcysteine (NAC) is the antidote for APAP toxicity and should be given if a toxic ingestion is suspected (based on ingested dose or APAP level and Rumack-Matthew nomogram).

▶ The priorities when dealing with a patient with an APAP overdose are to perform a rapid assessment, stabilize the ABCs, decontaminate, minimize absorption, and administer NAC if appropriate.

▶ In general, an APAP level should be drawn on any patient with an overdose history even when APAP ingestion is denied.

REFERENCES

Aghababian RV, Allison EJ Jr, Boyer EW, et al, eds. *Essentials of Emergency Medicine*. Sudbury, MA: Jones and Bartlett; 2006:792-794.

Bizovi KE, Hendrickson R. Acetaminophen. In: Marx JA, Hockberger RS, Walls RM, eds. *Rosen's Emergency Medicine: Concepts and Clinical Practice*. 7th ed. Philadelphia, PA: Mosby Elsevier; 2009.

Heard KJ. Acetylcysteine for Acetaminophen Poisoning. *N Engl J Med*. 2008;359:285-292.

Schaider J, Hayden SR, Wolfe R, Barkin R, Rosen P, eds. *Rosen and Barkin's 5-Minute Emergency Medicine Consult*. 3rd ed. Philadelphia, PA: Lippinott Williams & Wilkins; 2007:22-23.

Tintinalli JE, Kelen GD, Stapczynski JS, eds. *Emergency Medicine: A Comprehensive Study Guide*. 7th ed. New York, NY: McGraw-Hill; 2011.

Wolf SJ, Heard KH, Sloan EP, Jagoda AS. Clinical policy: critical issues in the management of patients presenting to the emergency department with acetaminophen overdose. *Ann Emerg Med*; 2007;50:292-313.

A 30-year-old woman with a history of sickle cell disease presents to the emergency department (ED) complaining of chest pain for 2 days. She states that the pain is right sided, worse with inspiration, and is more severe than her usual "crisis pain." She has subjective fevers, mild shortness of breath, and a productive cough. She denies vomiting, hemoptysis, or lower extremity swelling. Her last pain crisis was 3 months ago. She usually takes acetaminophen and hydrocodone for pain control during her crises, however, neither have been able to provide sufficient relief during this episode. On physical examination, her temperature is 38.3 °C (101°F), blood pressure is 126/65 mm Hg, heart rate is 98 beats per minute, respiratory rate is 22 breaths per minute, and oxygen saturation is 94% on room air. Lung examination reveals crackles in the right lower lung field. She does not have any jugular venous distension, calf tenderness, or lower extremity edema.

▶ What is the most concerning issue regarding this patient?
▶ What is the initial management?

ANSWERS TO CASE 41:
Sickle Cell Crisis

Summary: This is a 30-year-old woman with a history of sickle cell disease who presents with chest pain, shortness of breath, and cough. She is febrile, tachypneic, and hypoxic.

- **Most concerning issue:** Acute chest syndrome.

- **Initial management:** Supplemental oxygen, IV hydration, analgesia, and antibiotics.

ANALYSIS

Objectives

1. Recognize the clinical signs and symptoms of sickle cell crisis and its associated complications.

2. Understand the diagnosis and treatment of acute chest syndrome.

3. Understand the treatment of pain crises in patients with sickle cell disease.

Considerations

Sickle cell disease is common, affecting approximately 1 in every 400 African Americans and 1 in 16,000 Asian Americans. It can affect almost any organ system and has a wide variety of clinical presentations. Acute chest syndrome is the leading cause of death and second leading cause of hospitalization among patients with sickle cell disease. Acute chest syndrome can present primarily or develop after a sickle cell patient is hospitalized for a vasoocclusive crisis. The clinician's priorities are to differentiate the mild from the life-threatening crises and to treat them.

The patient in this case, a 30-year-old woman with known sickle cell disease, **has acute onset of chest pain, cough, fever, and subtle findings on the pulmonary examination.** Her **oxygen saturation is 94% on room air,** which is concerning, and should be followed up with an arterial blood gas. Pulmonary embolism, pneumonia, and **acute chest syndrome** should be considered as possible diagnoses, as individual or concomitant conditions. The chest radiograph can be helpful. Acute chest syndrome is a constellation of symptoms that includes chest pain and tachypnea. It can result from infectious or noninfectious (eg, pulmonary infarct) causes. It usually presents with some combination of chest pain, fever, hypoxia, and a new pulmonary infiltrate on chest radiography. Often, acute chest syndrome and pneumonia cannot be distinguished initially. Therefore, it is prudent to treat these patients with antibiotics, obtain a Gram stain and culture of the sputum, and admit them to the hospital. The treatment for acute chest syndrome is supportive and includes oxygen, intravenous fluid hydration, and analgesia. All patients with sickle cell disease who present to the ED require close follow-up with a hematologist.

DEFINITIONS

ACUTE CHEST SYNDROME: The presence of a new lobar or segmental infiltrate on chest radiography in the presence of fever, respiratory symptoms, and/or chest pain in patient with sickle cell disease.

VASOOCLUSIVE CRISIS: Painful episodes resulting from intravascular sickling causing obstruction of blood flow in the microcirculation leading to tissue ischemia and microinfarction.

SPLENIC SEQUESTRATION: Occurs when red cells become trapped in the spleen, resulting in a rapidly enlarging spleen, a sudden drop in hemoglobin, and the potential for shock.

APLASTIC CRISIS: A transient cessation of erythropoiesis resulting in the acute onset of anemia and reticulocytopenia. The most common cause of aplastic crisis appears to be infection, specifically parvovirus.

APPROACH TO:
Sickle Cell Crisis

CLINICAL APPROACH

Sickle cell disease is caused by abnormal hemoglobin production. In humans, hemoglobin is composed of two alpha and two beta chains. However, in sickle cell disease, hemoglobin S (HbS) results when a valine is substituted for glutamine in the sixth position of the beta chain. Under hypoxic or acidotic conditions, this abnormal hemoglobin polymerizes and sickles, resulting in sludging in the microcirculation. In turn, this causes tissue hypoxia, ischemia, acidosis, and more sickling.

The gene for HbS is autosomal recessive. Patients who are **heterozygous** (sickle cell trait) are generally asymptomatic except under extreme stress (eg, severe dehydration, temperature, or pressure change), but do tend to be more **susceptible than the general population to urinary tract infections.** Those who have sickle cell disease (homozygous), in contrast, are highly susceptible to vasoocclusion and pain crises.

Potential triggers for sickle cell crises are numerous. Some common triggers include infections (bacterial and viral), dehydration, exposure to cold temperatures, low oxygen environments such as airplane travel or smoke-filled rooms, and trauma. It should be recognized, however, that spontaneous, unexplained crises are common. Because these patients are functionally asplenic after early childhood, they are also at significant risk for bacterial infections, especially by **encapsulated organisms** such as *Salmonella typhi, Haemophilus influenza* type B, *Streptoccoccus pneumoniae, Neisseria meningitides,* and Group B *streptococci.* In fact, **the highest rate of mortality occurs in children between the ages of 1 and 3 years as a consequence of sepsis.**

COMMON COMPLICATIONS

Sickle cell crisis can affect multiple organ systems (see Table 41–1). During the assessment of patients with sickle cell disease, the history should focus on **identifying any precipitating causes and complications.** Pain that is different from previous pain crises may be an indicator of a potentially life-threatening event. A rapid assessment of the vital signs and a careful physical examination are important, because severe complications in sickle cell crisis often present with nonspecific manifestations. The clinician's concern should be heightened if the patient has a fever, severe abdominal pain, respiratory or neurological symptoms, joint swelling, priapism, or pain that is not relieved by usual measures.

Vasoocclusive Crisis

Acute vasoocclusive events (VOEs) or "painful crisis" are the **most common complications of sickle cell disease (SCD)** and the most frequent cause of ED visits in this patient population. Polymerization of the sickle cell hemoglobin causes the red blood cells to become rigid and sticky and formed into shapes that sometimes have the appearance of a sickle, hence the name. These sickled cells subsequently will cause obstruction of the microvasculature. It is probable that a multitude of factors contribute to VOEs, including red cell function, blood viscosity, adherence of sickled cells to endothelium, and environmental factors. Patients may live in a homeostatic balance with circulating sickle cells, but a seemingly minor event such as a viral illness, dehydration, trauma, or exercise may tip this balance resulting in a full-blown VOE.

Dactylitis, or hand-foot syndrome, may be the first clinical manifestation of SCD. Infarctions in the metacarpals result in episodes of pain and swelling involving the hands and feet. Infants and toddlers with dactylitis may become irritable, refuse to walk, or cry when touched or held. As children with SCD get older, pain shifts to the arms, legs, back, and pelvis, whereas adolescents may also complain of involvement of the chest and abdomen. These vasoocclusive episodes usually last from 3 to 9 days, but it is not atypical for those patients with longer episodes to continue to have patterns where their episodes remain prolonged.

Infection

Infection is the major cause of mortality in SCD. Virtually all patients with SCD are asplenic, predisposing them to overwhelming infections from **encapsulated microorganisms.** In addition to sepsis, patients are susceptible to other infections such as pneumonia, meningitis, and osteomyelitis. Although prophylactic penicillin and vaccines for pneumococci and *Haemophilus influenzae* type B have reduced the incidence of sepsis in this patient population, **pneumococcal sepsis remains a significant cause of death in children with SCD.** Adults are less vulnerable because their immune systems have matured to allow for type-specific antibody production; however, fever must be taken very seriously in all patients with SCD.

Acute Chest Syndrome

Acute chest syndrome (ACS) is the presence of a **new lobar or segmental pulmonary infiltrate in the presence of fever, respiratory symptoms, or chest pain.** Various causes may contribute to ACS including infection, pulmonary infarction

Table 41–1 • SICKLE CELL CRISES

Type Of Crisis	Comments	Diagnosis	Treatment
Vaso-occlusive crises: Precipitants are infection, dehydration, stress, fatigue, cold, high altitude			
Musculoskeletal pain	Commonly in low back, femur, tibia, humerus	Examination: Normal or may have local tenderness	Hydration, analgesia
Abdominal pain	Pain usually acute onset, poorly localized, and recurrent; broad differential includes hepatobiliary, splenic, or renal disease	Examination: No peritoneal signs; complete blood count, liver function tests	Treat underlying etiology, supportive care[a]
Acute chest syndrome	Pleuritic chest pain, cough, dyspnea	Examination: Fever, tachypnea, rales; pulse oximetry, chest x-ray, arterial blood gas, V/Q scan, angiography	Treat underlying etiology, supportive care, supplemental oxygen, antibiotics, anticoagulation
Central nervous system crisis	Headache, neurological deficit, seizure, mental status changes; usually infarct in children and hemorrhage in adults	CT scan, lumbar puncture, MRI	Exchange transfusion
Priapism	Painful erection without sexual stimulation caused by sickling in corpus cavernosum	Examination: engorged, painful penis	Supportive care, exchange transfusion, aspiration of corpus cavernosum, intrapenile injection of vasodilator, urologic consultation
Dactylitis	Swelling of hands and/or feet; usually occurs before 2 years of age	Painful edema of hands and/or feet	Supportive care, warm compresses
Renal crisis	Usually asymptomatic; may have flank pain	Urinalysis shows hematuria or tissue	Supportive care

(Continued)

Table 41–1 • SICKLE CELL CRISES (CONTINUED)

Type Of Crisis	Comments	Diagnosis	Treatment
Hematological crises			
Splenic sequestration	Rapid onset of fatigue, listlessness, pallor, abdominal pain; most common in children <6 years of age	Examination: hypovolemia, splenomegaly; severe anemia or significant drop in hemoglobin	Correction of hypovolemia, PRBC transfusion, exchange transfusion, splenectomy
Aplastic crisis	Precipitants: Parvovirus B19 infection, folic acid deficiency, phenylbutazone	Significant drop in hemoglobin with low reticulocyte count	IV fluids, PRBC transfusion; usually self-limited
Infectious crises			
	Common organisms: encapsulated (*Haemophilus influenzae, Streptococcus pneumoniae*), *Salmonella typhi, Mycoplasma pneumoniae, Escherichia coli, Staphylococcus aureus*	Examination: fever; complete blood count, urinalysis, blood and sputum and urine cultures (as indicated), chest x-ray	Broad-spectrum antibiotics

Abbreviations: CT = Computed tomography; IV = intravenous; V/Q ventilation = perfusion; PRBC = packed red blood cell.
ªSupportive care includes hydration and analgesia.

due to vasoocclusion, and fat emboli from marrow infarction. Chest pain from vaso-occlusion may cause splinting and hypoventilation, leading to the development of ACS in a patient who initially presents with a painful episode. Infectious organisms associated with ACS include S Pneumoniae in younger children and Mycoplasma or Chlamydia in adolescents. Acute chest syndrome carries a high risk of progression to respiratory failure and should be considered in all SCD patients with respiratory signs or symptoms.

All patients with ACS should be admitted to the hospital. The finding of an infiltrate on chest radiograph is diagnostically significant, but it should be recognized that it is common for the initial radiograph to be normal. Laboratory evaluation should include a CBC, reticulocyte count, blood and sputum cultures, and type and screen. A baseline arterial blood gas (ABG) measurement should be obtained, followed by serial ABG measurements to evaluate for worsening A-a gradient. In patients with ACS and hypoxemia (Pao_2 = 70 to 80 mm Hg, O_2 saturation of 92%-95%), **supplemental oxygen** should be administered via nasal cannula at a rate of 2 liters per minute. **Exchange (or conventional) transfusion** should be initiated in patients with hypoxia or a drop in hemoglobin >2 g below baseline. All patients should receive **empiric antibiotics** that cover typical and atypical microorganisms, (most commonly with a macrolide and third generation cephalosporin). Analgesia for chest pain should be provided but managed carefully to prevent hypoventilation. Regular use of an incentive spirometer has shown to significantly reduce the frequency of subsequent episodes of chest pain. Intravenous fluids given to patients with ACS should not exceed 1.5 times maintenance in order to prevent volume overload.

Stroke (Cerebrovascular Accidents)

Patients with SCD are at **greatly increased risk for both ischemic and hemorrhagic stroke.** Most strokes in children are ischemic events, usually involving large arteries, whereas hemorrhagic strokes are more common in adults. Common presenting signs and symptoms include hemiparesis, aphasia, dysphasia, cranial nerve palsies, seizure, or coma. A noncontrast enhanced CT scan should be obtained as soon as possible, followed by MRI and MRA with diffusion weighted imaging. The treatment for ischemic stroke in **children is exchange transfusion,** as conventional therapies (tissue plasminogen activator and antiplatelet agents) are not indicated. Ischemic strokes in **adults** with SCD are thought to be more likely due to common ischemic stroke mechanisms; therefore **conventional therapies are recommended.**

Splenic Sequestration

Acute splenic sequestration is the **most common cause of acute exacerbation of anemia in patients with SCD.** This occurs when red cells become trapped in the spleen, resulting in a sudden drop in hemoglobin and the potential for shock. It typically occurs between the ages of 3 months to 5 years. Patients typically present with sudden weakness, pallor, tachycardia, or abdominal fullness. The mortality of this condition is high, and death can occur within a matter of hours without aggressive management. All patients should be transfused with packed red blood cells emergently. **Splenectomy may be necessary** in children with recurrent splenic sequestration.

Aplastic Crisis

Patients with SCD are susceptible to transient red cell aplasia (TRCA). The majority of TRCA are caused by Parvovirus B19 infection. The virus is directly cytotoxic to erythroid precursors, which can cause transient suppression of erythropoiesis and reticulocytopenia. This will present as significant anemia after an illness without signs of hemolysis, usually 5 days postexposure and continuing 7 to10 days. Intravenous immunoglobulin (IVIG) infusion is the standard treatment once the diagnosis is made.

Priapism

Priapism, a prolonged painful erection of the penis, is a well-recognized complication of SCD that can result in fibrosis and impotence. Approximately 50% of patients with SCD reported having at least one episode of priapism before 21 years of age. In addition to pain management, effective strategies for immediate and sustained detumescence consist of aspiration of blood from the corpora cavernosa followed by irrigation of the corpora cavernosa with dilute epinephrine. In all cases, early urologic consultation should be obtained.

Treatment

It is important to note that **pain** is often the primary presenting complaint of all sickle cell–associated crises. It is thought that pain is caused by ischemia secondary to sickling. This causes sludging and local acidosis, which in turn engenders more sickling and the pain worsens.

Unfortunately, recent evidence shows that **patients with sickle cell disease are regularly undertreated for their pain.** This is likely due to sociocultural factors as well as the challenges of navigating the subjectivity of pain. Adequately treating pain is a vital component in the treatment of sickle cell patients who present to the emergency department.

The mainstay of **treatment for a pain crisis is supportive care: supplemental oxygen, hydration, and analgesia.** Due to the chronicity of these pain crises, and the long-standing pain that results from sickle cell complications (eg, avascular necrosis), adequate analgesia plays a pivotal role in patient care. Patients with moderate to severe pain typically require **intravenous opiates.** In patients with poor vascular access secondary to chronic intravenous line placement, subcutaneous and intramuscular administration is a suitable alternative. Oral opiates are used for patients in less severe pain. Although there are no definitive studies that show which opioid is superior in treating a pain crisis, morphine sulfate or hydromorphone are commonly used as first-line agents. Hydromorphone is a good option for patients who cannot tolerate the side effects of morphine (eg, nausea and pruritus). Meperidine, a commonly prescribed opioid, should be avoided due to its increased risk of causing seizures and serotonin syndrome. Adjunctive therapy with nonsteroidals, particularly ketorolac, should be considered. However, long-term use of these medications increases the risk of renal failure and peptic ulcer disease. Dosing of analgesics should be individualized for each patient and should be titrated to pain relief. Many patients will know which medication, dose, and frequency of administration are most beneficial to them. Many sickle cell patients with recurrent pain crises and other complications are started on **hydroxyurea,** a myelosuppressive agent shown to reduce these crises.

COMPREHENSION QUESTIONS

41.1 A 3-year-old girl is brought into the ED by her mother for being pale and irritable. The girl is known to have sickle cell disease. Which of the following tests would help to differentiate an aplastic crisis from a vasoocclusive crisis?

A. Reticulocyte count

B. Bone marrow biopsy

C. Peripheral smear

D. Hemoglobin level

E. Haptoglobin level

41.2 A 2-year-old boy with sickle cell disease is being seen by his pediatrician. Which of the following would make the most impact on mortality risk?

A. Screening urine culture

B. Bone radiograph to assess for osteomyelitis

C. Pneumococcal vaccination

D. Chest radiograph to assess for acute chest syndrome

E. Bone marrow biopsy to assess anemia

41.3 A 12-year-old girl is brought into the ED at the direction of her pediatrician. The patient's mother informs you that the patient has sickle cell disease. Which of the following findings would be most concerning to you?

A. Fever

B. Pain that is typical of past crises

C. Mild abdominal pain

D. Hematuria

E. Strabismus

41.4 Which of the following is most accurate concerning acute chest syndrome?

A. It is an uncommon complication of sickle cell disease.

B. It can be caused by pulmonary infection or infarct.

C. It can be ruled out with a normal chest x-ray.

D. Antibiotics should not be given until the patient is proven to have an infection.

ANSWERS

41.1 **A.** The **reticulocyte count** is low in aplastic crisis, but elevated or normal with a vaso-occlusive crisis. A bone marrow biopsy is invasive and causes a delay in diagnosis. Neither a smear nor a haptoglobin level would differentiate between the two diagnoses. A hemoglobin level may not show a difference in the acute setting.

41.2 **C.** Pneumococcal sepsis is the leading cause of death in children aged 1 to 3 years. Thus, **pneumococcal vaccine** is critical in its prevention.

41.3 **A.** The clinician should be worried if the patient has a **fever,** severe abdominal pain, respiratory or neurological symptoms, joint swelling, pain that is not relieved by usual measures, or priapism. The other signs and symptoms here require additional workup, but are not harbingers of the same level of morbidity as a fever.

41.4 **B.** Acute chest syndrome is caused by **pulmonary infection or infarct.** It is a common complication of sickle cell disease that is difficult to confirm simply by a chest radiograph. Because it is difficult to differentiate it from infectious pneumonia, patients are empirically started on antibiotics.

CLINICAL PEARLS

▶ Sickle cell disease can manifest in any organ system and has a variety of clinical presentations ranging from mild to life-threatening.

▶ Because patients with sickle cell disease are functionally asplenic after early childhood, they are at risk for infection by encapsulated organisms (eg, *Haemophilus influenzae, Streptococcus pneumoniae*), and therefore must be immunized with the appropriate vaccines.

▶ Acute chest syndrome is the leading cause of premature death in patients with sickle cell disease. Having a low threshold of suspicion in patients presenting with respiratory complaints, abnormal oxygen saturation, or findings on lung examination, is critical.

▶ Treatment of acute chest syndrome involves supplemental oxygen, hydration, analgesia, empiric antibiotics, and possibly exchange transfusion.

▶ Splenic sequestration has a very high mortality. Patients present with an abrupt drop in hemoglobin and the potential for shock, requiring emergent transfusion and spleenectomy.

▶ Aplastic crisis occurs from a transient suppression of erythropoiesis. It is characterized by significant anemia accompanied by a low reticulocyte count. It is most commonly caused by parvovirus B19.

▶ Patients in pain crises require prompt attention and treatment of their pain. Intravenous opiates, such as morphine or hydromorphone, are the mainstay of pain management in the ED.

REFERENCES

DeBaun MR, Vichinsky E. Sickle cell disease. In: *Nelson Textbook of Pediatrics*. 18th ed. New York, NY: Saunders; 2007:2026-2031.

Givens M, Rutherford C, Joshi G, et al. Impact of an emergency department pain management protocol on the pattern of visits by patients with sickle cell disease. *J Emerg Med*. 2007;32:239-243.

Glassberg J. Current guidelines for sickle cell disease: management of acute complications. *Emergency Medicine Practice Guidelines Update*. 2009;1(3):1-3.

McCreight A, Wickiser J. Sickle Cell Disease. In: Strange GR, Ahrens WR, Schfermeyer R, Wiebe R, eds. *Pediatric Emergency Medicine*. 3rd ed; 2009:Chapter 100.

Zempsky W. Evaluation and treatment of sickle cell pain in the emergency department: paths to a better future. *Clin Pediatr Emerg Med*. 2010;11:265-273.

A 44-year-old undomiciled man is found on a park bench in the middle of winter. He is cold and wet from the falling snow. A concerned citizen called EMS to transport the patient to the Emergency Department. The patient is minimally arousable and his clothes are soaked from the waist down. A pack of cigarettes and a small bottle of whiskey are found in his jacket pocket. On examination, he is thin, disheveled, malodorous, and his extremities are pale and cold. His blood pressure is 110/70 mm Hg, heart rate is 90 beats per minute and irregular, respiratory rate is 18 breaths per minute, and his rectal temperature is 30°C (86°F). There is no evidence of trauma and the patient is not shivering.

▶ What is your next step?
▶ What is the most likely diagnosis?
▶ What is your next step in treatment?

ANSWERS TO CASE 42:
Frostbite and Hypothermia

Summary: A 44-year-old undomiciled man with poor nutrition and a history of ethanol abuse and cigarette smoking was exposed to freezing temperatures and now has a decreased level of consciousness. The patient has an irregular heart rhythm, likely atrial fibrillation. He is not shivering and his rectal temperature is 30°C (86°F).

- **Next step:** Transfer to the ED and prevent further systemic heat loss. Remove any wet or constrictive clothing. Wrap the patient in warm, dry blankets. The affected areas should be immobilized, insulated, and kept away from dry heat sources

- **Most likely diagnosis:** Cold exposure injury leading to frostbite and hypothermia

- **Next step in treatment:** Rapid core rewarming

ANALYSIS

Objectives

1. Recognize the spectrum of cold exposure injuries.

2. Understand the pathophysiology of frostbite and hypothermia and how it affects various organ systems.

3. Know the treatments for frostbite and hypothermia.

Considerations

Accidental hypothermia is a multifaceted entity encompassing a range of clinical features. Frostbite occurs when the skin and body tissues are exposed to cold temperature for a prolonged period of time. To minimize soft tissue injury in this patient, the rewarming process should not be delayed. Evaluation of core body temperature is necessary to determine if hypothermia exists and to what degree. Once his wet and constrictive clothing are removed, passive rewarming techniques can be used to increase the core body temperature. Individuals who are at greatest risk for hypothermia include the elderly, diabetics, smokers, alcoholics, people with peripheral vascular disease, peripheral neuropathy, Raynaud disease, and those who are exposed to windy weather, which increases the rate of heat loss from skin.

APPROACH TO:
Frostbite and Hypothermia

DEFINITIONS

HYPOTHERMIA: Condition in which the core body temperature drops below that required for normal metabolism, which is less than 35°C (95°F).

FROSTNIP: Deposition of superficial ice crystals on the skin. It can be a warning sign for impending frostbite. Typically it is a retrospective diagnosis because it is defined by the absence of tissue damage upon rewarming.

FROSTBITE: Occurs when the skin tissue freezes. Superficial frostbite involves the skin; whereas deep frostbite involves deeper structures such as muscle, tendon, and bone.

TRENCH FOOT: Results from prolonged exposure of the extremities to a cold, wet environment, without freezing. Prolonged exposure to this environment leads to decreased peripheral circulation. This was a common condition in trench warfare during World War I.

CHILBLAINS (PERNIO): A nonfreezing cold-related injury that occurs in cool, humid environments. It is characterized by red, scaly lesions, often on the face, hands, or feet.

CLINICAL APPROACH

Physiology

The human cold response is aimed at maintaining the core body temperature and the viability of the extremities. The skin's thermoreceptors are densest on the upper torso. These peripheral thermoreceptors signal a central thermostat, located in the preoptic region of the anterior hypothalamus to activate autonomic as well as behavioral heat loss and gain mechanisms. Peripheral cooling of the blood leads to a cascade of events including catecholamine release, thyroid stimulation, shivering thermogenesis, and peripheral vasoconstriction. Heat loss is reduced by peripheral vasoconstriction mediated by sympathetic stimulation and catecholamine release. By using stored glycogen, shivering thermogenesis can provide several hours of heat, however once glycogen stores are depleted shivering stops. The extremities are protected by the **hunting reaction,** which consists of irregular, 5- to 10-minute cycles of alternating periods of vasodilation and vasoconstriction that protect the extremities against sustained periods of vasoconstriction. If the body is exposed to cold of prolonged duration or magnitude and the core body temperature is threatened, this mechanism is abandoned—the so-called life-versus-limb mechanism. Once the body has physiologically lost the ability to compensate for the cold, injury is inevitable. The physiologic consequences of cold injury are thus considered by a systems approach.

Heat loss occurs through four basic mechanisms: conduction, convection, radiation, and evaporation. Conduction occurs through heat transfer from the warmer body to a cooler object; in a wet environment, this occurs at a much greater rate. Convection is the transfer of heat from movement, where wind acts as a confounding

Table 42–1 • HYPOTHERMIA RISK FACTORS	
Disrupted Circulation	**Increased Heat Loss**
Tight-fitting clothing	Cold, windy environments
Medications	Medications
Smoking	Ethanol
Diabetes	Extremes of age
Peripheral vascular disease	Burns
Dehydration	
Decreased Heat Production	**Impaired Thermoregulation**
Hypothyroidism	Stroke
Hypoadrenalism	Tumor
Hypoglycemia	Ethanol
Malnutrition	Benzodiazepines
β-blockers	Opioids
Neuroleptics	Barbiturates
Extremes of age	Phenothiazines Atypical antipsychotics Alpha blockers Extremes of age

factor that draws heat away from the body. Radiation is heat transfer by electromagnetic waves from the noninsulated areas on the body. Evaporation of water leads to heat loss through exhalation of warm air.

There are many predisposing factors for the development of hypothermia (see Table 42–1). These can be generalized into four overlapping categories: disrupted circulation, increased heat loss, decreased heat production, and impaired thermoregulation.

Two high-risk populations include individuals who consume ethanol and the elderly. Ethanol use predisposes to hypothermia in many ways. First, it impairs judgment and thermal perception, therefore, increasing the risk to cold exposure. Ethanol predisposes to hypoglycemia, impedes shivering (ie, lack of fuel interferes with shivering), and causes peripheral vasodilation (ie, increases heat loss). In addition, ethanol's affect on the hypothalamus results in a lower thermoregulatory set point, resulting in a reduction of the core temperature. The elderly exhibit age-related impairments in many of the systems of thermoregulation. The elderly often have an impaired shivering response, decreased mobility, and malnutrition. They are less able to discriminate cold environments and often lack the ability to vasoconstrict adequately. Their risks are also increased secondary to their medications, particular cardiac medications, which may impede thermoregulation. The risk of falls is increased in the elderly. It is also critical to rule out sepsis as the cause of hypothermia in the elderly; particularly hypothermic individuals who are found indoors. For systemic effects of hypothermia, see Table 42–2.

Table 42–2 • SYSTEMIC EFFECTS OF HYPOTHERMIA		
Stage	Core Temp (°C)	Characteristic
Mild	37.6	Normal rectal temperature
	36	Increase in metabolic rate, BP, and preshivering muscle tone
	35	Maximal shivering response
	34	Development of the "umbles: bumble, stumble, tumble"; amnesia, dysarthria, poor judgment, maximum respiratory stimulation, tachycardia
	33.3	Development of ataxia and apathy, decreasing minute ventilation, cold diuresis
Moderate	32	Stupor, 25% decrease in oxygen consumption
	31	Extinguished shivering reflex
	30	Development of atrial fibrillation
	29	Progressive decrease in level of consciousness, pupils dilated
Severe	28	Decreased ventricular fibrillation threshold; decrease in oxygen consumption and pulse, hypoventilation
	27	Loss of reflexes and voluntary movement
	26	Anesthesia and areflexia
	25	Cerebral blood flow and cardiac output falls
	24	Hypotension and bradycardia
	23	Loss of corneal reflexes, areflexia
	22	Maximal risk of ventricular fibrillation
Profound	20	Lowest resumption of cardiac electromechanical activity
	19	EEG silent
	18	Asystole
	13.7	Lowest adult accidental hypothermia survival
	15	Lowest infant accidental hypothermia survival
	9	Lowest therapeutic hypothermia survival

Abbreviations: BP = blood pressure; CT = computed tomography; EEG = electroencephalogram.

Cardiovascular

Cardiovascular complications are common throughout the spectrum of cold injury. Initially during mild cold stress, tachycardia is noted, as temperatures decline, the response of the cardiovascular system shifts from tachycardia to progressive bradycardia that is refractory to atropine. A multitude of cardiac dysrhythmias are seen in hypothermia with atrial fibrillation being the most common. The Osborn or J wave is a well-known manifestation of hypothermia seen on ECGs (see Figure 42–1). It is characterized by elevation at the junction of the QRS complex and the ST-segment and is typically seen at temperatures below 32°C (89.6°F). As temperatures drop below 28°C (82.4°F), ventricular fibrillation occurs. As the core body temperature drops so does oxygen consumption. It is thought that in some people this decline in oxygen consumption may explain why profoundly hypothermic patients have been successfully resuscitated.

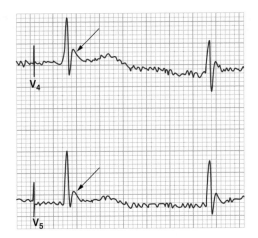

Figure 42–1. The J (Osborn) wave (arrows) appears on electrocardiograms of approximately 80% of hypothermic patients. In general, the amplitude and duration of the Osborn wave are inversely related to core temperature. (Reproduced, with permission, from Hall JB, Schmidt GA, Wood LDH, eds. *Principles of Clinical Care.* 3rd ed. New York, NY: McGraw-Hill; 2005:1681.)

Respiratory

Initially in response to cold, respirations increase and similarly to the cardiovascular system with continued cold exposure the hyperactivation of the system begins to slow down. Respiratory depression occurs with resultant respiratory acidosis from carbon dioxide retention. Protective airway mechanisms are impaired due to decreased ciliary motility, bronchorrhea, and thickening of respiratory secretions.

Renal

Mild dehydration and hypotension cause a decrease in renal blood flow and glomerular filtration rate. However, central hypervolemia from peripheral vasoconstriction, inhibition of ADH, impaired renal tubular function, and the loss of concentrating abilities result in large-volume cold diuresis.

Gastrointestinal

Poor perfusion to the liver results in the inability to clear toxins, the retention of lactate, and the formation of a metabolic acidosis.

Neurological

As temperature declines, an individual's level of conscious also declines. Pupillary light response and deep tendon reflexes also decline while muscular tone tends to increase.

Hematologic

Hypothermia leads to many hematologic changes. The most common include a progressive hemoconcentration of the blood resulting in an increase in hematocrit. In addition, low temperature inhibits enzymatic reactions of the clotting cascade, leading to a progressive coagulopathy.

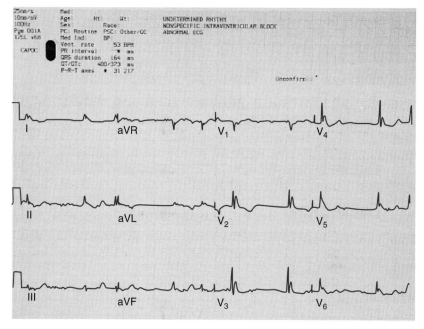

Figure 42–2. ECG shows J waves in a hypothermic patient. (Reproduced, with permission, from Knoop KJ, Stack LB, Storrow AB. *Atlas of Emergency Medicine.* 2nd ed. New York, NY: McGraw-Hill; 2002:516.)

FROSTBITE

Maintenance of core temperature takes precedence over rewarming of the extremities. When the body is exposed to a magnitude or duration of cold that is significant enough to disrupt the core body temperature, continuous and intense vasoconstriction occurs, promoting frostbite to the exposed tissue. **Frostbite occurs when tissue temperatures are less than 0°C (32°F).** There are two mechanisms for tissue damage: architectural cellular damage from ice-crystal formation and microvascular thrombosis and stasis. The initial phase of frostbite, the **"prefreeze phase,"** is characterized by tissue temperatures dropping below 10°C (50°F), and cutaneous sensation being lost. There is microvascular vasoconstriction and endothelial leakage of plasma into the interstitium. Crystal formation does not occur until tissue temperatures drop below 0°C (32°F). Areas of skin that experience a slow rate of cooling will develop ice crystals in the extracellular matrix, whereas cells that undergo rapid cooling develop intracellular ice crystals, the latter of which is less favorable to cell survival. During the **freeze–thaw phase,** extracellular ice crystals form. In an attempt to maintain osmotic equilibrium, water leaves the cells causing cellular dehydration and intracellular hyperosmolality. This leads to cellular collapse and demise. The third phase is the **progressive microvascular collapse phase.** Red cells sludge and form microthrombi during the first few hours after the tissues are thawed. The exact mechanism is unclear. Hypoxic vasospasm, hyperviscosity, and direct endothelial damage all adversely affect flow. Ultimately, there is plasma leakage and arteriovenous shunting resulting in thrombosis, increased tissue pressure, ischemia and necrosis also known as the **late ischemic phase**. In **superficial frost-bite, clear vesicles** may appear, whereas **hemorrhagic blisters** appear in **deep frost-bite injuries.**

MANAGEMENT

The ultimate goal of prehospital treatment is preservation of life. **Frostbite and hypothermia often coexist and prevention of further systemic heat loss is the priority.** Field rewarming should not be performed if there is any potential for inter-rupted or incomplete thawing, unless the possibility of evacuation does not exist, because **tissue refreezing is disastrous.** However, it is appropriate to remove wet, constricting clothing and replace with dry clothing. There is a direct relationship between the length of time the tissue is frozen and the extent of cellular damage.

As with all patients who present to the ED with serious conditions, evaluation and stabilization occurs simultaneously and the ABCs should always be promptly addressed. The patient should be placed on a cardiac monitor and have an intra-venous catheter placed. Once this occurs, a thorough history should be obtained including ambient temperature, wind velocity, duration of exposure, type of clothing worn, medication history, and preexisting medical problems that could affect heat loss. A core temperature needs to be determined. This is best achieved by obtain-ing a rectal temperature. Most standard hospital thermometers only read as low as 34°C (93.2°F). Therefore, in patients suspected to be hypothermic, it is critical to measure core temperature using a specialized thermometer that is capable of reading low temperatures.

Diagnostic studies that may be useful include a bedside capillary blood glucose. Correcting hypoglycemia early in presentation may prevent the need for more inva-sive rewarming techniques. As temperature declines, pulse oximetry may not be reli-able, so an arterial blood gas can determine oxygen saturation. An ECG should be obtained to evaluate cardiac dysrhythmias including atrial fibrillation. Laboratory studies may reveal an elevated hematocrit secondary to hemoconcentration, and low platelet counts due to splenic sequestration. Hyperkalemia is indicative of cel-lular acidosis and is a marker for a poor prognosis. Elevation in the blood urea nitro-gen (BUN) and creatinine (Cr) is commonly encountered in hypothermic patients. Low thyroid and cortisol levels may reveal a person predisposed to hypothermia. A high index of suspicion must be maintained for an occult traumatic injury as trauma and hypothermia commonly occur together. Consider a head CT scan and other radiographic studies on patients who have an altered mental status or who do not improve with rewarming.

After stabilizing the core temperature and addressing associated conditions, **rapid thawing** should be initiated. The core temperature will continue to fall even after the patient is extricated from the cold environment due to temperature equili-bration between the core and peripheral blood. Most patients are **dehydrated.** Warm intravenous fluids (crystalloid) should be administered. For frostbite, **rapid rewarm-ing of frozen or partially thawed tissue is accomplished by immersion in gen-tly circulating water that is carefully maintained at a temperature of 37°C to 41°C (99°F-106°F).** Rewarming is continued until the tissue is pliable and distal erythema is noted, usually about 10 to 30 minutes. Active, gentle motion is encouraged but direct tissue massage should be avoided. Parenteral analgesics should be administered because tissue rewarming causes throbbing, burning pain, and tenderness. Sensation is often diminished after thawing and then disappears with bleb formation. Sensation does not normalize until healing is complete.

After thawing, the injured extremities should be elevated to minimize swelling. Sterile dressings should be applied and involved areas handled gently. Digital exercises are encouraged to help avoid venous stasis. Treatment also includes NSAIDs, topical aloe vera, debridement of clear blisters (hemorrhagic blisters should be left alone), and tetanus vaccine if indicated. Antibiotics are also often given. In cases of gangrene, amputation is often delayed for up to 3 weeks, because the extent of tissue injury is difficult to initially assess.

Based on the severity of hypothermia, various rewarming schemes are followed. These include passive rewarming, active external rewarming for moderate hypothermia, and active core rewarming in severe hypothermia.

Passive external rewarming allows patients to warm by endogenous heat production. This requires the ability to shiver. Individuals who are malnourished, hypoglycemic, or have a core temperature below 30°C are not candidates for passive external rewarming. Therefore, this is a good option in healthy patients with a mild degree of hypothermia. The patient should be removed from the cold or wet environment, and be wrapped in blankets, sleeping bags, or other insulating materials.

The decision to actively rewarm a patient implies a greater degree of hypothermia and possibly a coexisting medical condition. Active external rewarming involves the application of heat directly to the skin by way of forced air surface warming, warm water immersion, radiant heat sources, and warm water bottles. In the hospital setting, forced air rewarming is most practical.

Active core rewarming refers to techniques that warm the patient from the inside out and are used to rewarm severely hypothermic patients. There are several methods used in active core rewarming including positive pressure ventilation using warm air, peritoneal and pleural irrigation with warmed saline, and extracorporeal blood rewarming. These methods are reserved for severely hypothermic patients and those presenting with cardiac arrest.

Hypothermic patients may experience complications secondary to rewarming. **Afterdrop** refers to the continual decline in core body temperature after the patient is removed from the cold environment. The current theory holds that rewarming causes disequilibrium across a gradient such that the body is cooled from the periphery to the inside and the core body temperature will continue to drop until core temperature is equal to peripheral temperature. This was thought to predispose to ventricular fibrillation. However, there is little evidence to support this. Nonetheless, ventricular fibrillation is typically resistant to defibrillation until core temperatures are above 28°C (82.4°F).

For patients who are pulseless and show no signs of life, death pronouncement only occurs when the individual's core body temperature is greater than 35°C. Since the physiologic response to hypothermia is extremely varied, the well known adage, "no one is dead until they are warm and dead" is often valid.

COMPREHENSION QUESTIONS

42.1 A 72-year-old woman with dementia is reported missing by nursing home staff late one December night. The patient was found 2 hours after the police were called lying on a park bench, soaking wet, in a thin night gown with no shoes on. EMS has arrived on the scene. Which of the following is the most appropriate next step in management?

A. Check capillary blood glucose and try to feed the patient.

B. Immediately place the patient on a stretcher, start an IV, and give fluids.

C. Check for airway, breathing, circulation, and then maintain core body temperature by removing wet clothes and wrapping in warm, dry blankets.

D. Cover the patient with any available materials so that passive rewarming can start.

42.2 An avid outdoorsman was hiking in the mountains when his boot broke through the ice on the edge of a stream submerging one foot. The patient has a long history of diabetes with known peripheral neuropathy. He was able to hike out to the ranger's station but had lost complete sensation of his wet foot afterwards. The patient has frostbite on his cheeks, hands, and this wet foot shows evidence of trench foot. All wet clothing is removed, he is wrapped in blankets and on arrival to the emergency department, his vitals signs are stable except for a core body temperature of 34°C. Which of the following is the most appropriate next step in management?

A. Initiate extracorporeal blood warming until a core temp of 37°C is reached.

B. Begin rapid rewarming with water 40°C to 42°C (103°F-104°F).

C. Rub the skin dry where there is evidence of trench foot to decrease the chance of blisters developing.

D. Treat the patient's diabetes and peripheral neuropathy then reassess sensation in each extremity.

42.3 A 14-year-old adolescent boy wandered into the woods chasing after his dog and lost his bearings. When he was finally found, he was brought to the ED with severe frostbite of the fingers of both hands. Initially, they appeared very blue, but are beginning to look black. He has not regained sensation 24-hours after the exposure. Which of the following describes the most appropriate time to wait before deciding on amputation of the affected fingers?

A. 24 hours after the episode

B. 48 to 72 hours after the episode

C. 3 to 7 days after the episode

D. 7 to 10 days after the episode

E. 2 to 3 months after demarcation

42.4 An undomiciled man of unknown age presents to the ED unresponsive. Bystanders believe he was outside all night in a snow storm. His core temperature is 30°C. What is the most common cardiac dysrhythmia seen in hypothermia?

A. Sinus tachycardia

B. Sinus bradycardia

C. Ventricular fibrillation

D. Atrial fibrillation

E. Prolonged QT syndrome

42.5 A 35-year-old undomiciled woman, with a history of schizophrenia, presents to the ED complaining of tingling in her fingers. The nursing staff removes her wet clothes and places her in a warm hospital gown. Her vital signs include a blood pressure of 130/75 mm Hg, heart rate of 80 beats per minute, and temperature of 36.05°C (96.9°F). On examination, you note discolored, frost-bitten hands. Which of the following features is a poor prognostic indicator in frostbite?

A. Hemorrhagic blisters

B. Demarcation line of viable tissue

C. Clear fluid-filled blisters

D. Edematous subcutaneous tissue

ANSWERS

42.1 **C.** The first step in emergency care is always to address and stabilize the airway, breathing, and circulation (ABCs). Passive rewarming methods are appropriate including removing wet clothing. It is critical that rapid rewarming be avoided if the patient may be delayed to receiving definitive care. Incomplete thawing and refreezing is detrimental to tissue. Checking a blood glucose is important in a patient with altered mental status but should be done after ABCs are addressed.

42.2 **B.** Rapid rewarming in the field is rarely practical, however, in the Emergency department it should be started as soon as possible. It is critical to avoid the deleterious effects of incomplete thawing and prevent refreezing. Although comorbid conditions such as diabetes influence the management of a hypothermic patient, the patient's lack of sensation is due to cold injury and this should be rapidly treated, not just treating the diabetes.

42.3 **E.** Generally, 3 weeks is the minimum time required to assess the viability of tissue after frostbite to see whether amputation is required. Tissue thought to be necrotic sometimes turns out to be viable. The line of demarcation between viable and nonviable tissue becomes clear in 1 to 2 months after the initial cold injury, but surgery may be delayed until 2 to 3 months.

42.4 **D.** Atrial fibrillation is the most common dysrhythmia in hypothermia and is characteristically seen at a core temperature of 30°C. Prolongation of any interval, bradycardia, asystole, atrial fibrillation/flutter, and ventricular tachycardia may also be seen. In this patient a 12-lead ECG was obtained showing an Osborne (J) wave, which is indicative of a junctional rhythm and is consistent with hypothermia. J waves may be seen at any temperature below 32.2°C (89.9°F), most frequently in leads II and V6. Below a core temperature of 25°C (77°F), they are most commonly found in the precordial leads (especially V3 and V4) and their size increases. J waves are usually upright in aVL, aVF, and the precordial leads.

42.5 **A.** Hemorrhagic blisters are a poor prognostic indicator due to their association with deep tissue injury. These blisters should not be debrided or drained because it leads to tissue desiccation and worsening of the injury. Clear blisters, on the other hand, should be drained because the fluid contains thromboxane, which is thought to be destructive to healthy tissue. A demarcation line of healthy tissue is a late sign in hypothermia. Edematous soft tissue is not a prognostic indicator in frostbite.

CLINICAL PEARLS

▶ Because hypothermia and frostbite often occur simultaneously, prevention of further systemic heat loss is the highest priority.

▶ Field rewarming is rarely warranted because of the potential for incomplete or interrupted rewarming. Injured parts should be protected, core temperature stabilized and patient transferred to the ED for rapid rewarming. A rewarming bath should be maintained at a temperature of 37°C to 41°C (98.6°F-105.8°F).

▶ Standard hospital thermometers only read as low as 34°C (93°F), so a specialized low-temperature thermometer is required to obtain an accurate core body temperature.

▶ A severely hypothermic patient can present with rigidity, asystolic, and with fixed pupils; however, he or she should not be pronounced deceased until the core body temperature has been warmed to at least 35°C (95°F).

▶ Hypoglycemia, sepsis, and hypothyroidism are conditions that may mimic or coexist with hypothermia.

▶ Ethanol abusers and the elderly are at high risk for cold-exposure injuries.

REFERENCES

Ahya SN, Flood K, eds. *The Washington Manual of Medical Therapeutics*, 33rd ed. St Louis, MO: Lippincott Williams & Wilkins; 2010.

Aslam AS, Aslam AK, Vasavada BC, Khan IA. Hypothermia: evaluation, electrocardiographic manifestations, and management. *Am J Med*. 2006;199:297-301.

Bessen HA, Ngo B, Hypothermia. In: Tintinalli JE, Kelen GD, Stapczynski JS, eds. *Emergency Medicine: A Comprehensive Study Guide*. 7th ed. New York, NY: McGraw-Hill; 2011.

Danzl DF. Frostbite. In: Rosen P, Barkin R, eds. *Emergency Medicine, Concepts and Clinical Practice*. 7th ed. Philadelphia, PA: Mosby; 2009.

Danzl DF. Accidental hypothermia. In: Rosen P, Barkin R, eds. *Emergency Medicine, Concepts and Clinical Practice*. 7th ed. Philadelphia, PA: Mosby; 2009.

Hermann L, Weingart S. Hypothermia and other cold-related emergencies. *Emerg Med Pract*. 2003;5(12):1-22.

Ikaheimo TM, Junila J, Hirvonen J, Hassi J. Frostbite and other localized cold-related injuries. In: Tintinalli JE, Kelen GD, Stapczynski JS, eds. *Emergency Medicine: A Comprehensive Study Guide*. 7th ed. New York, NY: McGraw-Hill; 2011.

McCauley RL, Killyon GW, Smith DJ, Robson MC, Heggers JP. Frostbite. In: Auerbach PS, ed. *Wilderness Medicine*. 5th ed. Philadelphia, PA: Mosby Elsevier; 2007:195-210.

Olin JW. Other peripheral arterial diseases. In: Goldman L, Bennett JC, eds. *Cecil Textbook of Medicine*. 24th ed. Philadelphia, PA: WB Saunders; 2011.

Van der Ploeg GJ, Goslings JC, Walpoth BH, Bierens JJ. Accidental hypothermia: rewarming treatments, complications and outcomes from one university medical centre. *Resuscitiation*, 2010:1550-1555.

A group of teenagers was swimming at the lake, when one of the boys failed to surface after diving off a platform. He was quickly found and rescued by another swimmer from the lake bottom. The patient was noted to be apneic, and cardiopulmonary resuscitation (CPR) was initiated by one of the bystanders. After the paramedics arrived, the patient was noted to have spontaneous shallow respirations, a weak palpable pulse, and Glasgow coma scale (GCS) score of 7 (eyes 1, verbal 2, motor 4). The paramedics intubated the patient and transported him to the emergency department (ED). In the ED, the patient has an initial pulse of 70 beats per minute, blood pressure of 110/70 mm Hg, temperature of 35.6°C (96.1°F), GCS score of 6 (eyes 1, verbal 1, motor 4), and oxygen saturation of 92% on 100% FiO_2.

▶ What are the complications associated with this condition?
▶ What is the best treatment for this patient?

ANSWERS TO CASE 43:
Submersion Injury

Summary: A teenage boy presents with near-drowning following a diving accident at a lake.

- **Complications:** Submersion injury results in global hypoxia and tissue ischemia primarily affecting the brain, lungs, and heart. Early complications include non-cardiogenic pulmonary edema, hypoxic encephalopathy, respiratory and metabolic acidosis, dysrhythmias, and renal impairment. Coagulopathy, electrolyte abnormalities, and hemodilution or hemoconcentration are rare but possible sequela. Pneumonia and acute respiratory distress syndrome can occur later in the patient's hospital course.

- **Best treatment:** The most important treatment to optimize outcome is rapid initiation of resuscitation in the prehospital setting (ie, stabilizing the ABCs). To this end, bystander CPR can be vitally important. Victims of submersion injury often require aggressive respiratory support, which may range from administration of supplemental oxygen to intubation. If cervical spine injury is suspected (as in this patient who dove off a platform), cervical spine stabilization should be maintained until spinal trauma is ruled out.

ANALYSIS

Objectives

1. Learn the pathophysiology of submersion injury.

2. Become familiar with the epidemiology and prevention of drowning.

3. Learn the special problems associated with cold-water-submersion injury.

Considerations

The initial management of patients with submersion injury is stabilization of the ABCs and correction of hypoxemia. In the ED, all of these patients require continuous cardiac monitoring and pulse oximetry. Initial diagnostics may include a complete blood count, blood glucose, electrolytes, creatinine, arterial blood gas, and chest x-ray. This patient will need to be admitted to the ICU where continued cardiopulmonary monitoring and mechanical ventilation support can be provided.

When encountering a patient with a submersion injury, the ED physician must always consider whether any precipitants exist that also require treatment. These precipitants may include alcohol or drug intoxication, seizures, hypoglycemia, cardiac arrest, attempted suicide or homicide, and child abuse or neglect. In addition, if the submersion is associated with a history of trauma (eg, diving into water, motor vehicle collision), cervical spine and head injuries are considerations. Hypothermia should also be considered if the patient is submersed in cold water. After the patient is hemodynamically stable, radiographic imaging of the cervical spine (plain x-rays or computed tomography [CT]) and CT of the head may be necessary to rule out concomitant injury.

APPROACH TO:
Submersion Injury

DEFINITIONS

DROWNING: Death following a submersion event.

SUBMERSION VICTIM: Patient with some degree of submersion distress requiring medical evaluation and treatment.

IMMERSION SYNDROME: Syncope or sudden death that occurs after submersion in water that is at least 5°C less than body temperature. Due to dysrhythmias induced by vagal stimulation.

CLINICAL APPROACH

Epidemiology and Prevention

Drowning is the fourth most common cause of accidental death in the United States. In children 1 to 14 years old, it is the second leading cause of death (behind motor vehicle collisions). Risk factors for drowning include age, gender, and race. The incidence of submersion injuries peaks in toddlers and young children, adolescents and young adults, and in the elderly. However, drowning deaths are most common in toddlers and older teenagers. Males account for 80% of drowning victims older than 12 months. Between 15 to 19 years of age, black boys have drowning rates 12 to 15 times higher than those of white boys.

Alcohol use and other medical conditions have also been associated with an increased risk of submersion injuries. Among teenagers and adults, alcohol use may be a contributing factor in 30% to 50% of drownings. Seizures, autism, and other developmental and behavioral disorders also increase the risk of drowning. In patients with prolonged QT syndrome, immersion in cold water may further extend the QT interval.

Submersion injuries can occur in natural bodies of water (freshwater and saltwater) as well as in domestic settings (such as bathtubs and swimming pools). Infants may even drown in toilets or buckets of water. However, if the infant is less than 6 months old or has an atypical presentation, healthcare providers should maintain a high suspicion for abuse. Efforts to decrease the incidence of submersion injuries and drowning deaths have focused on educating the public and increasing awareness of preventive measures. Preventive measures include adequate fencing around pools, decreasing the use of alcohol when engaged in water sports, increasing the supervision of children playing in or near water, and increasing the number of citizens trained in CPR. Water safety education for children, teenagers, and parents that encourages wearing flotation devices and never swimming alone should be reinforced in the school, community, and physician's office.

Pathophysiology of Submersion Injuries

Victims of submersion injuries initially hold their breaths. As hypoxia and air hunger develop, they eventually involuntarily swallow and aspirate water. After aspiration of 1 to 3 mL/kg of water, dilution and washout of surfactant occurs, resulting in atelectasis, decreased gas exchange across the alveoli, non-cardiogenic pulmonary edema, and ventilation-perfusion mismatch. This leads to worsening hypoxia and respiratory and metabolic acidosis. If this process continues, neuronal death and cardiovascular collapse ensue.

"Dry drowning" is a term that was traditionally used to refer to drowning deaths that occurred without aspiration of a significant amount of water (perhaps due to severe laryngospasm, hypoxia, and loss of consciousness). However, the medical literature does not support this mechanism of injury. Dry drownings are probably due to causes besides simple submersion.

Management

Patients with submersion injuries may present with signs of pulmonary and central nervous system dysfunction or dysrhythmias. The patient may arrive in extremis with hypoxia, cyanosis, severe respiratory distress, or respiratory arrest. Other pulmonary findings may include tachypnea, wheezes, rales, or rhonchi. Neurologically, patient presentations may range from a mild alteration of consciousness to coma. Neurological deficits at the time of initial evaluation do not necessarily portend a poor patient outcome. Dysrhythmias are mainly the result of hypoxemia and acidosis and may include ventricular fibrillation, ventricular tachycardia, and bradycardia asystole. Patients with severe submersion injury may develop acute respiratory distress syndrome, hypoxic encephalopathy, or cardiac arrest.

All patients should be placed on continuous cardiac monitoring and pulse oximetry in the ED. An ECG is useful to rule out QT prolongation and dysrhythmias. A chest x-ray should also be performed to identify any infiltrates or pulmonary edema with the caveat that initial x-ray findings may progress over time. Although they are often normal at first, a baseline complete blood count, electrolytes, creatinine, and glucose should be obtained. Arterial blood gases may be helpful in monitoring for acidosis, hypercarbia, and hypoxemia. If a concern for rhabdomyolysis exists, serum creatinine kinase and urine myoglobin levels may be useful.

One of the most critical elements in the successful management of submersion victims is prompt and effective basic life support delivery in the prehospital setting. The Heimlich maneuver is no longer recommended to expel fluid from the lungs because of the high rate of aspiration induced by this maneuver and because of the delay it causes in initiation of ventilation. An awake patient with mild respiratory symptoms may benefit from noninvasive positive pressure ventilation (NIPPV) although a risk of gastric distention and vomiting does exist with the use of NIPPV. Indications for intubation include a lack of protective airway reflexes, respiratory distress, hypercarbia, hypoxia (despite noninvasive oxygen delivery), and apnea.

Intravenous fluids consisting of lactated Ringer solution or normal saline should be initiated in most victims. Glucose containing solutions are generally contraindicated except in hypoglycemic patients. Scientific investigations indicate that glucose solutions may worsen the neurological outcome in animals that have incomplete cerebral ischemia. In general, empiric antibiotics are not indicated for patients with submersion injuries. Antibiotics may benefit patients who were submerged in grossly contaminated water or manifest signs of infection.

Patients who are asymptomatic may be observed in the ED for 4 to 6 hours. If they maintain normal oxygen saturations on room air and have normal pulmonary examinations and chest x-rays, they may be discharged home. Admission is required for patients who are symptomatic, have been unconscious or hypoxic or apneic, have an abnormal chest x-ray, or have evidence of dysrhythmia.

Cold Water Submersion Injury

Submersion in cold water may be more advantageous than submersion in warm water due to induction of the diving reflex and hypothermia. In the diving reflex, blood is shunted away from the victim's peripheral tissues to the heart and brain, decreasing metabolism and reducing anoxic injury. This reflex is strongest in children less than 6 months old and decreases with age. The protective effects of this reflex may partially account for reports of complete neurological recovery in children after prolonged submersion. Hypothermia has been theorized to be neuroprotective because of the induction of global hypometabolic state, leading to the conservation of oxygen and glucose for brain metabolism. Cold water also has potentially deleterious effects, most significantly cardiac irritability (leading to dysrhythmias), exhaustion, and altered mental status. Although some case reports have described patients who survived prolonged submersion in cold water, hypothermia is usually a poor prognostic indicator.

COMPREHENSION QUESTIONS

43.1 Each of the following patients is being treated for a submersion experience. Which one of the following is most appropriate for discharge from the ED after several hours of observation?

A. A 3-year-old boy found face-down in the swimming pool, requiring 4 minutes of CPR, has a return of normal vital signs, with GCS score of 15, and mild respiratory distress.

B. A 12-year-old boy found unconscious and submerged in a swimming pool after striking his head on the bottom. His chest x-ray (CXR) and head CT are normal. His GCS score is 14. He is complaining of headache and no respiratory symptoms.

C. A 6-year-old boy who was washed into the ocean by a large wave and was rescued by a bystander. No CPR was required, and the boy had an initial GCS score of 14 and normal vital signs. CXR and physical examination are normal. Room air O_2 saturation is 95%.

D. A 3-month-old infant who was brought to the ED after accidental submersion in the bathtub. The physical examination is unremarkable except for bruising over both arms and ankles. His CXR is normal and his room air O_2 saturation is 98%.

43.2 Which of the following is a correct statement regarding submersion injuries?

A. Antibiotics may benefit patients who were submersed in grossly contaminated water.

B. The diving reflex is neuroprotective for adults who are submersed in cold water.

C. Neurological deficits on initial evaluation portend a poor prognosis.

D. A normal initial chest x-ray rules out pulmonary injury.

ANSWERS

43.1 **C.** Although the boy described in choice A is stable, his initial requirement for 4 minutes of CPR places him at a great risk for pulmonary and neurological sequelae. The patient described in B has mild respiratory symptoms, but his mechanism of injury and neurological findings are concerning for a closed head injury that requires further observation. The patient described in D is stable from the standpoint of a submersion injury, but the physical findings suggest possible intentional injury that may need further investigation.

43.2 **A.** Antibiotics may benefit patients who were submersed in grossly contaminated water or who have signs of infection on examination. The diving reflex is strongest in infants and children. Neurological deficits at the time of initial evaluation do not rule out the possibility of neurological recovery. Initial chest x-ray findings may progress over time.

CLINICAL PEARLS

▶ Precipitants (such as alcohol use, seizures, and hypoglycemia) and associated cervical spine and head injuries must be considered in any submersion victim.

▶ The most common complications involve pulmonary or central nervous system dysfunction or dysrhythmias.

▶ The most important treatment to optimize outcome is rapid initiation of resuscitation in the prehospital arena. Victims of submersion injury often require aggressive respiratory support.

REFERENCES

Bowers RC, Anderson TK. Chapter 44. Disorders due to physical and environmental agents. Stone CK, Humphries RL. eds. *Current Diagnosis and Treatment: Emergency Medicine*. 6th ed. Available at: http://www.accessmedicine.com/content.aspx?aID=3113673.

Causey AL, Nichter MA. Chapter 209. Drowning. In: Tintinalli JE, Stapczynski JS, Cline DM, Ma OJ, eds. *Emergency Medicine: A Comprehensive Study Guide*. 7th ed. New York, NY: McGraw-Hill; 2011. Available at: http://www.accessmedicine.com/content.aspx?aID=6379687.

Causey AL, Tilelli JA, Swanson ME. Predicting discharge in uncomplicated near-drowning. *Am J Emerg Med*. 2000;18:9-11.

Kuo DC, Jerrard DA. Environmental insults: smoke inhalation, submersion, diving, and high altitude. *Emerg Med Clin N Am*. 2003;21:475-497.

Richards DB, Knaut AL. Drowning. In: Marx JA, Hockberger RS, Walls RM, eds. *Rosen's Emergency Medicine: Concepts and Clinical Practice*. 7th ed. Philadelphia, PA: Mosby Elsevier; 2011: Chapter 143.

Volturo GA. Submersion injuries. In: Aaron CK, Abujamra L, eds. *Harwood Nuss' Clinical Practice of Emergency Medicine*. 4th ed. Lippincott Williams & Wilkins; 2005: Chapter 356.

Weinstein MD, Kriegr BP. Near-drowning: epidemiology, pathophysiology, and initial treatment. *J Emerg Med*. 1996;14:461-467.

A 50-year-old woman presents with a severe headache of abrupt onset of 10 hours duration. The pain is diffuse, throbbing, and worsened when she went outside into the sunlight. She denies any recent fever, neck pain, numbness, weakness, vomiting, and any change in vision. She was concerned because she has never had a headache as strong as this before. Her past medical and family histories are unremarkable. She does not take any medications, does not smoke, and only drinks alcohol socially.

On examination, her temperature is 36.9°C (98.4°F), blood pressure 136/72 mm Hg, heart rate 88 beats per minute, and respiratory rate of 16 breaths per minute. She is not in any acute distress but appears to be mildly uncomfortable. Her pupils are equal and reactive bilaterally. There is no evidence of papilledema on fundoscopic examination. Movement of her neck causes her some increased discomfort. Her neurological examination is normal, including cranial nerves, strength, light touch sensation, deep-tendon reflexes, and finger-to-nose. The computed tomography (CT) scan of her head is normal.

▶ What is the most likely diagnosis?
▶ What is the next diagnostic step?

ANSWERS TO CASE 44:

Headache

Summary: This is a 50-year-old woman with acute onset of "the worst headache of her life."

- **Most likely diagnosis:** Subarachnoid hemorrhage.

- **Next diagnostic step:** CT scan of the head followed by lumbar puncture.

ANALYSIS

Objectives

1. Learn to differentiate emergent, urgent, and less urgent causes of headache.

2. Understand the treatment of various types of headache.

Considerations

This 50-year-old woman has an acute onset of severe headache, described as the "worse headache of her life." The acute onset and severity of her symptoms are concerning for subarachnoid hemorrhage (SAH). Headache is a very common chief complaint in the emergency department (ED), accounting for up to 2.2% of all ED visits. When evaluating patients with headaches, the clinician's goals are to identify those with serious or life-threatening conditions and to alleviate pain. The physical examination should screen for non-neurological causes of headache including palpation of the sinuses (looking for tenderness consistent with sinusitis), palpation of the temporal arteries (for tenderness or reduced pulsations suggestive of temporal arteritis). A thorough eye examination is important and should consist of assessment of the pupils, visual acuity, and fundoscopy. A detailed neurological examination should also be performed. This patient's CT scan of the head is unremarkable, which does not definitively rule out subarachnoid hemorrhage. CT scan is often performed to rule out a cerebral mass before performing lumbar puncture (LP). Erythrocytes in the cerebral spinal fluid (CSF) or a xanthochromic CSF are considered diagnostic for SAH. However, xanthochromia may take up to 12 hours to appear. Therefore, a negative LP in the face of clinical suspicion for subarachnoid hemorrhage may necessitate repeat LP or other neuroimaging such as magnetic resonance imaging (MRI) or angiography.

APPROACH TO:
Headache

CLINICAL APPROACH

Headaches can be caused by many intracranial and extracranial processes. One of the easiest ways to classify them is to separate them into primary and secondary causes. Primary headaches are most common and include migraine, tension-type, and cluster headaches. Secondary headaches are the result of some other disease process (eg, infection, tumor). Headaches can also be subdivided into critical or emergent versus nonemergent causes. Critical and emergent headaches have an etiology that mandates immediate identification and treatment (Table 44–1). In contrast, nonemergent causes are benign and do not present any immediate threat to life. This category includes primary headache syndromes and postlumbar puncture headaches. Less than 1% of patients with headache have a potentially life-threatening etiology, but identification of these patients is paramount.

When evaluating patients with headaches, the history should focus on the nature of the pain (location, severity, character, onset), any associated symptoms, and aggravating or alleviating factors. Past medical history (including history of head trauma, medications) and family history are important to identify risk factors for serious disease. A history of prior headaches and any previous diagnostic studies can also be helpful. Potentially ominous historical findings include a sudden onset, the "worst headache of life," headaches dramatically different from past episodes, immunocompromised, new onset after age 50 years, and onset with exertion.

A complete physical examination with a detailed neurological evaluation can also help to separate the emergent from other causes. Abnormal vital signs can be a harbinger of life-threatening conditions. Other warning signs include altered mental status, abnormal fundi, meningeal signs, focal neurological deficits, and a rash suspicious for meningococcemia. Some types of headache have classic historical or examination findings that will aid in narrowing the differential (Table 44–2).

Table 44–1 • CRITICAL AND EMERGENT CAUSES OF HEADACHE
Anemia
Anoxia
Brain abscess
Carbon monoxide poisoning
Glaucoma
Hypertensive encephalopathy
Meningitis/encephalitis
Mountain sickness
Shunt failure
Subarachnoid/other intracranial hemorrhage
Temporal arteritis
Tumor/cerebral mass

Table 44–2 • CLASSIC HISTORICAL AND EXAMINATION FINDINGS

Etiology	History	Examination
Brain tumor	Headache with nausea and vomiting, gradual onset, worse in morning, most commonly metastatic	Papilledema, cognitive difficulties, focal neurological deficits
Cluster	Severe, unilateral periorbital pain with lacrimation, rhinorrhea; worse at night; attacks "clustered" in short time period; more common in men	Ipsilateral conjunctival injection, ptosis, miosis
Hypertensive encephalopathy	Diffuse, throbbing headache; worse in morning	Diastolic blood pressure >120-130 mm Hg, altered mental status, papilledema
Idiopathic intracranial hypertension (pseudotumor cerebri)	Headache with visual complaints, classically young obese females of childbearing age	Papilledema, visual field defects
Meningitis	Febrile illness	Fever, meningismus, altered mental status; Kernig and Brudzinski signs
Migraine	Unilateral, throbbing headache with nausea, vomiting, photophobia, phonophobia; may be accompanied by visual, motor, or sensory disturbances; more common in women	
Post lumbar puncture	Bilateral, throbbing headache; worse upon standing, better when lying down	
Subarachnoid hemorrhage	"Thunderclap" onset, "worst headache of life," nausea, vomiting	Retinal or subhyaloid hemorrhages, meningismus, third or sixth nerve palsy
Temporal arteritis	Pain over temporal artery; visual problems, jaw claudication; fever, malaise, weight loss; joint pains; worse at night; more common in women >50 years old	Tenderness or induration of temporal artery, decreased or absent pulse in temporal artery, optic nerve edema
Tension type	Dull, "band-like" headache	Pericranial muscle tenderness

Because there is no routine workup of headaches, testing must be based on clinical suspicion of serious illness (Table 44–3). Diagnostic imaging of the head should be considered for patients with sudden-onset severe headaches, HIV-positive patients with a new headache, and headaches with new abnormal findings (eg, focal deficit, altered mental status). Management includes stabilizing any life-threatening conditions, controlling pain, and addressing any underlying disease or specific etiologies.

SUBARACHNOID HEMORRHAGE

Subarachnoid hemorrhage (SAH) has an annual incidence of 1 in 10,000 Americans. Most cases occur in patients 40 to 60 years old. The presentation can be very subtle with a normal neurological examination, little or no nuchal rigidity, normal level of

Table 44–3 • DIAGNOSTIC TESTS AND TREATMENT		
Etiology	**Diagnostic Tests**	**Treatment**
Brain tumor	CT; consider CT with contrast or MRI	Neurosurgical consultation. If increased intracranial pressure, consider intubation and mild hyperventilation, osmotic agents, steroids
Cluster		High-flow oxygen, sumatriptan, DHE; consider intranasal lidocaine
Hypertensive encephalopathy	CT; rule out other end-organ damage	Control blood pressure (eg, nicardipine, labetalol)
Idiopathic intracranial hypertension	CT to rule out other causes of increased intracranial pressure; LP with opening pressure	Serial LPs, acetazolamide; surgical intervention may be required
Meningitis	CT may be needed prior to LP; LP	Intravenous antibiotics (without delay); consider steroids
Migraine		Acetaminophen, NSAIDs, antiemetics (eg, metoclopramide, prochlorper azine), serotonin agonists (sumatriptan), ergot alkaloids (DHE); narcotics if refractory pain; consider steroids
Post lumbar puncture		Hydration, bed rest, NSAIDs, narcotics, caffeine; consider epidural blood patch for severe, prolonged symptoms
Subarachnoid hemorrhage	CT, LP if CT negative; MRI or angiography may be required	Neurosurgical consult, control blood pressure, analgesia, nimodipine, antiemetics, antiseizure medications
Temporal arteritis	Erythrocyte sedimentation rate; consider temporal artery biopsy (may be done as outpatient)	Steroids
Tension type		Aspirin, acetaminophen, NSAIDs, stress reduction

Abbreviations: CT = computed tomography; MRI = magnetic resonance imaging; DHE = dihydroergotamine; LP = lumbar puncture; NSAIDs = nonsteroidal anti-inflammatory drugs.

consciousness, and normal vital signs. Nevertheless, the mortality associated with SAH approaches 50%. Thus, the ED physician must maintain a high index of suspicion in a patient with acute onset of severe headache. CT scan is usually the initial imaging test. Although the newer high-resolution CTs have higher sensitivity, no imaging procedure can definitively rule out SAH. Thus, many authorities advocate performing a lumbar puncture on all patients suspected of having SAH, even in the face of a normal CT scan. The lumbar puncture revealing xanthochromic CSF is considered the gold standard of diagnosis. Because xanthochromia may take up to 12 hours to develop, persistently bloody CSF is also worrisome for SAH. Neurosurgical evaluation is important once the diagnosis of SAH is established. Nimodipine may be helpful in decreasing cerebral arterial spasm and subsequent ischemia. Angiographic evaluation is usually undertaken to assess for possible need of surgical intervention of lesions such as berry aneurysms. Prognosis generally correlates with initial neurological status.

CEREBRAL CAUSES

Viral or bacterial meningitis can cause severe headache. Lumbar puncture is the best method of assessing for these infections. Immunocompromised states such as human immunodeficiency virus (HIV) infection may cause more subtle or atypical symptoms (eg, lack of fever or meningismus). Pre-LP CT does not necessarily need to be performed for a patient without risk factors for a mass lesion (such as HIV or cancer) and a normal neurological examination, normal level of consciousness, and absence of papilledema. Stroke or transient ischemic attack (TIA) may present as headache, but usually there is a history of or continued neurological deficit. The classic presentation of a brain tumor (headache associated with nausea or vomiting, sleep disturbances) is uncommon. Thus persistent atypical headache (such as new onset after age 50 years), severe pain, or associated with even subtle cognitive or neurological function should be investigated, usually with CT.

TEMPORAL ARTERITIS

Temporal arteritis (TA) almost always occurs in patients older than age 50 years and is more common in women. It is caused by systemic arteritis, which presents as severe and throbbing headache, located over the frontotemporal region. Often, the temporal artery has a diminished pulse or is tender or is pulsating. Patients are diagnosed with TA if they fulfill three of the following criteria: age older than 50 years, new-onset localized headache, decreased pulse or tenderness over the temporal artery, an erythrocyte sedimentation rate exceeding 50 mm/h, and/or abnormal temporal artery biopsy. Vision loss is a potential complication, and immediate treatment should include prednisone 40 to 60 mg/d and urgent referral.

PRIMARY HEADACHE SYNDROMES

Migraine headaches are common. Onset usually occurs during the teenage years, and women are more often affected than men. Family history is often positive. The most common variety is migraine without aura, which is usually slow in onset, unilateral, and throbbing. Photophobia, phonophobia, nausea, and vomiting frequently accompany the pain. Patients with migraines with aura have a similar type of headache that is preceded by reversible visual phenomena (most common), paresthesias, motor deficits, or language difficulties. Treatment includes intravenous hydration if the patient is dehydrated and placing the patient in a dark, quiet room. Pharmacological options include dihydroergotamine (a nonspecific serotonin agonist), sumatriptan (a selective serotonin agonist), or dopamine antagonists such as metoclopramide, chlorpromazine, or prochlorperazine. In general, opiates are used for patients with refractory pain.

Tension headaches are extremely common. They are usually characterized by bilateral, nonpulsating, "band-like" pain around the forehead to the occiput. Nausea and vomiting are uncommon. Treatment includes acetaminophen, nonsteroidal anti-inflammatory drugs (NSAIDs), and stress reduction techniques.

Cluster headaches are rarer than other types of primary headache syndromes. They occur more commonly in men and usually start after 20 years of age. Patients typically present with unilateral, severe, orbital or temporal pain, often associated with ipsilateral lacrimation, nasal congestion, rhinorrhea, miosis, and/or ptosis. The headaches tend to occur in "clusters" for several weeks and then remit for months or years. High-flow oxygen is usually effective. DHE and sumatriptan can also help relieve symptoms.

COMPREHENSION QUESTIONS

44.1 Several patients have been brought into the ED with a chief complaint of headache. Which of the following patients should be seen first (ie, which is most likely to have a potentially life-threatening condition)?

  A. A 52-year-old man with headache of 8-hour duration, and blood pressure of 210/120 mm Hg.

  B. A 32-year-old woman with severe throbbing headache involving the right side of her head.

  C. A 32-year-old woman who underwent an outpatient bilateral tubal ligation under spinal anesthesia and now complains of severe bilateral headache, especially with sitting up.

  D. A 35-year-old woman with severe headache and a diagnosis given to her of pseudotumor cerebri.

44.2 A 22-year-old woman complains of headache of 2 hours duration that is described as unilateral and throbbing with nausea, photophobia, and phonophobia. Which of the following is the most likely diagnosis?

  A. Cluster headache

  B. Brain tumor

  C. Migraine headache

  D. Tension-type headache

44.3 A 34-year-old woman is brought into the ED for "the worst headache of her life." She has some lethargy, photophobia, and nuchal rigidity. A lumbar puncture is performed after examining her eye grounds. Which of the following findings in cerebrospinal fluid is most concerning for subarachnoid hemorrhage?

  A. Red blood cells

  B. White blood cells

  C. Elevated opening pressure

  D. Xanthochromia

ANSWERS

44.1 **A.** The first patient is most likely to have a potentially life-threatening condition (hypertensive crisis).

44.2 **C.** Migraine headaches are described as unilateral and throbbing with nausea, photophobia, and phonophobia.

44.3 **D.** Xanthochromia in cerebrospinal fluid is most concerning for subarachnoid hemorrhage. Because it results from hemoglobin metabolism, xanthochromia may take up to 12 hours to develop.

CLINICAL PEARLS

▶ Potentially ominous historical findings include sudden onset, "the worst headache of life," headaches dramatically different from past episodes, immunocompromised, new onset after age 50 years, and onset with exertion.

▶ Diagnostic testing must be based on clinical suspicion. For example, if there is a concern for a subarachnoid hemorrhage, a CT scan of the head and lumbar puncture (if CT is negative) are warranted.

▶ In general, management includes stabilizing any life-threatening conditions, controlling pain, and addressing any underlying disease or specific etiologies.

REFERENCES

American College of Emergency Physicians. Clinical policy: critical issues in the evaluation and management of adult patients presenting to the emergency department with acute headache. *Ann Emerg Med*. 2008;52:407-436.

Godwin SA, Villa J. Acute headache in the ED: evidence-based evaluation and treatment options. *Emerg Med Pract*. 2001;3(6):1-32.

Goldstein JN, Camargo CA Jr, Pelletier AJ, et al. Headache in United States emergency departments: demographics, work-up and frequency of pathological diagnoses. *Cephalalgia*. 2006;26:684-690.

Hamilton GC, Sanders AB, Strange GR, Trott AT, eds. *Emergency Medicine: An Approach to Clinical Problem-Solving*. Philadelphia, PA: WB Saunders; 2003:535-551.

Marx JA, Hockberger RS, Walls RM, eds. *Rosen's Emergency Medicine: Concepts and Clinical Practice*. 7th ed. Philadelphia, PA: Mosby Elsevier; 2009.

Mick NW, Peters JR, Silvers SM. *Blueprints in Emergency Medicine*. Malden, MA: Blackwell Publishing; 2002:139-142.

Tintinalli JE, Kelen GD, Stapczynski JS, eds. *Emergency Medicine: A Comprehensive Study Guide*. 7th ed. New York, NY: McGraw-Hill; 2011.

A 74-year-old man is found in his small apartment after having a seizure on a hot summer day. The paramedics state they found him in a poorly ventilated apartment without any air conditioning. They established an IV of normal saline prior to arrival and obtained a fingerstick glucose of 146 mg/dL. Because he was postictal during transport, they were unable to obtain any other history about past medical problems, medications, or allergies.

On arrival in the emergency department (ED), his temperature is 41.1°C (106°F), blood pressure is 157/92 mm Hg, heart rate is 156 beats per minute, and respiratory rate is 28 breaths per minute. He is extremely warm to touch. He is combative, moaning, and flailing his arms and legs at staff. His pupils are mid-range and reactive to light. His mucous membranes are dry. His neck is supple. His skin is flushed, hot, and dry.

▶ What is the most likely diagnosis?
▶ What is the best initial treatment?

ANSWERS TO CASE 45:
Heat-Related Illnesses

Summary: This is a 74-year-old man with a seizure who is hyperthermic, tachycardic, tachypneic, and altered mental status.

- **Most likely diagnosis:** Seizure secondary to heat stroke, but is essential to rule out other causes such as sepsis and medications overdose.

- **Best initial treatment:** Management of the ABCs and rapid cooling

ANALYSIS

Objectives

1. Learn the clinical signs and symptoms associated with heat-related illness.

2. Learn the management and treatment of heat-related illness.

Considerations

When evaluating hyperthermic patients, the clinician must first determine if the patient has a fever or suffering from heat stroke. The presumptive diagnosis of heat stroke can be made on the basis of environmental conditions and circumstantial evidence (hot day, enclosed apartment without air conditioning or adequate ventilation), and the next step is to determine the severity of the patient's heat-related illness, which could be useful in guiding his treatment. Because **heat stroke has a mortality of 10% to 20% even with treatment,** it is essential to diagnose and begin therapy immediately. This patient has severe heatstroke, as evidenced by his altered mental status and seizure. Simultaneously, laboratory and radiographic studies should be performed to rule-out infectious etiologies and drug overdoses.

APPROACH TO:
Heat-Related Illnesses

DEFINITIONS

HEAT STRESS: Feeling of discomfort and physiologic strain with normal core temperatures. These patients exhibit decreased exercise tolerance and no other symptoms.

HEAT EXHAUSTION: Mild dehydration, with or without sodium abnormalities. Patients have profuse sweating, thirst, nausea, vomiting, confusion and headache, and may have collapsed. Core temperatures range from 38°C to 40°C (100°F-104°F). Generally, the victim is not able to continue his/her activities as the result of the environmental conditions.

HEAT STROKE: Severe dehydration with core temperature greater than 40°C. Patients are flushed, with hot, dry skin. Symptoms include those associated with CNS disturbances such as dizziness, vertigo, syncope, confusion, delirium, and unconsciousness. Classically, heat strokes develop slowly over days and occur more frequently in older individuals with chronic illnesses.

EXERTIONAL HEAT STROKE: Heat stroke affecting individuals involved in strenuous physical activities. This type of heat stroke can have a more rapid onset than non-exertional heat strokes. Weather conditions including high humidity and increased temperatures are risk factors. The at-risk individuals are highly motivated athletes, laborers, and soldiers.

CLINICAL APPROACH

The primary abnormality in heat-related illnesses is the individual's inability to adequately transfer heat (produced from normal metabolic activities) to the environment resulting in an increase in core temperature. Risk factors for developing heat illness include ambient heat and humidity, extremes of age, strenuous exercise, cardiovascular disease, dehydration, obesity, impaired mentation, and various medications (eg, diuretics, anticholinergics, antihistamines, phenothiazines, cyclic antidepressants, sympathomimetics, alcohol).

The spectrum of heat-related illness varies in severity from benign to severe. Table 45–1 describes the minor syndromes. In contrast to these benign entities, **heat stroke is characterized by a loss of thermoregulation, tissue damage, and multiorgan failure.** Classically, patients present with **hyperpyrexia (temperature >41°C [106°F])**, central nervous system (CNS) dysfunction (eg, altered mental status, seizure, focal neurological deficits), and anhidrosis.

Diagnosis

Diagnosing heat stroke is largely a matter of ruling out other causes of hyperthermia with concomitant CNS dysfunction. The differential includes alcohol withdrawal; salicylate toxicity; phencyclidine, cocaine, and amphetamine toxicity; tetanus; sepsis; neuroleptic malignant syndrome; encephalitis, meningitis, and brain abscess; malaria; typhoid fever; malignant hyperthermia; anticholinergic toxicity; status epilepticus; cerebral hemorrhage; diabetic ketoacidosis; and thyroid storm.

Laboratory studies should include complete blood count, electrolytes, blood urea nitrogen (BUN)/creatinine, glucose, liver enzymes, coagulation studies, urinalysis, urine myoglobin, and arterial blood gas. An electrocardiogram (ECG) should be considered if the patient has syncope or a history of cardiovascular disease. Chest radiographs are useful to rule out aspiration or any pulmonary infection. CT scan of the head and/or lumbar puncture may also be needed.

Treatment

In treating heat stroke, the clinician should strive to stabilize the **ABCs, commence rapid cooling, replace fluid and electrolyte losses, and treat any complications.** The goal is to cool the patient to 40°C (104°F) to avoid overshoot hypothermia. There are a number of cooling methods that are applied and these can be divided

Table 45-1 • MINOR HEAT ILLNESSES			
Diagnosis	Cause	Symptoms	Treatment
Heat edema	Vasodilation and pooling of fluids in dependent areas	Mild swelling of hands and feet	Self-limited; elevate legs, use of support hose; no diuretics
Heat rash	Blockage of sweat gland pores, may have secondary staphylococcal infection	Pruritic, erythematous, maculopapular rash on clothed areas	Antihistamines for itching, loose-fitting clothing; chlorhexidine cream, dicloxacillin, or erythromycin if infected
Heat cramps	Salt depletion (often from drinking only water)	Severe muscle cramps in fatigued skeletal muscles (usually calves, thighs, shoulders) during or after strenuous exercise	Fluid and salt replacement, rest
Heat syncope	Vasodilation, decreased vasomotor tone, volume depletion	Postural hypotension and syncope	Removal from heat source, rehydration, rest
Heat exhaustion	Water and salt depletion	Sweating, weakness, fatigue, headache, nausea, dizziness, malaise, lightheadedness, temperature usually <40°C (104°F)	Rest, volume, and salt replacement

categorically as evaporative techniques and conduction techniques. **Although there are strong proponents for the different cooling methods, there is no current consensus regarding which of the techniques is most effective. In all patients, the initial measures consist of removing the patient from the hot environment if possible and removing clothing.** Evaporative cooling using cool mist and fans is simple and effective approach to cooling in the field; the evaporative approach is advocated by a number of investigators because the physical cooling principle suggests that the evaporation of 1 ml of water is associated with seven times the amount of heat dissipation when compared to melting 1 g of ice. Alternative cooling methods also include ice packs to the groin and axillae, cooling blankets, ice water immersion, peritoneal lavage, and cardiopulmonary bypass. Antipyretics are not effective in this scenario.

In addition, **shivering can be controlled with benzodiazepines or phenothiazines.** Benzodiazepines can also be used to treat any seizures. If the laboratory studies reveal evidence of rhabdomyolysis, mannitol and alkalinization of the urine are other considerations. The most common complications of heat stroke are rhabdomyolysis, renal failure, liver failure, disseminated intravascular coagulation, heart failure, pulmonary edema, and cardiovascular collapse.

The following independent negative prognosticators for survival have been identified, and these include age >80 years, cardiac disease, cancer, core temperature >40°C, living in an institutions, previous diuretic use, systolic BP <100 mm Hg, GCS <12, and transport to hospital by ambulance.

COMPREHENSION QUESTIONS

45.1 A 33-year-old man is found comatose at a construction site in the noon-hour on a hot summer day. His core temperature is 41.7°C (107°F). The ED physician orders evaporative cooling measures and ice packs. The patient begins with intense shivering. Which of the following is the best next step?

   A. Continued observation.

   B. Short-acting benzodiazepine.

   C. Begin intravenous cooling solution.

   D. Increase the number of ice bags.

   E. Stop the cooling.

45.2 A 70-year-old man is brought into the ED complaining of headache and fatigue. His blood pressure is 100/70 mm Hg, heart rate is 100 beats per minute, and core temperature is 40.3°C (104.5°F). Upon using ice bags, his core temperature is down to 38°C (100.4°F). Which of the following is the best next step?

   A. Observation for 4 to 6 hours and then, if stable, discharge home.

   B. Continue ice bags until the core temperature is 36.7°C (98°F).

   C. Admission to the hospital for observation of complications.

   D. Administer cold gastric lavage.

   E. Discharge the patient only if he can be placed in a different environment after discharge.

ANSWERS

45.1 **B.** This patient most likely has exertional heatstroke where core temperature elevations may occur rapidly; therefore, measurement directed at reducing his core temperature are appropriate and must be continued. Benzodiazepines are first-line therapy for shivering or seizures in heat stroke.

45.2 **C.** All patients with severe heat exhaustion or heat stroke, particularly those who are older, should be admitted.

CLINICAL PEARLS

▶ Heat stroke is distinguished from other heat illnesses by a loss of thermoregulation, tissue damage, and multiorgan failure. Classically, these patients present with hyperpyrexia and CNS dysfunction.

▶ Because heat stroke has a mortality of 10% to 20% even with treatment, it is essential to diagnose and begin therapy immediately.

▶ The treatment of heat stroke consists of stabilizing the ABCs, rapid cooling, replacing fluid and electrolyte losses, and treating any complications (eg, shivering, seizures, rhabdomyolysis).

REFERENCES

Becker JA, Stewart LK. Heat-related illness. *Am Fam Physician*. 2011;83:1325-1330.

Hadad E, Rav-Acha M, Heled Y, Epstein Y, Moran DS. Heat stroke: a review of cooling methods. *Sports Med*. 2004;34:501-511.

Hausfater P, Megarbane B, Dautheville S, et al. Prognostic factors in non-exertional heatstroke. *Intensive Car Med*. 2010;36:272-280.

You are in the emergency center when two patients are brought in by paramedics. By report, the two men in their twenties were victims of lightning injury while playing golf. Eyewitnesses at the scene report that the victims were standing several feet apart, when one of the men was struck directly by lightning that resulted in both men falling to the ground immediately and becoming unconscious. One of the victims was found pulseless at the scene and cardiopulmonary resuscitation (CPR) was initiated by a bystander. The second man was noted to be unconscious for several minutes after the incident and has remained confused. On examination, one victim has extensive soft-tissue burn over his back, and he is intubated and ventilated without spontaneous respirations. No palpable pulse is identified and fine ventricular fibrillation appears on the electrocardiogram (ECG) monitor. The second victim is awake with a pulse rate of 80 beats per minute, blood pressure of 130/80 mm Hg, respirations of 18 breaths per minute, Glasgow coma scale (GCS) score of 13, with no identifiable external sign of injury.

▶ What are the complications of lightning injury?
▶ How are the complications identified?

ANSWERS TO CASE 46:
Lightning and Electrical Injury

Summary: Two adult victims present to the emergency center following lightning injuries. One patient with cardiac arrest appears to have been a victim of direct lightning strike, while the second victim appears to have minimal external signs of injury.

- **Lightning-related complications:** Cardiac injury, usually in the form of arrhythmia, neurological damage, burns, spinal cord injury, and respiratory arrest.

- **Identification of complications:** Thorough and careful physical examination and electrocardiography will identify arrhythmia and cutaneous burns. Computed tomography (CT) scan of the head is indicated in all patients with severe lighting injury and those with abnormal neurological examination. Spinal protection and immobilization are necessary until injury is ruled out, and aggressive, persistent resuscitation according to advanced life support protocol is indicated, including airway control and ventilation support until spontaneous respiration is restored.

ANALYSIS

Objectives

1. Learn to recognize and treat the immediate and late complications associated with electrical injury and lightning injury.

2. Learn to recognize the spectrum of injury associated with lightning and electrocution.

3. Understand the relationship between Ohm law and injuries produced by electric current.

Considerations

One patient suffered a direct lightning strike and is in cardiac arrest. Because of its massive direct current countershock, lightning strike can induce depolarization of the entire myocardium leading to cardiac standstill. **Immediate cardiac arrest is the most common cause of death after a lightning strike.** However, respiratory arrest may also occur, either due to paralysis of the respiratory center in the medulla, or as a result of tetany of the respiratory muscles from electric current passing through the thorax. Many patients will regain cardiopulmonary function if timely and appropriate resuscitation efforts are able to sustain oxygenation and circulation while the organ systems recover.

Given the first patient's young age and lack of comorbid factors, there is a greater likelihood for response to resuscitation efforts than in victims with cardiac arrest from other traumatic causes. The heart's inherent automaticity renders it possible for spontaneous recovery if immediate defibrillation and tissue oxygenation is maintained.

The second patient, although hemodynamically stable, has suffered a high-risk electrical injury with loss of consciousness. Head and/or spinal injury could be present as a consequence of being "thrown" by the lightning strike. He requires evaluation with CT scan of the head, ECG, spinal immobilization, and evaluation and initial observation in the ICU for close monitoring of the cardiopulmonary status.

APPROACH TO:
Lighting and Electrical Injury

CLINICAL APPROACH

Although lightning strike is a rare phenomenon, **this injury is associated with a 25% fatality rate, and more than 70% of those who survive have permanent injuries.** Lightning strike is responsible for approximately 100 deaths annually in the United States. Electrical injury, excluding lightning, is responsible for more than 500 deaths annually, with approximately 20% of its victims being younger than age 18 years. The effects of electrical injury are related to the intensity and magnitude of the electric current. According to **Ohm law,** the current flow (amperage) is directly related to the voltage and inversely related to the resistance in the current's pathway, represented by the following formula: **current (amperage) = voltage/resistance.** Because of their low resistance, **nerves, blood vessels, mucous membranes, and muscle are the preferred pathways for electric current passage and are most susceptible to electrical and lightning injury.** Bones, fat, tendon, and skin have relatively high resistance, and therefore sustain less damage during electric and lightning injuries. The probable path of the electrical current should be assessed; for example, **burns on both hands indicate a path likely through the heart, which has a poor prognosis.**

Electrical current exists in two forms: **alternating current (AC)** and **direct current (DC).** AC involves electrons flowing back and forth in cycles, whereas in DC, the electron flow occurs in only one direction. Alternating current (AC) is more dangerous because it may cause tetanic muscle contractions and the "locking on" phenomenon, preventing the victim from releasing the electrical source and prolonging the exposure to the current. Lightning strike is a form of DC electrical injury with extremely high voltage and amperage, but short duration of exposure. During lightning injury, the electrons flow in only one direction, thereby typically inducing a single intense muscle contraction that "throws" its victim and causes simultaneous fractures and spinal injury. There are four types of lightning injury (Table 46–1).

Pathophysiology

Electrical injury can cause direct necrosis of the myocardium, ischemic injury as a result of vasoconstriction caused by excess catecholamine release, or disturbances in the cardiac rhythm. Even low currents can produce arrhythmias, including asystole and ventricular tachycardia. Late dysrhythmias are uncommon in previously healthy patients, but can be produced by patchy myocardial necrosis and injury to the

Table 46–1 • TYPES OF LIGHTNING INJURY
Direct strike: The most serious type; when the major path of lightning current travels through the victim
Side flash (splash): When the current is discharged from a victim or object of direct strike onto a nearby person. In these cases, the current is traveling through paths of least resistance to the victim
Ground current or stride potential: When the lightning strikes the ground and then enters the victim's body from one foot and exits via the opposite foot
Flashover phenomenon: When the force of nearby lightning causes expansion and implosion of surrounding air, causing a blast effect
Blunt injury: This type of injury may occur when the victim is in close proximity to the shockwave produced by lightning, and the forces may result in the victim being thrown, causing tympanic membrane ruptures, and other contusive injuries

sinoatrial (SA) node. Lightning is able to induce cardiac standstill by depolarizing the entire myocardium. Because of the inherent automaticity of the heart, normal sinus rhythm often spontaneously returns.

Clinical Considerations

Cardiovascular Effects All victims of lightning strike and high-voltage electric injury should have immediate **ECG** monitoring and cardiopulmonary support to maintain tissue perfusion as needed. A cool, extremity with diminished sensation and pulse is usually caused by vasoconstriction and nerve ischemia, which may resolve spontaneously with time. Because extremity compartment syndrome may develop, reexamination with **compartment pressure** measurements is indicated in selective patients. Aggressive treatment by **fasciotomy** is indicated when elevated compartment pressures are identified. Victims of electrical injury with no loss of consciousness or physical findings who are asymptomatic and have normal ECG can be safely discharged home.

Neurological Effects Nerve damage is common after electrical injury, but no one condition is pathognomonic. Approximately 75% of patients struck by lightning will have transient loss of consciousness and brief extremity weakness or paresthesia. Lightning victims often have **keraunoparalysis**, a temporary paralysis with loss of sensation that typically involves lower limbs. Strength and sensation return to normal within a few hours. Other physical findings common in electrical injury are confusion, amnesia, headache, visual disturbance, and seizure. Direct spinal cord injury has been reported after hand-to-hand flow with damage to C_4-C_8.

The most serious effect, especially common after lightning strike, is injury to the respiratory control center in the medulla, resulting in respiratory arrest. In addition, lightning and electrical injury victims often have fixed and dilated pupils as a result of autonomic responses, and this should not be interpreted as a sign of nonsurvival until cerebral function is fully assessed.

As in any apneic trauma victim, the **airway, oxygenation, and ventilation** should be restored immediately. **CT scan of the head** is indicated in patients with neurological findings or loss of consciousness to evaluate for possible intracranial pathology. **Spinal immobilization** should be continued until neurological examination is normal or injury is ruled out radiographically. Most victims of electrical and lightning injury without cardiac arrest will survive, but should be counseled that persistent sequelae, including memory deficit, sleep disturbances, dizziness, fatigue, headaches, and attention deficits may occur.

Skin Burns are common after high-voltage electrical injury, but are less often seen after lightning strike because of instantaneous exposure time. Victims of electrical injury have "flush burns" caused by heat generated by the electrical current, or "flame burns," usually as a consequence of ignition of clothing. Because of its instantaneous exposure time, burns are less common after lightning injury. Lightning strike can cause partial-thickness linear burns in areas of high sweat concentration and low resistance, which result in a transient fern-like skin pattern called the **Lichtenberg figure** that is pathognomonic of lightning. In children, the most common mode of electrical injury is from chewing or biting electrical cords, which manifests as perioral edema and eschar formation.

Thorough **physical examination** will reveal any cutaneous manifestations of electrical injury. Early **intravenous access** should be established for fluid management as soon as possible in any burned patient. Fluids should be titrated to adequate urine output. Severe injuries will require admission to a specialized burn unit. Children may have excessive bleeding from the labial artery as a consequence of **perioral** burn.

Special Considerations

Other injuries associated with electrical and lightning injuries include **fractures** from severe muscle contraction or blunt trauma after exposure. Upper limb and spinal fractures are common. The kidneys are particularly vulnerable to anoxic damage that accompanies electrical injury, where **rhabdomyolysis** is common. However, rhabdomyolysis is rare after lightning injury. **Rupture of the tympanic membrane** occurs in up to 50% of lightning victims. **Cataracts** often present as a late sequelae of lightning strike. **Curling ulcers** are common in burn victims, and preventative treatment for these stress ulcers should be initiated at admission.

When lightning injuries are not witnessed, some victims may simply be found down, and in those situations, thorough evaluations need to be initiated to look for other causes (cerebral vascular accident, toxic ingestions, spinal cord injuries, closed head injuries, myocardial infractions, and primary seizure disorders) responsible for the unexplainable neurologic and cardiovascular deficits.

COMPREHENSION QUESTIONS

46.1 A 40-year-old man who is employed as an electrician is brought to the ED after he accidentally grabbed a high-voltage wire, and this caused him to fall from a 8-ft ladder onto his back on the pavement below. He was ambulatory at the scene but because of persistent pain in his left hand and arm, he presents to the ED for treatment. He is conscious and conversant but complains of intense pain in a 3-cm burn wound on his left hand and also pain throughout his left forearm. On examination, the patient has GCS of 15 and is stable from the cardiopulmonary view. He has dry eschar over the hand wound, the sensation and motor activities are diminished in his left hand, and he has firmness and tenderness throughout the left forearm. Which of the following next step is most appropriate?

A. Obtain x-rays to rule out fractures.

B. Measure forearm compartment pressures.

C. Administer systemic antibiotics to prevent skin infection.

D. Obtain electromyograms (EMGs) to rule out peripheral nerve injury.

E. Obtain a CT scan to evaluate the muscle and nerves.

46.2 A 49-year-old man was fixing the electrical wiring in his house as a remodeling project and neglected to shut off the electricity at the electrical box. He suffered a substantial electrical injury primarily on the right hand, and was taken by paramedics to the ED. Which of the following is most likely to be true regarding electrical injury?

A. Cataract formation usually only occurs when there is a contact point on the head.

B. Renal failure is usually a result of direct electrical injury to the kidney.

C. With high-voltage injuries, dysrhythmia usually develops 24 to 48 hours after injury.

D. Electrical burns commonly produce a fern-like skin burn pattern.

E. Even with minor cutaneous involvement, major internal injury can occur.

46.3 A 13-year-old adolescent boy and his friend were curious about the inner workings of high-voltage transformers. After scaling the fence around one such complex near their school, one of the boys touched the transformer, believing that because he was wearing rubber-soled tennis shoes, he would be immune to electrical shock. He suffered a significant jolt of electricity at 10,000 V. Which of the following organ systems is most susceptible to high-voltage injuries?

A. Bones, tendons, and muscles

B. Skin, brain, and fat

C. Fat, heart, and skeletal muscle

D. Blood, nerves, and mucous membranes

E. Hair

46.4 A 45-year-old accountant was getting into his car on the top of his high-rise office building during a thunderstorm. Suddenly, a lightning strike occurred, throwing him to the ground. Which of the following is most accurate regarding complications to his injuries?

    A. Tetanic contractions are commonly caused by AC current.

    B. The instantaneous duration of exposure lessens cutaneous burn risk compared to other high-voltage electrical injuries.

    C. Rhabdomyolysis is a common delayed sequelae.

    D. Respiratory arrest is caused by paralysis of thoracic muscles.

    E. Lightning strike carries 80% mortality.

ANSWERS

46.1 **B.** This patient's history of high-voltage injury and current complain of intense forearm pain, diminished motor and sensory function in the hand, and tenseness in the forearms are highly suspicious for compartment syndrome secondary to myonecrosis in the forearm. Direct compartment measurement is the most rapid and reliable approach to diagnosis. Even though fracture can occur from the fall, bony injury would not account for motor and sensory changes in the hand. Treatment of burn wounds with systemic antibiotics is not indicated. CT scan is not sensitive for identification of compartment syndrome.

46.2 **E.** Even with minor cutaneous involvement, major internal injury can occur. The renal failure following electrical shocks generally occurs as a result of myoglobinuria. Although dysrhythmia is common after electrical injury, it almost always develops *immediately* after exposure. Cataract formation may occur even when there is no contact point on the head. Lichtenberg figure is the transient fern-like pattern that occurs on the skin of lightning strike victim because the electricity is splashed onto skin based on the vascular and nerve distribution patterns of the skin.

46.3 **D.** In high-voltage injuries, the electricity tends to follow the path of least resistance. Blood, nerves, and mucous membranes are frequently injured after electrical exposure because of their low resistance. Fat, bones, and tendon have high resistance.

46.4 **B.** Because of instantaneous exposure, burns are relatively rare in lightning injury. Lightning is DC current, and respiratory arrest is usually a result of injury to the respiratory control center in the medulla. Rhabdomyolysis is common after high-voltage electrical injury, but rare after lightning strike. Contrary to popular beliefs, the mortality associated with lightning injuries are low with most recent series reporting rates of 5% to 10%.

CLINICAL PEARLS

▶ Victims of lightning strike should be treated with aggressive ventilatory and circulatory support until cerebral function can be assessed, because many patients will recover function with time.

▶ Typical signs of brain death, fixed/dilated pupils and apnea, do not necessarily indicate brain death in electrical victims. Moreover, typical triage criteria for mass casualty situations do not apply to electrical injury.

▶ Even with small outward sign of injury, major internal damage is common.

▶ Children may have excessive bleeding from chewing on electrical cords.

REFERENCES

Fish RM, Geddes LA. Conduction of electrical current to and through the human body: a review. *Journal of Plastic Surgery*; 2009. www.eplasty.com

Katz RD, Deune EG. Electrical and lightning injuries. In: Cameron JL, Cameron AM, eds. *Current Surgical Therapy*, 10th ed. Philadelphia, PA: Elsevier Saunders; 2011:1047-1057.

O'Keefe Gatewood M, Zane RD. Lightning injuries. *Emerg Med Clin N Am*. 2004;22:369-403.

Ritenour AE, Morton MJ, McManus JG, et al. Lightning injury: a review. *Burn*. 2008;34:585-594.

Zimmermann C, Cooper MA, Holle RL. Lightning safety guidelines. *Ann Emerg Med*. 2001;39: 660-664.

A 10-year-old boy with sickle cell disease presents to the emergency department (ED) in the midst of presumed sickle cell crisis manifested as severe abdominal pain, pleuritic chest pain, dyspnea, and fever. His initial hemoglobin is 9 g/dL, white blood cell count (WBC) is 15,500 cells per mm^3, and chest x-ray reveals a nonspecific infiltrate in the left lung field with a small left pleural effusion. The electrocardiogram reveals sinus tachycardia. Following treatment with intravenous fluid, supplemental oxygen by nasal canula, parenteral analgesics, and empiric broad-spectrum antibiotics therapy, the patient complained of worsening dyspnea and chest pain, requiring increased oxygen supplementation by face-mask and eventual endotracheal intubation. At this juncture, exchange transfusion therapy is contemplated.

▶ What are the complications associated with blood transfusions in this setting?
▶ What are the ways to reduce the incidence of transfusion-related complications?

ANSWERS TO CASE 47:
Transfusion Complications

Summary: A 10-year-old boy with sickle cell crisis associated with severe respiratory symptoms (acute chest syndrome). The patient continues to have significant respiratory symptoms despite supportive care, and therefore exchange transfusion therapy is considered.

- **Transfusion complications:** Transfusion reactions and transfusion-related infections.

- **Ways to reduce transfusion complications:** Strict adherence to patient identification, specimen handling, and blood product storage protocols, and thorough review of transfusion history. Transfuse blood products based on need rather than arbitrary transfusion triggers.

ANALYSIS

Objectives

1. Develop an understanding of the epidemiology and basic pathophysiology of transfusion reactions.

2. Learn the evaluation and treatment of acute, life-threatening transfusion complications.

3. Learn the indications for blood product transfusion.

Considerations

Because sickle cell disease predisposes the patient to chronic anemia, it is more than likely that this particular patient has had an extensive history of transfusions; therefore, a thorough review of the transfusion history is vital. If the patient or the medical records indicate prior occurrence of minor transfusion reactions, then premedication with antihistamines and/or antipyretics may be useful. As a group, patients who are homozygous for sickle hemoglobin are at markedly increased risk of suffering complications from transfusion therapy, including transfusion-related infections (approximately 10% are infected with hepatitis C virus), and non-infectious etiologies related to alloimmunization (affecting up to 50% of sickle cell patients). The increased risks of alloimmunization are primarily related to recurrent antigen exposure and phenotypic dissimilarities between blood cells in the predominately white-donated blood supply and African American sickle cell patients.

To reduce the risk of transfusion-related complications, blood banks have intensified the cross-matching process for transfusions in sickle cell patients, with a demonstrable decrease in rates of alloimmunization. **Leukocyte-reduced packed red blood cells (PRBC) are recommended for patients with sickle cell disease and other patients requiring recurrent transfusions.** Additional benefits include a reduced rate of human leukocyte antigen (HLA) alloimmunization, and possible decreased rates of febrile nonhemolytic transfusion reactions (FNHTRs).

| APPROACH TO: |
| Transfusion Complications |

CLINICAL APPROACH

Conceptually, transfusion complications are best categorized into acute immune-mediated reactions, delayed immune-mediated reactions, nonimmunologic complications, and infectious complications.

ACUTE IMMUNE-MEDIATED REACTIONS

Acute Hemolytic Transfusion Reactions

Acute hemolytic transfusion reactions occur in 1:25,000 transfusions and cause death in 1:470,000 transfusions. The **majority of acute hemolytic transfusion reactions** are due to **errors made during the processing of the blood,** either at the patient bedside or in the blood bank. The majority of these reactions may be avoided with meticulous specimen processing, patient identification, and transfusion guidelines. Onset of reaction is **immediate, presenting with a combination of hypotension, tachypnea (often with the sensation of chest constriction), tachycardia, fever, chills, nausea, hemoglobinuria, and body pain (joints, lower back, legs).** Hemolysis can be either intravascular (more severe) or extravascular and is directed toward donor red blood cells (RBCs), usually mediated by preformed antibodies (anti-A, anti-B) within the recipient's serum. Because the causative antibodies to ABO group antigens are pre-existing in susceptible individuals, no prior alloantigen exposure is necessary for acute hemolysis to occur. However, recent sensitization to other alloantigens (such as an Rh-negative patient being exposed to Rh-positive blood) can result in similar pathology if a subsequent blood transfusion contains the same alloantigen(s). Given the potential for new alloantibody formation, a blood sample from the recipient should only be used for cross-matching assays within 48 hours from the time of collection.

Immediate management of suspected cases includes stopping the transfusion and changing the IV tubing or using alternative access sites to initiate aggressive crystalloid infusions, aiming to **maintain urine output above 1 to 1.5 mL/kg/h for 24 hours.** The remainder of the transfusion and a sample of the patient's blood should be sent to the blood bank for testing. The sequelae of acute hemolysis include **acute tubular necrosis (ATN), disseminated intravascular coagulation (DIC), and myocardial ischemia** (as a consequence of hemodynamic instability). DIC may be confirmed by the presence of **hemoglobinuria and plasma-free hemoglobin.** The definitive diagnosis of acute hemolytic transfusion reactions is made with **direct antiglobulin test** (DAT, also known as the direct Coombs assay), which detects antibody or complement bound to the surface of donor RBCs in a sample of the recipient's blood.

Febrile Nonhemolytic Transfusion Reactions

These reactions occur with approximately 0.5% to 1% RBC units, 2% apheresis platelet unit, and 5% to 30% donor-pooled platelets. Febrile nonhemolytic transfusion reactions **(FNHTR) constitute the most common and least-worrisome** complications of blood product transfusion. Patients may present with fever, chills, rigors, headache, malaise, and tachycardia, but **without hemodynamic instability and respiratory compromise.** Because prior history of transfusion is required for this reaction, **fever in a first-time transfusion recipient should be treated as an acute hemolytic reaction until proven otherwise.** Conversely, prior episodes of FNHTR indicate an increased risk of recurrence.

Management may include stopping the transfusion, administration of an antipyretic, and patient reassurance. Patients with a history of febrile reactions can be premedicated with antipyretics. **Antipyretic premedication** is a matter of preference, but **should be generally avoided in first-time transfusion recipients, because fever is more likely to represent serious sequelae in these patients.** Because FNHTR is a diagnosis of exclusion, samples of patient's blood and the transfusate should be sent to rule out a hemolytic reaction or bacterial **contamination.**

Allergic Transfusion Reactions

The incidence of these allergic reactions is 1% to 3% of transfusions, and the reactions are caused by recipient antibodies (immunoglobulin [Ig] E) against donor serum proteins; symptoms may range from urticaria to frank anaphylaxis. Urticaria can be managed symptomatically with antihistamines and by briefly stopping the transfusion until symptoms resolve. Mild allergic reactions do not necessitate discontinuing the transfusion, as symptoms are not strictly dose related. Patients prone to develop these reactions can be premedicated with antihistamines to prevent the development of mild allergic reactions.

Frankly, anaphylactic reactions to blood products are rare (1:20,000 to 1:170,000) and can occur within seconds of transfusion initiation. Anaphylactic reactions are IgE-mediated and occur, in most cases, as the result of **genetic deficiency of IgA in the recipient,** resulting in the production of anti-IgA, -IgE. Other less-common causes of anaphylaxis include reactions caused by IgE against allergens in the transfused blood, and the passive transfer of reactive IgE from donor to the recipient. **Patients with known IgA deficiency should be given RBCs and platelets that have been thoroughly washed free of plasma proteins. Plasma component transfusions in IgA-deficient patients should be obtained from IgA-deficient donors.**

Anaphylaxis should be managed by immediately addressing the ABCs (airway, breathing, circulation), accompanied by the administration of **epinephrine, antihistamines, and corticosteroids,** along with the immediate discontinuation of the transfusion. **Patients taking angiotensin-converting enzyme (ACE) inhibitors** will have more severe anaphylactic reactions (ie, severe angioedema) because of their **inability to degrade bradykinin.**

Transfusion-Related Acute Lung Injury

Transfusion-related acute lung injury (TRALI), with an estimated incidence of 1:4500 transfusions, is an under-recognized **life-threatening complication of transfusion.** TRALI is thought to be **mediated by anti-leukocyte antibodies,** resulting in systemic inflammation and neutrophil-mediated lung injury. The onset is generally within 6 hours of exposure to plasma-containing transfusion products, with most cases occurring within 1 to 2 hours. Random donor platelet transfusions (pooled platelets) are responsible for the majority of cases. Patients with hematological malignancies and cardiac disease are at increased risk of developing TRALI. Fever, tachycardia, and dyspnea are the most common presenting symptoms. **The hallmark of this complication is respiratory distress with the presence of diffuse, bilateral alveolar and interstitial infiltrates on radiographic imaging.** TRALI may be easily confused with acute pulmonary edema secondary to volume overload. Because **TRALI patients have normal to low left-heart pressures, echocardiography may be useful to differentiate between TRALI and pulmonary edema.** The management of this condition consists of stopping the transfusion and immediate attention to the "ABCs," which may include intubation and mechanical ventilation. Respiratory compromise is usually self-limiting within 48 to 72 hours. The mortality rate associated with TRALI is about 10%.

DELAYED IMMUNE-MEDIATED REACTIONS

Delayed Hemolytic Transfusion Reactions

Delayed hemolytic transfusion reactions (DHTRs) are notably less severe than their acute hemolytic counterparts. The incidence is about 1:1000 transfusions. The mechanisms of DHTR are related to recipients having developed antibodies against RBC alloantigens from prior foreign RBC exposures, most often through transfusions or pregnancies.

Unlike acute hemolytic reactions, which require high circulating levels of reactive antibodies, the **alloantibodies responsible for DHTR are present only at low levels prior to transfusion.** Following exposure to these alloantigens, antibody generation is slowly increased over the following days, resulting in hemolysis of the donor RBCs. **Symptoms associated with DHTR are mild to nonexistent.** Patients typically present with a mild fever and recurrent anemia. No specific therapy is warranted aside from repeat transfusion.

Graft-Versus-Host Disease

Transfusion-related graft-versus-host disease (GVHD) is a rare disorder where donor lymphocytes engraft and proliferate in the recipient's bone marrow, which over time may lead to a severe graft-mediated reaction against the recipient's tissues, including the bone marrow. It is **fatal in more than 90% of cases.** Symptoms of GVHD develop on average 1 to 2 weeks following transfusion and include fevers, maculopapular rashes, hepatitis, diarrhea, nausea, vomiting, weight loss, and pancytopenia leading to sepsis and death. **Immunocompromised recipients are especially at risk for GVHD; therefore, blood products administered to these patients should be subjected to gamma irradiation** to render remaining leukocytes incapable of proliferation. Blood products donated by first-degree relatives or between patients with partially matched HLA haplotypes have an increased risk of donor lymphocyte engraftment because of homology between donor and recipient HLA genes; therefore, **blood product donated by first-degree relatives should be irradiated prior to transfusions.** The highest incidence of GVHD has been from regions where the population is racially homogeneous with highly likelihood of shared

HLA haplotype (eg, Japan). GVHD is most problematic when patients receive fresh blood that is processed within 7 days from time of collection. In the United States, blood products that are older than 7 days generally do not contain viable lymphocytes.

Post-transfusion Purpura

Post-transfusion purpura is a rare complication, characterized by sudden thrombocytopenia occurring 5 to 10 days following transfusion of any blood product. The pathophysiology involves native platelet destruction, mediated by antibodies to the platelet antigen (PLA)1. Anti-PLA1 antibodies develop in patients previously exposed to foreign platelets through transfusion or pregnancy. Patients usually present with spontaneous bleeding (mucous membranes, epistaxis, hematochezia, hematuria). **Nine percent of patients may develop intracranial hemorrhage**. Treatment involves administration of intravenous immunoglobulin, corticosteroids, plasma exchange therapy, and transfusion with **PLA1-negative platelets**. If left untreated, the thrombocytopenia usually resolves spontaneously within 2 weeks of onset.

Alloimmunization

Alloimmunization refers to the formation of new antibodies against antigens on donated cells. **The formation of alloantibodies against HLA surface molecules may render patients refractory to platelet transfusions**, thus supporting the administration of leukoreduced blood for patients who will likely need exogenous platelets in the future. The presence of alloantibodies is primarily responsible for the increased rates of transfusion complications seen in repeat transfusion recipients.

Infectious Complications

The most frequent and concerning infectious complication of transfusion therapy is bacterial contamination, which can be detected in up to 2% of blood products. The most commonly isolated organism in refrigerated products (ie, RBCs) is *Yersinia enterocolitica*, which can grow at temperatures as low as 1°C (33.8°F). Other cryophilic organisms include *Pseudomonas*, *Enterobacter* and *Flavobacterium*. Platelets, which are stored at room temperature (22°C-24°C [71.6°F-75.2°F]), are more likely to develop gross contamination than are refrigerated products. *Staphylococcus* and *Salmonella* are often reported in fatal cases of platelet transfusion-mediated sepsis. Signs and symptoms may include fevers, rigors, chills, rash, hypotension, and even shock accompanied by sepsis. Symptoms may develop immediately or over several hours. Suspected cases of contamination should be managed with respiratory and circulatory support, immediate discontinuation of the transfusion, and broad-spectrum antibiotic therapy. Because it is difficult to distinguish some of the immune-mediated transfusion reactions from bacterial transmission, **any transfusion that causes hypotension in the setting of fever warrants immediate testing of the donor blood with Gram stain and culture, in addition to standard workup for hemolytic reactions**.

Indications for Blood Products

Given the potential complications from blood product transfusion, it is imperative that physicians understand and follow the indications for blood transfusion. The transfusion of blood products is indicated in patients with acute blood loss associated with hemodynamic instability and those with large amount of ongoing blood loss in hemodynamically stable individuals. The use of transfusion triggers had been a common practice in the past; however, based on the findings of a randomized controlled clinical trial (TRICC trial), hospitalized patients maintained at a hemoglobin values of 7 to 9 g/dL had lower in-hospital mortality than those maintained at hemoglobin values of 10 to 12 g/dL. The findings of the TRICC trial demonstrated that critically ill patients (with the exception of patients with acute coronary syndrome) can tolerate much lower hemoglobin levels, and the transfusion of packed RBC should be determined based on patients' needs rather than an arbitrary laboratory value. Platelet transfusion is generally indicated in patients with platelet count of less than 10,000 μL, 10,000 to 20,000 with bleeding, less than 50,000 with a severe trauma, and those with bleeding time greater than 15 minutes. Fresh-frozen plasma transfusion is considered appropriate in bleeding patients with prothrombin time more than 17 seconds and following massive transfusion where replacement of 1 unit of fresh-frozen plasma and one single donor platelet unit for each unit of PRBC transfused is recommended as a strategy to improve clotting and hemostasis (hemostatic resuscitation).

COMPREHENSION QUESTIONS

47.1 A hemodynamically stable 40-year-old man with gastrointestinal (GI) bleeding and hemoglobin of 6 g/dL is receiving packed RBC transfusion. Soon after the initiation of blood transfusion, the patient becomes confused, develops urticaria, and subsequently unresponsive with a systolic blood pressure of 60 mm Hg. Which of the following agents may have worsened this patient's condition?

A. Lisinopril (an ACE inhibitor)

B. Atenolol

C. Lactated Ringer solution

D. Morphine sulfate

E. Salicylate

47.2 A 60-year-old woman with chronic anemia caused by a myelofibrosis presents to the emergency room from her oncologist's office with a hemoglobin of 6 g/dL. She notes feeling very lethargic over the past week, and had some mild chest discomfort while climbing stairs in her house last night. A type- and cross-match is performed for 2 units of packed erythrocytes, which are given without incident and marked improvement in her symptoms is seen. While going over discharge instructions with the emergency physician, the patient notes that she feels feverish and slightly short of breath. Over the next several minutes her dyspnea worsens markedly. Vital sign measurement reveals an oxygen saturation of 93%, a heart rate of 120 beats per minute, and a blood pressure of 95/55 mm Hg. The patient continues to deteriorate from a respiratory standpoint despite supplemental oxygen, requiring endotracheal intubation. A portable chest radiograph shows evidence of diffuse bilateral infiltrates. Which of the following statements is most accurate regarding this patient's condition?

A. This patient's left ventricular end-diastolic pressure is likely to be elevated.

B. This condition has a mortality rate of up to 90%.

C. Diuretic therapy is unlikely to be effective.

D. Radiographic abnormalities develop several days after the onset of clinical manifestations.

E. Mechanical ventilatory support is generally not helpful.

ANSWERS

47.1 **A.** Patients taking ACE inhibitors may experience a more severe anaphylactic reaction than other patients because of their inability to degrade bradykinin; however, these agents do not confer an increased risk of anaphylaxis. Patient misidentification is the leading preventable cause of transfusion reactions.

47.2 **C.** Patients with TRALI are not volume overloaded, but rather suffer from increased capillary permeability at the level of the pulmonary vasculature. As such, they have normal to low left-side heart pressures, and will only be harmed by diuretic therapy because of the potential to cause organ hypoperfusion. Mortality rates are around 10%. Radiographic abnormalities are present almost immediately, and persist for several days after the resolution of clinical manifestations. Mechanical ventilatory support is a mainstay of therapy for patients with suspected TRALI, as the process is generally self-limiting.

CLINICAL PEARLS

▶ TRALI, thought to be mediated by antileukocyte antibodies, presents with fever, tachycardia, and dyspnea as the most common presenting symptoms.

▶ The hallmark of TRALI is respiratory distress with the presence of diffuse, bilateral alveolar and interstitial infiltrates on radiographic imaging.

REFERENCES

Herbert PC, Wells G, Blajchman MA, et al. A multicenter, randomized, controlled clinical trial of transfusion requirement in critical care. Transfusion requirements in critical care investigators, Canadian Critical Care Trials Group. *N Engl J Med.* 1999;340:409-417.

Leo A, Pedal I. Diagnostic approaches to acute transfusion reactions. *Forensic Sci Med Pathol.* 2010;6: 135-145.

Vamvakas EC, Blajchman MA. Blood still kills: six strategies to further reduce allogeneic blood transfusion-related mortality. *Transfus Med Rev.* 2010;24:77-124.

A 17-year-old adolescent boy arrives at the emergency department (ED) after he developed the acute onset of severe right testicular pain about 4 hours ago while at soccer practice. The patient does not recall any recent trauma to the area and denies any fever, dysuria, or penile discharge. Although he is nauseous, he does not have any abdominal pain or vomiting.

On examination, his temperature is 99.5°F, blood pressure 138/84 mm Hg, heart rate 104 beats per minute, and respiratory rate of 22 breaths per minute. He is in acute distress due to pain. His abdomen is benign. On visual inspection, he has right scrotal erythema and swelling although no penile lesions or discharge. Because his scrotum is so diffusely tender, it is difficult to examine it more closely. However, there is no testicular rise when his inner thigh is stroked. His urinalysis shows 3 to 5 white blood cells (WBCs)/high power field (hpf).

▶ What is the most likely diagnosis?
▶ What is the next diagnostic step?

ANSWERS TO CASE 48:

Scrotal Pain

Summary: This is a 17-year-old adolescent boy who presents with acute onset right testicular pain without any preceding trauma.

- **Most likely diagnosis:** Testicular torsion

- **Next diagnostic step:** Urological consultation. Manual detorsion can be attempted while awaiting the consultant.

ANALYSIS

Objectives

1. Learn the differential diagnosis for acute scrotal pain.

2. Recognize the clinical signs and symptoms associated with testicular torsion.

3. Understand the diagnostic and therapeutic approach to suspected testicular torsion.

Considerations

The differential diagnosis of acute testicular pain includes testicular torsion, epididymitis, orchitis, torsion of the testicular appendages, hernia, hydrocele, and testicular tumor (Table 48–1). Because of the risk of ischemia and infarction of the testes, testicular torsion is the priority condition that must be promptly recognized and treated. This patient is 17 years old without a history of trauma. Adolescents during puberty are especially at risk of testicular torsion because of high hormonal stimulation. This patient's history of acute onset, especially associated with vigorous physical activity, is classic. The involved testis is firm, tender, and located higher in the scrotum on examination, and the cremasteric reflex is absent, again consistent with testicular torsion. When the clinical presentation is unclear, Doppler flow studies of the intratesticular blood flow may be helpful. This patient, however, has a clear-cut diagnosis, and time is of the essence.

Table 48–1 • DIFFERENTIAL DIAGNOSES FOR ACUTE SCROTAL PAIN

Diagnosis	Comments	Clinical Findings	Treatment
Epididymitis	Young boys: may be due to sterile reflux or coliform bacteria. <35 to 40 years old: usually due to *C trachomatis* or *N gonorrhoeae*. >35- to 40 years old: usually due to *E coli* and *Klebsiella*. More gradual onset. May be associated with fever and urinary symptoms	Tenderness, erythema, warmth of scrotum (may be isolated to epididymis/posterolateral testis initially). ± urethral discharge. Pain improves with scrotal elevation (Prehn sign). Doppler US: increased testicular blood flow, enlarged hypoechoic epididymis	Antibiotics, analgesia, bed rest with scrotal elevation, scrotal support, ice packs,
Fournier gangrene	Polymicrobial infection causing necrotizing fasciitis of perineal, genital, or perianal regions. Risk factors: diabetes, immuno-compromised, chronic alcoholism. 40% mortality	Systemically ill. Scrotal pain (initially pain out or proportion to examina-tion), perineal erythema and swelling. Induration, ecchymosis, crepitus as later findings. US: diffuse swelling and thickening of scrotum	Fluid resuscitation, intravenous antibiotics, surgical debridement. Consider hyperbaric oxygen therapy.
Hydrocele	Gradual onset	Scrotal swelling and transillumination. US: fluid-filled cavity	Urology follow-up
Inguinal hernia	Variable presentation depending on age and type of hernia	Inguinal and scrotal swelling and pain. ± Signs of intestinal obstruction if incarcerated or strangulated	Surgery
Orchitis	Most commonly viral etiology (eg, mumps). Bacterial orchitis usually associated with epididymitis. Gradual onset	Testicular tenderness and swelling. ± Systemic symptoms with bacterial orchitis or parotitis with mumps orchitis	Antibiotics if bacterial etiology. Otherwise symptomatic care (analgesia, bed rest, scrotal support, ice packs)
Testicular tumor	Most common malignancy in young men. Seminomas most common. Gradually progressive	Often painless swelling although pain may occur with hemorrhage into tumor. Testicular mass, firmness, swelling. US: intratesticular mass	Urgent urologic referral. Radical orchiectomy, radiation therapy, and chemotherapy may be needed
Appendageal torsion	Twisting of one of four vestigial structures of the testes (most commonly the appendix testes). Most common in boys 7 to 14 years old. Nausea and vomiting less common than with testicular torsion	Acute scrotal pain (although less severe than with testicular torsion), tender nodule (near head of testis or epididymis), "blue dot sign." Doppler US: normal or increased testicular blood flow	Analgesia, bed rest, scrotal support. Usually resolves within 3 to 10 days. Consider surgical excision if severe or refractory

Abbreviations: US = ultrasound

APPROACH TO:
Scrotal Pain

CLINICAL APPROACH

When any male presents with scrotal pain, testicular torsion must be considered. Prompt diagnosis and therapy are vital because delays can lead to ischemia, loss of the testicle, and impaired fertility. In general, the best salvage time of the testis is attained within 4 to 6 hours after the onset of pain, but clinical parameters are often unreliable. Patients with testicular torsion often have a congenital "bell clapper" deformity, which allows the epididymis and testicle to hang freely and rotate in the scrotum. When torsion occurs, the spermatic cord becomes twisted, cutting off the blood supply to the testicle. Although torsion can occur at any age, it is most common in children less than 1 year old and around puberty.

When obtaining the history, the clinician should focus on the onset and duration of pain, alleviating and aggravating factors, and any associated symptoms, such as nausea and vomiting, fever, urethral discharge, and dysuria. He/she should also remember that some patients may complain of abdominal rather than scrotal pain. In addition, it is important to inquire about any previous episodes and any recent trauma. A typical patient with **testicular torsion** presents with the **sudden onset of severe pain in the lower abdomen, inguinal area, or scrotum.** Associated nausea and vomiting are common. The pain is often preceded by strenuous physical activity or trauma although episodes can occur during sleep. Pain that persists for more than one hour after scrotal trauma is not normal and merits further investigation. Past episodes that resolved spontaneously are not uncommon.

On examination, the clinician should pay close attention to any abdominal findings, scrotal swelling or skin changes, penile discharge or rash, inguinal lymphadenopathy or hernia, and testicular tenderness or masses. Classically, a **torsed testicle is diffusely tender and swollen with an abnormal (horizontal) lie.** There is usually a loss of the cremasteric reflex on the affected side. However, no historical or examination findings can definitively distinguish testicular torsion from other disease processes. In addition, infants and children may lack the typical examination findings.

Testicular torsion is largely a clinical diagnosis, and no diagnostic tests should delay urological evaluation and surgical exploration. If the diagnosis is uncertain, color-flow Doppler ultrasound (US) or radionuclide scintigraphy may be helpful. With testicular torsion, Doppler US will reveal decreased or absent testicular blood flow. The utility of these studies may be limited by their availability and timeliness. In addition, scintigraphy does not provide any anatomical information, and therefore cannot differentiate epididymitis from torsion of the appendix testis. Many times, leukocytes are found in the urine of men with testicular torsion. This finding should not distract the clinician from the diagnosis.

TREATMENT

When the diagnosis of testicular torsion is considered, prompt urological consultation is mandatory. Definitive treatment involves emergent surgical exploration, detorsion, and orchiopexy. While awaiting urological consultation, the clinician may attempt manual detorsion. Because most torsions occur in a lateral to medial manner, the testis should initially be turned in a medial to lateral direction like "opening a book." Successful detorsion results in significant pain relief. If the pain worsens, however, the maneuver should be tried in the opposite direction. Intravenous access and analgesics are also necessary. The differential diagnosis for acute scrotal pain includes several benign and emergent conditions (Table 48–1).

COMPREHENSION QUESTIONS

48.1 A 22-year-old baseball player comes to the ED complaining of 10 hours of severe right testicular pain. He denies a history of trauma. On examination, his right testis is diffusely tender and indurated, and the pain does not change with patient position. He has a cremasteric reflex on the right side. Which of the following is the best next step?

    A. Continued observation

    B. Oral antibiotics

    C. Bed rest, ice to scrotum, and elevation of the scrotum

    D. Surgical exploration of the scrotum

48.2 A 32-year-old jogger is brought into the emergency room with the acute onset of severe left testicular pain. A diagnosis of testicular torsion is made, and manual detorsion is successfully accomplished. Which of the following is the most appropriate advice to this patient?

    A. Likely no further therapy is needed.

    B. Surgical exploration may be needed if another episode of torsion occurs.

    C. Surgical correction will be needed but does not necessarily need to be done urgently.

    D. Surgical exploration still needed to be performed and should occur within 24 hours.

Match the probable diagnoses (A-F) to the clinical scenario in questions 48.3 to 48.6:

    A. Torsion of the appendix testis

    B. Testicular torsion

    C. Epididymitis

    D. Orchitis

    E. Testicular tumor

    F. Acute prostatitis

48.3   A 24-year-old man complains of severe left scrotal pain increasing over 24 hours. Urinalysis shows 25 WBC/hpf, and Doppler flow shows increased intratesticular flow.

48.4   A 58-year-old man complains of urgency, dysuria, lower back pain, and pain with ejaculation.

48.5   A 14-year-old adolescent complains of 2 days of testicular pain. On examination, there appears to be a tender nodule of the testis. Transillumination reveals a small blue spot at the affected area.

48.6   A 28-year-old man complains of heaviness in his scrotum. On examination, there is a firm, nontender mass involving his right testis.

ANSWERS

48.1   **D.** The clinical history is consistent with testicular torsion. The presence of a cremasteric reflex does not rule out the disease. Emergency scrotal exploration is the procedure of choice when the history, physical examination, and imaging tests do not rule out testicular torsion.

48.2   **C.** Detorsion of the torsed testis converts an emergent condition into one that is amenable to elective correction. Manual detorsion is not definitive therapy.

48.3   **C.** The Doppler ultrasound finding consistent with epididymitis is increased or preserved blood flow. Also epididymitis usually has a more gradual onset of pain. Fifty percent of patients with epididymitis have pyuria or bacteriuria.

48.4   **F.** Acute prostatitis usually occurs in older patients. Urinary urgency, hesitancy, frequency, and perineal pain with ejaculation are common symptoms. The most common causative organism is *Escherichia coli*. Appropriate antibiotic choices include fluoroquinolones (ciprofloxacin, ofloxacin, norfloxacin) as well as trimethoprim-sulfamethoxazole.

48.5   **A.** Torsion of a testicular appendage classically presents as a tender testicular nodule, and upon transillumination, a "blue dot" may be seen. Color Doppler blood flow is increased or normal.

48.6   **E.** Testicular carcinoma classically presents as a painless scrotal mass.

CLINICAL PEARLS

▶ Testicular torsion should always be considered in the differential diagnoses of acute scrotal or abdominal pain.

▶ No single historical or examination finding can definitively distinguish testicular torsion from other processes.

▶ Time is testicle. If testicular torsion is suspected, prompt urological consultation is mandatory.

▶ Definitive treatment of testicular torsion is surgery. Manual detorsion may be attempted as a temporizing measure.

REFERENCES

Lewis AG, Bukowski TP, Jarvis PD, et al. Evaluation of acute scrotum in the emergency department. *J Pediatr Surg.* 1995;30:277-282.

Marx JA, Hockberger RS, Walls RM, eds. *Rosen's Emergency Medicine: Concepts and Clinical Practice.* 7th ed. Philadelphia, PA: Mosby Elsevier; 2009.

Mufti RA, Ogedegbe AK, Lafferty K. The use of Doppler ultrasound in the clinical management of acute testicular pain. *Br J Urol.* 1995;76:625-627.

Rabinowitz R. The importance of the cremasteric reflex in acute scrotal swelling in children. *J Urol.* 1984;132:89-90.

Ringdahl E. Testicular torsion. *Am Fam Physician.* 2006;74(10):1739-1743.

Tintinalli JE, Kelen GD, Stapczynski JS, eds. *Emergency Medicine: A Comprehensive Study Guide.* 7th ed. New York, NY: McGraw-Hill; 2011.

It is approximately 2 AM, when a woman presents to the emergency department (ED) with her 3-year-old son. According to the mother, the patient had been playing and fell off the upper level of his bunk bed earlier in the evening. On examination, the child is somnolent. His pulse rate is 110 beats per minute, blood pressure is 100/85 mm Hg, respiratory rate is 28 breaths per minute, and Glasgow coma scale (GCS) score is 11 (eye opening 2, verbal 5, motor 4). There is presence of soft-tissue contusion over the left frontal scalp and ecchymosis over the left periorbital region. The chest is clear with bilateral breath sounds. The abdomen is mildly distended and tender throughout. The patient's left thigh is markedly swollen and tender, and all his extremities are mottled and cool.

▶ What is the most likely mechanism responsible for this patient's clinical picture?
▶ What are the next steps in the management of this patient?

ANSWERS TO CASE 49:

Trauma and Extremes of Age

Summary: A 3-year-old boy presents several hours after an unwitnessed fall, with somnolence and external signs of head injury. In addition to the contusions on the scalp, his abdomen is distended and tender, left thigh is swollen and tender, and his skin is mottled and cool.

- **Most likely responsible mechanism:** This child has multiple injuries, possibly secondary to intentional trauma.

- **Next steps in management:** Pediatric trauma resuscitation and evaluation to include administration of intravenous fluids, a thorough examination, and a computed tomography (CT) scan of the head and abdomen. **Protection of the child by reporting potential child abuse, and admission to the hospital.**

ANALYSIS

Objectives

1. Become familiar with the evaluation and management of pediatric and geriatric patients with multiple severe injuries presenting in shock.

2. Recognize the signs in the presentation of children and elderly patients that are consistent with abuse and become familiar with the appropriate response.

Considerations

The presentation of this child should raise concerns for multiple reasons, and it is vitally important to appropriately prioritize your attention to these concerns. The first priority should be concern over his medical condition, not the mechanism of the injury. This patient's vital signs presented in the case scenario are not out of the range of normal for his age (Table 49–1). Despite the normal vital signs, his general presentation indicates the potential for multisystem injuries, and putting that together with the findings of mottled and cool skin indicate that this child is in **hemorrhagic shock until proven otherwise.** The vital signs of an injured child can be within normal ranges for an extended period of time secondary to an excellent ability to compensate physiologically for hypovolemia. However, when the limits of

Table 49–1 • NORMAL VITAL SIGNS BY AGE GROUP			
Age Group (Years)	Heart Rate (Beats/Min)	Blood Pressure (mm HG)	Respiratory Rate (Breaths/Min)
0-1	120	80/40	40
1-5	100	100/60	30
5-10	80	120/80	20

that compensatory reserve are reached, the ability of a child to tolerate shock is poor and his condition will likely decline very rapidly.

The secondary concern regarding this child is the manner in which he presented suggesting potential abuse. Factors that raise these concerns include the **delay in presentation**, the extent of **the injuries that appear much more severe than can be accounted for by the history**, the **age** of the child, and the **unwitnessed report** of the injury. All 50 states have mandatory child abuse reporting laws for the treating physician. Regardless of the management plan, this child should be placed in a protected environment (admission to the hospital), and a report of suspected abuse should be submitted. However, the treating physician's suspicions or emotions should not delay the child's medical care (which is the first responsibility). Accurate and complete evaluations and documentation of your findings in an unbiased manner is the first important step. Confrontations with family members in the midst of a trauma room evaluation are rarely fruitful, and can hamper your efforts to care for the child.

APPROACH TO:
The Pediatric Trauma Patient

CLINICAL APPROACH

A **systematic and expeditious approach** to children with unknown injury mechanisms or mechanisms capable of producing multisystem injury should include a rapid survey for all potential injuries, **consideration of the need for intubation, administration of intravenous fluids, and the prevention of heat loss. CT scan of the head and abdomen** may be obtained for further evaluation as needed, and the patient should be prepared for operative care as indicated. In those patients with multiple injuries identified, prioritizing the most life-threatening problem is of paramount importance. Even when intracranial hemorrhage may be suspected on the basis of physical presentation, the immediate threat to most children with multisystems injury is hypovolemic shock from abdominal injury and other hemorrhagic sources. Addressing blood loss source is critical not only for the correction of hemorrhagic shock but also for the prevention of secondary brain injury in these patients.

The guidelines found in the advanced trauma life support (ATLS) and advanced pediatric life support (APLS) manuals should be followed in the initial management of injured children. **The initial priorities** are the assessment and maintenance of **airway, oxygenation, and ventilation.** Determination for immediate intubation is dependent on the initial evaluation of the child and the resources available. Certainly, if there is any **airway compromise**, or if the **neurological status** raises concern of airway protection (a **GCS score <9**; Table 49–2), then **intubation is mandatory.** If the airway is not compromised and the GCS score is adequate, then the decision for elective intubation may be determined by the level of patient cooperation for the timely completion of potentially lifesaving diagnostic studies such as CT imaging.

The circulation and the neurological status should be the next priorities. Approximately 90% of pediatric patients presenting with blunt trauma are successfully

Table 49–2 • PEDIATRIC GCS VERBAL SCORES	
5	Appropriate words or social smile, fixes and follows
4	Cries, but consolable
3	Persistently irritable
2	Restless, agitated
1	None

managed without operative intervention. However, the **initial signs of shock, including tachycardia, skin changes, and lethargy, represent a loss of approximately 25% of the child's blood volume** (Table 49–3). The likelihood of injury requiring operative control of hemorrhage is much greater in these children, and careful attention should be paid to the amount of fluid or blood that is required to maintain stable vital signs. A large-bore IV should be started, and two sequential boluses of **20 mL/kg of warmed crystalloid solution** should be administered. If further fluids are required beyond this, then administration of packed red blood cells (10 mL/kg) should be considered. Evaluation of the **abdomen by ultrasound (if unstable) or CT scan** should be performed to determine the extent of injuries. **If the vital signs worsen** during the attempt to obtain a head and abdominal CT scan, this should be abandoned and a **laparotomy performed** to control any hemorrhage.

There is no doubt that the child presented in this case often presents a considerable challenge. Not only does the possibility of abuse evoke strong emotions that are difficult to ignore during the evaluation, there is potential of multiple life-threatening injuries that must be prioritized. A systematic and efficient approach, with focus on the most immediate of concerns, cannot be emphasized enough (Table 49–4).

THE BATTERED CHILD

There are very few other things encountered by physicians that will evoke such strong distasteful emotions as child abuse, making one think that reporting of these cases would not be a significant problem. However, to report a case of child abuse, the physician must first recognize that it is child abuse. The subtleties of recognizing

Table 49–3 • SYSTEMIC RESPONSES TO BLOOD LOSS IN THE PEDIATRIC PATIENT		
<25% Blood Volume Loss	**25%-45% Blood Volume Loss**	**>45% Blood Volume Loss**
Weak, thready pulse; increased heart rate	Increased heart rate	Hypotension, tachycardia to bradycardia
Lethargic, irritable, confused	Change in the level of consciousness, dulled response to pain	Comatose
Cool, clammy	Cyanotic, decreased capillary refill, cold extremities	Pale, cold
Minimal decrease in urinary output; increased specific gravity	Minimal urine output	No urine output

Data from ATLS Manual, American College of Surgeons. 1997:297.

Table 49–4 • INITIAL MANAGEMENT OF THE INJURED CHILD
Primary survey
• Establishment of a reliable airway
• Ventilation
• Establishment of large-bore IV lines
• Support of circulation
• Rapid assessment of neurological status
Secondary survey
• Diagnostic studies
• Establishment of surgical priorities
• Mass lesion in the brain
• Chest and abdominal injuries
• Peripheral vascular injuries
• Fractures

Data from O'Neill JA. Principles of Pediatric Surgery. *St Louis, MO: Mosby; 2003:783.*

child abuse, and the fear of making incorrect accusations of caregivers that appear well meaning can make this a difficult issue. The reporting and protection of the battered child is further confounded by the legal requirements for appropriate and complete documentation by the physician, which often is lacking if suspicions of abuse were not entertained upon initial presentation.

Intentional injury accounts for approximately 10% of all trauma cases in children younger than 5 years old. While this figure may be alarming, it also suggests that the vast majority of trauma in children is actually accidental. There are several key aspects of the history, physical examination, and presentation of the child that should alert the practitioner to the possibility that the trauma was not accidental. Table 49–5 lists suggestive characteristics that should alert the practitioner to abuse. Skin and soft-tissue injuries are the most common injuries encountered in child abuse cases. This is followed by fractures, which often are multiple or repetitive. The third most common problem with child abuse is head injury. Unfortunately, this is also the injury with the highest mortality.

Currently, there is no federal standard regarding the legal requirements for reporting of child abuse. However, all states have mandatory reporting legislation for suspected child abuse that includes healthcare workers, school personnel, social workers, and law enforcement officers. Very few states recognize the physician-patient communication privilege as exempt from these reporting requirements. Most states impose either a fine or imprisonment penalty to individuals that knowingly or willfully fail to report abuse. However, several states also impose penalties for false reports of child abuse.

When intentional injury is suspected in a pediatric trauma case, the appropriate child protective agency should be notified after the child's medical condition is addressed. During the investigational process, it is often incumbent on the medical personnel to provide a high-visibility protected environment for the child. Although it is often emotionally tempting for the physician to become involved in the investigational process, it is important at this stage to **maintain focus on the medical**

Table 49–5 • PATTERNS SUGGESTING PHYSICAL ABUSE	
Presentation	Age younger than 3 years (limited ability to communicate)
	Significant delay between injury and presentation
	Presence of risk factors
	• Chronic illness
	• Premature birth
	• Congenital deficiencies
	• Mental delay
History	Unwitnessed injury
	Injuries not consistent or more significant than suggested by the history
	Evasive responses
	Reported self-injury not consistent with the child's stage of development
Physical Examination	Multiple injuries
	Signs of prior injuries and fractures
	Injuries and different stages of healing
	Pattern of injuries
	• Demarcated buttock-scalding injuries
	• Retinal hemorrhage
	• Multiple bruises
	• Hand or whip marks
	• Cigarette burns

condition. This becomes particularly important in terms of adequate documentation. A **complete, unbiased, and well-recorded history and physical** examination can be vital in the protection of the child at a later date.

Particularly important information includes detailed descriptions of the reported mechanism of the injury, the time of the injury and any delay in presentation, the presence of witnesses, conflicts, and inconsistencies. A complete physical examination should be documented and should include pictures or diagrams of all bruises, documentation of the color of each bruise, a complete neurological examination, and a genital examination. An eye examination for retinal hemorrhages should be performed because this is often encountered with cerebral trauma and the "shaken baby syndrome." Radiographic evaluations should be performed on all extremities to search for patterns of previous injury (Table 49–6). Any reports from previous admissions (including from other hospitals) should be referenced.

Table 49–6 • MUSCULOSKELETAL MANIFESTATIONS OF ABUSE
Spiral fractures attributed to falls
Subperiosteal calcification with no history of injury
Multiple fractures in various stages of healing
Bucket-handle fractures or epiphyseal–metaphyseal separation and fragmentation from pulling or shaking forces
Unexplained fractures associated with chronic subdural hematomas

Data from, O'Neill JA. Principles of Pediatric Surgery. St Louis, MO: Mosby; 2003.

GERIATRIC TRAUMA

Older patients often have coexisting medical problems that may impact the response to the acute injuries. Details surrounding the initial injuring events are frequently relevant (eg, medication reactions, chest pains, strokes). Nevertheless, the basic approach to trauma in the elderly patient is the same as the approach to the adult patient.

When assessing the geriatric trauma patient, the possibility of elder abuse must be taken into consideration. If elder abuse is suspected, practitioners should follow the same steps used when assessing suspected child abuse.

Physiological Changes

The older age group is one of the fastest growing population sectors in the United States. Thus, the number of geriatric trauma incidents, arbitrarily defined as affecting those older than age 65 to 70 years, is expected to likewise increase. Injuries in these individuals are associated with higher mortality and longer hospital stay. Many physiological changes occur with aging (Table 49–7), including the progressive loss of myocyte number and increase in myocyte volume resulting in the ventricular stiffness and cardiac diastolic dysfunction. Furthermore, atherosclerotic changes cause large vessel stiffness and increased afterload. Additionally, aging contributes to diminution of cardiac β-adrenergic response, leading to diminished heart rate response. Because of the age-related cardiovascular changes, **the elderly patient is much less**

Table 49–7 • PHYSIOLOGICAL ALTERATIONS ASSOCIATED WITH AGING

Cardiovascular
- Loss of myocyte with reciprocal increase in myocyte volume and diminution in cardiac diastolic volume
- Large vessel calcification with increase in afterload
- Diminished cardiac chronotropic response to β-adrenergic stimulation
- Intimal hyperplasia and decreased vascular compliance result in decreased arterial perfusion

Pulmonary
- Decrease in forced expiratory volume in 1 second (FEV_1) due to decrease in respiratory muscle strength and increase in chest-wall rigidity
- Decrease in functional respiratory alveolar surface area

Renal
- Diminution in renal size after age 50
- Glomerulosclerosis may occur as the result of degenerative processes such as hypertension and diabetes, leading to loss of GFR

Hepatic
- Decrease in liver size after age 50
- Diminished and delayed regenerative capacity of the liver

Immunological
- Impairment in T-lymphocyte–mediated immunity resulting in increased infection risks
- Inflammatory mediated responses are diminished (TNF-alpha, IL-1, IL-6, and leukocyte adhesion molecule expression) leading to diminished inflammatory responses

capable of responding to increases in cardiac output demands. **Myocardial infarc-tion is the leading cause of death among 80-year-old patients in the postoperative and postinjury settings.** The elderly patient's limited ability to respond to stress and injuries has prompted some groups to apply age (>70 years) as the sole criteria for trauma-team activation, and by adapting to this approach, these investigators have demonstrated significant reduction in geriatric trauma mortality.

Outcome Predictors in Geriatric Patients

Various groups have attempted to identify outcome predictors in geriatric trauma patients (Table 49–8). "High-risk" patients can be identified based on mechanism, physiological parameter, and laboratory parameters. In the management of "high-risk" patients, early admission to the ICU, with earlier initiation of invasive hemo-dynamic monitoring, and aggressive resuscitation based on hemodynamic parameters are associated with a reduction in geriatric trauma patient mortality. Thus, **expedited patient disposition to allow early invasive monitoring** and **resuscitation** is helpful. Scalea and colleagues (1990) showed that early resuscitation of the "high-risk" elderly trauma patients, with **goals directed** at attaining **cardiac output** of more than 3.5 L/min and/or a **mixed venous saturation of greater than 50%,** led to an improve-ment in survival from 7% in historical control patients to 53% in the aggressively managed patients. More recent observations have not supported aggressive resuscita-tion measures based on predetermined parameters, because overly aggressive fluid resuscitation can contribute to pulmonary and cardiovascular complications. Close observations and monitoring directed toward the avoidance of tissue hypoperfusion and minimizing stresses related to hypothermia and pain are the important priorities during the initial management of older victims of traumatic injuries.

Given the overall poorer survival of geriatric trauma patients, some questions have been raised regarding the quality of life of the survivors. Long-term studies

Table 49–8 • PREDICTORS OF MORBIDITY AND MORTALITY
MORBIDITY PREDICTORS
Mechanisms
• Automobile-pedestrian collision
• Diffuse beating
Physiological parameters
• SBP <150
Laboratory parameters
• Base deficit (≤-6 mEq/L)
• Lactic acid (>2.4 mmol/L)
Anatomical injuries
• Blunt chest trauma with rib fractures
MORTALITY PREDICTORS
• SBP <90
• Hypoventilation (respiratory rate <10/minute)
• GCS = 3

of geriatric trauma patients indicate that majority of survivors return to a level of previous independence. Factors associated with long-term **reduced independence** include **hemodynamic shock upon admission, GCS score ≤7, age ≥75 years, head injury, and sepsis.**

COMPREHENSION QUESTIONS

49.1 A 3-year-old boy is brought into the ED with multiple bruises, abrasions, and several deep lacerations over the flank region. The parents state that he fell out of his bed. Which of the following is the most important next step in this patient?

A. Reporting these injuries to child protective services.

B. Firmly, but without judgment, confront the parents with the discrepancy of the story and the injuries.

C. Take accurate pictures of the injuries and seal them in an evidence envelope.

D. Evaluate the ABCs and any urgent injuries.

E. Station guards in front of the exits of the building to prevent the parents from leaving.

49.2 An 11-month-old infant is brought into the ED after rolling down a staircase while still buckled into the infant car seat. The baby is crying, but is consolable by his mother. His heart rate is 116 beats per minute and blood pressure 80/40 mm Hg at rest. The physical examination reveals only slight bruising over the knees. The abdomen is nontender. Which of the following is the best next step?

A. CT scan of the abdomen to assess for intraperitoneal hemorrhage

B. Chest radiograph to assess for pleural hemorrhage

C. Continued observation and reassurance

D. IV access and infusion of normal saline 10 mL/kg

E. Transfuse 10 mL/kg PRBC

49.3 An evaluation of an 80-year-old woman who was a pedestrian struck by an automobile traveling at a speed of 20 miles per hour identified right tibia and fibula fracture, right pubic ramus fracture, and facial lacerations. Her vital signs are a pulse of 80 beats per minute, blood pressure of 120/70 mm Hg, respiratory rate of 20 breaths per minute, and a GCS score of 15. Which of the following sequences of events is the most appropriate in management of this patient?

A. Computed tomography (CT) scan of the abdomen; plain x-rays of the pelvis, lower extremities, and spine; splinting of fractures; and invasive monitoring in the ICU.

B. CT scan of the abdomen; splinting of fractures; invasive monitoring in ICU; and x-rays of the pelvis and lower extremities.

C. Invasive monitoring in ICU; splinting of the fractures; and CT of abdomen.

D. Splinting of fractures; invasive monitoring in the ICU; and CT of abdomen; and x-rays of the extremities and pelvis.

E. Exploratory laparotomy, splinting of the femur fracture, and pelvic fixation.

ANSWERS

49.1 **D.** The first and foremost priority is the patient's medical condition, and as normal, initially addressing the ABCs. Child protective services probably do need to be notified, and the injuries do need to be documented. In general, the parents should not be confronted, but rather asked about their story.

49.2 **C.** The normal heart rate and blood pressure levels of a child are substantially different from that of any adult. These values are normal for this infant; therefore, more aggressive measures are not indicated at this time.

49.3 **B.** This sequence of events outlined is most appropriate for immediate identification of possible intra-abdominal hemorrhagic source in a patient with injury mechanism capable of producing multiple injuries. When this life-threatening problem is ruled out, the next steps are early invasive monitoring in the ICU and stabilization of fractures to decrease pain and injuries to adjacent soft tissue, while simultaneous efforts are made to identify other non–life-threatening injuries. Exploratory laparotomy is not indicated in this patient at this time because she is hemodynamically stable and without clear signs of intra-abdominal injuries.

CLINICAL PEARLS

▶ The first priority in evaluating a pediatric or geriatric trauma patient is the ABCs.

▶ The most life-threatening injury in intentional child injury is head injury.

▶ Soft-tissue and skin injuries are the most common child injury.

▶ Myocardial infarction is the leading cause of death among 80-year-old patients in the postinjury setting.

▶ Early management of geriatric trauma patient should be directed toward early monitoring of patients to avoid hypovolemia, inadequate treatment of pain, and hypothermia.

REFERENCES

Aalami OO, Fang TD, Song HM, et al. Physiologic features of aging persons. *Arch Surg.* 2003;138: 1068-1076.

Cooper A. Early assessment and management of trauma. In: Whitefield Holcomb III G, Murphy JP, Ostlie DJ, eds. *Ashcraft's Pediatric Surgery.* 5th ed. Philadelphia, PA: Saunders Elsevier; 2010:167-181.

DiScala C, Sege R, Li G, Reece R. Child abuse and unintentional injuries: a 10-year retrospective. *Arch Pediatr Adolesc Med.* 2000;154(1):16-22.

Victorino GP, Chong TJ, Pal JD. Trauma in the elderly patient. *Arch Surg.* 2003;138:1093-1098.

A 24-year-old Gravida 0, Para 0 woman is brought in the emergency center with a history of heavy vaginal bleeding for 8 days. The patient says that the bleeding has been heavier than normal and that she has used up to 20 pads per day that are soaked. She has been passing clots the size of "golf balls" also. She feels faint and lightheaded. The patient's mother states that her daughter has had irregular menses throughout her life, with menses every 30 to 70 days, and bleeding heavy at times and light at other times. On examination, the BP is 90/60 mm Hg, and HR is 120 beats per minute. Generally, she is anxious. The mucous membranes are moist and skin turgor is normal. There is a 2-second capillary refill. The heart and lung examinations are normal. The abdominal examination reveals slight obesity with no scars or tenderness. The pelvic examination shows active bright red bleeding. The vagina has 30 cc of blood in the vault. The cervix appears normal. Pelvic examination reveals a normal-sized uterus and no adnexal masses. There is slight tenderness but no cervical motion tenderness. The hemoglobin level is 8 g/dL, and platelet count 160 000/mm^3. The pregnancy test is negative.

▶ What is the most likely diagnosis?
▶ What is the initial management?
▶ What is the most likely etiology for the patient's condition?
▶ What are the options in treating the patient's hemorrhage?

ANSWERS TO CASE 50:

Dysfunctional Uterine Bleeding

Summary: A 24-year-old nulligravid woman is brought into the emergency center with significant menometrorrhagia for 8 days. The patient has had a long history of oligomenorrhea. On examination, the BP is 90/60 mm Hg, and HR is 120 beats per minute. Generally, she is anxious. The skin turgor, mucous membranes, and capillary refill are normal. The pelvic examination shows active bright red bleeding. The vagina has 30 cc of blood in the vault. There are no abnormalities noted on pelvic examination. The hemoglobin level is 8 g/dL, and platelet count 160 000/mm^3. The pregnancy test is negative.

- **Most likely diagnosis:** Dysfunctional uterine bleeding

- **Initial management:** ABCs—intravenous isotonic saline infusion, urgent pelvic ultrasound examination, gynecological consultation

- **Most likely etiology:** Anovulatory state leading to proliferative endometrium and fragmented endometrial desquamation

- **Treatment options of hemorrhage:** Intravenous estrogen versus dilatation and curettage

ANALYSIS

Objectives

1. Be able to define dysfunctional uterine bleeding (DUB) and be aware that it is associated with normal uterine anatomy.

2. List the common etiologies of abnormal vaginal bleeding.

3. Describe a logical approach to abnormal vaginal bleeding and be aware that dysfunctional uterine bleeding is the most common cause of non–pregnancy-related abnormal vaginal hemorrhage.

4. Be aware of common treatments for DUB.

Considerations

This is a 24-year-old woman with a long history of oligomenorrhea, possibly due to polycystic ovarian syndrome. The patient is noted to be obese but there is no mention of hirsutism or glucose intolerance. The initial attention should be toward assessment of the patient's volume status, and resuscitation of intravascular volume as needed. Pregnancy should be ruled out, since pregnancy-associated vaginal bleeding is usually incomplete abortion, and typically treated by dilatation and curettage (D and C) and not amenable to medical therapy. The emergency physician should also entertain coagulopathy as an etiology with questions about easy bruising and bleeding tendencies. Once pregnancy is ruled out, in the absence of significant contraindications (active liver disease, breast cancer, suspicion of endometrial cancer, thrombophilia), intravenous estrogen can be initiated. Typically, the bleeding will dissipate within several hours, and be markedly decreased within 8 hours. Gynecological consultation is paramount since consideration should be given for endometrial sampling when there is suspicion of endometrial hyperplasia or cancer. In this individual, her age makes these conditions less likely. After intravenous estrogen such as conjugated equine estrogen (Premarin) 25 mg intravenously every 6 hours is given for 3 to 4 doses, then the patient is usually transitioned to an oral contraceptive agent and menses regulated with these medications.

APPROACH TO:
Dysfunctional Uterine Bleeding

DEFINITIONS

MENORRHAGIA: Excessive vaginal bleeding, classically exceeding 80 mL during menses, or greater than 7 days in duration, which leads to anemia without iron supplementation. Menorrhagia is not associated with irregular menses but heavy menses.

MENOMETRORRHAGIA: Prolonged and/or excessive vaginal bleeding that occurs at irregular intervals, usually due to anovulation.

OLIGOMENORRHEA: Menses occurring at intervals of greater than 35 days.

AMENORRHEA: Absence of menses for greater than 6 months.

CLINICAL APPROACH

Initial Approach

The initial condition of the patient dictates the rapidity of the evaluation, and therapeutic maneuvers employed. A patient who presents to the emergency center in frank shock due to excessive vaginal bleeding should have urgent management of hypovolemia and blood products en route while very basic diagnostic information is sought. Establishing whether the patient is pregnant is critical, and this should be determined by a reliable hospital/office test, and not by patient history (contraception, abstinence, home pregnancy test). Screening questions and examination about amount of vaginal bleeding and presence or absence of clots, number of pads, and degree that each pad is soaked may be helpful, but multiple research studies have highlighted the unreliability of an individual's assessment of their menstrual bleeding. This initial patient assessment should address the following questions:

1. Is the patient in hypovolemia shock?

2. Is the patient pregnant?

3. Is the patient actively bleeding and to what degree?

4. Is there an obvious etiology for the vaginal bleeding (uterine fibroids, coagulopathy, cervical cancer, genital tract laceration)?

Because **the amount of vaginal bleeding is difficult to characterize,** women with DUB may sometimes present with profound anemia, or volume depletion that is well compensated. A systematic assessment of volume status will prevent undue delay in these patients. Also, in older women, myocardial infarction and stroke should be considered if hypotension is prolonged. The treatment for hypovolemic shock is the same as that of other conditions, such as trauma.

Pregnancy must be reliably ruled in or out early in the evaluation of patients with DUB. A complication of pregnancy usually indicates an incomplete abortion, such that a uterine dilation and curettage should be performed to stop the bleeding. Other conditions that should be considered include molar pregnancy, and antepartum vaginal bleeding such as placenta previa or placental abruption. When the uterus is above the level of the umbilicus in a pregnant woman with vaginal bleeding, a speculum examination or digital examination should be avoided since these actions may exacerbate placenta previa. An ultrasound examination instead is helpful in conditions of pregnancy-related vaginal hemorrhage.

Active vaginal bleeding necessitates more aggressive management. Upon examining the woman, **blood stains down the legs indicates significant bleeding,** and the probable need for transfusion. The speculum examination should be performed to assess for degree of bleeding, lesions of the vagina or cervix, and ascertaining whether the bleeding is coming from within the uterus (supracervical) versus the cervix or vagina. Lacerations of the vagina or cervix may indicate instrumentation or trauma. A digital pelvic examination is performed to assess for cervical pathology, and also uterine size and shape. In the face of DUB, once structural abnormalities of the genital tract are ruled out, active bleeding will usually necessitate high-dose estrogen parenteral therapy or uterine D and C. In situations of less active bleeding, oral hormonal therapy may be considered.

A systematic approach should be undertaken to assess for underlying causes of DUB. A history of medication use such as oral contraceptives, IUD use, depoprovera, family history of coagulopathy, structural lesions of the uterus or cervix (see Table 50–1), and differential diagnosis of ovulatory dysfunction should also be considered (see Table 50–2).

Dysfunctional Uterine Bleeding

The diagnosis of DUB is one of exclusion after other disorders are ruled out. The bleeding is due largely to anovulation, that is, unopposed estrogen effect on the endometrium leading to overgrowth of the endometrium without progesterone to arrest the growth. Fragments of endometrium slough off leading to bleeding from

Table 50–1 • DIFFERENTIAL DIAGNOSIS OF DUB
Pregnancy-related complications (incomplete abortion, placenta previa, placenta abruption)
Laceration/trauma
Coagulopathy
Structural disorders of the genital tract (uterine fibroids, endometrial or cervical polyps)
Endometrial hyperplasia or cancer
Infections of the genital tract

Table 50–2 • ETIOLOGIES OF OVULATORY DYSFUNCTION
Hypothyroidism
Hyperprolactinemia
Polycystic ovarian syndrome
Premature ovarian failure
Perimenopause, menarche
Excessive exercise
Stress
Excessive weight loss
Chronic illness
Androgen excess (Cushing's, adrenal tumor, ovarian tumor)
Hormonal therapy (contraception)

denuded endometrium. Polycystic ovarian syndrome (PCOS) is a common condition associated with DUB. PCOS is a constellation of obesity, anovulation, hirsutism, glucose intolerance, oligomenorrhea, and hyperandrogenism. In a woman older than age 35, or in a younger patient with persistent and prolonged unopposed estrogen, endometrium sampling should be performed to assess for endometrial hyperplasia or cancer. A reasonable workup for anovulatory DUB is listed in Table 50–3.

Acute treatment of DUB is principally estrogen-containing hormonal therapy. With significant bleeding, IV premarin causes re-epithelialization of the denuded endometrium to arrest bleeding from these "raw surfaces." Nevertheless, after three to four doses of parenteral estrogen, the bleeding should be significantly diminished, and the patient transitioned to an oral combination estrogen/progestin regimen. In most situations where there is less active bleeding, oral contraceptive agents can be used. Various regimens are used, and one common method is to use 3 tablets a day of a combination OC (such as ortho novum 1/35) for 7 days, and then after the 7 days, the patient should begin the same oral contraceptive 1 tablet a day. Bleeding should improve within 2 days, and be very minimal within 4 to 5 days. Follow-up should be arranged within a week. Hormonal therapy should not be initiated until pregnancy and structural lesions of the uterus are ruled out. Endometrial sampling should be performed prior to initiation of hormonal treatment if possible. Notably, bleeding due to uterine fibroids will typically not respond to hormonal manipulation.

Table 50–3 • WORKUP OF DUB
CBC and pregnancy test
Ultrasound examination of the uterus and pelvis
Consider endometrial sampling
Consider assessing for bleeding diathesis (PT, PTT, bleeding time, Von Willebrand work-up)
Consider assessing liver function tests
Consider assessing thyroid function

In some individuals, estrogen therapy will be contraindicated, such as those with active liver disease, active breast cancer, or high risk for thrombosis. In those women, inflation of a Foley balloon in the uterus has been described as a temporarizing measure, and may be life-saving for those patients who cannot receive estrogen and also are not suitable surgical candidates. However, most of these patients will undergo uterine D and C, both for diagnostic purposes, and also to acutely arrest the hemorrhage. It is important to note that the underlying pathological process that induced the bleeding is not addressed with a D and C, and the patient may return to the emergency center in several months if the cause is not addressed. Women who have PCOS for whom oral conceptive agent, or progestins are contraindicated may need surgical therapy for the bleeding, such as endometrial ablation or hysterectomy.

COMPREHENSION QUESTIONS

50.1 A 16-year-old adolescent girl is brought into the ED with complaints of significant vaginal bleeding with her menses. She bleeds 5 days each month with heavy flow, utilizing 25 to 30 pads. She is tired and gets dizzy during menses. On examination, her BP is 80/60 mm Hg and heart rate 120 beats per minute. Her external genitalia are normal; there are no lesions of the cervix or vagina. The uterus is normal sized and anteverted. There are no masses or tenderness. The pregnancy test is negative. Her hemoglobin level is 7 g/dL. The emergency physician orders a transfusion. Which of the following is the best next step?

A. Screen for sexually transmitted infections.

B. Begin intravenous progestin.

C. Consult a gynecologist for endometrial ablation.

D. Screen for coagulopathy.

50.2 A 32-year-old woman is seen in the ED with heavy vaginal bleeding. She states that she has had irregular menses for 3 years, and at times has "baseball-sized clots" pass vaginally. On examination, her BP is 120/70 mm Hg and heart rate 90 beats per minute. Her uterus is 4-week size and without tenderness. There are no abnormalities on pelvic examination including speculum examination of the cervix and vagina. Approximately 30 cc of dark blood is noted in the vaginal vault and a moderate flow of blood from the cervix. Her hemoglobin level is 10 g/dL. Which of the following is the next appropriate step?

A. Begin intravenous estrogen.

B. Administer intramuscular progestin.

C. Transfuse 2 units of packed erythrocytes.

D. Begin oral contraceptives at 3 pills per day.

50.3 A 42-year-old woman is seen in the with profuse vaginal bleeding. She has a history of diabetes mellitus. On examination, her BP is 100/60 and heart rate 105 beats per minute. Her uterus is irregular and enlarged and nontender. There is active bleeding arising from the uterus. Her hemoglobin level is 9 g/dL, glucose level 140 mg/dL and her pregnancy test is negative. Which of the following is the best management of this patient?

A. Begin IV estrogen therapy.

B. Begin oral progestin therapy.

C. Begin oral contraceptive therapy.

D. Lower the blood sugar.

E. Refer the patient for hysterectomy.

F. Perform endometrial sampling.

ANSWERS

50.1 **D.** In an adolescent who has significant menorrhagia requiring transfusion, the incidence of coagulopathy approaches 20% to 30%. Von Willebrand disease is the most common etiology, and will often respond to desmopressin (DDAVP). Coagulopathy should be ruled out prior to starting estrogen therapy, although sometimes this is impossible given laboratory constraints. IV progestin has no role in this condition. Endometrial ablation is appropriate for older women who have finished child bearing, and in whom the endometrium has been assessed for pathology. Endometrial ablation should not be performed on younger patients.

50.2 **D.** This patient is appropriate for oral combination contraceptive therapy. She does not have contraindications, does not seem to require sampling of the endometrium, and there does not seem to be a structural etiology for the bleeding. Intravenous estrogen is usually reserved for women with significant active bleeding and requires hospitalization.

50.3 **F.** This patient is 42 years old with **DUB** and hence, an endometrial sampling should be performed. In general, the endometrium should be assessed for women above age 35 years before any hormonal therapy is initiated. The blood sugar does not need to be acutely lowered. Although the uterus is enlarged and irregular indicating possible uterine fibroids, an evaluation should be performed prior to hysterectomy such as pelvic ultrasound and endometrial sampling.

CLINICAL PEARLS

▶ Dysfunctional uterine bleeding (DUB) is a diagnosis of exclusion and indicates excessive or prolonged bleeding without structural pathology of the genital tract.

▶ The most common reason for DUB is anovulation, the bleeding pattern is heavy and unpredictable.

▶ Therapeutic options of acute and active significant vaginal hemorrhage due to DUB include IV estrogen therapy and uterine D and C. A clinical effect from the estrogen can be seen within 4 hours.

▶ Pregnancy must be ruled out in any woman presenting with DUB.

▶ Endometrial sampling should be considered in any woman over the age of 35 with DUB and in individuals at risk for endometrial hyperplasia/cancer.

▶ Oral contraceptive agents are a reasonable option for the treatment of patients with DUB who are hemodynamically stable once pregnancy, coagulopathy, and structural lesions of the uterus are excluded.

▶ A teenager who presents with DUB may have a bleeding diathesis such as von Willebrand.

REFERENCES

American College of Obstetricians and Gynecologists. Endometrial ablation. ACOG *Practice Bulletin 81.* April 2007.

American College of Obstetricians and Gynecologists. Menstruation in girls and adolescents: using the menstrual cycle as a vital sign. ACOG Committee Opinion 349. November 2006.

American College of Obstetricians and Gynecologists. Polycystic ovarian syndrome. ACOG *Practice Bulletin 108.* December 2009.

Morrison LJ, Spence JM. Vaginal bleeding in the nonpregnant patient. In: Tintinalli JE, Stapczynski JS, Ma OJ, Cline D, Cydulka R, Meckler G, eds. *Emergency Medicine: A Comprehensive Guide.* 7th ed. New York, NY: McGraw-Hill; 2010:647-653.

A 28-year-old man arrives at the emergency department (ED) complaining of 3 days of chest pain that began after multiple episodes of retching and vomiting following a night of heavy drinking. He reported subjective fever and sweats the day following the initial vomiting. He has been unable to tolerate any swallowing and has urinated only twice since the onset of symptoms. He describes the lower anterior chest pain that is non-radiating and of moderately severe intensity. He has no history of prior chest pain. He also complains of an intermittent sore throat and painful swallowing. He does not appear short of breath but states that he has to control his breathing to avoid a "tight feeling in his throat". He states that his voice sounds "different" and that he feels weak and faint. The review of systems is otherwise negative. His temperature is 37°C, HR 132, blood pressure 168/94 and RR 22 with an O2 saturation of 98% on room air. Physical examination shows an ill and uncomfortable appearing man who is tachycardic, hypertensive, and afebrile. He has dry mucous membranes and faint bibasilar crackles. He has no past medical history and is taking no medications.

▶ What is the most likely diagnosis?
▶ What are the next diagnostic steps?
▶ What therapies should be instituted immediately?

ANSWERS TO CASE 51:

Noncardiac Chest Pain

Summary: This is a 28-year-old man presenting with acute severe chest pain, diaphoresis, and dyspnea after multiple episodes of vomiting.

- **Most likely diagnosis:** Spontaneous esophageal perforation or Boerhaave Syndrome

- **Next diagnostic steps:** Place the patient on a cardiac monitor, establish IV access and obtain an electrocardiogram (ECG) immediately. A chest x-ray (CXR) should be obtained as soon as possible.

- **Immediate therapies:** NPO, NGT, IV resuscitation with isotonic fluids, broad spectrum antibiotics, pain management and immediate surgical consultation

ANALYSIS

Objectives

1. Become familiar with the serious causes of noncardiac chest pain (NCCP).

2. Consider spontaneous esophageal perforation in the differential diagnosis of chest pain and recognize the key signs and symptoms of Boerhaave Syndrome.

3. Understand the therapeutic approach to NCCP in general and Boerhaave Syndrome in particular.

Considerations

This case presents a young male ED patient with chest pain who is severely ill. Failure to recognize, diagnose and treat the acuity and severity of this patient illness would be catastrophic. While the diagnosis in this case is Boerhaave Syndrome, the differential diagnosis in this case should also include: esophagitis, gastroesophageal reflux disease (GERD), esophageal spasm, esophageal foreign body, peptic ulcer disease, hepatitis, pancreatitis, pneumonia, pneumomediastinum, pulmonary embolism, pericarditis, aortic dissection/aneurysm and musculoskeletal disorders. Coronary artery disease would be very rare in a 28-year-old individual but should remain in the differential, especially in young diabetics or those with unusual risk factors.

APPROACH TO:
Noncardiac Chest Pain

DEFINITIONS

BOERHAAVE SYNDROME: Post-emetic barotrauma induced spontaneous rupture of the esophagus

GASTROGRAFIN: Water soluble iodinated radiographic contrast agent (each mL contains 660 mg diatrizoate meglumine and 100 mg diatrizoate sodium). Each 100 mL contains 37 g of elemental iodine.

BARIUM: Water insoluble particulate suspension of barium sulfate used as radiographic contrast agent

APPROACH TO SUSPECTED BOERHAAVE SYNDROME

Pathophysiology

Boerhaave syndrome results from an increased intraesophageal pressure alternating with a negative intrathoracic pressure due to straining or vomiting. In most cases, the tear occurs along the left posterolateral aspect of the distal esophagus, as it is the least supported portion of the esophagus. Localized cervical esophageal perforation may also occur and generally follows a benign course. The esophagus is especially vulnerable to rupture because it lacks a serosal layer, and therefore collagen and elastin fibers to provide support. It is most common among 40- to 60-year-old males.

Esophageal rupture from other causes is a related but different clinical entity. The majority of esophageal ruptures are iatrogenic due to endoscopy.

Morbidity and mortality associated with Boerhaave Syndrome are due to an overwhelming inflammatory response to mediastinal soilage caused by gastric contents and oropharyngeal bacteria deposited in the mediastinal and pleural spaces with subsequent development of pneumonia, mediastinitis, empyema, sepsis, and multiorgan failure. *Untreated Boerhaave Syndrome has a 100% case fatality rate.*

Evaluation

Mackler triad: vomiting, lower chest pain, and subcutaneous cervical emphysema are classically associated with Boerhaave Syndrome, but is seen in a minority of cases on early presentation. Important potential signs and symptoms include fever, chest pain, back pain, tachypnea, tachycardia, dyspnea, cervical subcutaneous emphysema and Hamman sign, a "mediastinal crunch" heard as the heart beats surrounded by mediastinal air. Breath sounds may be decreased on the side of perforation due to pleural effusion.

If esophageal perforation is suspected, a CT scan of the chest should be ordered promptly. A CXR will likely be the initial study performed and may show pleural effusion, pneumomediastinum, widened mediastinum or pneumothorax. It should be noted that on early presentation, the CXR can be negative. CT scan is far more sensitive and may show esophageal wall thickening, periesophageal fluid, extraesophageal air, and/or air and fluid in pleural spaces. Contrast radiographic studies of the esophagus may be necessary to localize the perforation. Although barium is superior to gastrografin when attempting to locate a small perforation, it causes a severe inflammatory reaction in the mediastinum or peritoneum. Small esophageal perforations are frequently missed by both contrast modalities. If a thoracentesis is performed, fluid should be evaluated for food particles, pH <6 and elevated amylase. Endoscopy has no role in the evaluation of Boerhaave Syndrome and may exacerbate the perforation due to insufflation during the procedure.

Treatment

An immediate surgical consult should be obtained. Definitive treatment will depend on the size and location of the perforation, whether preexisting disease is present, and whether or not it is contained. If the CT scan shows containment, treatment consists of NPO status, NGT placement with suction to remove gastric fluids and prevent further contamination, broad spectrum IV antibiotics and parenteral nutrition. If the perforation is not contained surgical repair is indicated. Liberal narcotic analgesia and anti-emetics to prevent additional valsalva induced barotrauma should be given as early as possible in the course of treatment.

Complications

Any delay in diagnosis or treatment will result in increased morbidity and mortality. Death due to spontaneous esophageal rupture is generally reported in 20% to 40% of treated cases. Complications of surgical repair include persistent esophageal leaks, mediastinitis, and sepsis. Despite adequate repair, continued leakage may occur in up to 30% of patients.

CLINICAL APPROACH

Chest pain (CP) is responsible for more than 6 million visits per year to the ED in the US. The evaluation of acute CP should always begin with a complete history focusing on quality, radiation of pain, context of onset, duration, risk factors, and exacerbating factors.

Due to the high morbidity and mortality of myocardial infarction, an ECG should be obtained immediately upon presentation to help assess the possibility of acute ischemia. Even when NCCP is suspected, reevaluation may be necessary if traditional cardiac risk factors suggest a high pretest probability of cardiac disease. One recent study showed that 2.8% of a study population diagnosed with NCCP had adverse cardiac events within 30 days. This correlates well with the reported missed diagnosis rate of 1% to 5% for patients presenting to the emergency department with acute myocardial infarction. The pretest probability of a cardiac etiology for an episode of CP increases with the patient age and positive risk factor profile.

How sensitive is ECG in predicting cardiac disease? That depends on how you ask the question. A meta-analysis of exercise tolerance test results reported a sensitivity of 68% and a specificity of 77% for cardiac ischemia. A single ECG cannot logically be any better than this result. Another study reported ECG abnormalities in 50% to 90% of patients who ultimately died of MI. In short, a work up including ECG with and without pain and serial cardiac enzymes is probably indicated at initial presentation for any patient with a moderate or greater pretest probability of cardiac disease before diagnosing them with NCCP.

NCCP is generally defined as CP occurring in the presence of normal large epicardial coronary artery anatomy and thus, not related to myocardial ischemia. A small percentage of these patients may have ischemia due to vasospasm or isolated distal arterial disease, but this does not change the general approach or differential diagnosis. The global differential diagnosis of NCCP for any patient should include the following etiologies in decreasing order of prevalence: musculoskeletal, esophageal/GI, psychiatric, pulmonary, other cardiac causes (pericarditis, etc), and other/nonspecific. Despite the preceding statement, the most common cause of NCCP seen in the ED is GERD.

Differential Diagnosis of Noncardiac Chest Pain

Musculoskeletal Chest Pain: Musculoskeletal CP is usually associated with a history of trauma, specific injury or repetitive use. It should be reproducible on careful examination by palpation or through specific motions or movements of the involved anatomic structures. The pain may also be pleuritic, or associated with deep breathing. Patients are frequently extremely anxious, making the diagnosis more difficult. Associated symptoms should be minimal once the effect of anxiety has been discounted. A detailed knowledge of the muscular and boney anatomy of the neck, thorax, and upper abdomen is necessary to fully evaluate this cause of NCCP. Frequently the only evaluation needed will be a careful and complete history and physical examination. Nonetheless, chest radiography (CXR) is appropriate if boney or pulmonary disease is being considered. Bedside ultrasound or formal echocardiography may be used to rule out pneumothorax, pericarditis, structural heart disease or aortic pathology. Liberal utilization of EKG is indicated and appropriate. Once the diagnosis has been made, appropriate care includes reassurance, analgesics, nonsteroidal anti-inflammatory drugs (NSAIDs), and temporary behavioral restrictions to minimize re-injury. Follow-up examination in 1 to 2 weeks is recommended with their PMD.

Esophageal and Gastrointestinal Causes of Chest Pain: Multiple pathologies of the esophagus may result in CP. These include reflux and chemical esophagitis, esophageal ulceration, foreign body, perforation and spasm. Esophageal perforation is discussed elsewhere in this chapter. Esophageal foreign body is usually obvious from the patient history except in young children and the elderly. In the case presented above, aspirated foreign body is certainly a possibility. CXR and neck films will identify radiopaque foreign bodies other objects require upper endoscopy for further evaluation. The remaining pathologic entities may be grouped under the label of GERD. The history in patients with GERD may include epigastric pain at night when lying supine and a correlation with large meals near bedtime. Caffeine, alcohol and tobacco use all decrease lower esophageal sphincter pressure, and thus increase the likelihood of reflux. NSAIDs and alcohol use both injure the esophageal mucosa. Long term reflux and esophagitis induce typical histologic changes in the distal esophageal mucosa and Barrett esophagus, that are diagnostic on biopsy. Physical examination is nonspecific and may show only subxiphoid or epigastric tenderness. Acute treatments are not helpful from the standpoint of narrowing the differential possibilities. Nitroglycerin relieves GERD associated esophageal spasm but also relieves cardiac CP. The classic "GI cocktail" of antacid, lidocaine and donnatal relieves GERD pain, but also anesthetizes nerves carrying pain sensations from other potentially lethal mediastinal pathologies. Thus, neither of these treatments should ever be used to rule out or rule in any single diagnosis. Long-term management of esophageal disorders includes behavior modification to prevent nocturnal reflux and various medications (PPI, H2 blocker, mucosal protectants) to allow healing of the esophageal mucosa. Peptic ulcer disease (PUD) is frequently associated with GERD. Triple therapy with PPI, H2 blockers, and antibiotics for eradication of *Helicobacter pylori* have resulted in >90% healing rate. Referral to a gastroenterologist for ongoing management is appropriate in more complicated cases.

Diseases of the upper abdominal organs may cause NCCP. Hepatitis can cause pain that radiates into the upper right chest due inflammation of the right hemidiaphragm. Cholecystitis can result in substernal CP and subxiphoid epigastric pain. Pancreatitis can cause pain that radiates from the epigastrum into the back and may radiate into the left chest in association with transudative pulmonary effusion. Splenic hematoma or infarction can result in CP that radiates to the left upper chest due to inflammation of the left hemidiaphragm.

Psychiatric Causes of Chest Pain: Depression frequently results in complaints of chest or abdominal pain. The patient may or may not be aware of the depression. Patients complaining of CP should be questioned about symptoms of depression such as anhedonia; early morning awakening, insomnia, and loss of interest or pleasure in normal activities. Physical examination in the organically depressed may reveal emotional lability, flattened affect, suicidal ideation, or psychomotor retardation but is generally negative for specific findings associated with other physical causes of CP. Somatization is the term applied to a specific type of conversion disorder where the patient depressive symptoms find focus in a specific physical complaint such as CP or abdominal pain. The patient may be fixated on the presenting physical complaint and unaware of the depressive component to their complaint. Diagnostic work up of this type of patient should be guided by a careful history and physical. A reasonably extensive initial diagnostic work up is indicated. Diagnosis of a psychiatric etiology for CP must be a diagnosis of exclusion. Recent meta-analysis has revealed a potential association between the diagnoses of panic attack with anxiety induced CP and CAD in the primary care and ED settings. The care provider should also keep in mind that depression may coexist with other organic causes of CP and that this risk increases with age. Also to be kept in mind is that depression alone may have lethal consequences and requires accurate diagnosis and aggressive therapy by a mental health care professional.

Pulmonary Causes of Chest Pain: The lungs, air passages and pleura can all cause chest discomfort. Irritation of the pleura can be caused by peripheral pneumonic inflammation from infectious causes, such as pneumonia; ischemia due pulmonary embolism or infarction; or mechanical irritation due to disruption of normal anatomy of the visceral and/or parietal pleural due to pneumothorax, pneumomediastinum, exudative effusions and some cancers. Infectious causes of CP will often be suspected if fever and hypoxia are present. Pneumothorax or pulmonary embolism should be suspected when the patient has acute unilateral pleuritic pain. Unilateral pleuritic CP ipsilateral to blunt chest trauma strongly suggests pneumothorax, but pneumothorax may occur spontaneously. Tracheal deviation, hypoxia, hypotension and hyper-resonance of the hemithorax contralateral to the tracheal deviation indicate the presence of tension pneumothorax. This is an immediately life threatening condition that requires emergency needle decompression of the hyper-resonant hemithorax with a large gauge needle or angiocath. If available, bedside ultrasound (US) may rapidly diagnose pneumothorax in trained hands. If the patient is unstable, treatment of tension pneumothorax should never be delayed for radiographic confirmation. Occult hypoxia may be uncovered by obtaining ambulatory pulse oximetry. Physical examination of the chest may reveal rales, rhonchi, wheezing, decreased breath sounds, signs of consolidation or effusion, and/or abnormalities of the chest wall. These finding may occur together or in isolation and should be correlated with the history and two view CXR to accurately determine the cause and scope of the patient pathology. If an infectious etiology is suspected in a patient likely to require admission to the hospital, then antibiotics should be administered as early as possible. Current nationwide quality improvement efforts sponsored by Centers for Medicaid and Medicare Services (CMS) specify ≤6 hour window, from time of patient arrival, for initial antibiotic administration in pneumonia patients admitted for inpatient care.

Other Causes of Chest Pain: Pericarditis is a non-ischemic cause of cardiac CP that results from inflammation of the pericardium, the connective tissue sack which envelopes the heart. The pain associated with this entity is worse when supine and improves with erect posture or sitting up. Auscultation of the heart may reveal a rough scratchy sound very different from a murmur associated with cardiac systole and diastole. This is known as a pericardial friction rub. ECG findings vary over the course of the disease but, in general, are characterized by diffuse ST segment elevations. Many causes of pericarditis exist. These include but are not limited to post-infarction (Dressler syndrome), autoimmune, infectious (viral, bacterial, fungal), and traumatic. Viral infection is the most common non-infarction cause. Evaluation should include ECG, serial cardiac enzymes, and echocardiography. Until proven otherwise, ischemic cardiac disease should remain high in the differential. Echocardiography can demonstrate a thickened pericardium or a pericardial effusion typical of the disease and rule out the potentially lethal complication of pericardial tamponade. Tamponade may develop if pressure from the effusion is great enough to significantly impair cardiac filling. Emergent treatment consists of immediate pericardial drainage by needle aspiration. Treatment of pericarditis is more subacute and consists of analgesics, NSAIDs and frequent follow up until improvement is achieved.

A high suspicion must be maintained for aneurysm/dissection and pulmonary embolism to avoid missed diagnosis and potentially catastrophic outcomes for the patients. In both diseases the onset of CP can be sudden and associated with syncope. In aortic aneurysm the patient complains of CP radiating to the back. If the dissection involves the root of the aorta, and thus the coronary arteries, the patient may also have CP due to cardiac ischemia. Early echocardiography and/ or CT imaging will result in timely diagnosis. It is imperative to not treat blindly as the treatment for pulmonary embolism can exacerbate aortic dissection and/or aneurysmal rupture with life threatening results.

Another consideration in a vomiting patient with CP is the less serious but still potentially life threatening Mallory-Weiss tear. This entity involves a traumatic mucosal disruption usually located either at the gastroesophageal junction or gastric cardia. These esophageal tears may result in significant GI hemorrhage and can perforate if intense vomiting or retching continues. Deeper tears of the esophageal mucosa may manifest as intramural esophageal hematomas which can develop into full esophageal perforations with delayed rupture during the inflammatory weakening that accompanies healing.

Spontaneous pneumomediastinum without evidence of gastrointestinal or pleural source has been reported. It is usually seen in patients who have suffered from a valsalva episode against a closed glottis such as may occur during powerful coughing. Chest pain is universal and on exam a loud crunching sound may be heard as mediastinal air is squeezed by the beating heart (Hamman crunch). It is hypothesized that the mediastinal air arises from pulmonary interstitial emphysema caused by bronchoalveolar barotrauma. Crack cocaine smokers appear to be at particular risk. Despite the ominous CXR findings, this entity has a generally benign course. Nonetheless, the diagnosis of pneumomediastinum requires a diligent and exhaustive search for both pulmonary and gastrointestinal sources.

Breast pathology should be considered in the differential of NCCP in women presenting to the ED. Causes of breast pain include infectious etiologies, mastitis or abscess, benign lumps, cysts, or inflammatory carcinoma. Physical examination may reveal an asymmetric breast mass with or without signs of significant local induration, erythema, and tenderness. The patient with more serious pathology is often febrile. Intravenous analgesics, antibiotics and early surgical consultation are appropriate.

The preceding list is not exhaustive and difficult clinical cases may require evaluation for more esoteric causes of NCCP. In the geriatric population, many patients may have more than one operative diagnosis causing their NCCP. As such, it is imperative that early primary care follow-up be arranged for patients given this diagnosis.

Presentation of Boerhaave Syndrome (Pressure Induced Esophageal Rupture)

The classical presentation of Boerhaave Syndrome follows an episode of forceful retching and vomiting and includes retrosternal CP and/or epigastric pain. Odynophagia, dyspnea, tachypnea, cyanosis, fever, and shock may all develop thereafter. In one review, 40% of patients had a history of heavy drinking, 41% suffered from PUD, 83% complained of pain, 79% had a history of vomiting, 32% presented with shock and 39% with dyspnea. The diagnosis of Boerhaave Syndrome may be delayed because the clinical presentation may not be typical and causes are broad: childbirth, defecation, seizures, and heavy lifting. Common misdiagnoses include: myocardial infarction, pancreatitis, lung abscess, pericarditis, and spontaneous pneumothorax. Concurrent alcohol intoxication may also delay diagnosis.

COMPREHENSION QUESTIONS

51.1 In the initial evaluation of most ED patient with CP, what is the most important diagnostic test?
A. Chest x-ray
B. ECG
C. Serum cardiac markers
D. Computed tomography
E. Cholesterol levels

51.2 Which of the following is the most common cause of NCCP?
A. Musculoskeletal
B. Gastrointestinal
C. Other–nonspecific
D. Psychiatric
E. Pulmonary

51.3 A 45-year-old man with a known history of Boerhaave syndrome and primary surgical repair 5 years ago presents to the ED complaining of 24 hours of increasing CP and shortness of breath, what diagnostic test should be ordered to rule out perforation?
A. ECG
B. CXR
C. CT thorax
D. Barium esophagram

ANSWERS

51.1 **B.** An ECG to evaluate the patient for evidence of acute ischemia is the first indicated test. The healthcare provider should always keep in mind that a negative ECG does not rule out cardiac pathology.

51.2 **A.** Musculoskeletal conditions is the most common cause. All the listed answers are causes of NCCP and are listed in decreasing order with respect to their prevalence in the general population. GERD is the most common cause of NCCP seen in ED patients.

51.3 **C.** CT of the thorax is by far the most sensitive and specific test in assessing for possible esophageal perforation, especially in this patient given the time course of the symptoms and the history of prior surgery.

CLINICAL PEARLS

▶ Boerhaave syndrome should always be considered in the differential diagnosis of acute CP and especially if the patient has been vomiting or performing any activity where barotrauma may have been sustained due to valsalva maneuver.

▶ Gastrografin should be used instead of barium to avoid severe medi-astinal and intra-pleural inflammatory reactions when doing contrast studies to locate the site of esophageal perforation.

▶ GI Cocktail can not be used to reliably rule out a cardiac etiology for an episode of CP.

▶ Response to a trial of sublingual nitroglycerin does not distinguish between coronary artery disease and GERD induced esophageal spasm.

▶ A single normal ECG can not be used to make the diagnosis of NCCP.

▶ A significant percentage of patients (2%-3%) labeled with a diagnosis of NCCP will have an adverse cardiac event within 30 days.

REFERENCES

Chambers J, Bass C, Mayou R. Non-cardiac chest pain: assessment and management. *Heart.* 1999;82: 656-657.

Dumville JC, MacPherson H, Griffith K, et al. Non-cardiac chest pain: a retrospective cohort study of patients who attended a Rapid Access Chest Pain Clinic. *Fam Pract.* 2007 Apr;24(2):152-157.

Glombiewski JA, Rief W, Bösner S, et al. The course of nonspecific chest pain in primary care: symptom persistence and health care usage. *Arch Intern Med.* 2010 8;170(3):251-255.

Herring N, Paterson DJ. ECG diagnosis of acute ischaemia and infarction: past, present and future. *QJM.* 2006;99(4):219-230.

Katerndahl DA. Chest pain and its importance in patients with panic disorder: an updated literature review. *Prim Care Companion J Clin Psychiatry.* 2008;10(5):376-383.

Kiev J, Amendola M. A management algorithm for esophageal perforation. *Am J Surg.* 2007;194: 103-106.

Klinkman MS, Stevens D, Gorenflo DW. Episodes of care for chest pain: a preliminary report from MIRNET. *J Fam Pract.* 1994;38(4):345-352.

Long CM, Ezenkwele UA. Esophageal Perforation, rupture and tears. Available at: www.emedicine.com. (Accessed June, 2010).

Martina B, Bucheli B, Stotz M, et al. First clinical judgment by primary care physicians distinguishes well between nonorganic and organic causes of abdominal or chest pain. *J Gen Intern Med.* 1997;12(8): 459-465.

Mayou RA, Bass C, Hart G, et al. Can clinical assessment of chest pain be made more therapeutic? *QJM.* 2000;93(12):805-811.

Mayou RA, Bass CM, Bryant BM. Management of non-cardiac chest pain: from research to clinical practice. *Heart.* 1999;81(4):387-392.

Newby DE, Fox KA, Flint LL, Boon NA. A "same day" direct-access chest pain clinic: improved manage-ment and reduced hospitalization. *QJM.* 1998;91(5):333-337.

Svavarsdóttir AE, Jónasson MR, Gudmundsson GH, Fjeldsted K. Chest pain in family practice. Diagnosis and long-term outcome in a community setting. *Can Fam Physician*. 1996 Jun;42:1122-1128. Erratum in: *Can Fam Physician*. 1996;42:1672.

Triadafilopoulos G, LaMont JT. Boerhaave syndrome: effort rupture of the esophagus. Available at: www.uptodate.com (Accessed June 2010).

Verdon F, Herzig L, Burnand B, Bischoff T, Pécoud A, Junod M, et al. Chest pain in daily practice: occurrence, causes and management. *Swiss Med Wkly*. 2008 14;138(23-24):340-347.

A 54-year-old man is brought to the emergency department with complaints of generalized weakness, nausea, and an overall sense of illness. The patient symptoms have progressed insidiously over the past 2 to 3 days. His past medical history is remarkable for longstanding diabetes and poorly controlled hypertension. He is currently taking many medications that include a sulfonylurea, a diuretic, and an angiotensin-converting enzyme (ACE) inhibitor. On physical examination, the patient appears lethargic and ill. His temperature is 36.0°C (96.8°F), pulse rate is 70 beats per minute, blood pressure is 154/105 mm Hg, and the respiratory rate is 22 breaths per minute. His head and neck examination shows normal conjunctiva and mucous membranes. There is moderate jugular venous distention. The lungs have minor bibasilar rales. The cardiac examination reveals normal rate, no murmurs or rubs, and a positive S_4. The abdomen is soft and nontender to palpation, with hypoactive bowel sounds and no organomegaly. The rectal examination is normal. Skin is cool and dry. Extremities demonstrate pitting edema to the knees bilaterally. On neurologic examination the patient moans and weakly localizes pain. He is oriented to person and place but cannot provide any further history. The initial rhythm strip is shown in Figure 52–1.

▶ What is the most likely diagnosis?
▶ What is the next step?

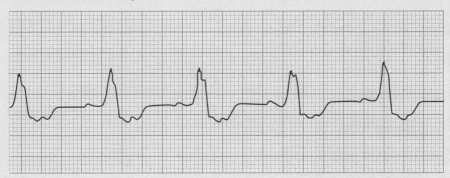

Figure 52–1. ECG rhythm strip.

ANSWERS TO CASE 52:
Hyperkalemia Due to Renal Failure

Summary: A 54-year-old man with hypertension and diabetes complains of weakness, nausea, and a general sense of illness. His symptoms have progressed slowly over 3 days. His medications include a sulfonylurea, a diuretic, and an ACE inhibitor. On examination, he appears lethargic and ill. His BP is 154/105 mm Hg, HR 70 bpm, temperature 36.0°C (96.8°F), and respiratory rate 22 breaths per minute. The physical examination reveals moderate jugular venous distension, some minor bibasilar rales, and lower extremity edema. He is oriented to person and place but is not able to give further history. The ECG confirms a wide complex rhythm (Figure 52–2).

- **Most likely diagnosis:** Hyperkalemia

- **Next step:** Management of the ABCs, including immediate vascular access and continuous cardiac monitoring, rapid stepwise administration of medication to reverse the effect of excess potassium (calcium), shift potassium into cells (insulin, sympathomimetics, possibly sodium bicarbonate), and remove potassium from the body (sodium polystyrene sulfonate or diuretics). Arrange for emergency dialysis and admit to the hospital.

ANALYSIS

Objectives

1. Recognize the clinical settings, the signs and symptoms, and complications of hyperkalemia.

2. Understand the diagnostic and therapeutic approach to suspected hyperkalemia.

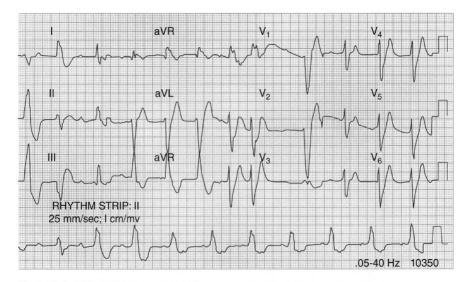

Figure 52–2. ECG.

Considerations

This patient has developed end-stage renal failure (also referred to as chronic kidney disease, stage 5), due to his longstanding hypertension and diabetes. His damaged kidneys have very little capacity to excrete potassium. ACE inhibitor therapy contributes to his potassium retention. Acidosis and blunted insulin response both lead to potassium shifts into the extracellular space. His cardiac cell membranes are destabilized by the high potassium level and he is at high risk of death by arrhythmia. His weakness and general sense of illness, while nonspecific, are very typical of untreated renal failure. Weakness can also be a prominent feature of severe hyperkalemia. It is important to suspect this condition from the history and ECG, because laboratory test results may be delayed and the patient could die before those test results become available.

Laboratory studies should be performed and in this patient case, the leukocyte count is 9000 cells/L, and the patient is mildly anemic with hemoglobin 10.5 and hematocrit 32%. Electrolytes show sodium of 134 mEq/L, potassium 7.8 mEq/L, chloride 101 mEq/L, and bicarbonate 18 mEq/L. BUN is 114 mg/dL and creatinine is 10.5. The serum glucose is 180 mg/dL (10 mmol/L). The serum amylase, bilirubin, AST, ALT, and alkaline phosphatase are within normal limits. A 12-lead ECG confirms the wide-complex rhythm shown previously. His CXR shows mild cardiomegaly and pulmonary vascular congestion.

This patient clinical presentation is fairly representative of hyperkalemia in renal failure. Hyperkalemia is a common complication of end-stage chronic kidney disease, though it can occur in many other clinical conditions. Symptoms of hyperkalemia may be nonspecific or even nonexistent, and are most often dominated by whatever illness has predisposed the patient to elevated potassium. Morbidity and mortality may result from delayed or inadequate treatment, since severe hyperkalemia may rapidly progress to arrhythmia and cardiac arrest. Early suspicion, prompt recognition of associated ECG changes, and prompt resuscitation with effective agent, are essential. Once resuscitated, the patient will require prompt consultation for emergent hemodialysis.

APPROACH TO:
Suspected Hyperkalemia

CLINICAL APPROACH

Hyperkalemia is a severe metabolic emergency. A delay in treatment may lead to significant mortality. Up to one-quarter of patients with end-stage chronic kidney disease will have at least one episode of life-threatening hyperkalemia. Hyperkalemia can occur from many other conditions, including medication side effects, ingestion of potassium-containing supplements, crush injuries and burns, and redistribution resulting from acidotic states such as diabetic ketoacidosis. Many cases of hyperkalemia are discovered as an incidental laboratory finding. Clinical findings associated with hyperkalemia are summarized in Table 52–1.

Table 52–1 • SYMPTOMS OF RENAL FAILURE AND HYPERKALEMIA		
	Hyperkalemia	**Chronic Renal Failure**
Fatigue	+	++
Weakness	++	+
Paresthesias	+	+
Paralysis	+	
Palpitations	+	
Anorexia, nausea, vomiting	+	+
Edema		+

Potassium Homeostasis

The average diet contains about 100 mEq of potassium per day, and most is excreted in the urine, with a smaller component excreted in the stool. Long-term balance is regulated in large part by the aldosterone system. Renal excretion can be markedly affected by any impairment of kidney function, and by a wide variety of medications. Two common and potent inhibitors of renal potassium excretion are the angiotensin-converting enzyme inhibitors and the potassium-sparing diuretics. The body has a very large intracellular store of potassium, with the serum potassium representing only about 2% of the total body store of approximately 3500 mEq. The serum level is tightly regulated to maintain appropriate gradients across cell membranes. Potassium is actively transported into cells in exchange for sodium by the Na-K-ATPase. Na-K-ATPase is a target of digitalis glycosides, so hyperkalemia is a prominent feature of severe digoxin poisoning. Potassium uptake into cells is stimulated by insulin and beta-adrenergic drugs. In states of increased hydrogen ion concentration (acidosis), potassium may shift out of cells. Also, potassium follows osmotic gradients, so hyperosmolar states such as DKA may cause increased serum potassium.

Classification of Hyperkalemia

From a laboratory perspective, the normal range for serum potassium is 3.5 to 5.0 mEq/L. Levels from 5.1 to 5.5 mEq/L are generally not significant elevations. The range from 5.5 to 6.0 mEq/L is mild hyperkalemia and significant ECG changes would be unusual. Levels of 7.0 mEq/L or greater constitute severe hyperkalemia; prompt aggressive treatment is almost always warranted even if ECG changes are not severe. Although pseudohyperkalemia can result from hemolysis of the blood specimen prior to measurement, most clinical laboratories are attuned to this problem and will note hemolysis when it is detected.

ECG Changes of Hyperkalemia

One of the earliest ECG changes of hyperkalemia is a "peaked" appearance to the T wave. Unfortunately, there is no widely accepted scientific definition of a peaked T wave, though some authors have suggested imagining the T wave as a seat. If it is too pointed to sit upon comfortably, then it is likely peaked. Other described changes of hyperkalemia include widening of the QRS, prolongation of the PR interval,

QT prolongation, ST changes (which may mimic myocardial infarction), wide P waves or the disappearance of P waves. Severe hyperkalemia generally causes a very wide QRS, which may progress to a sine wave pattern and asystole. A variety of blocks and dysrhythmias may also be seen.

Many textbooks describe a classic progression of ECG changes, and attempt to correlate those changes with usual levels of potassium. It is vitally important to understand that this correlation is poor. **Patients may have severe hyperkalemia with minimal ECG changes, and prominent ECG changes with mild hyperkalemia.** It is well described that patients with mild ECG changes may suddenly progress to severe changes, and a stepwise progression cannot be counted upon. Despite these caveats, the ECG remains the best available guide to the initial therapy of hyperkalemia.

Therapy

Calcium given intravenously is first-line lifesaving treatment. Calcium stabilizes cardiac cell membranes and can counteract hyperkalemia within seconds to minutes. Unfortunately the effect is not sustained and fades within 10 to 20 minutes, so additional agents are required. Because of the short-lived effect and potential downsides of hypercalcemia, this author reserves calcium for patients who demonstrate ECG changes suggestive of hyperkalemia. Calcium should be given to all dialysis patients who are in cardiac arrest, as hyperkalemia is very frequently a contributing cause of the arrest. Historically it was believed that calcium was contraindicated in potential digoxin toxicity, because the heart might undergo a tetanic contraction from which the patient could not be resuscitated. This historical concern has not been supported by current science (see Table 52–2).

Calcium is available in two forms, as calcium chloride and calcium gluconate. Calcium chloride contains approximately three times as much elemental calcium per unit volume, and is considerably more caustic to soft tissue. Thus, general practice is to use calcium chloride for patients in cardiac arrest or near-arrest situations, and calcium gluconate for patients with less severe ECG changes.

Table 52–2 • MEDICATIONS USED IN TREATMENT OF HYPERKALEMIA			
Medication	Available Forms	Dose	Duration Of Action
Calcium	Calcium chloride 10% (14 mEq/10 mL)	10-20 mL slow IV	minutes
	Calcium gluconate (4.65 mEq/10 mL)	20-30 mL slow IV	
Sodium bicarbonate	44.6 mEq/50 mL	50-150 mL	minutes-hour
Insulin	Regular	5-10 units IV	1-2 h
Dextrose	50% dextrose in water	25-50 g	1-2 h
Albuterol	5 mg/mL concentrate	10-20 mg nebulized	1-3 h
SPSS (Kayexelate)	15 g/60 mL suspension	15-60 g q6 h	hours

Sodium bicarbonate given intravenously is a traditional second-line agent for hyperkalemia. It is thought to shift K into cells by reversing acidosis. It also raises extracellular sodium levels, which may have beneficial effects on membrane potentials. Some research has called into question the benefit of sodium bicarbonate. In animal studies, no consistent K-lowering effect could be demonstrated. However, this may not be an adequate model of academic renal-failure patients, and even some nephrologists who have questioned the efficacy of bicarbonate continue to recommend it.

Insulin therapy is a mainstay in the acute management of hyperkalemia. Five to ten units of regular insulin given IV can reliably lower serum potassium approximately 0.5 mEq/L for 1 to 2 hours. Of course this therapy can cause hypoglycemia, so the insulin is usually given with 25 g or 50 g of 50% dextrose. Some have advocated giving just the D50, expecting the patient endogenous insulin stores to lower the potassium. However, many patients who experience hyperkalemia will be diabetic and may have impaired or absent insulin release. Furthermore, it has been shown in animal studies that large osmolar loads may transiently increase serum potassium.

Albuterol, administered as an aerosol in doses of 10 to 20 mg, reliably lowers the serum potassium by an average of 0.5 mEq/L for 1 to 3 hours. The effect is additive with the effect of insulin. Albuterol also reduces the incidence and severity of rebound hypoglycemia often seen after glucose and insulin therapy. Albuterol has the advantage of requiring no IV access, and therefore can be started quickly. Side effects of tremor and tachycardia may limit its use in some patients, especially those with severe cardiovascular disease. Note that this is a substantially higher dose than typically used for the initial treatment of asthma.

Sodium polystyrene sulfonate or SPSS (Kayexelate and others) is an ion-exchange resin that is usually administered orally. It can also be given rectally as an enema, but this is generally less effective and carries some risk of colonic injury. SPSS exchanges sodium for potassium across the gut, so patients who are severely volume overloaded may not tolerate this therapy. Onset of action takes several hours. This medication is contraindicated in cases of ileus or suspected bowel obstruction or perforation. It is more effective for maintenance therapy than for acute management.

If the patient is not completely anuric, diuresis is a remarkably effective way to excrete large quantities of potassium. This will not be effective for the end-stage kidney disease patient who has been on dialysis for years, but it is appropriate for many patients with acute hyperkalemia due to dehydration, rhabdomyolysis, or medication effects. Once intravascular volume is restored with crystalloid, loop diuretics such as furosemide can be given to promote potassium excretion.

Dialysis is the ultimate treatment of choice for all kidney disease patients with significant hyperkalemia. However, it is time-consuming and not always immediately available. Reliable vascular access and reasonably stable vital signs are prerequisites for hemodialysis, while the less-common peritoneal dialysis requires a peritoneal catheter.

COMPREHENSION QUESTIONS

52.1 A 55-year-old man presents in cardiac arrest. A dialysis fistula is present in the right arm. In addition to standard ACLS therapies, which of the following is most appropriate for this patient?

A. 25 g of 50% dextrose, IV push

B. Sodium bicarbonate, 50-mL IV push

C. Begin immediate hemodialysis

D. Calcium chloride, 20-mL slow intravenous push

52.2 A 45-year-old man is brought into the emergency center due to significant dehydration and weakness. His potassium level is noted to be 7.2 mEq/L. Which of the following statements is most accurate regarding his potassium level?

A. Hyperkalemia can usually be diagnosed by symptoms alone.

B. An ECG showing peaked T waves means the patient is stable and treatment can safely wait until laboratory results are obtained.

C. Hyperkalemia can mimic a myocardial infarction on the ECG.

D. Hyperkalemia is synonymous with kidney disease.

52.3 Which of the following statements regarding treatment of hyperkalemia in patients with some renal function is incorrect?

A. Administration of normal saline may hasten the excretion of potassium.

B. Administration of furosemide can hasten the excretion of potassium.

C. The combination of saline with a diuretic is often indicated because hyperkalemic patients are frequently dehydrated.

D. Patients with some renal function do not need dialysis even for severe hyperkalemia.

52.4 A patient with severe renal disease is found to have hyperkalemia, with tall, peaked T waves on ECG. Vascular access cannot be readily obtained, but vital signs are stable. Which of the following would be appropriate temporizing measures?

A. Inhaled albuterol 2.5 mg in 3 mL saline

B. Oral sodium bicarbonate with rectal sodium polystyrene sulfonate

C. Inhaled albuterol 20 mg, with oral or rectal sodium polystyrene sulfonate, 30 g

D. Oral dextrose 25 g

ANSWERS

52.1 **D.** Calcium is the only agent with rapid and reliable enough onset to potentially help this patient. Bicarbonate might be appropriate, but its onset is slower than calcium and its effect is more disputed. Dialysis requires a hemodynamically stable patient.

52.2 **C.** The ST-segment and T-wave changes of hyperkalemia may mimic the ECG appearance of myocardial infarction. The nonspecific symptoms typical of hyperkalemia are also often seen in patients with MI, particularly elderly patients. Peaked T waves indicate that the heart is significantly affected by hyperkalemia and the patient should not be considered stable. Many conditions and medications may cause hyperkalemia, not just renal failure.

52.3 **D.** Dialysis is definitive therapy for hyperkalemia. Patients who have some residual kidney function can sometimes be managed without resorting to dialysis, but it should always be available for those who fail to respond quickly.

52.4 **C.** High-dose inhaled albuterol (10-20 mg) can reliably lower serum potassium with reasonable safety. SPSS can remove potassium through the GI tract, but its effect is slow. Oral dextrose and oral bicarbonate have no role. Standard doses of albuterol have too slight an effect on potassium levels.

CLINICAL PEARLS

▶ In a patient with known or suspected renal failure, ECG changes consistent with hyperkalemia should be treated immediately as a life-threatening emergency. Do not await laboratory confirmation.

▶ The ECG findings of hyperkalemia can progress very rapidly, and do not reliably pass through all the stages of the "typical" textbook presentation.

▶ Intravenous calcium is the antidote of choice for life-threatening arrhythmias related to hyperkalemia, but its effect is brief and additional agents must be used.

▶ Symptoms of renal failure and hyperkalemia are usually nonspecific, so risk factors must be used to suspect the diagnosis.

REFERENCES

Evans KJ, Greenberg A. Hyperkalemia: a review. *J Intensive Care Med.* 2005;20(5):272-290.

Kamel KS, Wei C. Controversial issues in the treatment of hyperkalaemia. *Nephrol Dial Transplant.* 2003;18:2215-2218.

Levine M, Nikkanen H, Pallin DJ. The effects of intravenous calcium in patients with digoxin toxicity. *J Emerg Med.* 2011;40(1):41-46.

Mahoney BA, Smith WA, Lo DS, et al. Emergency interventions for hyperkalaemia. *Cochrane Database Syst Rev.* 2005;(2):CD003235.

Sood MM, Sood AR, Richardson R. Emergency management and commonly encountered outpatient scenarios in patients with hyperkalemia. *Mayo Clin Proc.* 2007;82(12):1553-1561.

Watson M, Abbott KC, Yuan CM. Damned if you do, damned if you don't: potassium binding resins in hyperkalemia. *Clin J Am Soc Nephrol.* 2010;5(10):1723-1726.

A 24-year-old woman presents to the emergency department (ED) with complaints of flank pain and fever for the last 1 to 2 days. She describes feeling pain with urination over the previous week. She is currently feeling febrile and nauseated, but has not vomited. The pain in her right flank is a dull, constant, nonradiating ache that she rates as 5/10 for pain. She took 600 mg of ibuprofen last night to help her sleep, but this morning the pain persisted so she came into the ED for evaluation. She reports that she is sexually active and her last menstrual period was 1 week ago. She denies any vaginal discharge or abdominal pain. Her vital signs include a temperature of 38.3°C (101°F), heart rate of 112 beats per minute, respiratory rate of 15 breaths per minute, and blood pressure of 119/68 mm Hg. Her examination is significant for tenderness to palpation on her right costovertebral angle (CVA).

▶ What is the most likely diagnosis?
▶ What is the best treatment?

ANSWERS TO CASE 53:

Acute Pyelonephritis

Summary: This otherwise healthy young woman presents with dysuria, flank pain, fever, and nausea. She is febrile, tachycardic, and has CVA tenderness.

- **Most likely diagnosis:** Urinary tract infection (UTI) complicated by pyelonephritis.

- **Treatment:** Antibiotics, hydration, analgesia, antipyretics, exclusion of other pathology.

ANALYSIS

Objectives

1. Recognize the clinical signs and symptoms of UTIs.

2. Understand the diagnosis and treatment of UTIs.

3. Understand the spectrum of UTIs and their variable treatment.

Considerations

Urinary tract infections are a spectrum of diseases that can affect any part of the urinary system. They are second only to respiratory tract infections as a problem encountered by physicians. Individuals who present to the ED with genitourinary complaints often warrant a rapid but thorough history and physical examination. This patient presentation (ie, dysuria, flank pain, nausea, and fever) is consistent with **acute pyelonephritis; an infection of the renal parenchyma.** Generally, the clinical features of acute pyelonephritis **include fever, chills, dysuria, and flank and costovertebral angle pain.** Patients may feel **nauseated** and **vomit.** The initial workup includes assessing the patient stability and immediately addressing any life threats. As the workup proceeds, the patient should receive an antipyretic (eg, acetaminophen), and intravenous fluids for hydration.

The differential diagnosis for patients with urinary complaints is broad and includes cystitis, pyelonephritis, urethritis, and vaginitis. In addition, patients who exhibit signs of systemic involvement (eg, fever) should be evaluated for other pathologies including ectopic pregnancy, perforated viscous, infected kidney stone, appendicitis, pancreatitis, colitis, and pneumonia. A good history and physical examination will help the physician narrow down these possibilities.

Laboratory studies are helpful in confirming the diagnosis. A urinalysis typically reveals leukocytes, red blood cells, and bacteria. A **urine culture is essential to guide antibiotic therapy.** Blood cultures should be obtained if the patient has a fever. A complete blood count, electrolytes, and renal function studies are also recommended. Patients with suspected pyelonephritis typically do not require imaging studies. However, patients who clinically exhibit pyelonephritis, but whose urinalysis is negative, and patients with a suspected urinary obstruction, should undergo imaging. In the ED, this is usually an ultrasound or contrast-enhanced CT scan. **Supportive care** consists of **IV hydration, analgesia, antipyretics, and anti-emetics.** In uncomplicated acute pyelonephritis, patients can receive a **10 to 14 day course of oral antibiotics** (eg, fluoroquinolone) and be discharged home. In more **severe cases,** patients should be **admitted to the hospital** and receive **intravenous antibiotics.**

APPROACH TO:
Urinary Tract Infections

DEFINITIONS

DYSURIA: Painful urination

CYSTITIS: Inflammation of the urinary bladder that generally results in dysuria, urinary frequency, urgency, and suprapubic pain.

ACUTE PYELONEPHRITIS: Inflammation of the kidney secondary to a UTI of the renal parenchyma and collecting system. It typically presents as the clinical syndrome of fever, chills, and flank pain.

BACTERIURIA: Presence of bacteria in the urine

HEMATURIA: Blood in the urine, may be micro- or macroscopic.

PYURIA: Pus in the urine

UNCOMPLICATED UTI: An infection of a structurally and functionally normal urinary tract that is generally eradicated by a 3- to 5-day course of antibiotics.

COMPLICATED UTI: An infection in patients with underlying immunological, structural, or neurological disease that diminish the efficacy of standard antimicrobial therapy.

URETHRITIS: Inflammation of the urethra

CLINICAL APPROACH

UTIs are a common diagnosis in the ED. They can range from simple cystitis to pyelonephritis resulting in sepsis and shock. Urinary tract infections affect women more commonly than men. However, in children, boys are affected more commonly until 1 year of age. Urinary tract infections in children warrant further sonographic evaluation of the urinary tract to rule out congenital anomalies. The lifetime prevalence of UTIs is estimated to be 14,000 per 100,000 men and 53,000 per 100,000 women.

UTIs can be divided into **lower tract (urethra and bladder) and upper tract (ureters and kidneys)** infections. The symptoms of lower infections are localized and are commonly crampy suprapubic pain, dysuria, foul-smelling or dark-colored urine, hematuria, urinary frequency and urgency. Patients with upper tract infections usually appear more ill and are more likely to have abnormal vital signs and systemic symptoms (eg, fever, chills, nausea and vomiting). It is important to distinguish lower- from upper-tract infections as the treatments differ vastly, as will be discussed later.

Commonly, the infecting organism gains access to the urinary tract by direct entry from the urethra. The human body evolved many defenses against UTIs including frequent urinary flow, urine urea concentration and acidification, and urethral epithelial lining. The normal periurethral flora includes the bacteria *lactobacillus* that provides a symbiotic protective mechanism. The perirectal area and the vagina are both potential sites of bacterial colonization and are in much closer proximity to the urethral meatus in women. The female urethra is also much shorter than in males and brings the urethral meatus in closer proximity to the bladder, thus increasing the risk of infection by external organisms. A UTI in a man is usually the result of benign prostatic hypertrophy, kidney stones that become infected, urethral instrumentation (surgery or catheterization), or immunocompromised states.

Care should be taken to exclude other etiologies in patients who present with urinary complaints. Cervicitis, vulvovaginitis and pelvic inflammatory disease are important conditions to exclude in women and are more likely to present with discharge, lack of bacteria on urinalysis, and lack of urinary frequency and urgency. In considering these diagnoses, the patient should undergo a pelvic examination. Sampling with DNA probes for gonococcus and *Chlamydia* should be obtained, a wet mount slide examination performed, and treatment for these conditions considered. Pregnancy should also be considered and tested for in all women of reproductive age with any urinary symptoms. In men, urethritis and prostatitis should be excluded before the diagnosis of cystitis or pyelonephritis is confirmed.

UTIs are typically caused by a single bacterial species. **Eighty percent of infections are caused by *Escherichia coli*, a gram-negative rod.** *Staphylococcus saprophyticus* is the second most common cause of UTI and is common in young women. Other organisms include *Proteus, Klebsiella, Enterococci,* and *Pseudomonas.* The identification of an exact organism is rarely indicated in the ED. The "gold standard" of quantitative culture takes several days, but will significantly assist in treatment if the patient is being admitted to the hospital or failed outpatient therapy.

Major risk factors for women aged 16 to 35 years include sexual intercourse, pregnancy, bladder catheterization, and diaphragm usage. Later in life, additional risk factors include gynecologic surgery and bladder prolapse. In both sexes, conditions resulting in urinary stasis increase with age, as does the incidence of UTIs. Benign prostatic hypertrophy is a major risk factor in older men.

Laboratory Studies

The **mainstay in the diagnosis of a UTI is urinalysis and culture.** Collection of sterile urine is critical because a contaminated specimen can result in a false-positive urinalysis. Suprapubic aspiration and catheterization provides the best sample; however, both are invasive and uncomfortable to the patient. Clean catch urine samples, obtained by the patient collecting urine in midstream is standard and provides an adequate sample if done properly. In children, "bag" urine collection, by placing a bag over the perineum, should be avoided due to the high rates of contamination. Condom catheterization collection of urine is not acceptable for urinalysis due to the contact of the male glands to the collection vessel. Typically, contaminated urine will exhibit cellular elements (eg, epithelial cells) and should not be used to determine the presence of a UTI.

Table 53–1 • URINALYSIS SENSITIVITY AND SPECIFICITY		
Diagnostic Test	**Sensitivity (%)**	**Specificity (%)**
Leukocyte esterase	83 (67-94)	78 (64-92)
Nitrite	53 (15-82)	98 (90-100)
LE or N	93 (90-100)	72 (58-91)
WBCs	73 (32-100)	81 (45-98)

Abbreviations: LE = leukocyte esterase; N = nitrite; WBCs = white blood cells.

Urinalysis can include urine dipstick testing, urine microscopy, and urine culture with sensitivities. Table 53–1 lists the sensitivity and specificity of different components of the urinalysis.

Urine dipstick It tests urine for infection by measuring two specific entities: leukocyte esterase, a compound released by white blood cell breakdown in the urinary tract, and nitrite, a compound produced by the reduction of dietary nitrates by some gram-negative bacteria (eg, *E coli*).

Urine microscopy It examines the urine for white blood cells, bacteria, and other visible structures. Classically, the criteria for diagnosis of UTI on microscopy include the presence of more than five leukocytes or red blood cells per high-powered field or 2+ bacteria. Microscopic criteria are highly debated and the presence of WBCs, RBCs, and bacteria should be used in conjunction with clinical presentation to confirm the diagnosis of a UTI.

Urine culture Diagnosis and treatment of a UTI based on the UA result is presumptive as the true diagnosis requires a culture with greater than $(10 \times 5)/mL$ colony count. ED urine cultures should be sent on high-risk populations including infants and children. Cultures are also obtained in the elderly, adult men, pregnant women, individuals with comorbid illness, or failing initial antimicrobial therapy. Gram staining of the urine can also be helpful, but is not routinely indicated.

Imaging

The majority of patients with urinary complaints do not require imaging in the ED. However, in certain clinical settings it is indicated. Patients who exhibit clinical signs or symptoms of a urinary infection, but have a negative urinalysis, those with a suspected urogenital obstruction, and complicated UTIs often require imaging studies. In addition, first episodes of UTIs in girls younger than 4 years and men, should undergo an imaging study.

Imaging of the urinary tract consists of ultrasound, computed tomography (CT) scans, intravenous pyelography (IVP), and radionucleotide scans. Ultrasound testing is an acceptable initial study in the ED because it is quick, noninvasive, and can detect many abnormalities including perinephric abscess, hydroureter, urinary tract stone, pyelonephritis, and congenital anomalies. CT scans are more sensitive at detecting these abnormalities, but expose the patient to higher levels of radiation and often require the administration of IV contrast. The use of IVP and radionucleotide scans are generally not performed during ED evaluation and reserved for inpatient or outpatient workups.

Treatment

The correct choice of antibiotic can be a difficult one for the emergency physician. There are many factors that affect this decision including patient drug allergies, bacterial susceptibility, community versus hospital flora, local antibiotic resistance rates, the presence of medical comorbidities, as well as the patient ability to pay for the prescription. Table 53–2 lists the most commonly used antibiotics for the treatment of UTIs.

Uncomplicated cystitis patients are treated as outpatients. Antibiotic choices must be effective against E coli and include trimethoprim-sulfamethoxazole (TMP-SMX), amoxicillin/clavulanate, nitrofurantoin, ciprofloxacin, and levofloxacin. Typically, patients are treated for 3 to 5 days. Longer therapy generally offers no benefit. However, in patients with suspected subclinical upper-tract infection, communities with high resistance rates, extremes of age, and comorbidities, a longer course (ie, 7-10 days) is recommended. For symptomatic relief, physicians often prescribe phenazopyridine, a drug that concentrates in the urine and often relieves the pain and irritation of urination. The drug causes a distinct color change in the urine; typically to a dark orange to reddish color. Phenazopyridine is contraindicated in patients with glucose-6-phosphate dehydrogenase deficiency because it can lead to drug-induced hemolysis of red blood cells.

Uncomplicated pyelonephritis can be treated as an outpatient, provided the patient can tolerate oral medications, has mild symptoms, gets good follow-up, and is not pregnant. TMP-SMX, amoxicillin/clavulanate, or a fluoroquinolone antibiotic should be prescribed for 10 to 14 days. All pregnant patients with pyelonephritis require admission (see Table 53–3).

Complicated pyelonephritis requires admission and IV antibiotics. The antibiotic choices are TMP-SMX, ceftriaxone, gentamycin (with or without ampicillin), and fluoroquinolones. In more severe cases where urovsepsis or a resistant organism is suspected, cefepime, ampicillin plus tobramycin, piperacillintazobactam may be indicated.

Table 53–2 • UTI TYPES AND TREATMENT CHOICES		
Infection Type	**Dosing Regimen**	**Considerations**
Lower, uncomplicated	TMP-SMX DS 1 tab bid for 3-5 d Ciprofloxacin 250 mg bid for 3-5 d Nitrofurantoin sustained-release 100 mg bid for 3-5 days Amoxicillin/clavulanate 875/125 mg bid for 3-5 d	No culture indicated[a] Tailor to community susceptibilities
Upper uncomplicated or complicated lower	Ciprofloxacin 500 mg bid for 7-14 d Nitrofurantoin sustained-release 100 mg bid for 7-14 d Amoxicillin/clavulanate 875/125 mg bid for 7-14 d	Cultures recommended Admit if severe

[a]Due to increasing resistance patterns, urine culture should be considered.

Table 53–3 • ADMISSION CRITERIA FOR PYELONEPHRITIS
Sepsis/shock (consider intensive care setting)
Inability to tolerate oral antibiotics
Obstruction of the UG Tract
Pregnant
Extremes of age
Failed outpatient management
Immunocompromised host
Inadequate follow-up/poor social setting

All children and men who are discharged with the diagnosis of UTI require urological follow-up to assess for underlying anatomical abnormalities. Adults with complicated UTIs also need follow-up and evaluation of the genitourinary system.

Pregnant patients require special attention. Simple, asymptomatic bacteriuria **necessitates treatment** due to the **increased risk of preterm labor, perinatal mortality, and maternal pyelonephritis.** It is important that the bacteriuria is eliminated despite the patient being clinically asymptomatic. First-line agents include penicillins (eg, amoxicillin, ampicillin), and cephalosporins. Fluoroquinolones and tetracyclines are contraindicated as they are known teratogens. Admission should be considered in patients in their third trimester, suspected pyelonephritis, or those who cannot tolerate fluids by mouth.

Some patients require chronic placement of **indwelling catheters,** which serve as a nidus for infection. Treatment of asymptomatic bacteriuria in these patients is not indicated because frequent antibiotic administration results in increased microorganism resistance. Generally, removal of the catheter results in elimination of bacteria. Symptomatic patients, who cannot be without the catheter, should be treated with antibiotics, have the catheter replaced, and be considered for admission to the hospital due to the high risk for systemic infection.

COMPREHENSION QUESTIONS

53.1 A 64-year-old woman is brought to the ED by her family for mental status changes. She has multiple sclerosis and self-catheterizes for urine. The family reports that over the past several days she has not been feeling well. They state that the patient vomited that day and was behaving bizarrely. Her vital signs are blood pressure of 83/38 mm Hg, heart rate of 135 beats per minute, respirations of 26 breaths per minute, and rectal temperature 38.8°C (101.9°F). After a history and physical examination, which of the following is the most appropriate next step in management?

A. Obtain a urinalysis and culture.

B. Start broad-spectrum antibiotics.

C. Perform a lumbar puncture.

D. Establish IV access and place the patient on a cardiac monitor.

E. Discharge the patient after close follow-up is arranged.

53.2 A 34-year-old woman complains of mild crampy suprapubic abdominal pain, dysuria, and urinary frequency for the last 3 days. She has no fever. Her blood pressure is 125/70 mm Hg, heart rate is 88 beats per minute, respiratory rate is 16 breaths per minute, and temperature is 36.8°C (98.3°F). She has no significant past medical history and is able to drink oral fluids with difficulty. She has a clean-catch urinalysis that reveals 2+ leukocyte esterase, 1+ nitrite, 1+ blood, and 2+ bacteria. Her β-hCG is negative. Which of the following organisms is most likely responsible for her presentation?

A. *Klebsiella* spp

B. *Escherichia coli*

C. *Pseudomonas aeruginosa*

D. *Proteus mirabilis*

E. *Enterobacter* spp

53.3 A 24-year-old woman presents to the ED for painful urination over the last 2 days that is associated with urinary urgency. She states that she is pregnant and the fetus is at 12-week gestational age as measured by ultrasound. On examination, she is well appearing, and sitting comfortably in bed. Her blood pressure is 115/70 mm Hg, heart rate is 81 beats per minute, respiratory rate is 16 breaths per minute, and temperature is 37.2°C (98.9°F). A urinalysis reveals 5 WBC/mm^3, 1+ leukocyte esterase, and 1+ bacteria. The urine is negative for nitrite and blood. As you return to the patient bed to tell her the results, she states that her pain has resolved, she is urinating without difficulty, and wants to go home. Which of the following is the most appropriate course of management?

A. Admit the patient for intravenous antibiotics.

B. Discharge the patient with a prescription for antibiotics and tell her to fill the prescription only if the culture results are positive.

C. Ask the patient to undergo another examination to evaluate for gonorrhea and *Chlamydia*.

D. Administer a dose of ciprofloxacin in the ED and have the patient call the hospital to find out her culture results.

E. Prescribe the patient nitrofurantoin for 5 to 7 days and have her follow-up with her obstetrician.

53.4 A 65-year-old man with hypertension and benign prostatic hyperplasia (BPH) presents to the ED with urinary retention and a UTI on a catheterized urine analysis. He was evaluated by the urologist and is being discharged home with an in-dwelling Foley catheter and follow-up in the urology clinic in 1 week. Which of the following is the most appropriate antibiotic for this patient?

A. TMP-SMX bid for 3 days

B. Nitrofurantoin 100 mg for 14 days

C. Amoxicillin 100 mg tid for 14 days

D. Ciprofloxacin 500 mg bid for 14 days

E. Levofloxacin 250 mg qd for 3 days

53.5 Which of the following patients with pyelonephritis can be safely discharged home with close follow-up?

A. A 23-year-old woman in her second trimester of pregnancy.

B. A 13-year-old woman who cannot tolerate her diet despite anti-emetics.

C. An 88-year-old man with urinary retention and dehydration.

D. A 67-year-old woman with 3+ bacteria, a sulfa allergy, and a history of lupus.

E. A 44-year-old woman with a kidney stone and hydroureter on CT scan.

ANSWERS

53.1 **D.** This woman may indeed have a urinary tract infection; however, her vital signs are unstable. The mainstay of treatment in emergency medicine is to first address the patient airway, breathing, and circulation (ABCs). This patient is hypotensive (eg, BP 83/38 mm Hg). The first step in her management is placing an IV line and administering fluids. She should also be placed on a cardiac monitor to monitor her blood pressure, heart rate, and rhythm. Once her ABCs are addressed, laboratory studies should be obtained, including a urinalysis and culture. She should also receive broad-spectrum antibiotics and an antipyretic. This patient may need a lumbar puncture, but not until her ABCs are addressed. This patient requires admission to the hospital.

53.2 **B.** *E coli* is the infecting organism in more than 80% of all UTIs. All of the other choices cause urinary tract infections, but are less common. *S saprophyticus* is a common organism in young, sexually active women. In hospitalized or nursing home patients, *Pseudomonas* spp and *Staphylococcus* spp are frequent pathogens. Lactobacilli are normal urethral flora and are not considered a causative organism. Complicated UTIs are more likely to be caused by other organisms.

53.3 **E.** The patient is pregnant and has evidence of a urinary tract infection on the urinalysis. Pregnant patients are at high risk for preterm labor and perinatal mortality if a urinary infection goes untreated. Therefore, this patient should receive a 5 to 7 days course of nitrofurantoin or a penicillin-based antibiotic and follow-up with her obstetrician. The patient does not need to be admitted to the hospital for intravenous antibiotics. This would likely be the case if she were diagnosed with pyelonephritis. The patient should not wait for culture results and delay receiving her antibiotics. It is important to eradicate the bacteriuria as quickly as possible. This patient does not report the symptoms of gonorrhea or *Chlamydia* (eg, vaginal discharge) at this time, and does not require further evaluation for these conditions. Fluoroquinolones (eg, ciprofloxacin) are contraindicated in pregnant patients due to the risk of fetal abnormalities (eg, tendon maldevelopment).

53.4 **D.** Men with urinary tract infections automatically fit into the "complicated" variety of UTIs. Therefore, the most appropriate therapy is ciprofloxacin for 14 days. With the exception of amoxicillin as monotherapy, all of the above choices are appropriate for treatment of certain types of UTIs. Complicated UTIs mandate 14 days of therapy with an appropriate antibiotic. The emergency physician should also consider sending urine cultures on this patient and provide good follow-up. Patients with benign prostatic hypertrophy or other lower urinary tract obstructions may be discharged with a Foley catheter if they have good follow-up, understand how to manage their catheter, and have to significant medical comorbidities.

53.5 **D.** Despite a chronic medical condition, this patient may be safely discharged home. Because this patient has a sulfa allergy, TMP-SMX should not be administered. Other treatment options include quinolones, amoxicillin/ clavulanate, and nitrofurantoin. All of the other patients should be admitted for treatment. All pregnant patients with pyelonephritis require admission. The 13-year-old and 88-year-old are not tolerating their diet and require intravenous hydration. The 44-year-old has a urinary obstruction with a UTI, which makes it a complicated UTI. These patients are at high risk for developing sepsis. For most admitted patients, urine cultures should be sent to guide antibiotic therapy.

CLINICAL PEARLS

▶ All urinary tract infections in men are considered complicated.

▶ The definitive diagnosis of a UTI is made on urine culture from a noncontaminated urine sample.

▶ Care should be taken to exclude other etiologies, such as cervicitis, vulvovaginitis, and pelvic inflammatory disease, in female patients who present with urinary complaints.

▶ All pregnant patients with bacteriuria require antibiotic treatment to prevent complications.

▶ Patients with a UTI and an obstructed kidney stone are at high risk for morbidity and require urgent urologic consultation.

▶ Antibiotic therapy should be tailored to the type of UTI, the community resistance rates, and the patient ability to tolerate the medications.

REFERENCES

Ban KM, Easter JS. Selected urologic problems. In: Marx JA, Hockberger RS, Walls RM, eds. *Rosen's Emergency Medicine: Concepts and Clinical Practice*. 6th ed. Philadelphia, PA: Mosby Elsevier; 2009.

Dielubanza EJ, Schaeffer AJ. Urinary tract infections in women. *Med Clin N Am*. 2011;95:27-41.

Howes DS, Bogner MP. Urinary tract infections and hematuria. Tintinalli JE, Stapczynski JS, Cline DM, Ma OJ, Cydulka RK, Meckler GD, eds. *Tintinalli's Emergency Medicine: A Comprehensive Study Guide.* 7th ed. New York, NY: McGraw-Hill; 2011.

Lane DR, Takhar SS. Diagnosis and management of urinary tract infection and pyelonephritis. *Emerg Med Clin N Am.* 2011;29:539-552.

Nicolle LE. Uncomplicated urinary tract infection in adults including uncomplicated pyelonephritis. *Urol Clin N Am.* 2008;35:1-12.

Schrock JW, Reznikova S, Weller S. The effect of an observation unit on the rate of ED admission and discharge for pyelonephritis. *Am J Emerg Med.* 2010;26:682-688.

An 87-year-old man with a past history of stroke is brought in by ambulance from a skilled nursing facility after being found unresponsive in bed with rapid, shallow breathing. In the past 3 to 4 days he has had a wet sounding cough. Paramedics report his room air saturation in the field was 67%. In the emergency department he is obtunded with sonorous respirations, labored breathing and copious thick yellow secretions. His vital signs are the following: temperature 38.7°C, BP 90/58 mm Hg, P 118 bpm, RR 29 breaths per minute and oxygen saturation 84% on a non-rebreather face mask.

▶ What is the immediate first step in the management of this patient?
▶ What special factors need to be considered?

ANSWERS TO CASE 54:
Airway Management/Respiratory Failure

Summary: This patient is an elderly male with a depressed level of consciousness, hypoxia, respiratory distress and pooling secretions. He is not oxygenating well or protecting his airway from aspiration.

- **First step:** This patient needs immediate airway management and endotracheal intubation.

- **Additional factors:** As a critically ill patient from a nursing facility, it is important to attempt to verify his code status before intubating. It is also important to consider the underlying causes for his altered mental status and respiratory distress.

ANALYSIS

Objectives

1. Learn how to evaluate the airway and indications for intervention.

2. Become more familiar with emergency airway procedures.

3. Understanding of the rationale for and the steps involved with rapid sequence intubation.

4. Recognize and anticipate the potentially difficult airway and special circumstances.

Considerations

In the case above, the patient has several concerning findings indicating he will need active airway management. He is hypoxic, tachypneic, and with his altered mental status he may not able to protect his airway from secretions or emesis. Because of his depressed level of consciousness and inability to protect his airway he is not an appropriate candidate for noninvasive positive pressure ventilation (such as BiPAP).

He likely has a pneumonia and/or aspiration event, but it is also important to consider that he may have had a separate preceding event such as a cerebral vascular accident or medication overdose which created the altered mental status before aspirating. His other vital signs indicate that he is probably septic and will need to be resuscitated after his airway is addressed.

> ## APPROACH TO:
> ## Airway Management

CLINICAL APPROACH

Evaluation

Assessing a patient airway and breathing are critical first steps in evaluating any patient in the emergency department. Begin by grossly observing the appearance of the patient paying particular attention to key markers of oxygenation and ventilation: skin color looking for the presence of cyanosis, evidence of severe bronchospasm such as intercostal retractions, difficulty speaking, low or falling oxygen saturation, increased or decreased respiratory rate. Evaluation of the airway includes not just the actual structures of the head and neck but also the patient mental status and amount of secretions or blood present in the airway.

Indications for active airway intervention:

Respiratory Failure: persistent and or worsening hypoxia, severe hypercarbia/respiratory acidosis.

Airway Protection: absent gag, depressed level of consciousness, excess secretions.

Impending or existing airway obstruction: mass, infection, angioedema, foreign matter or excess secretions, etc.

Facilitation of further studies or to protect the airway during transport when deterioration may be anticipated.

Airway Protection There are several signs of an inadequately protected airway which indicate need for intubation: pooling secretions (eg, gurgling sounds with respiration), an absent or weak cough reflex and depressed mental status often correlating with GCS of 8 or less. In general, a patient whose level of consciousness is depressed enough to tolerate insertion of an oropharyngeal airway is not protecting his or her airway and requires airway protection.

Reversible and or transient causes of a decreased level of consciousness must be considered prior to active airway intervention. Treating hypoglycemia or suspected opiate overdose before intubating can save the patient a major intervention. Additionally, providers should consider that the patient may be postictal because they may improve rapidly to a point where they can protect their airway.

Respiratory Failure Respiratory failure refers to either failure to oxygenate or failure to ventilate. Failure to oxygenate is reflected by hypoxia despite maximum supplemental oxygen administration. Failure to ventilate, indicated by elevated levels of carbon dioxide (measured on blood gas or capnography) can be equally life-threatening and requires intervention. Hypercapnea may manifest as somnolence, agitation or otherwise altered mental status.

In select patients who are awake and alert, noninvasive positive pressure ventilation (BiPAP) may be an option to delay or prevent intubation in the setting of hypoxic or hypercapneic respiratory failure.

Anticipated Clinical Deterioration There are several clinical scenarios in which awake patients without current respiratory failure may still require intubation. The emergency physician needs to anticipate the potential clinical course of a patient and may wish to "intubate early" to avoid less controlled intubation conditions later. Situations in which this may be considered include worsening airway obstruction such as in patients with anaphylaxis, angioedema, severe burns or smoke inhalation, penetrating neck trauma with an expanding neck hematoma, epiglottitis or deep space neck infections. Clinical scenarios that require the transfer of critically ill patients to a higher level of care requires a great deal of caution. If deterioration of the mental or respiratory status is anticipated it may be prudent to proceed with intubation prior to transfer.

Facilitation of Medical Evaluation Occasionally patients require intubation to safely complete necessary studies or procedures. One such scenario is that of a trauma patient who may be agitated or combative. These patients often require emergent CT imaging as part of their initial workup. If they require sedation to facilitate adequate imaging or procedures, intubation may be required for airway protection. Often these patients can be promptly extubated after completion if they are without respiratory issues.

Interventions Airway management is much more than just intubation. It can be as simple as providing supplemental oxygen or repositioning the patient. Knowledge of minimally invasive maneuvers and devices is critical and can be lifesaving.

Supplemental Oxygen Supplemental oxygen can be delivered (in order of increasing delivery) via nasal cannula, face mask, non-rebreather mask and high-flow nasal cannula. These are appropriate first steps for patients that are hypoxic but are otherwise protecting their airway. Supplemental oxygen is appropriate to treat hypoxemia and is indicated as part of one preparation for intubation should it become necessary.

Airway Positioning Positioning of patient with a depressed level of consciousness or with significant somnolence can be very important. The most common cause of airway obstruction in the semiconscious or unconscious patient is loss of muscle tone, causing the tongue and soft tissue to occlude the airway. The simplest corrective maneuver is the chin lift (see Sec I, Emergency Assessment and Management), opening the airway through neck hyperextension. This maneuver is contraindicated in patients with a suspected cervical spine injury. A jaw thrust (see Figure I–2) can also be performed by placing two or three fingers behind the angle of the mandible and lifting anteriorly. Since neck manipulation is not required, this maneuver can be safely performed in the context of cervical spine injury.

Other obstructive processes such as mediastinal masses, very large tonsils or morbid obesity may also require an upright position. A patient in respiratory failure from pulmonary edema will likely not tolerate laying flat and it is important to allow them to be upright.

Airway Adjuncts In addition to airway repositioning, placement of an oropharyngeal (OPA) and or nasopharyngeal airway (NPA) is required and may be highly effective. An OPA is designed to keep the tongue from obstructing the posterior pharynx. This device is only used in unconscious patients who do not have a cough or a gag reflex. Using an appropriately sized OPA is important: a device which is too small will be ineffective while an overly large OPA can worsen obstruction. It is particularly important to have an OPA in place when giving positive pressure ventilations (PPV) through a bag valve mask. Otherwise, external pressure on the patient chin may force the tongue into an obstructive position.

In the semiconscious patient with an intact gag reflex, insertion of an OPA can induce vomiting and possible aspiration. An NPA is the more appropriate adjunct for the semiconscious patient as it rarely induces gagging. The NPA functions by helping bypass tongue obstruction. It is contraindicated in patients with severe facial trauma due to the risk of brain intrusion.

Suctioning along the sides of the mouth is also important in patients with pooling secretions. The suction device should not be inserted deep into the oropharynx where it is likely to induce gagging and emesis.

Noninvasive Positive Pressure Ventilation Noninvasive positive pressure ventilation (NIPPV) is often used in the emergency department. NIPPV is the use of mechanical ventilatory support without an invasive airway in place such as an endotracheal tube. A tightly secured mask is the most common method used to deliver NIPPV. There are several varieties of masks and ventilatory modes used to deliver NIPPV. The two most commonly seen in the emergency department are continuous positive airway pressure (CPAP) and bi-level positive airway pressure (BiPAP). In the appropriately selected patient its use may prevent the need for intubation. Current evidence suggests the patients most likely to respond to NIPPV have conditions such as chronic obstructive pulmonary disease and cardiogenic pulmonary edema. Other clinical indications include severe respiratory acidosis, hypoxia, dyspnea, tachypnea and increased work of breathing.

Absolute contraindications to NIPPV include coma, cardiac arrest, respiratory arrest and any condition warranting immediate intubation. Relative contraindications include evidence of airway obstruction, cardiac instability (shock requiring pressors, ventricular dysrhythmias), GI bleeding, inability to protect airway, and status epilepticus.

Intubation As discussed above, the indications for endotracheal intubation may be straight forward and objective or subtle and vague. The need is obvious when there is clear failure to oxygenate or ventilate using less invasive means. Decision making is far more difficult when the clinical indications are less extreme.

Crash intubations are indicated in pulseless, and apneic patients, often without the use of preoxygenation or medications. Urgent intubations refer to patients needing intubation within minutes rather than seconds and do allow for the use of preoxygenation and induction medication. Stable patients who are likely to require active airway protection allow for a trial of alternative treatments and careful preparation.

RAPID SEQUENCE INTUBATION

What Is It?

Rapid sequence intubation (RSI) is a method that attempts to simultaneously sedate and paralyze a patient while creating optimum intubating conditions. The major goal is to leave the airway unprotected for the shortest time possible. The procedure assumes that the patient may have a full stomach and is at great risk of vomiting and aspiration. Rapid sequence intubation is one of the most important skills for the emergency physician and requires careful but quick preparation.

What Are the Steps of Rapid Sequence Intubation?

Once it has been determined a patient needs endotracheal intubation, if time allows, there are several key steps to follow. These are widely known as the "seven Ps" and are presented in temporal sequence below.

Step 1: Preparation:

Assess the Patient Is the patient a good candidate for RSI? Remember, the patient will be paralyzed and the physician is taking complete control over the airway. The question should always be asked how likely is the intubation to be successful? Can the patient be ventilated with a bag-valve-mask (BVM) if RSI should fail? Does the patient have dentures that need to be removed? Does the patient have signs of upper airway obstruction, such as drooling or stridor, due to edema, trauma, or mass? Is there any restriction of neck mobility? Heavy facial hair, a short thick neck, a recessed chin, or a large tongue should all be considered as potential impediments to bag-valve-mask ventilation or oral tracheal intubation. Examine the neck for surgical scars. A scar from a prior cricothyroidotomy is a concerning sign. Severe kyphosis or cervical spine immobilization will make intubation more difficult.

There are a few rules of airway evaluation that may be helpful in alert and cooperative patients. The first is the 3-3-2 rule. The patient should be able to insert at least 3 fingers into his/her mouth in the vertical orientation, between the upper and lower front teeth; the hyomental distance (from the hyoid cartilage to the chin) should be at least 3 fingers breadth; and there should be at least 2 fingers breadth between the floor of the mouth and the thyroid cartilage. The Mallampati score is another means of predicting intubation difficulty. The patient is asked to stick out his/her tongue while opening the mouth wide as possible. The amount of posterior pharynx visible is divided into four classes. The best view is referred to as "class one" including full visibility of the tonsils, uvula, and soft palate. The more limited class-three and class-four views may be associated with difficult intubations.

Concerns that the patient is not a good candidate for RSI should prompt immediate consultation with an anesthesiologist. A surgeon should also be emergently consulted if a cricothyroidotomy is likely.

Prepare Materials It is essential that all equipment is available and working before embarking on this procedure. Necessary pre-intubation equipment includes oral and nasal pharyngeal airways, suction, oxygen, and a bag valve mask. Basic intubation equipment includes a laryngoscope handle and several blades. The most commonly

Table 54–1 • MATERIALS FOR ENDOTRACHEAL INTUBATION
Suction Oxygen Airway adjuncts Pharmacology Monitoring Equipment IV

used laryngoscope blades are the curved Macintosh blade and the straight Miller blade. They should be tested for adequate light function before use.

Endotracheal tubes (ETT) of various sizes and stylets must also be ready for use. The ETT has a distal balloon that should be inflated and deflated before use to test for leaks. The ETT should be preloaded with an internal stylet and is typically bent in the shape of a hockey stick to allow it to pass more anteriorly. Several other ETTs, at least a 1/2 size larger and smaller, should also be available. The formula used to predict endotracheal tube size for children ages two and older: (age in years + 16)/4.

Airway "rescue" devices should be available and familiar to the provider to be used in difficult intubation scenarios. These devices include bougies, a video laryngoscope and several sizes of laryngeal mask airways (LMA). Cricothyroidotomy materials should always be nearby.

The medications selected for induction and paralysis should be drawn up and ready. The patient should be attached to a cardiac monitor with frequently cycling blood pressure, a pulse oximeter, and an end-tidal CO_2 monitor. Importantly, the patient must have a freely flowing IV. These steps are summarized by the mnemonic SOAP ME IV (Table 54–1).

Step 2: Preoxygenation Preoxygenation is a key part of RSI and should be started when one is even considering the need for active airway management. The purpose of preoxygenation is to allow for a greater reservoir of oxygen in the lungs via nitrogen washout. Three to five minutes of high-flow O_2 is adequate and allows for a substantial apneic period without oxygen desaturation in otherwise healthy patients (see Figure 54–1). Pre-oxygenating with high-flow oxygen requires that the patient is breathing. If the patient is apneic, studies have shown that 8 full-volume BVM ventilations over 1 minute are equivalent. Yet bag-valve-mask ventilation of the spontaneously breathing patient is contraindicated because it unnecessarily increases the risk of gastric distension and aspiration.

Step 3: Pretreatment Pretreatment is a controversial topic that deserves brief mention. Manipulation of the airway causes a transient increase in intracranial pressure (ICP). In patients who may already have increased ICP (eg, in intracerebral hemorrhage), any further increase could be potentially devastating. Several medications may be used in sequence in attempt to diminish the effect of airway manipulation on intracranial pressure. Starting a few minutes before induction, fentanyl (3-5 μg/kg) followed by lidocaine (1.5 mg/kg), and a defasciculating dose of the paralytic agent (1/10th the treatment dose) may be given. However, there are

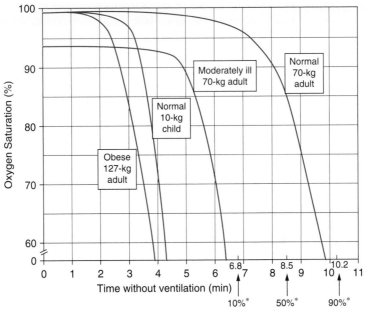

Figure 54–1. Hemoglobin Desaturation Curve.

conflicting data regarding the potential benefit with the use of these medications. In addition, pretreatment may lead to other complications and a delay in intubation.

Step 4: Induction and Paralysis Induction involves administering a medication that will quickly and reliably sedate the patient prior to paralysis. Ideally, the sedative agent will have little effect on heart rate or blood pressure or cause other adverse side effects.

The induction agent most commonly used in emergency medicine is etomidate (0.3 mg/kg) as it meets these criteria well. It is rapidly sedating and hemodynamically neutral. It is also thought to be cerebroprotective. A potential downside of etomidate is that it causes transient adrenal suppression. Although the clinical significance of this effect is uncertain, some physicians avoid etomidate when intubating septic patients.

Ketamine is another drug that may be used for induction, ideally suited for patients in status asthmaticus, anaphylactic shock, and sepsis. Ketamine is a derivative of PCP and acts as a dissociative agent. It has rapid onset of action (1.5 mg/kg IV) and causes increases in blood pressure and heart rate through catecholamine release. It is unique in that it leaves airway reflexes protected and does not induce apnea. Additionally, it has bronchodilatory and analgesic properties. It should be used with caution in patients with known coronary artery disease.

Propofol and thiopental are other fast-acting sedative agents of short duration, but less commonly used in RSI due to associated hypotension.

Table 54–2 • INDUCTION AGENTS					
Drug	**IV Dose**	**Class**	**BP**	**HR**	**Positive/Adverse Effects**
Etomidate	0.3 mg/kg	Imidazole derivative	$\varnothing$	$\varnothing$	**Rapid onset** **Hemodynamically neutral** **cerebroprotection** Adrenal suppression
Ketamine	1.5 mg/kg	Phencyclidine derivative	$\uparrow$	$\uparrow$	**Bronchodilator**/Increases ICP Avoid in pts with CAD
Propofol	1.5-2 mg/kg	Alkylphenol derivative	$\downarrow\downarrow$	$\varnothing$ or $\uparrow$	**Rapid onset** Hypotension Egg allergy
Thiopental	3-5 mg/kg	Barbiturate	$\downarrow$	$\varnothing$ or $\uparrow$	**Rapid onset, short acting** Hypotension Histamine release

Paralysis Paralytic drugs come in two basic types—depolarizing and nondepolarizing, describing their action at the neuromuscular junction. The only depolarizing agent in common clinical use is succinylcholine which has the most rapid onset and shortest duration of all paralytics. It is an analogue of acetylcholine and acts by transiently binding to ACh receptors, keeping ion channels open, leading to paralysis. Succinylcholine action at the motor endplate causes potassium efflux, and therefore should be avoided in patients with hyperkalemia. Succinylcholine and its effects on extracellular potassium levels may be pronounced and should be avoided in patients with recent or ongoing neuromuscular disorders, subacute burns, severe debilitation, crush injuries, or rhabdomyolysis. Acute head injury, acute burns, and acute strokes are not contraindications to the use of succinylcholine.

Nondepolarizing agents act by competitive inhibition of the postsynaptic acetylcholine receptor, thereby preventing depolarization and causing paralysis. The agents most commonly used are rocuronium and vecuronium. Rocuronium is preferred for RSI among the nondepolarizing agents as it has the most rapid onset and shortest duration.

Table 54–3 • PARALYTIC AGENTS					
Drug	**Dose**	**Class**	**Onset**	**Duration**	**Contraindications**
Succinylcholine	1.5 mg/kg	Depolarizing	45-60 sec	6-10 min	Hyperkalemia, neuromuscular disorders, rhabdomyolysis
Rocuronium	1 mg/kg	Nondepolarizing	45-60 sec	30 min	Anticipated difficult airway
Vecuronium	0.01 mg/kg priming dose then 0.15 mg/kg	Nondepolarizing	2-3 min	20-40 min	Anticipated difficult airway

Step 5: Positioning and Protection Patient positioning for RSI is an extremely important but often overlooked step in the emergency department. The proper head position in adults is the "sniffing" position, with the base of the neck flexed forward and the head hyperextended. When done properly, the patient ear should be at the level of the sternum. This position greatly enhances the view of the vocal cords from the mouth. Prior to administration of medications, the patient head should be positioned at the very end of the bed, and the bed height should be adequate for the operator. Once induction agents are given, firm downward pressure to the cricoid cartilage (known as the Sellick maneuver) is often done to prevent gastric distention and possible aspiration. However, recent studies have suggested that this may not be necessary and can worsen the view of the operator.

Step 6: Placement with Proof Once the patient is paralyzed and positioned, the ETT should be placed without delay. The first step is to open the patient mouth and insert the laryngoscope blade along the right side deep into the posterior oropharynx, then move to the center sweeping the tongue out of the way while lifting up and out. This usually provides a view of the vocal cords. The ETT is advanced until the balloon is just beyond the vocal cords, then the operator must **stop,** inflate the balloon, and remove the stylet.

The next step is to confirm that the endotracheal tube is in the right place. The absolute best way to do this is to watch it pass through the cords. Other confirmatory measures (end-tidal CO_2 change, fogging of the tube, and listening for breath sounds) should always be performed. However, these are nonspecific signs and can all be misleading in various circumstances.

Step 7: Postintubation Management Once placed and confirmed, the endotracheal tube must be secured. A chest x-ray is obtained to assess appropriate depth of the ETT. The chest x-ray is not useful for differentiating tracheal from esophageal intubation. Next, orders should be given for a longer acting sedative agent as well as analgesia. Finally, ventilator settings should be established which include the mode, respiratory rate, Fio_2, tidal volume, and peak-end expiratory pressure. The 7 Ps for RSI are summarized in Table 54–4.

Table 54–4 • THE 7 Ps FOR RSI		
Step	**Name**	**Time to Intubation**
1	Preparation	10 min
2	Preoxygenation	3-5 min
3	Pretreatment	3 min
4	Paralysis with induction	1 min
5	Positioning and protection	45 sec
6	Placement with proof	Time 0
7	Postintubation management	+ 1 min

COMPREHENSION QUESTIONS

54.1 The best way to confirm endotracheal tube placement is
   A. Chest x-ray
   B. End tidal CO_2
   C. Breath sounds heard in both lung fields
   D. Watching the ETT pass through the vocal cords

54.2 Which of the following is a contraindication to succinylcholine?
   A. Acute burns
   B. Acute renal failure
   C. History of coronary artery disease
   D. Sepsis

54.3 A 20-year-old man presents to the emergency department after being stung by
   a bee. His skin is red and covered with welts. He has obvious swelling of his lips
   and tongue, but no wheezes. After treatment with appropriate medications, he
   complains of throat swelling and his voice is hoarse. He has stridorous inspira-
   tions but a normal respiratory rate and oxygen saturation. What is the most
   appropriate management of this patient airway?
   A. Continued observation as long as oxygen saturation remains normal
   B. Call anesthesia and prepare for RSI.
   C. Begin high-dose nebulized albuterol and continue to observe.
   D. Prepare for cricothyroidotomy.

54.4 You are the first person on scene to a code blue in your hospital. You arrive
   to find an elderly woman who is unconscious, has a weak pulse and does not
   appear to be breathing. Your first steps are
   A. Wait for the code cart to arrive and then intubate the patient.
   B. Begin chest compressions and mouth-to-mouth resuscitation.
   C. Attempt to remove any foreign body from the mouth and reposition the
       airway with chin lift or jaw thrust.
   D. Begin bagging the patient immediately.

ANSWERS

54.1 **D.** Watching the ETT pass through the vocal cords is the best way to assure
   proper placement. CXR has no role in differentiating between endotracheal
   and esophageal intubation. The other choices are helpful but not failsafe.

54.2 **B.** Succinylcholine transiently increases serum potassium levels. It is presumptively contraindicated in renal failure patients who often have elevated potassium levels. Acute burns are not a contraindication. Beginning 2 to 3 days after a burn, acetylcholine receptor upregulation can lead to hyperkalemia. Neither coronary artery disease nor sepsis is a contraindication to the use of succinylcholine.

54.3 **B.** This patient displays signs of impending airway obstruction. His worsening airway edema, despite appropriate medical therapy, dictates intubation before complete airway occlusion and a cricothyroidotomy is required. There is no wheezing to suggest bronchoconstriction that could be treated with a bronchodilator such as albuterol. Stridor is a worrisome sign of upper airway obstruction. Normal respiratory rate and oxygen saturation should not delay intubation as falling oxygen saturation is a late sign of respiratory failure. Cricothyroidotomy is only indicated after all other measures have failed.

54.4 **C.** The most common cause of airway obstruction is the tongue and/or soft tissues of the upper airway. No other adjuncts may be necessary for initial management except relieving the obstruction with airway repositioning. This should certainly be the first step, and there is no need to wait for the code cart before performing this maneuver. There is no indication for chest compressions in a patient with palpable pulses. The patient will require BVM ventilation after airway repositioning and placement of an oral airway. If the patient is easy to ventilate, reversible causes of respiratory depression, such as a narcotic overdose, should be investigated and may eliminate the need for RSI.

CLINICAL PEARLS

▶ Remember the noninvasive maneuvers and interventions that may eliminate the need for intubation: nasopharyngeal airways, chin lift, suction, BiPAP.

▶ Always have suction available.

▶ Bag-valve-mask ventilation is a lifesaving intervention for almost all patients with respiratory failure—know how to do it!

▶ Use an oral airway when bagging a patient.

▶ Head position is key for both basic and advanced airway management.

▶ Take time to thoroughly prepare for RSI. Poor preparation should never be the reason for a failed airway.

▶ Call anesthesia and/or surgery early if a difficult airway is anticipated.

▶ Always anticipate the difficult airway and have back-up airway devices immediately available.

REFERENCES

Baraka AS, Taha SK, Aouad MT, et al. Preoxygenation: comparison of maximal breathing and tidal volume breathing techniques. *Anesthesiology*. 1999;91(3):612-616.

Benumof JL, Dagg R, Benumof R. Critical hemoglobin destauration will occur before return to an unparalyzed state following 1 mg/kg intravenous succinylcholine. *Anesthesiology*. 1997;87(4):979-982.

Butler J, Sen A. Best evidence topic report. Cricoid pressure in emeceny rapid sequence induction. *Emerg Med J*. 2005;22(11):815-816.

Ellis DY, Harris T, Zideman D. Cricoid pressure in emergency department rapid sequence intubations: a risk-benefit analysis. *Ann Emerg Med*. 2007;50(6):653-665.

Ray DC, McKeown DW. Effect of induction agent on vasopressor and steroid use, and outcome in patients with septic shock. *Crit Care*. 2007;11(3):R56.

Robinson N, Clancy M. In patients with head injury undergoing rapid sequence intubation, does pretreatment with intravenous lidocaine lead to an improved neurological outcome? A review of the literature. *Emerg Med J*. 2001;18(6):453-457.

Walls, R M. Rapid Sequence Intubation in Manual of emergency airway management, Phildelphia Lipencott Williams & Wilkens; 2004.

Yeung JK, Zed PJ. A review of etomidate for rapid sequence intubation in the emergency department. *CJEM*. 2002;4(3):194-198.

A 50-year-old man presents to the emergency department (ED) with anxiety, insomnia, and nausea. He denies having any hallucinations or seizures. He states that he had been drinking about a half bottle of hard liquor each day for years. After his wife threatened to divorce him and he was fired as a result of his alcoholism, he decided to stop drinking "cold turkey." His last alcohol intake was two days ago. He has a history of hypertension, for which he takes hydrochlorothiazide. He does not smoke or use illicit drugs.

On examination, his temperature is (100.4°F), blood pressure is 175/95, heart rate is 120 beats per minute, and respiratory rate is 24 breaths per minute. He is tremulous and diaphoretic. He appears mildly dehydrated with dry mucous membranes. The lungs are clear to auscultation, and the heart sounds are regular although tachycardic. He is alert and oriented, and he does not have any focal neurologic deficits except for bilateral distal sensory loss in the hands and feet (in a stocking-glove distribution).

▶ What are potential complications?
▶ What is the best treatment for this patient?

ANSWERS TO CASE 55:

Ethanol Withdrawal

Summary: This is a 50-year-old man with acute alcohol withdrawal as evidenced by his anxiety, tremor, and signs of autonomic hyperactivity (hyperthermia, hypertension, tachycardia, tachypnea, diaphoresis). However, he does not currently exhibit the more serious signs of alcohol withdrawal, such as seizure, hallucinations, or delirium.

- **Potential complications:** seizures, hallucinations (auditory, visual, or tactile), delirium (delirium tremens or DTs).

- **Treatment:** Intravenous (IV) fluids, repletion of electrolytes as needed, benzodiazepines to control symptoms and prevent more serious manifestations of withdrawal (listed above).

ANALYSIS

Objectives

1. Recognize the clinical signs and symptoms of ethanol withdrawal (including seizures, hallucinations, and delirium).

2. Understand the evaluation and treatment of patients with ethanol withdrawal.

Considerations

Because ethanol abuse is prevalent in the community, emergency physicians need to be prepared to treat those who present with alcohol withdrawal. Symptoms may range from mild anxiety, nausea or vomiting, insomnia, and tremor to hallucinations, seizures, and delirium. Mild cases of withdrawal may be treated with oral benzodiazepines; however, patients with more serious symptomatology may require large doses of IV benzodiazepines, IV hydration, repletion of electrolytes, and hospital admission.

APPROACH TO:
Ethanol Withdrawal

CLINICAL APPROACH

Among patients presenting to the ED for any complaint, the prevalence of alcoholism or inappropriate drinking is estimated to be between 8% to 40%. Some patients arrive at the ED due to a desire to stop drinking; others have already ceased their alcohol intake and require relief of the symptoms of withdrawal. In addition, alcohol-dependent patients with prolonged ED stays may be unable to maintain their usual ethanol intake and begin to manifest anxiety or tremors. Thus, emergency physicians will encounter many patients with alcohol withdrawal and must be prepared to treat this syndrome.

Because ethanol has a depressant effect on the central nervous system (CNS), withdrawal leads to CNS excitation. Symptoms may range from mild anxiety, nausea or vomiting, insomnia, and tremor to agitation, hallucinations, seizures, and delirium. Patients often manifest signs of autonomic hyperactivity (hyperthermia, hypertension, tachycardia, tachypnea, diaphoresis, hyperreflexia). Withdrawal may occur as soon as the blood alcohol level starts to fall following an abrupt reduction in or cessation of alcohol intake. Minor withdrawal tends to begin earlier with a peak at 24 to 36 hours while major withdrawal usually occurs after 24 hours with a peak at 50 hours.

Alcohol withdrawal hallucinations may be auditory, visual, or tactile although auditory ones are most common. Patients with this condition have a clear sensorium. Alcohol withdrawal seizures are tonic-clonic and may occur singly or multiply. Up to one-third of these patients progress to DTs. Delirium tremens is the most severe form of alcohol withdrawal. It is characterized by fluctuating levels of consciousness, cognitive disturbances, profound confusion, and severe autonomic hyperactivity. With treatment, the mortality of DTs is 1% to 10%.

The differential diagnosis of alcohol withdrawal is broad and includes infections (eg, meningitis, encephalitis), other seizure disorders (eg, epilepsy), endocrine disorders (eg, thyrotoxicosis or thyroid storm), trauma (eg, subdural hemorrhage), metabolic abnormalities (eg, hypoglycemia), psychiatric disorders (eg, schizophrenia), drug intoxications (eg, sympathomimetics, antihistamines), and other types of withdrawal syndromes (eg, benzodiazepines). Benzodiazepines are widely used as anxiolytics, sleep aids, anticonvulsants, and muscle relaxants. Because benzodiazepines are also CNS depressants, withdrawal from these agents may be clinically indistinguishable from alcohol withdrawal. A history of prolonged or high dose benzodiazepine use may be helpful to differentiate between the two. Abrupt discontinuance of short-acting benzodiazepines may be symptomatic after 2 to 3 days while withdrawal from long-acting agents may present up to 7 days after cessation.

Important historical information includes current symptomatology, usual amount of alcohol consumption, timing of last alcohol intake, comorbidities, and any other medication or other drug use. The initial evaluation of the patient should involve the assessment (and stabilization if necessary) of the ABCs. A complete set of vital signs is paramount in order to identify any autonomic hyperactivity. The patient should be examined from head to toe looking for evidence of alternative etiologies for the patient symptoms (eg, signs of trauma associated with intracranial hemorrhage, nuchal rigidity with meningitis, thyromegaly with thyrotoxicosis, etc). In addition, a thorough neurologic examination should be performed to identify any alterations in level of consciousness or mental status as well as any focal deficits.

Diagnostic studies are largely useful in ruling out alternative diagnoses and concomitant medical conditions. Patients with mild alcohol withdrawal may not require any laboratory studies or imaging. Those with severe withdrawal may require a more extensive workup including any or all of the following: complete blood count, electrolytes, renal function tests, glucose, liver enzymes, blood gas, thyroid function studies, cardiac enzymes, urinalysis, urine drug screen, ECG, chest x-ray, computed tomography of the head, and/or lumbar puncture.

Treatment

Treatment of alcohol withdrawal serves several purposes: symptomatic relief, calming of the patient to allow an adequate evaluation, and prevention of progression of symptoms. The mainstay of treatment is benzodiazepines, most commonly chlordiazepoxide, diazepam, and lorazepam. These medications are titrated to control the patient agitation, and very high doses may be required. Neuroleptics such as haloperidol or ziprasidone may be considered for patients who do not respond adequately to benzodiazepines. In addition, a continuous propofol infusion may be beneficial in patients with severe withdrawal who are refractory to high dose benzodiazepines. The alpha-agonist clonidine may be a useful adjunct to counteract the autonomic hyperactivity associated with alcohol withdrawal. β-Blockers may also help control tachycardia and hypertension; however, they may mask some of the earlier signs of impending DTs. Depending on the patient fluid and nutrition status, IV hydration and repletion of electrolytes (eg, potassium, magnesium, and phosphorus) may be needed. Malnourished patients should also be given thiamine and folate replacement.

The disposition of patients with alcohol withdrawal depends on the severity of symptoms, response to treatment, and availability of outpatient support. If the patient responds well to therapy in the ED, he/she may be discharged with an oral benzodiazepine taper, abstinence from alcohol, and participation in a rehabilitation program. However, patients who require high doses of benzodiazepines and those who have more severe symptoms or DTs must be admitted.

COMPREHENSION QUESTIONS

55.1 A 25-year-old woman has been taking clonazepam every day for 3 years for generalized anxiety disorder. She is in town on vacation but forgot her medication at home. When is she most likely to start showing symptoms of withdrawal?

A. 12 hours

B. 2 days

C. 6 days

D. 10 days

55.2 A 50-year-old man is admitted for a femur fracture following a motor vehicle collision. Two days after admission, he becomes very agitated, tremulous, diaphoretic, tachycardic, and hypertensive. From what substance might he be withdrawing?

  A. Alcohol

  B. Cocaine

  C. Marijuana

  D. Oxycodone

55.3 A 60-year-old homeless man presents to the ED with acute alcohol withdrawal. He has been given 2 mg of lorazepam IV, but still appears very agitated and anxious. What is the most appropriate next step?

  A. Clonidine 0.2 mg PO

  B. Haloperidol 5 mg IV

  C. Lorazepam 2 mg IV

  D. Propanolol 100 mg PO

ANSWERS

55.1 **C. Clonazepam is a long-acting benzodiazepine.** Abrupt discontinuance of short-acting benzodiazepines may be symptomatic after 2 to 3 days while withdrawal from long-acting agents may present up to 7 days after cessation. Treatment of benozodiazepine withdrawal involves reinstitution of a benzodiazepine followed by a gradual taper.

55.2 **A.** The agitation, tremor, and autonomic hyperactivity point towards alcohol withdrawal. All patients admitted to the hospital for medical or traumatic conditions should be asked about drug and alcohol use. After admission, they may not have access to the drugs and/or alcohol they regularly use and may present with withdrawal syndromes.

55.3 **C.** While all are appropriate treatments for alcohol withdrawal, benzodiazepine dosing is tapered to the patient agitation. It may be redosed at 10 to 30 minute intervals for patients in severe withdrawal. Very high doses may be required especially if the patient has DTs.

CLINICAL PEARLS

▶ Alcohol is a CNS depressant. Withdrawal leads to CNS stimulation and autonomic hyperactivity.

▶ The differential diagnosis of alcohol withdrawal includes infections, other seizure disorders, endocrine disorders, trauma, metabolic abnormalities, psychiatric disorders, drug intoxications, and other types of withdrawal syndromes.

▶ The mainstay of treatment for alcohol withdrawal is benzodiazepines.

REFERENCES

Marx JA, Hockberger RS, Walls RM, eds. *Rosen's Emergency Medicine: Concepts and Clinical Practice*. 7th ed. Philadelphia, PA: Mosby Elsevier; 2009.

Kelly JF, Renner JA. Alcohol-related disorders. In: Stern TA, Rosenbaum JF, Fava M, Biederman J, Rauch SL, eds. *Stern: Massachusetts General Hospital Comprehensive Clinical Psychiatry*. 1st ed. Philadelphia, PA: Mosby Elsevier; 2006:2858-2882.

Kosten TR, O'Connor PG. Management of drug and alcohol withdrawal. *N Engl J Med*. 2003;348(18): 1786-1795.

Tintinalli JE, Stapczynski JS. *Tintinall'si Emergency Medicine: A Comprehensive Study Guide*. 7th ed. New York, NY: McGraw-Hill; 2011.

An 18-year-old man presents to the emergency department (ED) agitated, confused and hallucinating. The patient friends state that the group was walking around in the woods looking for some "weeds to smoke" in order to get "high." The patient was first to smoke one of the weeds and subsequently became agitated. His friends decided to bring him to the ED for evaluation. On arrival to the ED, the patient vital signs are BP 180/100 mm Hg, HR 120 beats per minute, RR 18 breaths per minute, temperature 101°F, and pulse ox 98% on room air. On physical examination, his pupils are 6 mm, skin is erythematous and warm to the touch, axillae are dry, abdomen has decreased bowel sounds, and the patient is grabbing at things that are not there.

▶ What is the most likely diagnosis?
▶ What is the next step in treatment?

ANSWERS TO CASE 56:

Anti-muscarinic Toxidrome

Summary: This is a case of an unknown plant ingestion in a patient who presents with several signs of toxicity. The key features of this case include recognizing signs and symptoms of a toxidrome and knowing how to stabilize and manage poisoned patients. The patient presents with anti-muscarinic toxicity after smoking jimson weed, which contains belladonna alkaloids. These alkaloids possess strong anti-muscarinic properties.

- **Most likely diagnosis:** Jimson weed (anti-muscarinic) toxicity

- **Best initial treatment:** Benzodiazepines and consider physostigmine

ANALYSIS

Objectives

1. Develop an initial approach to the poisoned patient.

2. Learn the 5 basic classes of toxidromes.

3. Understand how to classify a patient into a toxidrome.

4. Understand the initial steps for stabilization of a symptomatic overdose.

5. Review the basic treatment for each of the toxidromes.

Considerations

This patient has several classic features of an anti-muscarinic toxidrome. The primary treatment efforts for the poisoned patient are the same as any other patient: maintenance and stabilization of the airway, breathing, and circulatory systems (ABCs). For **any intentional overdose, levels of acetaminophen and salicylate levels should be checked** due to their ubiquity in medications and great potential for morbidity and mortality.

In this case, the patient is febrile. Fever in the setting of a toxicologic problem is a predictor of increased morbidity and mortality. The cause of the fever is usually secondary to increased muscle activity. Initial treatment should include administration of benzodiazepines (eg diazepam, lorazepam) and intravenous fluids for hydration.

In general, symptomatic poisoned patients require hospital admission for continued monitoring. However, the majority does well with simple supportive care.

The local poison control center should be contacted early in the work-up of all symptomatic overdoses. This is critical both for epidemiologic purposes as well as management of complex patients and continuity of care. The national phone number for the nearest **poison control center is 1-800-222-1222.**

APPROACH TO:
Toxidromes

DEFINITIONS

TOXIDROME: A clinical syndrome that is essential for the successful recognition of poisoning patterns. A toxidrome is the constellation of signs and symptoms that suggest a specific class of poisoning.

DECONTAMINATION: Prevention of the continued absorption of a toxicant.

DRUG ABSORPTION: The movement of drug from its site of administration into the bloodstream.

ADSORPTION: The binding of a chemical (eg, drug or poison) to a solid material such as activated charcoal.

ANTIDOTE: A remedy to counteract a poison or injury.

OPIATE: A compound found in opium poppies (eg, morphine, codeine, thebane, etc) that binds to the opiate receptor.

OPIOID: A synthetic (eg, fentanyl, methadone, tramadol, etc) or semi-synthetic (eg, heroin, oxycodone, hydrocodone, etc) compound that binds to the opiate receptor.

BODY PACKER: An individual who ingests wrapped packets of illicit drugs such as cocaine, heroin, amphetamines, ecstasy, marijuana, or hashish to transport them.

BODY STUFFER: Someone who admits to or is strongly suspected of ingesting illegal drugs in order to escape detection by authorities, and not for recreational purposes or to transport the drug across borders. Cocaine is the drug most commonly involved in the body stuffer syndrome.

CLINICAL APPROACH

General Overdose Management

Airway and Breathing The general approach to the overdose patient is to start with an initial assessment that includes evaluation of the patient **airway, breathing, and circulation (ABCs).** The most easily correctable cause of toxicologic death is airway support. Sedate patients may have a partially obstructed airway due to a relaxed tongue. In addition, obtunded patients may loose their gag reflex. Understand also, that breathing consists of both oxygenation and ventilation. A hypoxic patient with a suspected overdose and no history of known medical problems, is also at risk for poor ventilation. Masking this hypoventilation and hypoxia by applying supplemental oxygen may actually decrease the patient intrinsic respiratory drive and lead to further hypoventilation. **Definitive airway management includes endotracheal or nasotracheal intubation.**

Circulation Toxidromes can lead to both extreme hypertension and hypotension. Extreme hypertension (sympathomimetics) may require the use of a direct alpha$_1$-receptor antagonist, such as phentermine. Hypotension should first be treated with intravenous fluids. Other agents such as vasopressors (norepinephrine, dopamine) may be required. Often, cardiac function is also affected in toxidromes. Tachy- and bradydysrhythmias are both common. Treatment depends on the underlying etiology of the dysrhythmia.

Decontamination In addition to the ABCs, it is also essential to consider **decontamination** and **elimination** (or ABCDE) in the management of a poisoned patient. Decontamination involves preventing further absorption into the system. For topical contaminations, removing the patient clothing, as well as washing off the affected area, may be all that is required. Another way of preventing absorption into the system is the administration of activated charcoal. **Activated charcoal** comes in two forms; with and without sorbitol. Sorbitol is thought to facilitate the movement of activated charcoal through the gastrointestinal (GI) tract. It is, however, a GI irritant and more than one dose of activated charcoal with sorbitol is not recommended. Patients who have the greatest benefit from activated charcoal include those who present early in their ingestion (<1 hour), are awake and can drink the activated charcoal without risk of aspiration, and ingestions whose chemicals are well absorbed by activated charcoal.

One main concern with the administration of activated charcoal is the potential for aspiration and subsequent charcoal pneumonitis. This risk can be decreased by administering activated charcoal only to patients who are awake and protecting their airway. In addition to this complication, activated charcoal poorly adsorbs certain chemicals (see Table 56–1), and therefore will have little benefit in these ingestions. Moreover, patients with caustic injuries often undergo endoscopy. Prior administration of activated charcoal may complicate the procedure.

Another method of decontamination is **gastric lavage.** This is accomplished by inserting a large oral gastric tube (eg, 40 French) into the stomach for the rapid administration and removal of large volumes (several liters) of fluid in an attempt to try to remove whole pills before they are dissolved and absorbed. One potential adverse effect is lavaging the lungs instead of the stomach. This can be avoided by intubating the patient prior to lavage. In addition, given the increasing number of bariatric surgery patients, a complication can occur if the tube gets stuck in the gastric band or causes gastric perforation. Given the large number of treatment options that are available for a wide variety of ingestions, gastric lavage should only be performed on patients who present early (<1 hour) and

Table 56–1 • POORLY ADSORBED COMPOUNDS BY ACTIVATED CHARCOAL
Ethanol
Methanol
Isopropyl alcohol
Ethylene glycol
Hydrocarbons
Caustics (acid and base)
Lithium and other salts

have a potentially life-threatening ingestion for which there are limited treatment options. This technique is not to be confused with nasogastric lavage (the administration and subsequent removal of fluid from an NG tube), which has **not** been shown to substantially alter the course of *any* substantially poisoned patient and usually ends at just removing some of the excipients (starches, waxes, and binding agents).

Another method of decontamination is **whole bowel irrigation.** In this method, a large amount of polyethylene glycol electrolyte lavage solution (PEG-ELS) is administered through an NG tube at a rate of approximately 1 L an hour. The goal of this therapy is to push whole pills through the GI tract to prevent absorption. This method is especially helpful in treatment of body packers and body stuffers as well as with sustained release medications.

Elimination Once the drug is absorbed into the body, there are options that may help to increase elimination from the body. These options include multidose charcoal, hemodialysis, charcoal hemoperfusion, and urinary alkalinization. **Multidose charcoal** has been shown to be effective with certain drugs, namely dapsone, carbamazepine, phenobarbital, quinine, and theophylline. While the first dose of charcoal with these patients can be given with sorbitol, subsequent doses should not contain sorbitol as it is a GI irritant and can lead to dehydration and GI upset.

Hemodialysis is effective for certain drugs that have a **low volume of distribution** (ie, water soluble) and may be used if there is no better antidote or if the patient is critically ill. Examples of these drugs include lithium, methanol, and aspirin. Acetaminophen technically is also amenable to dialysis but there is a noninvasive antidote that is more commonly used.

Charcoal hemoperfusion is similar to arterial venous hemodialysis, except that the drug is passed through a charcoal filter prior to systemic return. This is particularly effective in phenobarbital and theophylline overdoses as they adsorb well to charcoal.

Urinary alkalinization is a treatment regimen that increases poison elimination by the administration of intravenous sodium bicarbonate to produce urine with a pH >7.5. Alkaline urine facilitates ion trapping and excretion. This method is particularly useful for aspirin and phenobarbital toxicities.

Supplemental Testing

For any intentional overdose, an acetaminophen and salicylate level should be obtained. These medications are readily accessible and carry a high morbidity and mortality while being fairly easy to treat if caught early.

For **acetaminophen,** if the time of ingestion is known and it is a single acute ingestion, use of the **Rumack-Matthew nomogram** for acetaminophen toxicity can determine if the patient requires treatment. If the time of ingestion is unknown and any detectable acetaminophen level is found then strong consideration should be given towards treatment. Consideration should also be made with unexplained elevations in transaminases.

For **salicylates,** levels above 30 mg/dL should be treated with bicarbonate infusion and potassium supplementation to increase urinary elimination (prevent reabsorption). Certain patients may require dialysis. These include but are not limited to salicylate-induced pulmonary edema, salicylate-induced encephalopathy, severe acidosis, and levels greater than 80 mg/dL in the correct clinical setting.

Twelve-lead ECG may be helpful in early identification of **sodium channel blocking drugs** (eg, tricyclic antidepressants, diphenhydramine, and various other antidepressants and antipsychotics). Sodium channel blockade is manifested by a prolonged QRS complex. The first manifestation of this may be in lead aVR where it is possible to see an R-R-prime pattern and slurring of the terminal 30 msec of the QRS complex. Administering intravenous sodium bicarbonate until the QRS complex narrows helps treat this condition.

Patients with a wide QRS may also have QT prolongation. One should be careful to distinguish QRS prolongation from QT prolongation. Drugs that affect potassium efflux or influx or drugs that affect calcium influx will also cause QT prolongation. Treatment with sodium bicarbonate for a prolonged QRS can worsen a prolonged QT interval by pushing potassium into cells, which may lead to torsade de pointes.

Routine urine drug screen testing is not necessary for treatment of an acute overdose. Most urine drug screen testing is an immunoassay that tests for the presence of drug metabolites and are tailored to a specific core molecule. They do not necessarily detect the presence of the active compound and they do not tell you if the patient is under the effects of that particular compound. There are many false positives and false negatives in any given class of drugs tested on the urine drug screen. Treatment of an overdose should not wait until the return of the urine drug screen.

Toxidromes

Sedative Hypnotic This is a large class of drugs, which includes alcohols, benzodiazepines, barbiturates, chloral hydrate, propofol, carisoprodol, and many others. In general, the sedative hypnotic toxidrome is characterized by relatively **normal vital signs** (see Table 56–2) and a relatively normal examination except for a markedly **decreased level of consciousness.** The patient may be hypothermic but this would be due to environmental heat loss and loss of the shiver response. Treatment for this toxidrome is largely **support of airway and breathing.** In the undifferentiated sedative hypnotic patient, administration of **flumazenil, a benzodiazepine antagonist, is not indicated as it may precipitate a benzodiazepine resistant seizure.**

Opioid/Opiate This class of drugs includes synthetics and semi-synthetics such as fentanyl and meperidine, as well as compounds found in nature and close derivatives such as morphine and codeine. These agonize the opiate receptors in the body. Agonism at these receptors induces **euphoria, analgesia, antidepressant effects, and sedation** as well as **respiratory depression, miosis, decreased GI motility, and dependence.**

Vital signs in these patients may demonstrate decreased respirations and a **low pulse ox.** In severe overdoses the patient may be hypotensive or bradycardic or

Table 56–2 • PHYSICAL EXAM CHARACTERISTICS SEEN IN TOXIDROMES

	Sedative Hypnotic	Opiate	Sympathomimetic	Anti-muscarinic	Cholinergic
Vital signs	+/– (usually relatively normal, maybe hypotensive, bradycardic in severe overdoses; sometimes hypothermic if prolonged exposure	↓ (decreased respiratory rate and pulse ox, sometimes hypotensive or bradycardic, sometimes hypothermic if prolonged exposure)	↑ (febrile, tachycardic, hypertensive, tachypneic)	↑ (febrile, tachycardic, hypertensive, tachypneic)	↓ (bradycardic, sometimes tachypneic or bradypneic, sometimes hypotensive, sometimes hypoxic)
Bowel sounds	+/–	↓	↓	↓	↑
Skin moisture (axilla)	+/–	+/–	↑	↓	↑
CNS	↓	↓	↑	↑	↓
Treatment	Airway and breathing	Airway and breathing (consider naloxone)	Benzodiazepines	Benzodiazepines and consider physostigmine	Atropine and pralidoxime

both. On physical examination the pupils will be small (**miotic**), **bowel sounds are decreased,** reflexes are decreased, and overall level of consciousness is decreased. Unless the patient has hypotension or bradycardia, the focus is maintaining ventilation and oxygenation. Treatment for hypoxia in the opiate or opioid overdose patient is either **naloxone** (Narcan) administration or **endotracheal intubation.** In the non-critically ill patient, the amount of naloxone administered should be based on the patient response. The goal of treatment is to get the patient breathing again, not necessarily to make the patient awake and conversant. Nalaxone administration should be avoided in an intubated patient with opiate or opioid overdose since this will lead to significant vomiting.

Sympathomimetic   This class of drugs includes stimulants such as cocaine, ecstasy and methamphetamine, but may also include therapeutic medications such as albuterol, pseudoephedrine, and many others. Their mechanisms of action may vary, but the end result is increased **stimulation of the α- and β-adrenergic receptors.** This alpha and beta stimulation results in **tachycardia, hypertension,** and **hyperthermia.** Physical examination often reveals dilated pupils (**mydriasis**), increased CNS activity (**hallucinations or seizures**), increased reflexes, and **diaphoretic skin.** This toxidrome can look very similar to the anti-muscarinic toxidrome, but is usually distinguished by the presence of diaphoresis.

Mortality in these patients is typically from **hyperthermia,** so it is critical to **keep them cool.** Physically restraining a patient who is agitated or delirious without a sedative medication may lead to rhabdomyolysis and a dangerous increase in temperature. The mainstay in treatment includes the administration of benzodiazepines and intravenous fluids. If the patient is still agitated after receiving large doses of benzodiazepines, **consideration should be given to administering barbiturates or paralysis and intubation.**

Antimuscarinic   There are a large variety of drugs that fall under the anti-muscarinic toxidrome. These may also be referred to as **anticholinergic drugs,** but very few medications have anti-nicotinic activity, and thus we should correctly refer to this as the anti-muscarinic toxidrome. Antagonism at the muscarinic receptors leads a physical examination that is **very similar to the sympathomimetic toxidrome.** The area in which the sympathomimetic toxidrome differs from the anti-muscarinic toxidrome is that the **antimuscarinic toxidrome will have dry skin** while the sympathomimetic toxidrome will have wet skin. Patients tend to be tachycardic, hypertensive, and febrile. On physical examination they will have mydriatic pupils, an altered level of consciousness (hallucinating or seizing), **urinary retention,** and decreased bowel sounds. There is a mnemonic for this toxidrome: Mad as a hatter (hallucinations), dry as a bone (anhydrosis), red as a beet (increased agitation and fever), and blind as a bat (mydriasis).

Treatment of the anti-muscarinic toxidrome varies depending on the severity of effects and whether the effects are acting more peripherally (anhydrosis) or centrally (seizure, heart rate, and blood pressure). Peripheral anti-muscarinic toxicity can be treated with benzodiazepines. Central anti-muscarinic toxicity should also be treated with benzodiazepines, and consideration to use a medication that increases levels of acetylcholine, such as **physostigmine,** an **acetylcholinesterase inhibitor.**

Cholinergic Cholinergic drugs are drugs that increase the level of acetylcholine. This is usually through inhibition of acetylcholinesterase. Examples of these medications include edrophonium and physostigmine. Other sources for cholinergic toxicity include **insecticides** such as carbamates and organophosphates. Organophosphates are notable in that they have the potential to irreversibly bind and inhibit acetylcholinesterase–this process is called aging and is highly dependent upon the type of organophosphate such that significant aging varies between 2 to 36 hours after initial binding.

Excess acetylcholine can cause effects at both muscarinic and nicotinic receptors and its effects depend on the time course and severity of toxicity. Classically, it is associated with **bradycardia** and hypoxia secondary to either increased fluid in the lungs or diaphragmatic paralysis. Other findings on physical examination include **miotic pupils** (pinpoint), **hyperactive bowel sounds, and excessive secretions from the mouth, GI tract, and skin.**

The mnemonic SLUDGE (Salivation, Lacrimation, Urination, Defecation, GI upset, and Emesis) covers some but not all aspects of this toxidrome. It does not account for the bradycardia, bronchospasm, and bronchorrhea or the miotic pupils that are noted on physical examination. An alternative mnemonic is **DUMBBELLS** (Defecation, Urination, Miosis, Bradycardia, Bronchorrhea/Bronchospasm, Emesis, Lacrimation, Lethargy, and Salivation).

Treatment involves the administration of anticholinergic medication such as **atropine** as well as **pralidoxime (2-PAM).** Atropine should be administered to help **control bronchorrhea.** Pralidoxime should be administered to prevent binding and aging of the acetylcholinesterase in the case of organophosphate poisoning.

COMPREHENSION QUESTIONS

56.1 A farmer presents to the ED with difficulty in breathing. His vitals are BP 85/55, HR 50, T 97.8°F, RR 28, and pulse ox 91% room air. His examination reveals wheezing; excessive perspiration, vomiting, and tearing, and 1 mm pupils. Which is the best treatment for this patient toxicity?

   A. Benzodiazepines

   B. Physostigmine

   C. Pyridoxine

   D. Pralidoxime

   E. Naloxone

56.2 A teenager comes home after visiting his grandmother who is sick with cancer. His parents call 911 because he is minimally responsive. They find him with a BP 90/60, HR 65, T 98.5°F, RR 6, pulse ox 89% on room air. His examination includes 2 mm pupils, decreased bowel sounds, hyporeflexia, and responsiveness only to noxious stimuli. The paramedics check his blood sugar, which is normal, and administer which of the following?

A. Charcoal

B. Naloxone

C. Flumazenil

D. Lorazepam

E. Atropine

56.3 A college student with a history rhinorrhea comes in after being found by her roommate with an altered mental status. Her vitals are BP 160/90, HR 120, RR 18, T 100.5°F, pulse ox 100%. On examination she is picking at the air, has decreased bowel sounds, 6-mm pupils and no moisture in her axilla. Her blood sugar is normal. Which medication should they give her?

A. Atropine

B. Pralidoxime

C. Physostigmine

D. Flumazenil

E. Fomepizole

56.4 A 55-year-old homeless woman presents to the ED brought by ambulance. The police found her seizing in the street. Her vital signs are BP 220/150, HR 140, T 101°F, RR 16, pulse ox 100% on room air. On examination she has 6 mm pupils, very wet skin, decreased bowel sounds and is having uncontrollable limb movements. A check of her blood sugar is normal. What medication should this patient be administered?

A. Physostigmine

B. Lorazepam

C. Labetalol

D. Atropine then pralidoxime

E. Phytonadione

ANSWERS

56.1 **D.** This patient is exhibiting a **cholinergic toxidrome.** The mnemonic for this is **DUMBBELLS** (Defecation, Urination, Miosis, Bradycardia, Bronchorrhea, Emesis, Lacrimation, Lethargy, and Salivation). The treatment is to prevent the patient from drowning in his or her own saliva by administering atropine 1 mg at a time until the secretions dry up. In addition, **pralidoxime (2-PAM)** is administered to increase acetylcholinesterase availability and reduce acetylcholine. Benzodiazepines would not help with this patient. Physostigmine is a treatment for anti-muscarinic toxicity and would worsen this patient condition. Pyridoxine is vitamin B6 and can be useful in treating seizures if they are caused by isoniazid (INH). Naloxone is an opiate antagonist and while this presentation has some overlap with the opiate toxidrome, this patient is tachypneic and has excessive secretions that are not seen in the opiate toxidrome. His exposure was from the **pesticides** on the farm.

56.2 **B.** This patient is exhibiting an **opiate toxidrome.** He has miotic pupils and decreased respirations, GI motility and mental status. The treatment for this is patient should include **a trial of naloxone; enough to increase his oxygenation.** This patient likely stole opiate medication from his grandmother. Charcoal would not help this patient as he is already severely symptomatic. Additionally, **charcoal would be contraindicated** in this patient because of the risk of aspiration. Flumazenil is a benzodiazepine antagonist. Lorazepam is a benzodiazepine. Atropine is a strong anti-muscarinic drug and would not be helpful in treating this patient.

56.3 **C.** This patient is exhibiting an **antimuscarinic toxidrome.** This is characterized by **tachycardia, fever, hallucinosis, dilated pupils, hypoactive bowel sounds, and dry axilla.** The mnemonic is: **mad as a hatter (hallucinations), dry as a bone (anhydrosis), red as a beet (increased agitation and fever), and blind as a bat (mydriasis).** Treatment should be either decreasing the agitation and temperature through benzodiazepines or increasing acetylcholine by preventing its metabolism (physostigmine, an acetylcholinesterase inhibitor). Atropine is an anti-muscarinic drug and would worsen this patient toxidrome. Pralidoxime is a drug which makes acetylcholinesterase work again after exposure to an organophosphate. This patient does not have signs of cholinergic excess, therefore, pralidoxime would not be helpful. Flumazenil should not be given to adult patients because, as acting benzodiazepine antagonist, it may precipitate seizures that are not responsive to benzodiazepines. Fomepizole is an inhibitor of alcohol dehydrogenase and is helpful in the treatment of patients poisoned with ethylene glycol, methanol or other toxic alcohols. This patient had an accidental overdose of her **diphenhydramine** for her seasonal allergies.

56.4 **B.** This patient is exhibiting a **sympathomimetic toxidrome.** Her presentation is very similar to the patient in question 3. However, the key difference is that this patient has wet skin, while the patient in question 3 has dry skin. **The patient should receive as much lorazepam as is needed to stop the seizure and allow the temperature to fall.** Physostigmine is a treatment for anti-muscarinic toxicity and would not be helpful in this patient. Labetalol is a β-blocker. This patient has signs of active sympathomimetic excess. Treatment with a β-blocker **may lead to unopposed α-1 agonism and potentially may worsen a patient tissue perfusion.** While this patient is wet, she has none of the other signs of a cholinergic toxicity. Therefore, atropine and pralidoxime are not recommended. Phytonadione is vitamin K and is the treatment for warfarin toxicity. This patient recently used crack cocaine.

CLINICAL PEARLS

▶ Patients who are hypoxic from an overdose typically will require a definitive airway such as endotracheal or nasotracheal intubation.

▶ Fever from an overdose is a poor prognostic indicator and should usually be addressed with large doses of benzodiazepines and intravenous fluids.

▶ Symptomatic patients require observation or admission until they are asymptomatic.

▶ In the undifferentiated altered mental status patient, blood sugar level should immediately be checked.

▶ The nearest poison control center should be contacted (1-800-222-1222) for overdoses, accidental ingestions, and adverse drug effects.

REFERENCES

Aaron CK, Bora KM. Toxin ingestions in children. BMJ Point-of-Care. 2010; Available at: https://online.epocrates.com/u/2911885/Toxic+ingestions+in+children

Chyka PA, Seger D, Krenzelok EP, Vala JA. American Academy of Clinical Toxicology, European Association of Poisons Centres, Clinical Toxicologists. Position paper: single-dose activated charcoal. Clin Toxicol (Phila). 2005;43:61-87.

Goldfrank L, Flomenbaum N, Lewin N, et al. Goldfrank's Toxicologic Emergencies. 9th ed. New York, NY: McGraw-Hill; 2010.

Roberts DM, Aaron CK. Management of acute organophosphorus pesticide poisoning. BMJ. 2007;334:629-634.

Wu AH, McKay C, Broussard LA, et al. National academy of clinical biochemistry laboratory medicine practice guidelines: recommendations for the use of laboratory tests to support poisoned patients who present to the emergency department. Clin Chem. 2003;49:357-379.

A 45-year-old man presents to the ED complaining of left shoulder pain. Past history includes numerous skin abscesses, hepatitis C and injection drug use. He injected black tar heroin into the left upper extremity 2 days ago. On examination the patient is in mild distress. There is a low-grade fever, the heart rate is 115 bpm and blood pressure is 120/60 mm Hg. The dorsum of the upper arm is erythematous, indurated and tender. There is no obvious area of fluctuance. Edema extends to the shoulder and pectoralis region of the trunk.

▶ What is the most likely diagnosis?
▶ What are the next diagnostic and treatment steps?

ANSWERS TO CASE 57:
Skin and Soft Tissue Infections

Summary: This is an injection drug user with a fever and a skin and soft tissue infection (SSTI) of the upper extremity and shoulder.

- **Most likely diagnosis:** Soft tissue abscess from injection drug use. However, necrotizing soft tissue infection (NSTI) is a distinct possibility, and the differential diagnosis also includes cellulitis and septic shoulder joint.

- **Next steps:** Establish IV access. IV antibiotics are generally indicated when a SSTI produces a fever. Establish a definitive diagnosis as quickly as possible, beginning with a careful search for a pus pocket. If an abscess is found it must be drained. If not, NSTI remains a possibility and immediate surgical exploration is indicated. Search for signs of sepsis, and if present begin early goal directed therapy.

ANALYSIS

Objectives

1. Recognize the range of SSTIs, which can look remarkably similar on first inspection.

2. Become familiar with the usual pathogens responsible for SSTIs and the antimicrobial agents that are commonly used for empirical therapy.

3. Understand that NSTIs can be life threatening, rapidly progressive and difficult to diagnose.

4. Recognize the risk factors associated with necrotizing infections and with unusual pathogens.

5. Appreciate that uncomplicated abscesses often require only incision and drainage, and no antibiotics, for cure.

Considerations

SSTIs are among the most common problems seen in the ED, accounting for 3.4 million annual visits in the United States alone. There has been a recent rise in the incidence of these infections linked to the emergence of community-associated methicillin resistant *Staphylococcus aureus*. While simple abscesses predominate, there is a range of distinct SSTI types, which includes deep abscesses, nonpurulent cellulitis and NSTIs. NSTIs can be rapidly life-threatening and timely diagnosis is often difficult. SSTIs of all types are extremely common in injection drug users, and thus in emergency departments that serve an injection drug use population. Red flags can alert the astute clinician to a necrotizing infection as well as to unusual pathogens that require special antibiotics. To complicate matters, other diseases affecting the skin and underlying tissues can be confused with infection, particularly gout and other forms of arthritis and bursitis, allergic reactions to insect bites and deep vein thrombosis.

Diagnosis and management of SSTIs can be tricky. Different types of SSTIs, that require different approaches to management, can appear similar. While diagnostic tests such as bedside ultrasound, CT scan and blood lactate levels can be helpful, in most cases correct diagnosis relies solely on the bedside exam and judgment of the emergency physician. Many of these infections are primarily a surgical disease. Effective management often requires only the skillful administration of anesthetic and incision and drainage in the ED, but occasionally, immediate exploration and debridement in the operating room is required. Similarly, while judicious use of antibiotics is an important principal in the management of most simple SSTIs, serious SSTIs will occasionally cause sepsis syndrome, in which case immediate antibiotic administration and aggressive resuscitation is imperative.

APPROACH TO:
Skin and Soft Tissue Infections

DEFINITIONS

SKIN AND SOFT TISSUE INFECTION (SSTI): An infection, usually bacterial, of the skin and/or underlying soft tissues.

NECROTIZING SKIN AND SOFT TISSUE INFECTION (NSTI): A rapidly spreading bacterial infection (monomicrobial or polymicrobial) of the soft tissue below the skin surface including fat, fascia (fasciitis), and muscle (myositis).

PURULENT (CULTURABLE) CELLULITIS: Infection and/or inflammatory changes of the skin surrounding a purulent focus (usually an abscess).

NONPURULENT (NON-CULTURABLE) CELLULITIS: An infection of the skin and underlying dermis without an identifiable purulent focus.

ERYSIPELAS: Nonpurulent cellulitis restricted to the superficial skin layers with a sharply demarcated border.

CLINICAL APPROACH

Diagnosis

Clinical evaluation of SSTIs always begins with a search for a pus pocket, because both the differential diagnosis and clinical management depend on whether or not there is pus (Figure 57–1). Circular infections (as opposed to circumferential) on the buttock, groin and lower extremity almost always harbor pus near the center. First look for a visible spot of purulence or necrosis. Then palpate carefully for fluctuance, which can be subtle. Fluctuance may be absent if the abscess is deep, as often occurs in the pannus of the buttock or thigh, or if the abscess is early in its course. Very deep intramuscular abscesses can occur with injection drug use. Bedside ultrasound, using a high frequency linear transducer, can identify deep abscesses that are not appreciated on physical examination. On ultrasound, the abscess cavity typically appears

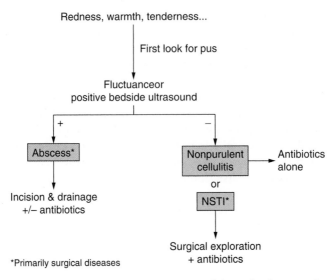

Figure 57–1. Approach to the diagnosis and management of skin and soft tissue infections. NSTI, necrotizing skin and soft tissue infection; * primarily surgical diseases.

anechoic (black with no echo). CT scan is considered the gold standard for abscess diagnosis, and is used to identify those near the neck, groin and perineum.

Spontaneous, superficial skin abscesses are called furuncles and patients often assume these are spider bites. Skin abscesses are usually caused by S aureus–over half by MRSA–and less commonly β-hemolytic streptococcal species. Abscesses associated with injection drug use, and those occurring near the perineum may contain gram negative and anaerobic bacteria. Abscesses are typically surrounded by a variable amount of cellulitis (so-called purulent cellulitis), and large abscesses may cause fever.

If an abscess is not present; the main diagnostic considerations are cellulitis versus NSTI (Figure 57–1).

Nonpurulent cellulitis tends to occur on the lower extremities in a circumferential pattern, often in an area of preexisting edema. The etiology is usually β-hemolytic streptococcal species, such as S pyogenes. Cellulitis may be associated with lymphangitis and fever. Erysipelas is a superficial, sharply demarcated cellulitis caused by S pyogenes that often occurs in elderly patients on the face or lower extremities, and causes fever and leukocytosis.

Cellulitis in certain settings is always considered high risk, either because it is caused by esoteric or resistant pathogens, or because of the likelihood of severe disease requiring admission or an operation. Infected puncture wounds of any kind are high risk and likely to involve deep structures like bone, joint or tendon, and to respond poorly to conventional antibiotics alone. Tenosynovitis, an orthopedic emergency, can complicate puncture wounds on the palmar hand and fingers. Diabetic foot ulcers, when infected, tend to harbor multiple resistant pathogens, can lead to NSTI, and generally require specialized podiatric care. Infected mammalian bite wounds, covered elsewhere in this textbook, are high risk, often harbor *Pasteurella* species or *Eikinella* (human bites) and generally require admission. Unusual pathogens that cause SSTIs in the setting of water exposure include *Vibrio vulnificus*, which often causes a necrotizing infection and sepsis, *Erysipelothrix*, and *Aeromonas*.

NSTIs are among the most feared infections in medicine. These infections typically spread rapidly along subcutaneous and muscular facial planes and produce toxins and trigger an intense cytokine response that lead to septic shock. Classically, NSTIs occur in the setting of devitalized tissue, such as from a shrapnel wound, and the etiology is polymicrobial, with C *perfringens* among the pathogens. A spontaneous, monomicrobial form of NSTI also occurs, typically caused by S *pyogenes*, but occasionally by Clostridial species or MRSA. Rapid diagnosis requires that the clinician be familiar with the risk factors for NSTI and red flags on physical examination (see Table 57–1).

An important risk factor for community onset necrotizing fasciitis is injection drug use, particularly subcutaneous and intramuscular injection ("skin popping") of black tar heroin. Other infection patterns that should raise a red flag are neglected diabetic foot ulcers and infections of the perineum, particularly in men. Classical skin signs such as necrosis, bullae or crepitance are often absent. The Clostridial infections associated with injection drug use may produce dramatic tissue edema and extreme leukocytosis. The combination of extreme leukocytosis and hyponatremia is suggestive of an NSTI. Diagnostic imaging can be helpful. Plane x-ray and CT scan may demonstrate gas along facial planes or within muscle, or an unsuspected abscess may be seen. When NSTI is suspected, however, the best diagnostic approach is prompt surgical exploration. The diagnosis is made when subcutaneous devitalized tissue, muscle necrosis and "dishwater pus" are found.

The bacteriology of the major forms of SSTI, are listed in Table 57–2, along with recommended antibiotics.

Table 57–1 • NECROTIZING SKIN AND SOFT TISSUE "RED FLAGS"
Risk Factors
Injection drug use Neglected diabetic foot ulcer Infection of scrotum or perineum
Skin signs
Tense edema Vullae Skin necrosis Crepitus
Diagnostic tests
Gas in tissues on x-ray or CT Extreme leukocytosis Hyponatremia

Table 57–2 • **THE 3 MAIN TYPES OF SKIN AND SOFT TISSUE INFECTIONS: USUAL ETIOLOGIC PATHOGENS AND COMMONLY RECOMMENDED ANTIBIOTICS**

SSTI Type	Pathogens	Recommended Antibiotics
Abscess	S aureus (often MRSA)	TMP-SMX clindamycin vancomycin
Nonpurulent cellulitis	β-hemolytic Streptococcus (such as S pygenes)	Cephalexin cefazolin
NSTI	S aureus (incl. MRSA) β-hemolytic Streptococcus Clostridial species (often C perfringens)	Clindamycin vancomycin pipercillin-tazobactam

Abbreviations: SSTI = skin and soft tissue infection; MRSA = methicillin-resistant Staphylococcus aureus; NSTI = necrotizing skin and soft tissue infection.

Management

Abscesses require drainage. Management begins with providing complete analgesia for the procedure. Options include local anesthetic, regional nerve block, and procedural sedation. In most cases drainage is best accomplished by incision with a scalpel and exploration of the cavity with a clamp, although needle aspiration is a good option for small abscesses on the face. Delaying drainage for a follow up visit is rarely the right plan. Small abscesses do not require packing. Large abscesses should be packed and the packing can be changed at 24-hour, either upon emergency department follow-up or by the patient themselves. Most simple abscesses do not require any antibiotics after incision and drainage. Small and uncomplicated abscesses rarely cause fever. If fever is present in these patient alternative sources should be considered. Antibiotics should be reserved for complicated abscesses, defined as >5cm, having a large area of surrounding cellulitis, or occurring in an immunosuppressed host. Admission for IV antibiotics should be considered for large abscesses accompanied by fever. Staphylococcal coverage, including MRSA, is required. Recommended agents include trimethoprim-sulfamethoxazole for oral therapy and vancomycin for IV therapy.

Nonpurulent cellulitis requires antibiotics for cure. Most cases can be treated with oral antibiotics and elevation of the affected part. Good Streptococcal coverage is required, usually with a first generation cephalosporin. (Therapy for purulent cellulitis must cover Staphylococcus as well; see above.) Admission for IV antibiotics is usually required if there is fever, lymphangitis or poorly controlled diabetes.

The biggest challenge with NSTIs is timely diagnosis. Once the suspicion for necrotizing infection reaches a reasonable threshold, the emergency physician should immediately consult a surgeon and request operative exploration for both definitive diagnosis and treatment. Immediate broad-spectrum antibiotic therapy is also important, and must cover streptococcal species, anaerobes and MRSA. Good choices are vancomycin plus clindamycin or piperacillin-tazobactam. If signs of sepsis are present (hypotension or lactate >4 mg/dL), central access and early goal directed therapy should be initiated.

COMPREHENSIVE QUESTIONS

57.1 A 40-year-old woman complains of a spider bite on her leg. What is the most likely diagnosis and etiologic organism?

A. Spider bite from a dermonecrotic spider species

B. Impetigo from Group A *Streptococcus*

C. Abscess from a polymicrobial mix of species including *Streptococcus milleri*

D. Furuncle from methicillin-resistant *S aureus*

57.2 A 35-year-old HIV-positive injection drug user presents complaining of a hip abscess where he injects heroin. The temperature is 38.1°C and there is a 10 × 10 cm circular area of erythema and induration on the lateral buttock without fluctuance. Which is the correct management?

A. Prescribe oral cephalexin for cellulitis and instruct the patient to return in 24 hours to assess whether an abscess has developed.

B. Attempt needle aspiration at the center of the infection, and if negative, cover with oral antibiotics.

C. Search for an abscess with bedside ultrasound and establish an IV in anticipation of a drainage procedure and admission for IV antibiotics.

D. Consult a surgeon immediately for suspected necrotizing skin and soft tissue infection.

57.3 An otherwise healthy young man presents with a 5 cm abscess on the lateral buttock. He is afebrile. The correct management includes all of the following except:

A. Pack the abscess and have the patient remove the packing himself within 24 hours and soak or bathe twice per day.

B. Treat with an oral first generation cephalosporin.

C. Incise with a scalpel and explore and open the cavity with a clamp.

D. Provide analgesia with oral ibuprofen and a ring of local anesthetic around the abscess.

57.4 Which of the following is true about necrotizing soft tissue infections?

A. Blood pressure in the normal range and normal renal function are strong evidence against this diagnosis.

B. In suspected cases, admission to a medical service for IV antibiotics with surgical consultation as needed is reasonable management.

C. Skin bullae or necrosis or subcutaneous crepitus or tissue gas on x-ray are usually found.

D. Poorly controlled diabetes is the most common risk factor in community onset infection.

E. Vancomycin to cover MRSA is recommended component of empirical antibiotics.

ANSWERS

57.1 **A.** Necrotic spider bites are unusual, whereas spontaneous furuncles (superficial skin abscesses) are extremely common in emergency practice. Patients with furuncles often complain of a "spider bite". MRSA accounts for 50% to 60% of all SSTIs in US emergency departments and may be even more common in spontaneous furuncles. While most of these simple infections are cured by incision and drainage alone, if antibiotics are deemed necessary, MRSA coverage is a must, with either trimethoprim-sulfamethoxazole, doxycycline or clindamycin.

57.2 **C.** This case is a classical presentation for a deep buttock or thigh abscess related to heroin injection. A septic hip or necrotizing infection should also be considered, although consultation for suspected NSTI is premature at this point. Nonpurulent cellulitis is very unlikely and simply treating with antibiotics is incorrect management. These abscesses can be very large and may cause a low-grade fever. When there is no obvious fluctuance, imaging with should be pursued with ultrasound, or occasionally CT, to confirm the diagnosis and guide drainage. Needle aspiration is reserved for small facial abscesses, and has no proven diagnostic role. Given the fever, this patient will likely require IV antibiotics and admission, as well procedural sedation via IV.

57.3 **B.** In a healthy host, an abscess 5 cm or less with only minimal to moderate surrounding cellulitis does not require antibiotics. This is supported by multiple studies. Long acting local anesthetic, such as bupivicaine, should be deposited in a ring around the abscess several minutes before incision and drainage. Packing is advised for abscesses that are more than a cm or so below the skin surface, as is commonly encountered in the buttocks, but it can be removed by the patient, with or without repacking. Soaking and scrubbing with soapy water is also recommended.

57.4 **E.** Necrotizing soft tissue infections are uncommon but potentially devastating and the diagnosis is rarely obvious at first presentation. Shock or organ dysfunction is initially evident in only 0% to 40% of cases. Classical skin signs are important red flags to recognize, but are frequently absent, and gas on plane x-ray is seen in 30% of cases, at most. Risk factors include diabetic foot ulcer, infections of the scrotum and perineum in men and injection drug use—which, in urban centers, is the leading cause of community onset necrotizing infections. Importantly, group A streptococcal NSTIs can occur spontaneously. NSTIs caused by community-associated MRSA have been reported.

REFERENCES

Chen JL, Fullerton KE, Flynn NM. Necrotizing fasciitis associated with injection drug use. *Clin Infect Dis.* 2001;33(1):6-15.

Jeng A, Beheshti M, Li J, et al. The role of beta-hemolytic streptococci in causing diffuse, nonculturable cellulitis: a prospective investigation. *Medicine (Baltimore).* 2010;89(4):217-226.

Moran GJ, Krishnadasan A, Gorwitz RJ, et al. Methicillin-resistant *S aureus* infections among patients in the emergency department. *N Engl J Med.* 2006 17;355(7):666-674.

Napolitano LM. Severe soft tissue infections. *Infect Dis Clin North Am.* 2009;23(3):571-591.

Talan DA. Lack of antibiotic efficacy for simple abscesses: have matters come to a head? *Ann Emerg Med.* 2010;55(5):412-414.

A 3-year-old boy is brought to the emergency department (ED) by his parents because of a rash that developed yesterday evening. The rash began on his neck and chest, then gradually spread to include his entire body except for his face. It does not seem to be painful nor pruritic. Although the child has had a fever and mild cough recently, he states that he "feels fine" and has not had any change in his behavior or oral intake. His parents deny any recent travel, camping or contact with animals. However, the boy does attend daycare, and several other children there have been ill recently. He is an otherwise healthy child with no history of major illness or medication allergies. He is taking acetaminophen as needed for the fever, and his immunizations are up to date.

On examination, his temperature is 38.9°C (102.1°F), blood pressure is 96/50 mm Hg, heart rate is 112 beats per minute, respiratory rate is 18 breaths per minute, and oxygen saturation is 98% on room air. The boy is sleeping comfortably in his mother arms but awakes easily during the examination. He does not appear acutely ill. His examination is unremarkable except for an erythematous maculo-papular rash covering his neck, torso and extremities.

► What is the most likely diagnosis?
► How should this patient be managed?

ANSWERS TO CASE 58:

Rash With Fever

Summary: This is a 3-year-old boy that presents with a rash, fever, and mild upper respiratory symptoms. On examination, he appears well and hydrated. He has a generalized maculopapular rash that spares the face.

- **Most likely diagnosis:** Viral exanthem

- **Management:** Symptomatic relief (eg, fever control) and follow up with his primary care physician as needed

ANALYSIS

Objectives

1. Define terminology used to describe rashes.

2. Review several causes of rash with fever.

3. Identify "red flags" associated with serious causes of rash.

Considerations

This 3-year-old boy has a maculopapular rash associated with fever and mild cough. The differential diagnosis is broad but can be focused by taking a detailed history and performing a thorough examination (that includes noting the appearance and distribution of skin lesions). Identifying specific etiologies may be difficult as multiple organisms and disease processes often cause similar types of rashes. Although most rashes are not associated with serious or life-threatening disorders, the ED physician must be able to identify those that are.

APPROACH TO:

Rash With Fever

CLINICAL APPROACH

Patients presenting with rash and fever have a broad differential diagnosis that includes relatively minor as well as life-threatening etiologies. A thorough history and physical examination and familiarity with common patterns of skin lesions and their potential causes will help the emergency physician make a quick diagnosis and accurate treatment plan.

Important historical questions include initial appearance and location of skin lesions, direction and rate of progression, duration of rash, and associated features such as pain or pruritis. The clinician should also inquire about systemic complaints (eg, fever, cough, sore throat, vomiting, diarrhea, seizures, mental status changes, and joint pain) and recent exposures (eg, medications, known allergens, animals, chemicals, foods, travel, and sick contacts). Past medical, family, and sexual histories may also provide clues as to the etiology of the rash.

Table 58–1 • DESCRIPTORS OF COMMON SKIN LESIONS	
Macule	Flat, circumscribed area ≤1 cm of discoloration
Patch	Flat, circumscribed area >1 cm of discoloration
Papule	Solid, raised lesion <0.5 cm in diameter
Nodule	Similar to papule but located deeper in the dermis or subcutaneous tissue; >0.5cm in diameter
Plaque	Solid, raised lesion >0.5 cm in diameter, often formed by confluence of papules
Pustule	Circumscribed, raised, containing purulent fluid
Vesicle	Circumscribed, raised, fluid-containing lesion, <0.5 cm
Bullae	Same as vesicle, except >0.5 cm in diameter
Petechiae	Small(<2-3 mm), flat, nonblanching red or purple spots caused by capillary hemorrhage
Purpura	Larger (>2-3 mm), flat, nonblanching purple discoloration
Wheal	Edematous, transient plaque

Patients with abnormal vital signs or evidence of toxicity may require initial stabilization before a detailed examination can be performed. If the patient is stable, care should be taken to inspect the entire body including mucous membranes. It is important to identify the color, morphology (listed in Table 58–1), location, and pattern of arrangement (including symmetry and configuration) of any lesions. A complete physical examination can help elicit additional diagnostic clues (eg, neck examination for nuchal rigidity and neurologic exam in patients with suspected meningococcemia [see Figure 58–1] or pelvic examination in those with possible disseminated gonococcemia). Although laboratory testing is not required for the evaluation of most rashes, it may be useful in some specific circumstances such

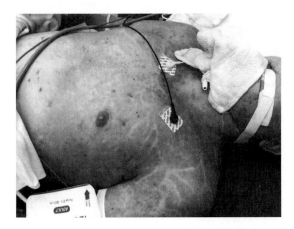

Figure 58–1. Fulminant meningococcemia with extensive purpuric patches.

as coagulation studies and platelet counts in patients with petechia or purpura or VDRL testing for suspected syphilis.

When developing a differential diagnosis, the clinician should consider three main categories: infectious, allergic, and rheumatologic. Table 58–2 includes

Table 58–2 • INFECTIOUS CAUSES OF RASH WITH FEVER		
Disease	**Rash**	**Diagnostic**
Rubella	Pink macular rash beginning on face, spreading to truck and extremities	Rash before fever. Upper respiratory symptoms. Forschheimer spots (soft palate petechiae)
Rubeola (Measles)	Red to brown maculopapular rash begins on face, neck, and shoulders, then spreads	The 3 Cs: cough, coryza, conjunctivitis. Associated with upper respiratory infection. Fever before rash, Koplik spots (bluish-white papules on red base on buccal mucosa)
Roseola (Human herpes virus 6)	Face-sparing pink maculopapular rash	Classically described as sudden onset of rash after resolution of high fever
Fifth disease (Erythema infectiosum)	Bright red facial rash or/with lacy reticular rash	Children: "slapped cheek" appearance. Adults: rash after fever associated arthralgias and myalgias. May be associated with aplastic crisis. Caused by Parvovirus B19
Hand, foot and mouth disease	Ulcer-like eruption in mouth with macular rash on palms and soles	1 to 2 days of fever followed by mouth ulcers and rash. Caused by enteroviruses
Scarlet fever	Erythematous "sandpaper" rash with increased redness in skin folds	Recent acute tonsillar or skin infection. "Strawberry tongue," Pastia sign (confluent petechiae in skin folds)
Varicella (chicken pox)	Papules to vesicles ("dewdrops on a rose petal") to pustules that eventually crust	Viral prodrome. Typically starts on trunk and spreads outward. Crops of lesions found in different stages. May include mucosal involvement. Consider acyclovir if complications or in immunocompromised patients
Lyme disease	Erythema migrans primary, macular rash secondary	Initial "bullseye" lesion associated with tick bite (caused by *Borrelia burgdorferi*). Associated fever, arthralgias, myalgias, malaise. Treat with doxycycline, amoxicillin, cefuroxime, ceftriaxone, erythromycin
Rocky Mountain spotted fever	Pink macules to red papules to petechiae. Begins on wrists, forearms, and ankles and spreads	Headache, myalgias, and rash with recent tick exposure. Possible bradycardia and leukopenia. Treat with doxycycline
Secondary syphilis	Red-pink maculopapular rash. Begins on trunk and spreads to palms and sole	Appears 2-3 months after initial chancre. Treat with penicillin or doxycycline

descriptions of several infectious causes of rash with fever. Differentiating an infectious from allergic rash can be difficult. Classically allergic rashes are pruritic rather than painful. They may be associated with the recent addition of a new medication or ingestion of an offending agent or appear in the area of contact with an environmental allergen. Wheals and urticaria are often associated with an allergic reaction. Rheumatologic rashes may appear similar to infectious or allergic ones but usually present with other systemic symptoms such as fever, fatigue, or arthralgias.

"Red flags" for potentially serious or life-threatening causes of rash include history of immunocompromised, fever, toxic appearance, hypotension, petechiae or purpura, diffuse erythema, severe or localized pain, and mucosal lesions. Petechiae and purpura can be associated with infectious conditions such as Rocky Mountain spotted fever or meningococcemia as well as coagulopathies such as disseminated intravascular coagulation. Diffuse erythema can be a harbinger of toxic shock syndrome, Staphylococcal scalded skin syndrome, or necrotizing fasciitis. Mucosal lesions may be a sign of Stevens-Johnson syndrome or toxic epidermal necrolysis (TEN). These conditions are classically associated with drug exposures (such as sulfa, phenytoin, and carbamazepine) or viral infections although many cases are idiopathic. Both conditions involve systemic symptoms (eg, fever), mucosal erosions, and diffuse cutaneous vesiculobullous lesions with epidermal detachment. They are differentiated by the amount of body surface area (BSA) involved (TEN: >30% BSA epidermal detachment). Patients with Stevens-Johnson syndrome and TEN are prone to infection and dehydration.

Treatment

Treatment is based on identification of the underlying process. The specific cause of many viral exanthems remains unidentified. These patients are usually treated symptomatically if they are otherwise well-appearing and hydrated. Rashes caused by bacteriologic organisms generally require antibiotic therapy. Table 58–2 lists some common disease processes with their appropriate diagnostic findings and treatments. Mild allergic reactions may be treated with removal of the offending allergen and antihistamines with or without corticosteroids. Patients with Steven-Johnson syndrome or TEN require admission for IV hydration and other supportive care.

COMPREHENSION QUESTIONS

58.1 A 6-year-old boy presents with a 3-day history of fever up to 102.2°F and rash. The mother reports associated cough, drainage from the right eye, and nasal irritation. What is the most likely diagnosis?

A. Rubeola

B. Roseola

C. Hand, foot, and mouth disease

D. Rubella

58.2 An 8-year-old boy presents with a pruritic rash and subjective fever after a weekend camping trip with the local Boy Scout troop. On examination, notice a linear, confluent maculopapular rash on the child leg. Which of the following findings is most specific for contact dermatitis secondary to an environmental exposure?

A. Fever

B. Maculopapular appearance

C. Pruritis

D. Linear confluence

58.3 A 2-year-old girl is brought to the ED by her parents for fever up to 103°F, decreased oral intake, and "not acting herself." On examination, the child is lethargic. She has pain with flexion of her neck. Note small, nonblanching red dots on her legs and torso. What is the best management option?

A. PO challenge and reassess

B. Begin IV hydration and empiric antibiotic treatment

C. Fever control and discharge home

D. Obtain laboratory testing to narrow the differential diagnosis

58.4 A 4-year-old girl presents with a fever, desquamating bullous rash covering her torso, and ulcers in her mouth and vaginal area. Her parents want to know what caused her condition. Which is the best answer?

A. Viral infection

B. Medication use

C. Idiopathic

D. Any of the above

ANSWERS

58.1 **A.** The boy symptoms are consistent with rubeola (measles). He displays the classic rash and "three Cs" (cough, conjunctivitis, and coryza).

58.2 **D.** Fever, pruritis, and maculopapular rash can be seen with numerous conditions. However, the linear confluence is more consistent with an allergic reaction secondary to an environmental exposure (eg, pattern due to an object, such as poison ivy, brushing against the boy leg).

58.3 **B.** This girl is lethargic. She has fever, meningeal signs, and a rash concerning for meningococcemia. Empiric antibiotic therapy should be started immediately.

58.4 **D.** The girl presentation is worrisome for Stevens-Johnsons syndrome, which can be caused by any of the aforementioned etiologies.

CLINICAL PEARLS

▶ A careful history and physical examination are useful in narrowing the differential diagnosis in patients with skin rashes.

▶ Patients with rashes should be examined from head to toe, including mucous membranes.

▶ "Red flags" for potentially serious or life-threatening causes of rash include history of immunocompromised, fever, toxic appearance, hypotension, petechiae or purpura, diffuse erythema, severe or localized pain, and mucosal lesions.

REFERENCES

Centers for Disease Control and Prevention. Diseases and Conditions. Available at: cdc.gov/DiseasesConditions/Accessed: March 31, 2012.

Cydulka RK, Garber B. Dermatologic Presentations. In: GL Mandell, JE Bennett, RD Douglas, eds. *Mandell, Douglas, and Bennett's Principles and Practice of Infectious Diseases.* Philadelphia, PA: Churchill Livingstone/Elsevier; 2010.

Kliegman, R, Nelson WE. *Nelson Textbook of Pediatrics.* Philadelphia: Saunders; 2007.

Letko E, Papaliodis DN, Papaliodis GN, et al. Stevens-Johnson syndrome and toxic epidermal necrolysis: A review of the literature. *Ann Allergy Asthma Immunol.* 2005;94(4):419-436.

Marx JA, Hockberger RS, Walls RM, et al. *Rosen's Emergency Medicine: Concepts and Clinical Practice.* 7th ed. Philadelphia: Mosby/Elsevier; 2009.

Schlossberg D. Fever and rash. *Infect Dis Clin North Am.* 1996;10:101-10.

Tintinalli JE, Stapczynski JS. *Tintinalli's Emergency Medicine: A Comprehensive Study Guide.* New York: McGraw-Hill; 2011.

Wolff K, Johnson RA, Fitzpatrick TB. *Fitzpatrick's Color Atlas and Synopsis of Clinical Dermatology.* New York: McGraw-Hill Medical; 2009.

Listing of Cases

Listing by Case Number

Listing by Disorder (Alphabetical)

Listing by Case Number

CASE NO.	DISEASE	CASE PAGE
1	Streptococcal Pharyngitis ("Strep Throat")	18
2	Myocardial Infarction, Acute	30
3	Atrial Fibrillation	40
4	Regular Rate Tachycardia	54
5	Diabetic Ketoacidosis	62
6	Severe Sepsis	70
7	Hemorrhagic Shock	82
8	Penetrating Trauma to the Chest, Abdomen, and Extremities	94
9	Extremity Fracture and Neck Pain	104
10	Anaphylaxis	114
11	Acute Exacerbation of Asthma	124
12	Facial Laceration	136
13	Rabies/Animal Bite	150
14	Stroke	158
15	Syncope	170
16	Pulmonary Embolism	182
17	Hypertensive Encephalopathy	196
18	Acute Abdominal Pain	208
19	Swallowed Foreign Body	220
20	Intestinal Obstruction	226
21	Acute Diarrhea	236
22	Nephrolithiasis	244
23	Acute Urinary Retention	252
24	Acute Pelvic Inflammatory Disease	260
25	Bell Palsy (Idiopathic Facial Paralysis)	268
26	Ectopic Pregnancy	274
27	Hyperemesis Gravidarum and OB Emergencies less than 26 Weeks' Gestation	282
28	Fever Without a Source in the 1- to 3-Month-Old Infant	296
29	Red Eye	304
30	Bacterial Meningitis	314
31	Seizure Induced by Traumatic Brain Injury	322
32	Altered Mental Status	334
33	Transient Synovitis	346
34	Febrile Seizure	358
35	Low Back Pain	366
36	Bacterial Pneumonia	372
37	Gastrointestinal Bleeding	380
38	Congestive Heart Failure/Pulmonary Edema	388

39	Cocaine Intoxication	396
40	Acetaminophen Toxicity	402
41	Sickle Cell Crisis	412
42	Frostbite and Hypothermia	424
43	Submersion Injury	438
44	Headache	446
45	Heat-Related Illnesses	454
46	Lightning and Electrical Injury	460
47	Transfusion Complications	468
48	Scrotal Pain	478
49	Trauma and Extremes of Age	486
50	Dysfunctional Uterine Bleeding	498
51	Noncardiac Chest Pain	506
52	Hyperkalemia due to Renal Failure	518
53	Acute Pyelonephritis	528
54	Airway Management/Respiratory Failure	540
55	Ethanol Withdrawal	554
56	Anti-muscarinic Toxidrome	560
57	Skin and Soft Tissue Infections	572
58	Rash With Fever	582

Listing by Disorder (Alphabetical)

CASE NO.	DISEASE	CASE PAGE
40	Acetaminophen Toxicity	402
18	Acute Abdominal Pain	208
21	Acute Diarrhea	236
11	Acute Exacerbation of Asthma	124
24	Acute Pelvic Inflammatory Disease	260
53	Acute Pyelonephritis	528
23	Acute Urinary Retention	252
54	Airway Management/Respiratory Failure	540
32	Altered Mental Status	334
10	Anaphylaxis	114
56	Anti-muscarinic Toxidrome	560
3	Atrial Fibrillation	40
30	Bacterial Meningitis	314
36	Bacterial Pneumonia	372
25	Bell Palsy (Idiopathic Facial Paralysis)	268
39	Cocaine Intoxication	396
38	Congestive Heart Failure/Pulmonary Edema	388

5	Diabetic Ketoacidosis	62
50	Dysfunctional Uterine Bleeding	498
26	Ectopic Pregnancy	274
55	Ethanol Withdrawal	554
9	Extremity Fracture and Neck Pain	104
12	Facial Laceration	136
34	Febrile Seizure	358
28	Fever Without a Source in the 1- to 3-Month-Old Infant	296
42	Frostbite and Hypothermia	424
37	Gastrointestinal Bleeding	380
44	Headache	446
45	Heat-Related Illnesses	454
7	Hemorrhagic Shock	82
27	Hyperemesis Gravidarum and OB Emergencies less than 26 Weeks' Gestation	282
52	Hyperkalemia due to Renal Failure	518
17	Hypertensive Encephalopathy	196
20	Intestinal Obstruction	226
46	Lightning and Electrical Injury	460
35	Low Back Pain	366
2	Myocardial Infarction, Acute	30
22	Nephrolithiasis	244
51	Noncardiac Chest Pain	506
8	Penetrating Trauma to the Chest, Abdomen, and Extremities	94
16	Pulmonary Embolism	182
13	Rabies/Animal Bite	150
58	Rash With Fever	582
29	Red Eye	304
4	Regular Rate Tachycardia	54
48	Scrotal Pain	478
31	Seizure Induced by Traumatic Brain Injury	322
6	Severe Sepsis	70
41	Sickle Cell Crisis	412
57	Skin and Soft Tissue Infections	572
1	Streptococcal Pharyngitis ("Strep Throat")	18
14	Stroke	158
43	Submersion Injury	438
19	Swallowed Foreign Body	220
15	Syncope	170
47	Transfusion Complications	468
33	Transient Synovitis	346
49	Trauma and Extremes of Age	486

Page numbers followed by *f* or *t* indicate figures or tables, respectively.

A

ABCDE, in trauma evaluation, 94
ABCs
  in anti-muscarinic toxidrome, 561
  in initial assessment, 7*f*, 8, 9*t*
  in trauma assessment, 82, 83*f*
Abdominal, infection, 72*t*
Abdominal examination, 4
Abdominal pain
  acute
    clinical approach, 210-214, 216
    clinical pearls, 216
    clinical presentation, 207-208
    differential diagnosis, 265
    in elderly patients, 211-212
    nonsurgical causes, 210-211
    surgical causes, 210
    in women, 207-209, 211, 279
  in acute pancreatitis, 212-214
  in bowel obstruction. *See* Bowel
    obstruction
  chronic or recurrent, 214
  in ectopic pregnancy, 274. *See also*
    Ectopic pregnancy
  in nephrolithiasis, 244. *See also*
    Nephrolithiasis
  in pelvic inflammatory disease,
    260
Abdominal trauma, 96*t*, 98
Abortion
  inevitable, 284
  spontaneous, 283-284
Abscess
  retropharyngeal and peritonsillar,
    23*t*
  tubo-ovarian, 261
ACE inhibitors. *See* Angiotensin-
    converting enzyme inhibitors

Acetaminophen (APAP) toxicity,
  563
  clinical pearls, 410
  clinical phases, 403*t*, 407*f*
  clinical presentation, 401-402
  complications, 402
  evaluation, 403-404
  pathophysiology, 403
  treatment, 404, 406-407
Acidosis
  in diabetic ketoacidosis, 65
  differential diagnosis, 64*t*
  in hemorrhagic shock, 87
ACS. *See* Acute coronary syndrome
Activated charcoal, 405*t*, 562, 562*t*
Activated protein C, for sepsis,
  75-76
Acute angle-closure glaucoma
  clinical presentation, 303-304,
    306*f*
  diagnosis, 305
  pathophysiology, 305, 311
  treatment, 305-306
Acute cerebral infarction/hemorrhage,
  203
Acute chest syndrome, 412, 413, 414,
  415*t*, 417, 420
Acute coronary syndrome (ACS)
  clinical pearls, 38
  clinical presentation, 29-30
  definition, 31
  evaluation, 31-34
    ECG findings, 31-32, 32*t*
    history and physical findings, 33*t*
  pathophysiology, 30-31
  risk factors, 33*t*
  TIMI risk score, 34*t*
  treatment, 34-36, 35*t*

Acute hemolytic transfusion reactions, 469

Acute lung injury (ALI)
in sepsis, 76
transfusion-related, 470-471, 474

Acute myocardial infarction, 203.
See also Acute coronary syndrome
clinical presentation, 29-30
complications, 36-37, 36t
pathophysiology, 30-31
treatment, 30, 34-36, 35t

Acute otitis media, 359, 360

Acute respiratory distress syndrome (ARDS), 76

Acyclovir, 270

Adjunctive therapy, 418

AEIOU TIPS mnemonic, in altered mental status, 337, 338t

Afterdrop (in hypothermia), 431

Agitation, 335

Airway complications
in anaphylaxis, 114-115, 120
infection-related, 18, 23, 23t, 26
obstruction, 539-540, 550

Airway management
airway adjuncts, 543
airway positioning in, 542
airway protection, 541
anticipated clinical deterioration, 542
clinical pearls, 550
evaluation of, 541-543
facilitation of medical evaluation, 542
indications for intubation, 543
interventions, 542
noninvasive positive pressure ventilation in, 543
rapid sequence intubation for.
See Rapid sequence intubation
respiratory failure, 541
supplemental oxygen, 542

Albuterol
for anaphylaxis, 118t
for asthma exacerbation, 127
for hyperkalemia, 521t, 522, 524

Alcohol withdrawal
clinical approach, 555-556
clinical pearls, 558
clinical presentation, 553-554
complications, 554
diagnosis, 556
differential diagnosis, 555
seizures induced by, 327
treatment, 554, 556

ALI. *See* Acute lung injury

Allergic reactions. *See also* Anaphylaxis
history of, 3
transfusion-related, 470

Alloimmunization, 472

Alteplase, 164

Altered mental status
in bacterial meningitis, 314-315.
See also Meningitis, bacterial
clinical approach, 335-339
clinical pearls, 343
clinical presentation, 333-334
diagnosis of, 338t
initial evaluation, 339-340
management, 339-341, 339t, 343
physical examination findings for, 336-337t

Alternating current (AC), 461

Amenorrhea, 499

Amides, 139t

Aminophylline, 129

Amiodarone
for atrial fibrillation, 44t, 47
for pharmacologic cardioversion, 46t

Amoxicillin/clavulanate, 532, 532t

Ampicillin, 318t

Ampicillin/sulbactam, 263t

AMPLE guide, in trauma, 84t

Amyl nitrate, 405t

Anaphylaxis
causes, 116
clinical criteria for diagnosis, 117
clinical pearls, 121
clinical pitfalls, 116t

clinical presentation, 113-114, 120
diagnosis, 116-117
epidemiology, 115
pathophysiology, 115-116
prevention, 117
transfusion-related, 470
treatment, 115, 117-119, 120
Anesthesia
isoflurane, 326, 329t
local, 138, 139t
Angiodysplasia, 383t
Angiotensin-converting enzyme
(ACE) inhibitors
for heart failure, 391
transfusion reactions and, 470
Animal bite
bacterial infections from, 151-152
clinical pearls, 155
clinical presentation, 149-150
general management, 151, 154
skin and soft tissue infections from,
575
Ankle-brachial indexes (ABI), 99
Anterior abdomen, 95, 98-99
Anterior uveitis, 308, 311
Antibiotics
for acute chest syndrome, 417
after animal bite, 151-152
for bacterial meningitis, 318t
C difficile infection following, 239
for necrotizing skin and soft tissue
infections, 576
for pelvic inflammatory disease,
262-263, 263t
for pneumonia, 375, 377
for sepsis, 74
for skin abscesses, 576
for skin and soft tissue infections,
573, 576t
in submersion injury, 441, 442
for traveler's diarrhea, 239
for urinary tract infections, 532,
532t
Anticholinergic agents
for asthma exacerbation, 128
overdose, 404t

Anticoagulants
for deep venous thrombosis/
pulmonary embolism, 184, 186,
186t
pre-cardioversion, 45-47, 45t
Antidotes, 405-406t, 561
Anti-muscarinic drugs, 566
Anti-muscarinic toxidrome. See also
Toxidromes
clinical presentation, 559-560,
565t
treatment of, 560, 565t, 566-567,
569
Aortic aneurysm, 511
Aortic dissection, 203, 511
Aortoenteric fistula, 383t
APAP toxicity. See Acetaminophen
toxicity
Aplastic crisis, 413, 416t, 418
Aspirin
in acute coronary syndrome, 35
in atrial fibrillation, 48, 48t
Asthma
acute exacerbation, 284-285
admission/discharge criteria,
130-131
clinical pearls, 133
clinical presentation, 123-124
diagnosis, 125-126
indications for ancillary tests,
127t
initial management, 124
risk factors, 126t
treatment, 124, 126-130, 132
epidemiology, 124-125
pathophysiology, 125
phases, 125
triggers, 126t
Atenolol, 44t, 287
ATLS classification, hemorrhage, 86t
Atrial fibrillation, 434
clinical approach, 41-42, 43f
clinical pearls, 50
clinical presentation, 39-41
complications, 42, 49
diseases associated with, 41-42, 41t

Atrial fibrillation (*Cont.*):
    pathophysiology, 42
    thromboembolic risk in, 42, 47-48,
        48t
    treatment, 42-43, 44t
Atropine, 569
Auricular hematoma, 137
Autoregulation, 199-200
Azotemia, 253

B
Back, penetrating injury to, 95, 99
Bacterial meningitis. *See* Meningitis,
        bacterial
Bacterial pneumonia. *See* Pneumonia,
        bacterial
Bacteriuria, 529
Barbiturates, for seizures, 326
Barium, 507
Basilar artery occlusion, 159t
Bat bite, 149-150, 155.
        See also Animal bite
Battered child. *See* Child abuse
Bees, allergy to, 116
Bell palsy
    alarm signals, 268t
    clinical approach, 269
    clinical pearls, 272
    clinical presentation, 267-268, 271
    differential diagnosis, 269, 271
    treatment, 268, 270
Benign prostatic hyperplasia, 253
Benzodiazepines, 555
    for alcohol withdrawal, 556, 557
    for altered mental status, 341
    for anti-muscarinic toxidrome,
        560, 565t, 567
    in cocaine intoxication, 398, 399
    for heat stroke, 456, 457
    overdose, 404t
    for seizure, 325, 326
    for sympathomimetic toxidrome,
        565t, 566
β-blockers
    for acute angle-closure glaucoma,
        306

for acute coronary syndrome, 35
for atrial fibrillation, 44t
contraindications, 398, 399
for hyperthyroidism, 287-288
overdose, 405t, 406t
for regular rate tachycardia, 58
Beta-2-agonist, 285
Bi-level positive airway pressure
        (BiPAP), 130, 541
Bismuth subsalicylate, 240
Blood transfusion
    complications of
        acute lung injury, 470-471
        allergic reactions, 470
        alloimmunization, 472
        clinical presentation, 467-468
        delayed hemolytic, 471
        febrile nonhemolytic reactions,
            469-470
        graft-versus-host disease,
            471-472
        infectious, 472
        post-transfusion purpura, 472
        prevention, 468
        risk factors, 468
    for hemorrhagic shock, 88
    indications, 473
Body packer, 561
Body packing, 221t, 397, 398
Body stuffer, 561
Boerhaave syndrome
    clinical approach, 508-512
    clinical pearls, 514
    clinical presentation, 505-506, 512
    complications, 508
    definition, 507
    differential diagnosis, 506
    evaluation, 507-508, 513
    pathophysiology, 507
    treatment, 508
Bone scan, in child with a limp, 349
Bowel necrosis, 230
Bowel obstruction
    clinical pearls, 233
    clinical presentation, 225-226, 229,
        233

closed-loop, 227
complications, 227, 231
differential diagnosis, 226
functional, 227
initial evaluation, 226
small vs large, 228t
management of, 230-231
mechanical, 227
neurogenic, 227
open-loop, 227
pathophysiology, 228
simple, 227
treatment, 230-231
Bradydysrhythmias, 171
Brain, anatomy of, 160f
Brain tumor, 448t, 449t, 450
Breast examination, 4
Breast pain, 512
Brown-Séquard syndrome, 111
B-type natriuretic peptide, 390-391
Bumetanide, 391
Bupivacaine, 139t, 578
Button battery, ingestion, 221t, 224

C
Calcium channel blockers, 44t
Calcium chloride, 405t, 521, 521t
Calcium gluconate, 405t, 409, 521,
521t
Calcium oxalate stones, 245, 246.
See also Nephrolithiasis
Campylobacter, 237t
Canadian C-spine rule (CCR), 105
Carbapenem, 375
Carbonic anhydrase inhibitors, 306
Cardiac arrest, after lightning strike,
460
Cardiac box, 95
Cardiac examination, 4
Cardiac failure, in sepsis, 77
Cardiac markers, 34
Cardiac syncope, 171. See also
Syncope
Cardiac tamponade, 511
Cardiogenic shock, 37
Cardiomyopathy, 41, 42

Cardioversion
anticoagulation prior to, 45-47, 45t
for atrial fibrillation, 43-47, 46t,
49
Carpal bone fractures, 108-109
Catheter, urinary, 533t
Cauda equina syndrome, 365-367,
368t
Cefotaxime, 263t, 317, 318t
Cefotetan, 263t
Cefoxitin, 263t
Ceftizoxime, 263t
Ceftriaxone
for bacterial meningitis, 317
for fever without a source, 298
for pelvic inflammatory disease,
263t
for urinary tract infections, 532
Centor criteria, for streptococcal
pharyngitis, 20f, 20t, 26
Central venous oxygen saturation
(ScvO$_2$), in sepsis, 74-75
Central venous pressure (CVP), in
sepsis, 74
Cephalosporins, 318t, 375
Cerebellar hemorrhage, 160t
Cerebral edema, in diabetic
ketoacidosis, 65
Cerebrospinal fluid, 317t
Cerebrovascular accident. See Stroke
Cervical motion tenderness, 261,
265
CHADS2 score, 47-48t
Charcoal hemoperfusion, in drug
elimination, 563
Cheek, 142, 143f
Chest, 95
Chest compressions, 7f
Chest pain
in acute coronary syndrome, 34t
evaluation, 508
in myocardial infarction, 29-30
noncardiac
clinical approach, 508-509
clinical pearls, 514
clinical presentation, 505-506

Chest pain, noncardiac (*Cont.*):
  differential diagnosis, 506,
    509-512
  esophageal and gastrointestinal
    causes, 509-510
  evaluation, 507-508
  musculoskeletal causes, 509
  psychiatric causes, 510
  pulmonary causes, 186-187,
    510-511
Chest radiography
  in acute coronary syndrome, 34
  in chest trauma, 100
  in congestive heart failure, 390
  in pneumonia, 374-375
  in pulmonary embolism, 188, 193
  in submersion injury, 440
Chest trauma, 96t, 97
Chest X rays. *See* Chest radiography
Chief complaint, 2-3
Chilblains (Pernio), 425
Child abuse, 355
  clinical presentation, 485-487
  incidence, 489
  musculoskeletal manifestations,
    490, 490t
  patterns suggestive of, 487, 489-490,
    490t
  reporting requirements, 489
Children
  abuse. *See* Child abuse
  foreign body ingestion in, 219-220
  limp in
    clinical pearls, 355
    differential diagnosis, 347, 354
    history taking, 347-348
    laboratory studies in, 349
    in Legg-Calve-Perthes disease,
      348, 351, 352f, 354
    in Osgood-Schlatter disease, 353
    osteomyelitis, 348, 350, 351f
    physical examination of, 348-349
    septic arthritis, 350
    in slipped capital femoral
      epiphysis, 348, 351-352,
      352f, 354

    toddler's fracture, 352
    in transient synovitis, 345-346
  trauma in
    clinical pearls, 495
    GCS verbal scores, 488t
    hemorrhagic shock and, 488,
      488t
    initial evaluation and management,
      487, 488t
    intentional. *See* Child abuse
    vital signs by age group, 486t
Chlamydia, pneumonia caused by,
    374t
Chlamydia trachomatis
  ectopic pregnancy and, 275
  in pelvic inflammatory disease, 260
Chloroprocaine, 139t
Cholecystitis, 510
Cholelithiasis, 265
Cholinergic agents, 404t, 567
Cholinergic toxidrome, 565t, 567,
    569
Cimetidine, 118t
Ciprofloxacin, 240, 532, 532t
Clenched-fist injury, 151
Clindamycin, 263t
Clinical problem solving
  assessing disease severity, 9-10
  emergency assessment and
    management, 7f, 8, 9t
  making diagnosis, 8-9
  monitoring response to treatment,
    10
  treatment selection based on stage,
    10
Clinical questions
  complications, 13-14
  confirmation of diagnosis, 11, 12
  determination of best therapy, 14
  determination of likely diagnosis,
    11
  determination of next step, 12
  disease mechanisms, 13
  risk factors, 13
Clonazepam, 557
Clonidine, 556

Clopidogrel
    in acute coronary syndrome, 35
    in atrial fibrillation, 48
Closed-loop obstruction, 227. *See also*
        Bowel obstruction
Clostridium difficile, 237t
Clostridium perfringens, 237t, 238
Clostridium tetani, 142
Cluster headache, 448t, 449t, 451
Cocaine intoxication
    clinical pearls, 400
    clinical presentation, 395-396, 398
    complications, 397-398, 397t
    differential diagnosis, 396
    evaluation, 398
    seizures in, 326
    symptoms, 397
    treatment, 398
Coin, ingestion, 221t
Cold water submersion injury, 441.
        See also Submersion injury
Colonic perforation, 231
Colorectal cancer
    bleeding in, 383t
    bowel obstruction in, 231
Coma, 335
Community onset necrotizing fasciitis,
        575
Community-acquired pneumonia, 373.
        See also Pneumonia
Compartment syndrome, 465
Compensated shock, 85
Complex febrile seizure, 359. *See also*
        Febrile seizure
Computed tomography (CT)
    in abdominal pain, 216
    in acute pancreatitis, 213-214, 213t
    in acute renal colic, 247
    in bacterial meningitis, 316t
    in bowel obstruction, 226-227, 230
    in headache, 446
    high resolution angiography, 188
    in hypertensive emergencies, 196
    indications, in lightning injury,
        460
    multidetector, 183-184

    multidetector angiography, 188
    in nephrolithiasis, 247
    in penetrating trauma, 97, 100
    pulmonary angiography, 184
    in seizure, 324
    in stroke, 162-163
    in subarachnoid hemorrhage, 449
    venography, 188-189
Conduction, 425
Confusion, 335, 338t
Congestive heart failure
    clinical approach, 388-389
    clinical pearls, 392
    clinical presentation, 387-388,
        389t
    differential diagnosis, 389-390,
        390t
    etiologies, 389, 392
    evaluation, 389-391, 392
    left-sided, 389t, 392
    pathophysiology, 388-389
    right-sided, 389t, 392
    treatment, 388, 391, 392
Conjunctival injection, 308
Conjunctivitis, 307
Contrast dye, nephrotoxicity, 247t
Controlling hemorrhage, for hemor-
        rhagic shock, 88-89
Convection, 425-426
Coral snakebites, 153
Corneal ulcer, 307-308
Coronary heart disease, 33t. *See also*
        Acute coronary syndrome
Corticosteroids
    for asthma exacerbation, 128-129
    for bacterial meningitis, 317-318
    for Bell palsy, 270
    for sepsis, 75
Cough
    in pneumonia, 373
    in pulmonary embolism, 186-187
    in sickle cell crisis, 412
Coumadin. *See* Warfarin
Crackles, in pulmonary embolism,
        186
Cricothyroidotomy, emergency, 24f

Crystalloid solution, for hemorrhagic shock, 87-88
C-spine injury
clearing in the blunt trauma patient, 106-107
clinical pearls, 111
emergency department management of, 107
management of, 110
role of corticosteroids, 107-108
CT. *See* Computed tomography
Culturable cellulitis, 573, 574
Curling ulcers, 463
Cyanide antidote kit, 405t
Cystitis, 529, 532

D
Dabigatran, in atrial fibrillation, 47-48, 48t
Dactylitis, 414, 415t
Dalteparin, 186t. *See also* Low-molecular-weight heparin
D-dimer assay, 183, 184, 189, 193
Decontamination, 561
Deep venous thrombosis (DVT), 193. *See also* Pulmonary embolism
definition, 183
diagnosis, 184, 185f, 192
risk factors, 185t
Deferoxamine, 405t
Delayed hemolytic transfusion reactions, 471
Delirium, 335, 339t
Delirium tremens, 327, 555
Dementia, 335, 339t
Depression, 510
Dexamethasone, 317-318
Dextrose, 405t, 521t, 522
Diabetic ketoacidosis (DKA)
clinical approach, 63-65
clinical pearls, 67
clinical presentation, 61-62
complications, 65
diagnosis, 62t, 63-64, 64t, 66
illnesses causing, 67

pathophysiology, 63
treatment, 64-65
Diagnostic peritoneal lavage (DPL), 99
Diaphoresis, in pulmonary embolism, 186
Diarrhea
acute
clinical pearls, 241
clinical presentation, 235-236, 238-239
definition, 238
etiologies, 237t, 238
initial management, 236-237
treatment, 239-240
in bowel obstruction, 229
chronic, 238
definition, 238
persistent, 238
Diazepam, 325, 329t
DIC. *See* Disseminated intravascular coagulation
Digoxin, 44t
Digoxin immune Fab, 405t
Dihydroergotamine, 450
Diltiazem, 44t
Diphenhydramine, 118t
Direct antiglobulin test, 469
Direct current (DC), 461
Disseminated intravascular coagulation (DIC)
in sepsis, 76-77
transfusion-related, 469
Distal radius fractures, 108
Diverticulosis, 383t
DKA. *See* Diabetic ketoacidosis
Dobutamine, 391
Dofetilide, 46t
Dopamine, 391
Doxycycline, 263t
Dronedarone, for atrial fibrillation, 44t, 47
Drowning, 439. *See also* Submersion injury
Drug absorption, 561
Dry drowning, 440

DUMBBELLS mnemonic, in cholinergic toxidrome, 567, 569

DVT. *See* Deep venous thrombosis

Dysfunctional uterine bleeding
clinical pearls, 504
clinical presentation, 497-498
coagulopathy and, 503
differential diagnosis, 500*t*
etiologies, 501*t*
initial evaluation, 499-500
pathophysiology, 500-501
treatment, 501-502, 501*t*, 503

Dyspnea
in acute myocardial infarction, 29-30
in atrial fibrillation, 39-40
definition, 41
in pulmonary embolism, 186-187
in transfusion-related acute lung injury, 471

Dysuria, 529

E

Ears, trauma to, 142

ECG. *See* Electrocardiogram

Eclampsia, 197, 199, 203

Ectopic pregnancy
clinical approach, 275-277
clinical pearls, 280
clinical presentation, 273-274
definition, 275
diagnosis, 274, 276
differential diagnosis, 275-276
incidence, 275
as medical complications before 26 weeks of pregnancy, 284, 292
occurrence, 275
risk factors, 275
ruptured, 275
treatment, 276, 277*f*

Elderly patients
abdominal pain in, 211-212
hypothermia in, 426
physiological changes, 491-492, 491*t*
trauma in, outcome predictors of, 492-493, 492*t*

Electric injury
clinical approach, 461
complications, 462-463, 465
pathophysiology, 461-462
treatment, 462-463

Electrocardiogram (ECG)
in acetaminophen overdose, 403
in acute coronary syndrome, 31-32, 32*t*, 33*t*, 38
in hyperkalemia, 517*f*, 518*f*, 520-521, 524
in hypothermia, 427, 428-429*f*
in lightning and electric injury, 462
in pulmonary embolism, 182, 192
in regular rate tachycardia, 55, 56*f*, 57*t*, 59
sensitivity in prediction of cardiac disease, 508-509
in submersion injury, 440

Emesis, 229

Enalaprilat, 201*t*, 202

Encephalopathy, hypertensive, 195-197, 203, 204. *See also* Hypertensive emergencies

Endophthalmitis, traumatic, 308

Endotracheal intubation. *See* Rapid sequence intubation

Enoxaparin, 186, 186*t*. *See also* Low-molecular-weight heparin

Entamoeba histolytica, 237*t*

Envenomation, 153

Epididymitis, 479*t*, 482

Epiglottis, 23*t*

Epilepsy, 322. *See also* Seizure(s)

Epinephrine
for anaphylaxis, 117-118, 118*t*, 120
for asthma exacerbation, 127
in local anesthetics, 138, 139*t*

Erysipelas, 573, 574

Erythema migrans, 585*f*

Escherichia coli
in diarrhea, 237*t*, 238, 241
in urinary tract infections, 530

Esmolol, 44*t*, 200, 201*t*

Esophageal perforation.
See Boerhaave syndrome

Esophageal varices, 383*t*
Esters, 139*t*
Estrogen, 499, 501
Ethanol
    as antidote, 405*t*
    hypothermia and, 426
    intoxication of, 341
    withdrawal of. *See* Alcohol
        withdrawal
Ethylene glycol ingestion, 405*t*
Etomidate, 546, 547*t*
Eutectic mixture of local anesthetics
        (EMLA), 138
Evaporation, 426
Exertional heat stroke, 455
Extracorporeal membrane
        oxygenation, for sepsis, 76
Extracorporeal shock wave lithotripsy,
        245
Extremities, penetrating injury to, 99
Extremity fracture and neck pain,
        103-105
Eyelids, lacerations of, 140. *See also*
        Lacerations

F
Facial lacerations. *See also* Lacerations
    anatomic considerations, 143*f*
    clinical pearls, 147
    clinical presentation, 135-136
    initial evaluation, 136
    treatment, 141*f*, 142, 146
Facial nerve
    palsy, 268*t*, 269. *See also* Bell palsy
    trauma, 136, 143*f*
Facial trauma, 137. *See also* Facial
        lacerations
Family history, 3
Fasciotomy, 462
Febrile nonhemolytic transfusion
        reactions, 469-470
Febrile seizure. *See also* Seizure(s)
    clinical approach, 359-360
    clinical presentation, 357-358
    complex, 359
    prevention, 360

recurrence risk, 360
simple, 359
treatment, 361, 363
Fenoldopam, 201*t*, 202
Fever low-grade, in pulmonary
        embolism, 186
Fever without a source (FWS)
    clinical presentation, 295-296
    definition, 297
    diagnosis, 297
    evaluation, 297-298
    pathogens, 298
    treatment, 298
Fight bite, 151
Flame burns, 463
Flank, 95, 96*t*, 99
Flash burns, 463
Flashover phenomenon, 462*t*
Flecainide, 46*t*
Fluid resuscitation
    in anaphylaxis, 117, 118*t*
    for bowel obstruction, 231
    for diabetic ketoacidosis, 64-65,
        66
    in gastrointestinal bleeding, 383
    in hemorrhagic shock, 87-88
Flumazenil, 406*t*, 569
Fluoroquinolones, 375
Focused abdominal sonography for
        trauma (FAST), 85, 97, 98*f*
Folic acid, 405*t*
Fomepizole, 405*t*, 569
Fondaparinux, 186*t*
Food allergies, 116
Forced expiratory volume (FEV$_1$),
        284
Forearm fractures, 108
Foregut, 209
Forehead lacerations, 139-140. *See also*
        Lacerations
Foreign body
    aspirated, 509
    ingested
        vs aspirated, 222*t*
        clinical approach, 220-223
        clinical pearls, 224

clinical presentation, 219-220
diagnosis, 222
treatment, 221t, 222-223, 224
types, 221t
Fosphenytoin, 325
Fournier gangrene, 479t
Fractures, hemorrhagic shock and, 86
Fresh-frozen plasma, 383
Frostbite
clinical pearls, 434
clinical presentation, 423-424
definition, 425
pathophysiology, 429-430
phases, 429-430
risk factors, 424
treatment, 424, 430-431
Frostnip, 425
Fulminant meningococcemia, 583f
Furosemide, 391
Furuncles, 574, 578
FWS. See Fever without a source

G
Gastric lavage, 562-563
Gastric varices, 383t
Gastritis, 383t
Gastroesophageal reflux disease
(GERD), 509-510
Gastrografin, 507
Gastrointestinal bleeding
clinical approach, 381-383
clinical pearls, 385
clinical presentation, 379-380
etiologies, 381, 383t, 385
initial evaluation, 380-381, 385
lower, 382f
treatment, 383-384, 385
upper, 381f
Generalized seizures, 323. See also
Seizure(s)
Genital examination, 5
Gentamycin, 263t
Giardia, 237t
Glasgow coma scale, 6t, 339, 339t
Glaucoma, acute angle-closure. See
Acute angle-closure glaucoma

Glomerulonephritis, poststreptococcal,
22
Glucagon
for anaphylaxis, 118, 118t
as antidote, 405t, 409
Glucose control, in sepsis, 76
Graft-versus-host disease,
transfusion-related, 471-472
Graves disease, 288-289
Group A β-hemolytic streptococcus
(GAβS), 19-22. See also
Pharyngitis, streptococcal
Guillain-Barré syndrome, 271

H
Haemophilus influenzae, 374t
Haloperidol, 398, 556
Hampton hump, 188, 193
Head and neck examination, 4
Headache
alarm signals, 447
cerebral causes, 450
clinical approach, 447-448
clinical pearls, 452
diagnostic tests and treatment, 449t
etiologies, 447t, 448t
evaluation, 446, 447-448
history and examination findings,
448t
primary, 447, 450-451
severe, 445-446
in subarachnoid hemorrhage,
448-450
Healthcare-associated pneumonia,
373. See also Pneumonia
Heart failure. See Congestive heart
failure
Heat cramps, 456t
Heat edema, 456t
Heat exhaustion, 454, 456t
Heat loss, 425-426
Heat rash, 456t
Heat stress, 454
Heat stroke
clinical pearls, 458
clinical presentation, 453-454, 455

Heat stroke (*Cont.*):
  complications, 456
  definition, 455
  diagnosis, 455
  treatment, 455-456
Heat syncope, 456t
Heat-related illness
  clinical approach, 455
  clinical presentation, 453-454
  minor, 456t
  risk factors, 455
Heliox, for asthma exacerbation,
    126-127
HELLP syndrome, 199
Hematemesis, 381, 382. *See also*
    Gastrointestinal bleeding
Hematoma
  auricular, 142
  septal, 140, 146
Hematuria, 246-247, 529
Hemodialysis, 563
Hemoglobin desaturation curve,
    546f
Hemorrhagic shock
  in children, 488, 488t
  classification, 86t, 90
  clinical approach, 84-86
  clinical pearls, 90
  clinical presentation, 81-82
  definition, 84
  diagnostic approach
    central monitoring, 87
    identification of source of
      bleeding, 86
    laboratory evaluation, 86-87
  pathophysiology, 85-86
  treatment, 87-89
Hemorrhagic stroke, 159, 160t, 164.
    See also Stroke
Hepatic failure, in sepsis, 77
Hepatitis, chest pain in, 510
Hindgut, 209
History, patient approach and, 2-4
HMG Co-A reductase inhibitors, 76
Hospital-acquired pneumonia, 373.
    See also Pneumonia

Human bites, 151, 154
Human chorionic gonadotropin
    (hCG), 274, 276
Hunting reaction, 425
Hydralazine, 199, 201t, 202
Hydrocele, 479t
Hydrocortisone, 118t
Hydromorphone, 418
Hydronephrosis, 253
Hydrophobia, 150, 152
Hydroxycobalamin, 406t
Hydroxyurea, 418
Hypercalcemia, 340
Hyperemesis gravidarum, 283, 293
Hyperkalemia
  classification, 520
  clinical pearls, 524
  clinical presentation, 517-519,
    517f, 518f
  ECG changes in, 520-521, 524
  in hypothermia, 430
  in renal failure, 517-518
  treatment, 519, 521-522, 521t
Hypertension, 197
Hypertensive emergencies
  clinical approach, 197-203
  clinical pearls, 205
  clinical presentation, 195-196
  conditions associated with, 203
  definition, 197
  diagnosis, 198
  headache in, 448t, 449t, 452
  initial management, 196-197
  pathophysiology, 198
  in pregnancy, 199
  treatment, 199-202, 201t
Hypertensive encephalopathy,
    195-197, 203, 204
Hypertensive urgency, 197, 198, 204
Hyperthermia. *See* Heat-related
    illness
Hyperthyroidism, 287-289
Hyphema, 309
Hypocalcemia, 340
Hypopyon, 308
Hypotension, syncope, and, 172

Hypothermia
    clinical pearls, 434
    definition, 425
    evaluation, 430
    pathophysiology, 425-426
    risk factors, 426, 426t
    systemic effects, 427-428, 427t, 428f
    treatment, 430-431, 433

I

Ibutilide, 46t
Idiopathic intracranial hypertension,
        448t, 449t
Immersion syndrome, 439
Immune response
    in anaphylaxis, 115-116
    in sepsis, 71-72
Immunocompetent adult, suspected
        infection, 72t
In vitro fertilization, ectopic
        pregnancy, and, 276, 279
Incompetent cervix, 284
Induction agents, 546, 547t
Inevitable abortion, 284
Inferior vena cava (IVC) filters, 186
Inflammatory bowel disease, 265
Inguinal hernia, 479t
Inhaled corticosteroids (ICS), 131
Insulin
    for diabetic ketoacidosis, 64
    for hyperkalemia, 521t, 522
Intestinal obstruction. See Bowel
        obstruction
Intracerebral hemorrhage, 160t
Intraocular pressure (IOP), 305
Intravenous immunoglobulin (IVIG),
        76
Intravenous pyelogram (IVP), 247
Intubation, indications for, 543.
        See also Airway management
Ipratropium bromide
    for anaphylaxis, 118t
    for asthma exacerbation, 28
Iritis, 308
Iron overdose, 405t
Irreversible shock, 85

Irrigation, wound, 137
Ischemic stroke. See also Stroke
    clinical presentation, 159
    hypertensive emergency in, 203
    incidence, 159
    syndromes, 159t
    thrombolytic therapy for, 163t, 164
Isoflurane anesthesia, 326, 329t
Isoniazid, seizures induced by, 326-327

J

Jaw-thrust maneuver, 7f

K

Kayexalate. See Sodium polystyrene
        sulfonate
Keraunoparalysis, 462
Ketamine, 130, 546, 547t
Kingella kingae, 347
Klebsiella pneumoniae, 374t

L

Labetalol hydrochloride
    dosage, 201t
    for hypertensive emergencies,
        196-197, 200, 201t
    side effects and contraindications,
        201t
Lacerations
    clinical approach, 137-142
    clinical pearls, 147
    facial. See Facial lacerations
    treatment
        anesthesia, 138, 139t
        irrigation, 137
        suture size, 138t
        wound closure, 139
Lactate clearance, in sepsis, 75
Left ventricular end-diastolic volume,
        87
Legg-Calve-Perthes disease, 348,
        351, 352f, 354
Legionella, 374t
Leucovorin, 405t
Leukocyte-reduced packed red blood
        cells, 468

Leukotriene antagonists, 129

Levalbuterol, 128

Levetiracetam, 326

Levofloxacin, 532

Lichtenberg figure, 463

Lidocaine, 58, 139*t*, 545

Lightning injury
  clinical approach, 461
  clinical pearls, 466
  clinical presentation, 459-461
  complications, 460, 462-463
  pathophysiology, 461-462
  types, 462*t*

Limp, 347, 348*t*. *See also* Children,
  limp in

Lip laceration, 140-141, 141*f*, 146

Lipid emulsion, IV, 406*t*

Liver failure, in sepsis, 77

Local anesthesia, 138, 139*t*

Log roll test, 348

Lorazepam, 325, 329*t*, 556, 560, 569,
  570

Low back pain
  alarm symptoms, 366*t*
  clinical approach, 367-369
  clinical pearls, 370
  clinical presentation, 365-367
  differential diagnosis, 367, 368*t*
  etiologies, 368*t*
  treatment, 369

Low-molecular-weight heparin
  for acute coronary syndrome, 35
  for deep venous thrombosis/
    pulmonary embolism, 186

Ludwig angina, 23*t*

Lumbar puncture
  in bacterial meningitis, 315, 317*t*
  in headache evaluation, 446
  headache following, 448*t*, 449*t*
  in subarachnoid hemorrhage, 449

M

Mackler triad, 507

Magnesium ammonium phosphate
  stones, 246, 249. *See also*
  Nephrolithiasis

Magnesium sulfate
  for anaphylaxis, 118*t*
  for asthma exacerbation, 129

Magnetic resonance imaging (MRI)
  in child with a limp, 349
  indications, 6

Malignant hypertension. *See*
  Hypertensive emergencies

Mallampati score, 544

Mallory-Weiss tear, 381*f*, 383*t*, 512

Mean arterial pressure (MAP), in
  sepsis, 74

Medical history, 3

Melena, 381, 382. *See also*
  Gastrointestinal bleeding

Meningitis, bacterial
  clinical pearls, 319
  clinical presentation, 313-314
  common pathogens and antibiotic
    recommendations, 72*t*
  diagnosis, 315-316, 316*t*, 319
  headache in, 448*t*, 449*t*
  treatment, 316-318, 318*t*, 319

Menometrorrhagia, 499. *See also*
  Dysfunctional uterine bleeding

Menorrhagia, 499. *See also*
  Dysfunctional uterine bleeding

Meperidine, 418

Mepivacaine, 139*t*

Metabolic acidosis, 87

Metacarpal and phalangeal fractures,
  109

Methanol poisoning, 405*t*

Methotrexate
  complications, 279
  for ectopic pregnancy, 276

Methylene blue, 406*t*

Methylprednisolone, 118, 118*t*

Metoprolol, 35, 44*t*, 287

Metronidazole, 263*t*

Midazolam, 329*t*

Midgut, 209

Migraine headache, 448*t*, 449*t*, 450,
  452

Mitotics, 306

MONA mnemonic, for chest pain, 34

Mononucleosis, splenic rupture in, 26
Morphine, 37
Morphine sulfate
  in acute coronary syndrome, 34
  in sickle cell crisis, 418
MRI. *See* Magnetic resonance
    imaging
Multidose charcoal, in drug
    elimination, 563
Multiorgan dysfunction syndrome
    (MODS), 71, 77
Multiple sclerosis, 257, 271
Myasthenia gravis, 271
Mycoplasma pneumonia, 374t
Myocardial infarction
  clinical presentation, 29-30
  in cocaine intoxication, 398
  complications, 36-37, 36t
  definition, 31
  diagnosis, 32-33, 34t, 38
  ST-elevation, 31
  treatment, 30, 34-36, 35t

N
N-Acetylcysteine, for acetaminophen
    overdose, 402, 404, 405t,
    406-407, 409
Naloxone, 340, 406t, 410, 566, 569
Nasopharyngeal airway, 543
National Institutes of Health stroke
    scale (NIHSS), 159, 160-162,
    161-162t
Near-drowning. *See* Submersion
    injury
Necrotizing skin and soft tissue
    infections (NSTI), 572-576,
    575t, 576t, 578
Neisseria gonorrhoeae, 260, 347
Nephrolithiasis
  alarm signals, 248
  clinical pearls, 250
  clinical presentation, 243-244,
    246-247, 249
  definition, 245
  differential diagnosis, 244, 245t
  epidemiology, 245-246

  management, 247-248
  risk factors, 245-246, 246t
  treatment, 248, 249
Neurocysticercosis, 327
Neurogenic seizures, 323. *See also*
    Seizure(s)
Neuroleptics, 556
Neurological examination, 5
Nexus low-risk criteria, 105
Nicardipine, 201t, 202
Nimodipine, 449
NIPPV. *See* Noninvasive positive
    pressure ventilation
Nitrofurantoin, 532, 532t
Nitroglycerin
  for acute coronary syndrome,
    34, 37
  dosage, 201t
  for heart failure, 391, 392
  for hypertensive emergencies, 202
  indications, 201t
  side effects and contraindications,
    201t
Nonculturable cellulitis, 573
Nonepileptic seizures, 323. *See also*
    Seizure(s)
Noninvasive positive pressure
    ventilation (NIPPV), 440
  for asthma exacerbation, 130
  for heart failure, 391
  in respiratory failure, 543
Nonpurulent cellulitis, 573, 574, 576,
    576t
Non-ST-elevation myocardial
    infarction (NSTEMI), 31,
    35-36. *See also* Acute
    coronary syndrome
Nose, trauma to, 140

O
Obtunded, 335
Octreotide, 383, 406t
Ohm law, 461
Oligomenorrhea, 499
Open-loop obstruction, 227. *See also*
    Bowel obstruction

Opiates, 561, 564, 565t, 566
  intoxication, 400
  for migraine headache, 450
  overdose, 404t
  in sickle cell crisis, 418
Opioid, 561, 564, 565t, 566
Optic neuritis, 309
Oral contraceptives, for dysfunctional
    uterine bleeding, 499, 501
Orbital cellulitis, 308
Orchitis, 479t
Oropharyngeal airway, 543
Orthostasis, 172
Osgood-Schlatter disease, 353
Osservatorio Epidemiologico sulla
    Sincope nel Lazio (OESIL),
    175, 176t, 177f
Osteomyelitis, 348, 350, 351f
Ovarian torsion, 265
Oxygen therapy, for asthma
    exacerbation, 126

P
Pancreatitis, 265, 510
Paralytic agents, 547, 547t
Partial cord syndromes, 105
Partial seizures, 323. See also Seizure(s)
Patient, approach to. See also
    Clinical problem solving;
    Clinical questions
  history in, 2-4
  physical examination, 4-8, 6t
Pediatric autoimmune neuropsychiatric
    disorder associated with group
    A streptococci (PANDAS), 22
Pelvic inflammatory disease (PID)
  clinical approach, 261-263
  clinical pearls, 266
  clinical presentation, 259-260
  complications, 263
  definition, 261
  diagnosis, 261
  etiologies, 260, 261-262
  pathogenesis, 262
  treatment, 262-263, 262t, 263t
Pelvis trauma, 96t

Penicillin
  allergy to, 116
  for GAβS pharyngitis, 22
Pentobarbital, 329t
Peptic ulcer disease, 383t, 385, 510
Percutaneous coronary intervention
    (PCI), 34-35
Perfusion and ventilation (V/Q)
    scan, 183-184, 188
Pericardial friction rub, 511
Pericarditis, 511
Peritonsillar abscess, 23t
Pharyngitis
  clinical pearls, 26
  streptococcal, 17-26
    clinical approach, 19-24, 20f,
      20t, 25
    clinical presentation, 17-19
    complications, 21-23
    differential diagnosis, 19
    treatment, 22
Phenazopyridine, 532
Phencyclidine intoxication, 399
Phenobarbital
  mechanisms of action, 325
  for seizures, 325, 329t
  side effects, 325
Phenothiazines, 398, 456
Phentermine, 562
Phentolamine, 398, 399
Phenytoin, 325, 329t
Physical examination, patient
    approach and, 4-8, 6t
Physostigmine, 406t, 565t, 567
PID. See Pelvic inflammatory disease
Pilocarpine, 306
Platelet transfusion, 472
Pneumonia
  bacterial, 371-373, 374t
  clinical pearls, 377
  community-acquired, 373
  diagnosis, 373-374
  disposition, 375
  healthcare-associated, 371-372, 373
  hospital-acquired, 373
  pathophysiology, 373, 374t

risk factors, 373
treatment, 375, 377
Pneumothorax
chest pain in, 510-511
clinical presentation, 100
tension, 97
Poisoning
acetaminophen. *See* Acetaminophen
toxicity
antidotes, 405-406*t*
toxidromes, 404*t*
Polycystic ovarian syndrome (PCOS),
501
Pork tapeworm, 327
Poststreptococcal glomerulonephritis,
22
Posttransfusion purpura, 472
Potassium balance, 520
Pralidoxime, 406*t*, 565*t*, 567, 569
Prednisone
for anaphylaxis, 118, 118*t*
for asthma exacerbation, 128-129
for Bell palsy, 270
for temporal arteritis, 450
Preeclampsia, 197, 199, 203
Pregnancy
arterial blood gas findings in, 285*t*
ectopic. *See* Ectopic pregnancy
hypertensive disease in, 197, 199,
203
medical complications before 26
weeks, 283-290
urinary tract infections in, 533, 535
Preload, 87
Premature rupture of membranes
(PROM), 285-287
Pressure induced esophageal rupture,
512
Presyncope, 171
Preterm premature rupture of
membranes (PPROM), 285-287
Priapism, in sickle cell crisis, 415*t*, 418
Prilocaine, 139*t*
Probenecid, 263*t*
Procaine, 139*t*
Progressive shock, 85

Propafenone, 46*t*, 47
Propofol, 326, 546, 547*t*, 556
Propranolol, 44*t*
Propylthiouracil (PTU), 288
Prostatitis, 482
Protamine, 406*t*
Proton pump inhibitors, 383
Pseudomonas aeruginosa, 374*t*
Pseudoseizures, 327-328
Pseudotumor cerebri, 448*t*
Psychogenic seizures, 323. *See also*
Seizure(s)
Pulmonary angiography, 184
Pulmonary artery catheter, in
hemorrhagic shock, 87
Pulmonary edema
after myocardial infarction, 37
cardiogenic. *See* Congestive heart
failure
Pulmonary embolism
clinical pearls, 194
clinical presentation, 181-182,
186-187
definition, 183
diagnosis, 187-189, 187*t*, 190*f*,
192-193
initial evaluation, 182
risk factors, 193
treatment, 186*t*, 189
Pulmonary Embolism Rule-Out
Criteria (PERC), 187-188, 187*t*
Pulmonary examination, 4
Purulent cellulitis, 573, 574
Pyelonephritis. *See also* Urinary tract
infections
admission criteria, 533*t*
clinical presentation, 527-528
definition, 529
evaluation, 528-529
as medical complications before 26
weeks of pregnancy, 289-290,
290*f*, 292
in nephrolithiasis, 246
treatment, 532, 532*t*
Pyridoxine, 326-327, 406*t*
Pyuria, 529

R
Rabies
    clinical presentation, 152
    immunization, 152-153
    postexposure prophylaxis, 150,
        152-153
    transmission, 152, 155
Radiation, 426
Radiofrequency catheter ablation, 47
Rales, in pulmonary embolism, 186
Ranitidine, 118*t*
Rapid respiratory syncytial virus
        (RSV) test, 300
Rapid sequence intubation (RSI),
        544-548
    induction and paralysis, 546-547,
        547*t*
    materials, 545*t*
    placement with proof, 548
    positioning and protection, 548
    postintubation management, 548
    preoxygenation, 545, 546*f*
    preparation, 544-545
    pretreatment, 545-546
    summary, 548*t*
Rapid-antigen test (RAT), 20-21, 21*f*
Rash with fever
    clinical approach, 582-585
    clinical pearls, 587
    clinical presentation, 581-582, 583*f*
    differential diagnosis, 584-585, 584*t*
    etiologies, 584*t*
    treatment, 585-586
Reading, approach to, 10-14
Recombinant tissue-type plasminogen
        activator (rt-PA), 164
Red eye
    clinical pearls, 311
    clinical presentation, 303-304
    differential diagnosis, 307-309, 307*t*
Referred pain, 209
Reflex-mediated syncope, 171.
        See also Syncope
Regular rate tachycardia
    clinical approach, 55-58
    clinical pearls, 60

clinical presentation, 53-54
    diagnosis, 55-56, 59
    ECG findings, 55, 56*f*, 57*t*, 59
    pathophysiology, 55
    treatment, 56, 58, 59
Renal failure
    hyperkalemia in, 517-518, 520*t*
    in sepsis, 77
Renal tubular acidosis, 254*t*
Respiratory failure, 539-540, 541
Reticulocyte count, in sickle cell
        crisis, 420
Retropharyngeal abscess, 23*t*
Rhabdomyolysis
    in cocaine intoxication, 398
    in electrical injury, 463
Rhabdovirus, 152
Right ventricular infarction, 37
Risk Stratification of Syncope in
        the Emergency Department
        (ROSE), 175-176, 176*t*, 177*f*
Rocuronium, 547, 547*t*
Ropivacaine, 139*t*
Rotavirus, 241
RSI. *See* Rapid sequence intubation
Rumack-Matthew nomogram, 563
Ruptured ectopic pregnancy, 275.
        See also Ectopic pregnancy

S
Saddle nose deformity, 137, 140
Salicylates toxicity, 563-564
Salmonella, 237*t*, 238
Salpingectomy, 275
Salpingostomy, 275
San Francisco Syncope Rule,
        175-176, 176*t*
Scalp lacerations, 139. *See also*
        Lacerations
Scleritis, 309
Scrotal pain
    clinical pearls, 483
    clinical presentation, 477-478
    differential diagnosis, 478, 479*t*
Sedative hypnotic toxidrome, 564,
        565*t*

Sedative-hypnotics, 404*t*, 564
Seizure(s)
　in alcohol withdrawal, 327, 555
　classification, 323
　clinical pearls, 331
　definition, 322
　diagnosis, 324, 330
　drug-induced, 326-327
　etiologies, 323-324, 328*t*
　long-term management, 328
　in neurocysticercosis infection, 327
　patient disposition, 328
　psychogenic, 323, 327-328
　status epilepticus, 323, 326, 330
　in traumatic brain injury, 321-322
　treatment, 325-326, 329*t*
Sellick maneuver, 548
Sengstaken-Blakemore tube, 383
Sepsis
　clinical pearls, 79
　clinical presentation, 69-70, 72-73
　complications, 76-77
　definition, 71
　evaluation, 73-76
　incidence, 70
　pathophysiology, 71-72, 72*t*
　severe, 71
　in sickle cell disease, 413
　treatment, 74-76, 78, 79
Septal hematoma, 140, 146
Septic arthritis, 346-347, 350
Septic shock, 71. *See also* Sepsis
Serious bacterial illness (SBI),
　297-298, 301
Severe preeclampsia, 197
Shigella, 237*t*, 238
Shock
　definition, 84
　hemorrhagic. *See* Hemorrhagic
　　shock
　pathophysiology, 84
　stages, 85
Sickle cell crisis
　clinical approach, 413
　clinical pearls, 420
　clinical presentation, 411-412, 420

complications, 414-418
　diagnosis, 415-416*t*
　hematological, 416*t*
　infectious, 416*t*
　pain management in, 418-419
　transfusion complications in,
　　467-468
　treatment, 415-416*t*
　triggers, 413
　vaso-occlusive, 413, 415-416*t*
Sickle cell disease, 412
Side flash, 462*t*
Skin abscesses, 574, 576, 576*t*
Skin and soft tissue infections (SSTIs)
　clinical presentation, 571-572
　definition, 573
　diagnosis of, 573-576, 574*f*
　etiologies, 576*t*
　management of, 574*f*, 576, 576*t*
Skin lesions, descriptors of, 583*t*
Slipped capital femoral epiphysis
　(SCFE), 348, 351-352, 352*f*,
　354
Slit-lamp examination, 304
SLUDGE mnemonic, in cholinergic
　toxidrome, 567
Snakebites, 153-154, 155
SOAP ME IV mnemonic, 545*t*
Social history, 3
Sodium bicarbonate, 398, 406*t*, 521*t*,
　522
Sodium channel blockade, 564
Sodium nitrate, 405*t*
Sodium nitroprusside, 196-197, 200,
　201*t*
Sodium polystyrene sulfonate, 521*t*,
　522
Somatic pain, 209, 216
Somatization, 510
Spinal fracture, 368*t*
Spinal infection, 368*t*
Spleen
　hematoma, 510
　rupture, in mononucleosis, 26
Splenic sequestration, 413, 416*t*, 417
Spontaneous abortion, 283-284

Spontaneous pneumomediastinum, 512

SSTIs. *See* Skin and soft tissue infections

ST-elevation myocardial infarction (STEMI). *See also* Acute coronary syndrome
definition, 31
ECG findings, 32, 32*t*, 33*t*
treatment, 34-35, 35*t*

Staphylococcus aureus
in diarrhea, 237*t*, 238, 241
pneumonia caused by, 374*t*
in septic arthritis, 347
in skin and soft tissue infections, 572

Statins, for sepsis, 76

Status epilepticus, 323, 326, 330

STEMI. *See* ST-elevation myocardial infarction

Stevens-Johnson syndrome, 585, 586

Stone composition analysis, 245

Straight-leg raise (SLR) testing, 367-368

Streptococcus pneumoniae
pneumonia caused by, 374*t*
in sickle cell disease, 417

Streptococcus pyogenes, 574

Stroke
clinical approach, 159-164
clinical pearls, 166
clinical presentation, 157-158, 159
definition, 158
diagnostic studies, 162-163, 166
differential diagnosis, 163-164
headache in, 450
hemorrhagic, 159, 160*t*
hypertensive emergency in, 203
initial evaluation, 158
ischemic, 159, 159*t*
in sickle cell disease, 417
treatment, 164

Stupor, 335

Subarachnoid hemorrhage, 448-450, 448*t*, 449*t*

Subconjunctival hemorrhage, 309

Submersion injury
clinical pearls, 442
clinical presentation, 437-439
cold water, 441
complications, 438
epidemiology, 439
patient disposition, 441, 442
prevention, 439
treatment, 438, 440-441

Submersion victim, 439

Succinylcholine, 547, 547*t*, 550

Suctioning, 543

Sumatriptan, 450

Supplemental testing, in overdose management, 563-564

Supraventricular tachycardia (SVT), 55

Surgical history, 3

Sutures, 138, 138*t*

Sympathomimetic toxidrome, 565*t*, 566, 570

Sympathomimetics, 404*t*, 566

Syncope
clinical approach, 171-177
clinical decision rules, 176*t*
clinical pearls, 179
clinical presentation, 169-170
definition, 170
diagnosis, 173-174, 179
etiologies, 171-173, 178
heat-related, 456*t*
management, 174-175, 175*f*, 179

Synovial fluid analysis, 349

Systemic inflammatory response syndrome (SIRS), 70-71, 85

T

Tachycardia
in acute hemolytic transfusion reactions, 469
in hypothermia, 427
in pulmonary embolism, 186
regular rate
clinical approach, 55-58
clinical pearls, 60

clinical presentation, 53-54
diagnosis, 55-56, 59
ECG findings, 55, 56*f*, 57*t*, 59
pathophysiology, 55
treatment, 56, 58, 59
Tachypnea
in acute hemolytic transfusion
reactions, 469
in pulmonary embolism, 186
Taenia solium, 327
Temporal arteritis, 309, 448*t*, 449*t*,
450
Tension headache, 448*t*, 449*t*,
450-451
Tension pneumothorax, 97, 511
Terbutaline, 127-128
Testicular torsion
clinical pearls, 483
clinical presentation, 477-478,
479*t*, 482
diagnosis, 480
treatment, 479*t*, 481
Testicular tumor, 479*t*, 482
Tetanospasmin, 142
Tetanus, 137, 142-143
Tetanus immunization, 142-143,
144*t*, 146
Tetanus immunoglobulin (TIG), 143
Tetracaine, 139*t*
Theophylline, 409
Thermoregulation, 425. *See also*
Hypothermia
Thiamine, 406*t*
Thioamides, 288
Thiopental, 546, 547*t*
Thiosulfate, 405*t*
Thoracoabdominal region, 95, 98
Thoracotomy, resuscitative, 97
3-2-2 rule, 544
Thromboembolism
atrial fibrillation and, 42, 47-48,
48*t*
definition, 41
Thrombolytics
complications, 37
contraindications, 398

definition, 158
for myocardial infarction, 34-35,
35*t*, 37
for pulmonary embolism, 189
for stroke, 163*t*, 164, 166
Thyroid storm, 289, 293
TIMI risk score, 34*t*
Timolol, 306
Toddler's fracture, 352
Toxic epidermal necrolysis (TEN),
585, 586
Toxidromes, 404*t*
airway management in, 561
anti-muscarinic, 565*t*, 566-567
cholinergic, 565*t*, 567, 569
clinical pearls, 570
decontamination in, 562-563
definition, 561
elimination in, 563
hypertension in, 561-562
hypotension in, 562
opioid/opiate, 564-566, 565*t*
overdose management in, 561-563
sedative-hypnotic, 564, 565*t*
supplemental testing, 563-564
sympathomimetic, 565*t*, 566
Transfusion complications. *See* Blood
transfusion, complications
Transient ischemic attack (TIA), 158,
159*t*
Transient red cell aplasia (TRCA),
418
Transient synovitis, 345-346, 354
Trauma
in children. *See* Children, trauma in
clinical pearls, 90
in elderly patients, 491-493, 492*t*
in extremities, 96*t*
facial, 137. *See also* Facial
lacerations
hemorrhagic shock in.
See Hemorrhagic shock
initial assessment, 82, 83-84, 83*f*,
84*t*, 90
lacerations. *See* Lacerations
patients, 106-107

Trauma (*Cont.*):
  penetrating
    anterior abdomen, 98-99
    chest, 97
    clinical pearls, 101
    clinical presentation, 93-94
    complications, 94
    initial evaluation, 94, 95-97, 96t
    initial management, 96-97
    thoracoabdominal, 98
  wound closure, 139
  wound irrigation, 137
Traumatic brain injury, 321-322
Traveler's diarrhea, 240
Trench foot, 425
Trendelenburg gait, 354
Tricyclic antidepressants
  overdose, 404t
  seizures induced by, 326
Trimethoprim-sulfamethoxazole
    (TMP-SMX), 532, 532t
Tubo-ovarian abscess, 261
Tympanic membrane rupture, in
    lightning injury, 463
Type 1 hypersensitivity reaction, 115.
    See also Anaphylaxis

U

Ultrasonography
  in child with a limp, 349-350, 350f
  indications, 8
  pelvic, 209
  for sepsis, 75
  for skin and soft tissue infections,
    573-574
  transvaginal, 276
  venous duplex, 183
Unfractionated heparin (UFH), 186t
Unstable angina (UA), 31, 35-36.
    See also Acute coronary
    syndrome
Upper extremity injuries, 108-109
Upper GI-small-bowel follow through,
    227
Urethritis, 529
Urinalysis, 531, 531t

Urinary alkalinization, in drug
    elimination, 563
Urinary retention, acute
  causes, 253t, 257
  clinical approach, 253-256
  clinical pearls, 257
  clinical presentation, 251-252
  definition, 253
  medications causing, 255t
  physical examination, 254-255
  symptoms, 254
  treatment, 255-256, 257
Urinary tract infections. *See also*
    Pyelonephritis
  cause of serious bacterial illness,
    301
  classification, 529
  clinical pearls, 536
  complicated, 529
  differential diagnosis, 528, 530
  imaging, 531-532
  laboratory studies, 530-531, 531t
  pathophysiology, 530, 535
  in pregnancy, 533, 535
  prevalence, 529
  risk factors, 530
  treatment, 532-533, 532t, 535,
    536
  uncomplicated, 529
Urine culture, 531
Urine dipstick, 531
Urine microscopy, 531

V

Vagal reflex, 171
Valproic acid, 325-326
Vancomycin, 318t
Varices, 383, 383t
Vascular necrosis of femoral head,
    351, 352f
Vasoocclusive crisis, 413-414
Vasopressin, 383
Vasovagal syncope, 171, 173-174.
    See also Syncope
Vecuronium, 547t
Venom, 151, 153

Venous duplex ultrasonography, 183, 184, 192
Venous thromboembolism. *See* Deep venous thrombosis
Ventilation and perfusion (V/Q) scan, 183-184, 188
Ventricular fibrillation, 36, 36t
Ventricular tachycardia (VT), 36, 36t, 55
Verapamil, 44t
Vermillion border, 137, 141f
Vernakalant, 46t
Vertebrobasilar syndrome, 159t
Vibrio cholerae, 237t, 241
Visceral pain, 209
Vision loss, acute, 307t, 309
Vital signs, by age group, 486t
Vitamin K, 383, 410
Vitamin K$_1$, 406t
Vomiting, in bowel obstruction, 229

W
Warfarin
    in atrial fibrillation, 47
    in chronic atrial fibrillation, 48t

for deep venous thrombosis/ pulmonary embolism, 186t
pre-cardioversion, 45, 45t
Well-appearing infant, 359
Wells criteria, pulmonary embolism, 187t
Westermark sign, 188, 193
Whole bowel irrigation, 563
Wolff-Parkinsons-White syndrome, 44f
Women, abdominal pain in, 207-209, 211
Wound(s). *See also* Trauma
    animal bite; Animal bite
    closure, 139
    irrigation, 137

X
Xanthochromia, 449, 452

Y
Yersinia enterocolitica, 472

Z
Ziprasidone, 556